Theory and Concepts of Biomechanics

Theory and Concepts of Biomechanics

Edited by **Randall Calloway**

hayle medical

New York

Published by Hayle Medical,
30 West, 37th Street, Suite 612,
New York, NY 10018, USA
www.haylemedical.com

Theory and Concepts of Biomechanics
Edited by Randall Calloway

International Standard Book Number: 978-1-63241-367-3 (Hardback)

Printed in China.

Contents

	Preface	**VII**
Part 1	**General Notes on Biomechanics and Mechanobiology**	**1**
Chapter 1	**Mechanobiology of Fracture Healing: Basic Principles and Applications in Orthodontics and Orthopaedics** Antonio Boccaccio and Carmine Pappalettere	**3**
Chapter 2	**Evolution of Locomotor Trends in Extinct Terrestrial Giants Affected by Body Mass** Valery B. Kokshenev and Per Christiansen	**31**
Chapter 3	**Mechanical Properties of Living Cells and Tissues Related to Thermodynamics, Experiments and Quantitative Morphology – A Review** Miroslav Holeček, Petra Kochová and Zbyněk Tonar	**57**
Part 2	**Biomechanical Modelling**	**75**
Chapter 4	**Biomechanical Computer Models** K. Engel, R. Herpers and U. Hartmann	**77**
Chapter 5	**Biomechanics and Modeling of Skeletal Soft Tissues** Rami K. Korhonen and Simo Saarakkala	**97**
Chapter 6	**Functional Data Analysis for Biomechanics** Elizabeth Crane, David Childers, Geoffrey Gerstner and Edward Rothman	**117**
Chapter 7	**Biomechanical Models of Endodontic Restorations** Antonio Pérez-González, Carmen González-Lluch, Joaquín L. Sancho-Bru, Pablo J. Rodríguez-Cervantes and José L. Iserte-Vilar	**133**
Chapter 8	**Development and Validation of a Three-Dimensional Biomechanical Model of the Lower Extremity** Shihab Asfour and Moataz Eltoukhy	**161**

Chapter 9 **Towards a Realistic and Self-Contained Biomechanical Model of the Hand** 187
Joaquín L. Sancho-Bru, Antonio Pérez-González, Marta C. Mora, Beatriz E. León, Margarita Vergara, José L. Iserte, Pablo J. Rodríguez-Cervantes and Antonio Morales

Chapter 10 **Feasible Simulation of Diseases Related to Bone Remodelling and of Their Treatment** 217
Václav Klika and František Maršík

Part 3 Locomotion and Joint Biomechanics 241

Chapter 11 **Physical Insights Into Dynamic Similarity in Animal Locomotion. I. Theoretical Principles and Concepts** 243
Valery B. Kokshenev

Chapter 12 **Physical Insights Into Dynamic Similarity in Animal Locomotion. II. Observation of Continues Similarity States** 261
Valery B. Kokshenev

Chapter 13 **Estimating Lower Limb Skeletal Loading** 279
Timo Rantalainen and Adam Kłodowski

Chapter 14 **Induced Acceleration Analysis of Three-Dimensional Multi-Joint Movements and Its Application to Sports Movements** 303
Masaya Hirashima

Chapter 15 **Stability During Arboreal Locomotion** 319
Andrew R. Lammers and Ulrich Zurcher

Chapter 16 **The Biomechanics of the Anterior Cruciate Ligament and Its Reconstruction** 335
Christopher D. S. Jones and Paul N. Grimshaw

Chapter 17 **Biomechanical Assessments in Sports and Ergonomics** 359
Pascal Madeleine, Afshin Samani, Mark de Zee and Uwe Kersting

Chapter 18 **Biomechanics of the Neck** 385
Haibin Chen, Liying Zhang, Zhengguo Wang, King H. Yang and Albert I. King

Permissions

List of Contributors

Preface

This book was inspired by the evolution of our times; to answer the curiosity of inquisitive minds. Many developments have occurred across the globe in the recent past which has transformed the progress in the field.

In the past few years, there has been an increasing awareness that issues emerging from biology or medicine require an interdisciplinary approach. Hence, certain forms of mathematics and applied physics have arisen; like biomechanics, mathematical biology and mechanobiology among others. This book discusses some general topics regarding biomechanics and mechanobiology, inclusive of theoretical contributions which provide explanations for certain aspects that experiments or clinical studies are unable to do. The book also discusses biomechanical modeling, a speedily growing field of biomechanical models and modeling methods utilized to increase the comprehension of various procedures occurring in the human body. Finally, this book also considers locomotion and joint biomechanics, which describe and analyze human movement, and the stability of the joints.

This book was developed from a mere concept to drafts to chapters and finally compiled together as a complete text to benefit the readers across all nations. To ensure the quality of the content we instilled two significant steps in our procedure. The first was to appoint an editorial team that would verify the data and statistics provided in the book and also select the most appropriate and valuable contributions from the plentiful contributions we received from authors worldwide. The next step was to appoint an expert of the topic as the Editor-in-Chief, who would head the project and finally make the necessary amendments and modifications to make the text reader-friendly. I was then commissioned to examine all the material to present the topics in the most comprehensible and productive format.

I would like to take this opportunity to thank all the contributing authors who were supportive enough to contribute their time and knowledge to this project. I also wish to convey my regards to my family who have been extremely supportive during the entire project.

Editor

Part 1

General Notes on Biomechanics and Mechanobiology

Mechanobiology of Fracture Healing: Basic Principles and Applications in Orthodontics and Orthopaedics

Antonio Boccaccio and Carmine Pappalettere
Dipartimento di Ingegneria Meccanica e Gestionale, Politecnico di Bari
Italy

1. Introduction

The Chapter describes how mechanobiological models can be utilized to predict the spatial and temporal patterns of the tissues differentiating within a fracture site during the healing process. It will be structured in four main Sections. Firstly, the basic principles of mechanobiology, the main theories and the principal models utilized to simulate the cellular processes involved in fracture healing will be illustrated. Second, two examples will be given showing how a mechano-regulation model, - where the bone callus is modeled as a biphasic poroelastic material and the stimulus regulating tissue differentiation is hypothesized to be a function of the strain and fluid flow-, can be utilized to assess bone regeneration in an ostetomized mandible submitted to distraction osteogenesis and in a fractured lumbar vertebra. Finally, the main limitations of the model utilized and, in general, of mechanobiological algorithms as well as the future perspectives will be outlined.
Fracture healing is a physiological process that initiates immediately after the fracture event and occurs by following two different modalities: by primary fracture healing or by secondary fracture healing. Primary healing involves a direct attempt by the cortex to re-establish itself once it has become interrupted. When stabilisation is not adequate to permit primary healing, the abundant capillaries required for bone repair are constantly ruptured and secondary healing takes place. Secondary healing involves responses within the periosteum and external soft tissues and subsequent formation of an external callus. Secondary fracture healing occurs in the following stages. Blood emanates from the ruptured vessels and a haemorrhage quickly fills the fracture gap space. Macrophages remove the dead tissue and generate initial granulation tissue for the migration of undifferentiated mesenchymal stem cells (MSCs), originating an initial stabilizing callus. These cells proliferate and migrate from the surrounding soft tissue (Einhorn, 1998, McKibbin, 1978) (Fig. 1a). Then, stem cells disperse into the fracture callus, divide (mitosis) and simultaneously migrate within the fracture site (Fig. 1b). In the next stage, mesenchymal cells may differentiate into chondrocytes, osteoblasts or fibroblasts, depending on the biological and mechanical conditions (Fig. 1c). These differentiated cells begin to synthesize the extracellular matrix of their corresponding tissue (Doblaré et al., 2004) (Fig. 1d). Intramembranous woven bone is produced by direct differentiation of the stem cells into osteoblasts. Endochondral ossification occurs when chondrocytes are replaced by osteoblasts.

2. Mechanobiology: Basic principles

Comparing patterns of differentiation during tissue repair to predictions of the mechanical environment within the mesenchymal tissue has led to the development of a number of hypothesis for mechano-regulated tissue differentiation. Theories on the relationship between mechanics and biology were originally proposed in relation to fracture healing. These theories later evolved into 'mechanobiological algorithms'; a finite set of rules that govern the effects of mechanical loading on stem cells and tissues. Mechanobiology merges the older science of mechanics with the newer and emerging disciplines of molecular biology and genetics.

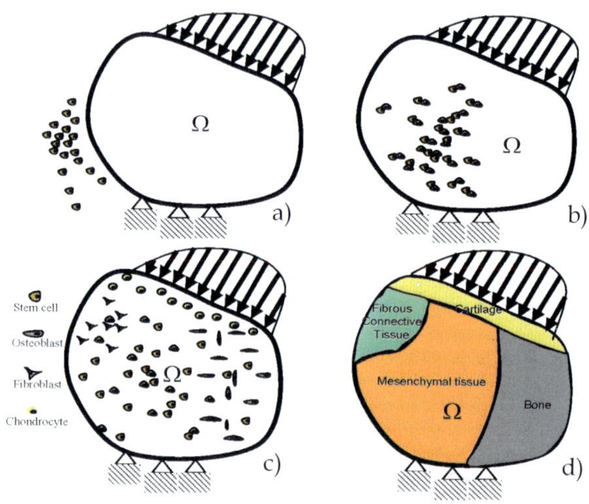

Fig. 1. Let Ω be an arbitrary fracture domain loaded and constrained over part of the surface. Immediately after the fracture event the mesenchymal stem cells (MSCs) reside outside the domain in the surrounding soft tissue (a). Then, stem cells disperse into the domain, divide (mitosis) and simultaneously migrate within the domain (b). Depending on the biological and mechanical conditions MSCs differentiate into fibroblasts, chondrocytes and osteoblasts (c). These differentiated cells begin to synthesize the extracellular matrix of their corresponding tissue (d).

At the centre of mechanobiology is the cellular process of mechano-transduction, or the way by which the cells sense and respond to mechanical forces or, in general to biophysical stimuli. Experimental and analytical models are often integrated in mechanobiology to gain a deeper understanding of the cells' response to mechanical factors. Experiments provide insights and measurements, which can then be interpreted within the context of analytical frameworks. Analytical simulations permit investigation of possible explanations that require in vivo validation and will suggest further experimental investigations (van der Meulen and Huiskes, 2002).

2.2 Mechanobiology of mesenchymal stem cells

Mesenchymal stem cells (MSCs) are nonhematopoietic progenitor cells found in adult tissues. They posses an extensive proliferative ability in an uncommitted state and hold the potential to differentiate along various lineages of mesenchymal origin in response to appropriate stimuli (Chen et al., 2007). Bone marrow is the most important source for MSCs (Simmons, 1985, Brighton and Hunt, 1991, Glowacki, 1998). However, MSCs have been also identified in different other tissues such as adipose, periosteum, trabecular bone, synovium, skeletal muscle, dental pulp and periodontal ligament (Barry and Murphy, 2004, Ballini et al., 2007, Ballini et al., 2010). Quiescent MSCs become mobilised during repair and remodelling through regulation by external chemical and physical signals that control their activation, proliferation, migration, differentiation and survival i.e. their fate (Byrne, 2008). One key aspect in mechanobiology of MSCs is the modelling of the cellular processes such as the cellular dispersal, the proliferation, the apoptosis, etc.

Concerning the process of cellular dispersal, it has been suggested that the movement of stem cells can be thought of as an assemblage of particles, with each particle moving around in a random way (Murray, 1989). In a number of studies (Lacroix and Prendergast, 2002, Geris et al., 2004, Andreykiv et al., 2005), a diffusion equation has been used to simulate the movement of cells through regenerating tissues. If c is the concentration of stem cells in a given volume and D the diffusion coefficient, the derivative of c with respect to the time is given by:

$$\frac{\mathrm{d}c}{\mathrm{d}t} = D\nabla^2 c \qquad (1)$$

However such a modelling of cellular dispersal presents the limitation that the diffusion coefficient assumes a value that does not depend on the cell phenotype or the tissue through which the cell is moving. Furthermore, this approach implicitly assumes that cells attempt to achieve a homogenous population density within the area of analysis. Lacroix et al. (2002) developed further the diffusion equation (1) by including the processes of cellular mitosis and apoptosis (programmed cell death). Therefore, the rate of change in cell concentration assumes the form:

$$\frac{\mathrm{d}c}{\mathrm{d}t} = D\nabla^2 c + cs(c_c) - kc \qquad (2)$$

The first term on the right-hand side of equation (2) describes cell migration by simple linear diffusion; the second term describes cell mitosis, where $c_c(x,t)$ is the chemical concentration of a mitosis-inducing factor; $s(c_c)$ is a function describing the mitosis rate per cell; and k is a constant describing the cell death or removal rate (Sherratt et al., 1992). Since the mesenchymal stem cells can differentiate into cells of different phenotypes i (i.e. fibroblasts, chondrocytes and osteoblasts) that produce different tissues j (i.e. fibrous tissue, cartilage and bone), a logical progression of the idea proposed by Lacroix et al., (Lacroix et al., 2002), would be that the diffusion coefficient D would depend on the cell phenotype i and the tissue type j through which the cell is moving. This modelling has been adopted in Kelly and Prendergast (Kelly and Prendergast, 2005, 2006). Boccaccio et al. (Boccaccio et al., 2007, 2008a), modelled the cellular dispersal by using the diffusion equation (1) however, they accounted for the fact that MSCs not only require time to differentiate, but that the differentiated cell types require time to synthesise and remodel new tissue. To this purpose, based on the results of Richardson et al. (Richardson et al., 1992) who observed an exponential increase in stiffness during tibial fracture healing, they assumed that the Young's modulus of all tissues within the fracture callus increases exponentially with time.

In reality, diffusion is not the mechanism of stem cell dispersal; cells disperse by crawling or proliferation or are transported in a moving fluid (Prendergast et al., 2009). In order to better simulate the cellular processes involved during the fracture healing process, Pérez and Prendergast (Pérez and Prendergast , 2007) developed a 'random-walk' model to describe cell proliferation and migration, with and without a preferred direction. In this approach, a regular lattice of points is superimposed on the fracture domain. Each lattice point is either empty, or occupied by a stem cell. Cell movement can be simulated by moving a cell from one lattice point to another; cell proliferation, by dividing a cell so that the daughter cell takes up a neighbouring lattice point; cell apoptosis, by removing a cell at a lattice point.

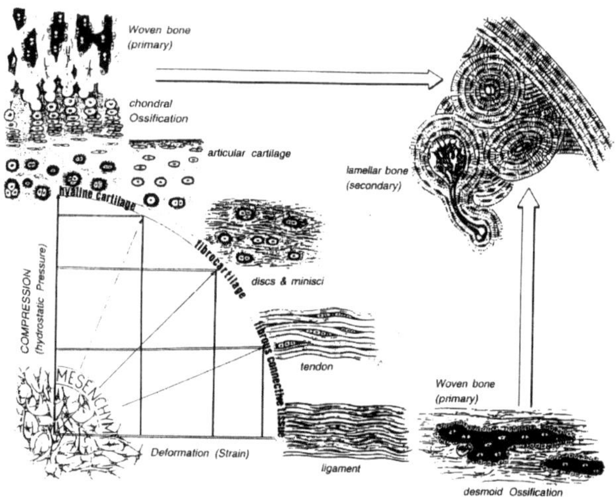

Fig. 2. Diagram showing the mechano-regulation model developed by Pauwels (Pauwels, 1960). The combination of two biophysical stimuli, shear strain and hydrostatic pressure, will act on the mesenchymal cell pool leading to either hyaline cartilage, fibrocartilage or fibrous tissue as represented on the perimeter of the quadrant. The larger arrows indicate that, as time passes, ossification of these soft tissues occurs, provided that the soft tissue has stabilized the environment. Reprinted from Bone, Vol. 19, Issue 2, Weinans H, Prendergast PJ, Tissue adaptation as a dynamical process far from equilibrium, Pages No. 143-149, Copyright (1996) with permission from Elsevier.

2.3 Principal mechano-regulation models

Pauwels, (Pauwels, 1960), who was the first to propose the hypothesis of a mechano-regulated tissue differentiation, suggested that the distortional shear stress is a specific stimulus for the development of collagenous fibres and that hydrostatic compressive stress is a specific stimulus for cartilage formation. When a soft tissue has stabilized the environment, differentiation of MSCs into osteoblasts is favoured leading to the formation of bone (Fig. 2).

Based on a qualitative analysis of clinical results of fracture healing, Perren (Perren, 1979) proposed that tissue differentiation is controlled by the tolerance of various tissues to strain. The basis of this theory, - normally known as 'the interfragmentary strain theory' - is that a tissue that ruptures or fails at a certain strain level cannot be formed in a region experiencing strains greater than this level. Based on the framework of Pauwels (Pauwels, 1960), Carter et al. (Carter et al., 1988, Carter and Wong, 1988) expanded the concepts relating tissue differentiation to mechanical loading. They proposed that local stress or strain history influences tissue differentiation over time (Carter et al., 1988). These ideas were later developed further and a more general mechano-regulation theory was proposed (Carter et al., 1998) (Fig. 3). They postulated that: (i) compressive hydrostatic stress history guides the formation of cartilaginous matrix constituents; (ii) tensile strain history guides connective tissue cells in their production and turnover of fibrous matrix constituents; (iii) fibrocartilage is formed when a tissue loading history consists of a combination of high levels of hydrostatic compressive stress and high levels of tensile strain; (iv) direct bone formation is permitted, in regions exposed to neither significant compressive hydrostatic stress nor significant tensile strain, provided there is an adequate blood supply; (v) pre-osseous tissue can be diverted down a chondrogenic pathway in regions of low oxygen tension. The mechano-regulation theory of Claes and Heigele (Claes and Heigele, 1999) was initially presented in quantitative terms, and although the resulting concept is similar to that of Carter et al. (Carter et al., 1998), they based their mechano-regulation theory on the observation that bone formation occurs mainly near calcified surfaces and that both intramembranous and endochondral ossification exist in fracture healing. Depending on local strain and hydrostatic pressure different cellular reactions and tissue differentiation processes were predicted to occur (Claes et al., 1998; Claes and Heigele, 1999).

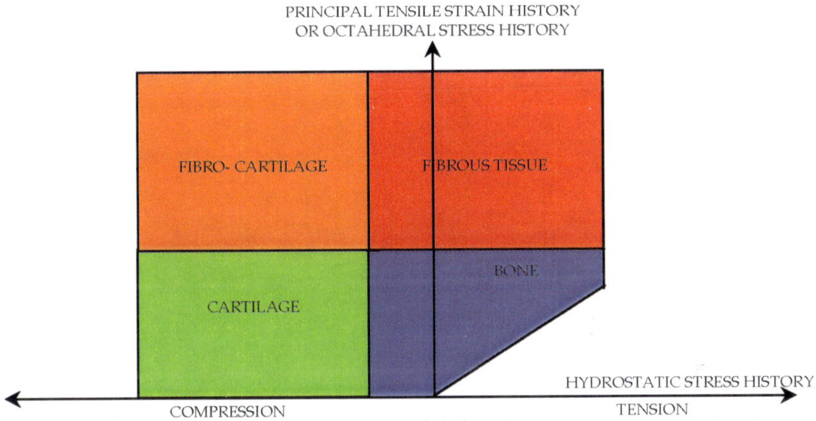

Fig. 3. Schematic of the mechano-regulation model developed by Carter and colleagues representing the role of the hydrostatic stress history and the maximum principle tensile strain history on the differentiation of mesenchymal stem cells in a well-vascularised environment (Carter et al., 1998)

Prendergast and Huiskes (Prendergast and Huiskes, 1995) and Prendergast et al. (Prendergast et al., 1997), created a poroelastic finite element model of a bone-implant interface to analyse the mechanical environment on differentiating cells. They found that the biophysical stimuli experienced by the regenerating tissue at the implant interface are not only generated by the tissue matrix, but also to a large extent by the drag forces from the interstitial flow. Based on this study, a new mechano-regulation theory was developed taking into consideration that connective tissues are poroelastic and comprise both fluid and solid. They proposed a mechano-regulatory pathway composed of two biophysical stimuli; octahedral strain of the solid phase and interstitial fluid velocity relative to the solid. Fluid flow and substrate strain in the tissue, are used as a basis for the stimulus S for cell differentiation as follows:

$$S = \frac{\gamma}{a} + \frac{v}{b} \tag{3}$$

where γ is the octahedral shear strain, v is the interstitial fluid flow velocity, a=3.75% and b=3μms^{-1} are empirical constants. High stimulus levels (S>3) promote the differentiation of mesenchymal cells into fibroblasts, intermediate levels (1<S<3) stimulate the differentiation into chondrocytes, and low levels of these stimuli (S<1) promote the differentiation into osteoblasts. Simulation of the time-course of tissue differentiation was presented by Huiskes et al., (Huiskes et al., 1997) (Fig. 4). The solid line shows what would occur in an environment where a high shear persists (i.e. maintenance of fibrous tissue and inhibition of ossification) whereas the dashed line shows what would occur if the presence of the soft tissue could progressively reduce the micromotions (i.e ossification would occur). Recently, the mechano-regulation model of Prendergast et al., (Prendergast et al., 1997) has been further developed to include factors such as angiogenesis (Checa and Prendergast, 2009), and the role of the mechanical environment on the collagen architecture in regenerating soft tissues (Nagel and Kelly, 2010). Gómez-Benito et al. (Gómez-Benito et al., 2005), presented a mathematical model to simulate the effect of mechanical stimuli on most of the cellular processes that occur during fracture healing, namely proliferation, migration and differentiation. They simulated the process of bone healing as a process driven by a mechanical stimulus, $\Psi(x,t)$ assumed to be the second invariant of the deviatoric strain tensor.

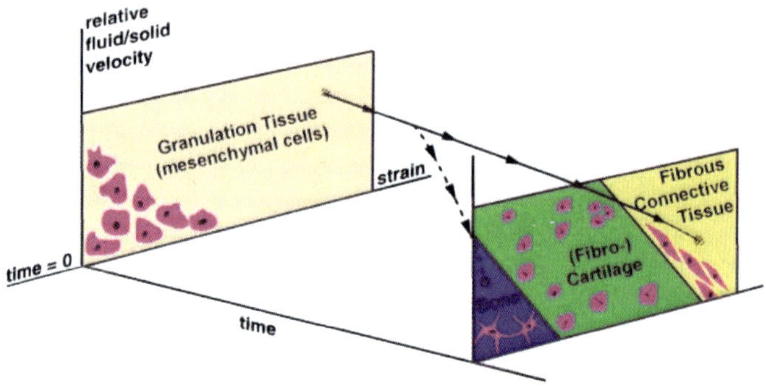

Fig. 4. Schematic of the mechano-regulation model proposed by Prendergast et al. (Prendergast et al., 1997). The solid line shows what would occur in an environment where a high shear persists (i.e. maintenance of fibrous tissue and inhibition of ossification) whereas the dashed line shows what would occur if the presence of the soft tissue could progressively reduce the micromotions (i.e ossification would occur).

The models above reviewed are based on theories of mechano-transduction, the way in which cells sense and respond to mechanical forces or displacements. Other bio-regulatory theories are reported in literature that put in relationship biochemical factors with the spatial and temporal patterns of tissue differentiation observed during the healing process of a fractured bone (Bailón-Plaza and van der Meulen, 2001, Geris et al., 2008).

2.4 Mechanobiology: Domains of applicability

Applications of mechanobiology can be found in three main areas:

i. In the development of new clinical therapies, for example in bone fracture healing, or osteoporosis. Different studies are reported in literature in which mechanobiological models are utilized to pursue this aim: Lacroix and Prendergast (Lacroix and Prendergast, 2002) predicted the patterns of tissue differentiation during fracture healing of long bones; Shefelbine et al. (Shefelbine et al., 2005) simulated the fracture healing process in cancellous bone.

ii. In the improvement of implant design. With implants such as prostheses, cells migrate up to the implant surface and begin to synthesis matrix, but if the micromotion is too high bone will not form to stabilise the implant – instead a soft tissue layer will form (Huiskes, 1993, Prendergast, 2006). A number of articles can be found in literature where mechanobiological models are utilized to predict the patterns of tissue differentiation at the tissue-implant interface: Andreykiv et al. (Andreykiv et al., 2005) simulated the bone ingrowth on the surface of a glenoid component; Moreo et al., (Moreo et al., 2009a,b) developed a mechano-regulation algorithm that models the main biological interactions occurring at the surface of endosseous implants and is able to reproduce most of the biological features of the osseointegration phenomenon.

iii. In bone tissue engineering and regenerative medicine. Appropriate biophysical stimuli are needed in bone scaffolds, in addition to nutrients and appropriate levels of oxygen supply, to favour an appropriate tissue differentiation process (Martin et al., 2004, Prendergast et al., 2009). A number of studies (Byrne et al., 2007, Milan et al., 2009; Olivares et al., 2009, Sanz-Herrera et al., 2009) are reported in literature that through a combined use of finite element method and mechano-regulation algorithms described the possible patterns of the tissues differentiating within biomimetic scaffolds for tissue engineering (Boccaccio et al., 2011a).

In this Chapter we will focus on the first domain of applicability (i) and, specifically, two examples will be illustrated that show how mechanobiology can be used to predict the patterns of tissue differentiation in a human mandible osteotomized and submitted to distraction osteogenesis as well the regrowth and the remodelling process of the cancellous bone in a vertebral fracture. Predictions were conducted by implementing the mechano-regulation model of Prendergast and colleagues (Prendergast et al., 1997).

3. Mechanobiology of mandibular symphyseal distraction osteogenesis

Mandibular Symphyseal Distraction Osteogenesis (MSDOG) is a common clinical procedure aimed to modify the geometrical shape of the mandible for correcting problems of dental overcrowding and arch shrinkage. Such problems are usually solved by tooth extraction or expansion protocols. However, these clinical procedures are unstable and tend to relapse towards the original dimension (McNamara and Brudon, 1993). Mandibular distraction osteogenesis may solve transverse mandibular deficiency problems. With this clinical procedure the mandibular geometry is definitively changed so that the risk of a relapsing towards the original dimension is avoided. In spite of consolidated clinical use, the process of tissue differentiation and bone regrowth in an osteotomized mandible remains poorly understood. Clinically, MSDOG can be divided into four stages: firstly the mandible is osteotomized and then instrumented with a distraction appliance; secondly a seven to ten day latency period is waited after the surgical operation in order to allow the formation of a good quality bone callus; thirdly the distraction device is progressively expanded with a well defined rate for seven-ten day time period; the final stage is the maturation period during which the patient is maintained in rigid external fixation. At the end of this period, more space is available on the inferior arch so that the teeth which are initially in intimate contact, can be repositioned (through orthodontic treatments) in the correct locations.

The second stage is crucial for successful MSDOG. If the latency period is too short, a weak and insufficient callus will form, and without a good callus not enough new bone may form and complications may arise such as fibrous union, non-union, tooth loss and periodontal defects (Conley and Legan, 2003). On the other hand, too long a latency period may substantially increase the risk of premature bone union, which can hinder the subsequent expansion process. Furthermore, the duration of latency period depends strictly on the aging of patient (Conley and Legan, 2003). In the case of young children, the accelerated healing process allows clinical protocols with shorter latency period to be adopted while, in the case of elder patients, as the healing process progresses slowly, longer latency periods are required. The distraction period (i.e., the third stage) is also critical. Too fast a rate of expansion of the appliance can lead to poor bone quality within the distraction gap, partial union, fibrous union or atrophic non-union. Conversely, too slow a rate can lead to premature consolidation hence hindering the distraction process (Conley and Legan, 2003).

Such issues have been investigated by developing a mechano-regulation model of a human mandible osteotomized and submitted to distraction osteogenesis.

3.1 Finite element model

The 3D model of a human mandible has been reconstructed from CT scan data and the processing of the CT files was made by means of the *Mimics® Version 7.2* software (Materialise Inc.) (Fig. 5(a-c)). The model also includes an orthodontic distractor tooth-borne

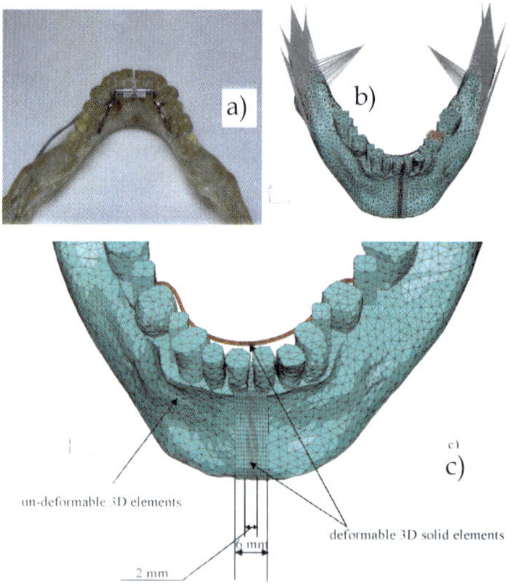

Fig. 5. (a) Epoxy resin model of the osteotomized mandible with a tooth-borne device; (b) mandible-distractor orthodontic device FEM model; (c) details of the osteotomized region and of the tooth-borne device

device. Since the stiffness of the mandibular bone is orders of magnitude greater than the callus, we modelled the portion of bone and of the device far from the osteotomized region as a rigid body. Conversely, the portion of the bone, of bone callus and of the device near to the middle sagittal plane was modelled with 3D deformable elements. With this strategy we reduced the computational cost of the analysis without introducing significant alterations with respect to the anatomo-physiological behaviour of the mandibular district. The finite element model consists of about 12000 3-node un-deformable triangular elements (see Fig. 5b) and about 5400 8-node hexahedral elements for meshing the osteotomized region and the deformable portion of the distractor device (Fig. 5c).

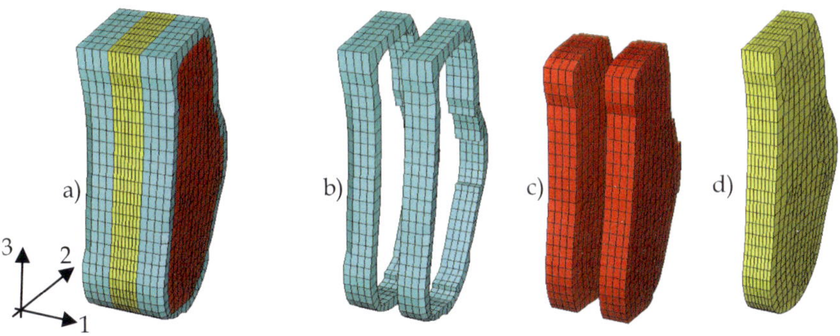

Fig. 6. (a) FEM model of the osteotomized region. Different regions and materials included in the model: (b) cortical bone (in light blue), (c) cancellous bone (in red), (d) fracture callus (in yellow).

Following Meyer et al., (Meyer et al., 2004), a 2 mm thick gap between the two mandibular *ramus* was created. The gap, surrounded by cortical and cancellous bone (Fig. 6) was hypothesized to be initially occupied by granulation tissue. The callus and bone tissue forming the portion of mandible near to the middle sagittal plane were modelled as biphasic poroelastic materials. Following Schwartz-Dabney and Dechow, (Schwartz-Dabney and Dechow, 2003) the cortical bone was modelled as an orthotropic material. The material properties used for all the other tissues are the same as used in previous models (Lacroix and Prendergast, 2002, Kelly and Prendergast, 2005).

3.2 Boundary and loading conditions

The FEM model is subjected to three boundary conditions applied simultaneously (Fig. 5b). Boundary condition (i) simulates the temporomandibular joint. The condyles are represented by two reference points at the locations of articulation. These reference points are connected to the mandible arms through coupling constraints. The behaviour of the temporomandibular joint disc is modelled by constraining these reference points to three fixed points by means of spring elements aligned to the coordinate system. The mandible hence can rotate about an axis defined by the line connecting the two condyles and translate along the coordinate directions. Boundary condition (ii) models the mastication. The action of the most important muscles involved in the mastication process, was simulated. Force intensity and direction are those used in a previous study (Boccaccio et al., 2006). Boundary condition (iii) simulates the unilateral occlusion on one tooth on the right mandibular arm.

The occlusion is modelled by constraining, with simple-supports preventing u_3-displacements (see direction 3 in Fig. 6), the second premolar.

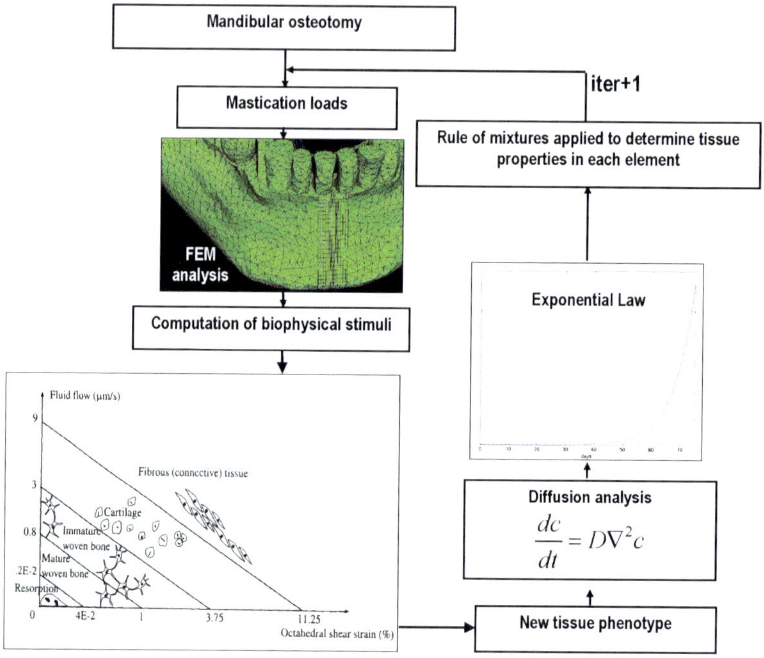

Fig. 7. Schematic of the implemented mechano-regulation algorithm

3.3 Determination of the optimal duration of the latency period

The mechano-regulation model of Prendergast and colleagues (Prendergast et al., 1997), combined with the above described finite element model was utilized to investigate the tissue differentiation process after osteotomy and to carry out an investigation on the optimal duration of the latency period and on its effects on the bone regeneration process. The spreading of mesenchymal stem cells throughout the bone callus was simulated with the diffusion equation (1) (Boccaccio et al., 2008a). The diffusion coefficient D was set so that the complete cell coverage in the callus is achieved two weeks after the osteotomy. As MSCs disperse from the bone marrow throughout the callus, they will differentiate into different cell phenotypes based on the value of a biophysical stimulus S computed with the equation (3). After the calculation of the new tissue phenotype and of the number of the MSCs invading the bone callus domain, the algorithm evaluates the mechanical properties for every element based on the exponential law described above (Section 2.2) and a simple rule of mixtures. The diffusion equation, the formulation for the calculation of the stimulus, the exponential law as well as the rule of mixtures were implemented into an algorithm a graphical summary of which is depicted in Fig. 7. If $\bar{E}$ is the Young's modulus for a given element averaged over the previous 10 iterations and c is the concentration of cells invading the domain in the current iteration *iter*, then the Young's modulus for that element and for next iteration *iter+1* can be computed as follows:

$$E(iter+1)=\frac{c}{c_{\max}}\cdot\overline{E}+\frac{(c_{\max}-c)}{c_{\max}}\cdot E_{granulation} \quad (4)$$

where c_{max} is the highest concentration of cells which may occupy any one element domain, $E_{granulation}$ is the Young's modulus of the granulation tissue. This rule of mixtures has been successfully adopted by Lacroix and Prendergast (Lacroix and Prendergast, 2002), to describe the delay between the time when stimulus first acts on the cells and the process of differentiation into a new phenotype. The algorithm was written in FORTRAN environment and each iteration corresponds to 4.8 hours, that is, the diffusion equation (1) computes the change of cells concentration occurring every 4.8 hours. Therefore, with 5 iterations a time period of 1 day is covered. This algorithm has been used to predict the patterns of the tissues differentiating within the bone callus of the osteotomized mandible during a ten day latency period.

The analyses carried out revealed that the Young's modulus of the bone, cartilage and fibrous tissue decreases towards the centre of the callus as we move away from the adjacent bone marrow (Fig. 8a). In order to investigate if premature bone bridging between the two sides of the fracture callus could hinder the subsequent distraction process, the amounts of new bone within the callus with a predicted Young's modulus greater than 0.7 MPa were isolated (see Fig. 8b which illustrates the process of bone formation in the frontal plane 1-3). After eight days, portions of bone tissue linking the left with the right side of the callus are predicted to form. The presence of bone bridges will hinder the distraction process. This suggests that is better to apply clinical protocols with a latency period not longer than seven-eight days so that the risk of a premature bone union is avoided. This is in agreement with Conley and Legan, (Conley and Legan, 2003) who suggest a latency period of seven days.

3.4 Determination of the optimal duration of the latency period for differently aged patients

The mechano-regulation model schematically illustrated in Figure 7 has been further developed to investigate how the optimal duration of the latency period changes for differently aged patients (Boccaccio et al., 2008b). Three different cases were considered: young (up to 20 years old), adult (about 55 years old) and elder (more than 70 years old) patients. Based on the histological analyses conducted by Chen et al., (Chen et al., 2005), Baxter et al., (Baxter et al., 2004), Mendes et al. (Mendes et al., 2002), and Park et al. (Park et al., 2005), the diffusion coefficient *D* was hypothesized to be a function of the patient's age. Let t_{elder}, t_{adult} and t_{young} be the time periods required by MSCs for recovering completely the bone callus domain respectively for the elder, adult and young patients. Following Chen et al. (Chen et al., 2005) who measured the proliferation of MSCs in an *in vitro* culture at different time intervals (4, 8, 12 16 and 20 days) the diffusion coefficient *D* for the differently aged patients has been set: t_{elder} =3 weeks, t_{adult} =2 weeks and t_{young}=1 week. Patterns of tissue differentiation were predicted for each case (Fig. 9).

A bony bridge between the left and right sides of the fracture callus forms after 5, 8 and 9 days for the young, adult and elder patients, respectively (Fig. 9). Such results lead us to conclude that the optimal duration of the latency period is: 5-6 days for the young patient, 7-8 and 9-10 days for the adult and the elder patients, respectively. These evaluations are in agreement with literature. For instance, Conley & Legan (Conley and Legan, 2003) suggest a latency period not longer than 7 days. Mattik et al. (Mattik et al., 2001), reported three clinical cases of young patients 18, 19 and 28 years old, for whom a latency period of 5 days was adopted. Lazar et al. (Lazar et al., 2003) submitted a 62-years old patient to mandibular distraction osteogenesis. The first distraction was given to the mandible following a delayed latency period of 10 days.

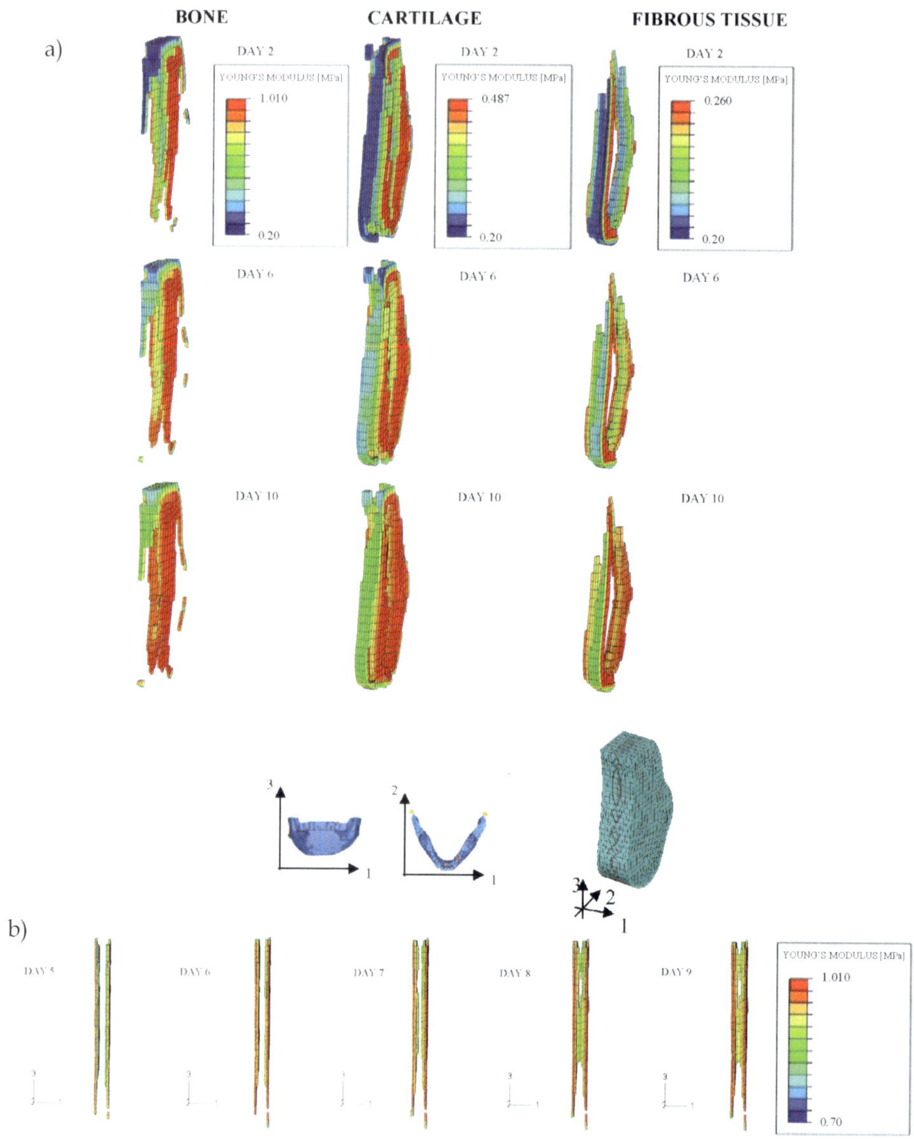

Fig. 8. (a) 3D visualization of tissue differentiation in the bone callus; (b) 3D visualization of the bone regeneration process in the frontal plane 1-3

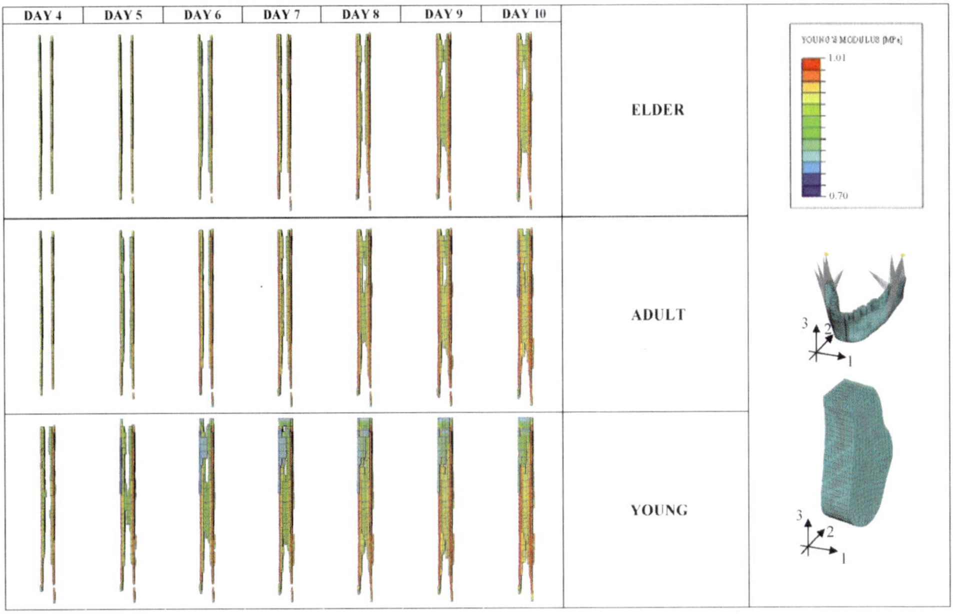

Fig. 9. Bone regeneration process for the young, adult and elder patients

3.5 Influence of expansion rates on mandibular distraction osteogenesis

Another important issue investigated with the mechano-regulation model of Prendergast and colleagues (Prendergast et al., 1997) and the above described finite element model, is the influence of expansion rates on the distraction process. The algorithm shown in Fig. 7 has been expanded to include the modelling of the distraction of the orthodontic appliance. Two different protocols of expansion were investigated: the first one where the device is distracted by 0.6mm/day for a period of ten days, the second where the device is distracted at 1.2 mm/day for five days. The final result with the aforementioned protocols is a widening of mandibular arch by about 6 mm corresponding to the space occupied by a lower incisor. The total number of iterations was set in order to cover a time period of 43 days, consisting of a one week latency period and a 37 day distraction and maturation period. In the case of the 0.6 mm/day distraction rate, this latter period included ten days of distraction and a 27 day maturation period, while the 1.2 mm/day distraction rate consisted of five days of distraction and a 32 day maturation period. In each iteration which simulates a distraction process, a structural FE analysis was run in order to model just the expansion of the appliance. In this analysis a given displacement was imposed to the arms of the distractor. Further details about the implemented algorithm are reported in Boccaccio et al. (Boccaccio et al., 2007). The spatial and temporal changes in tissue differentiation produced with these two different protocols were predicted and compared (Fig.10).

The computational analyses revealed that the lower expansion rate of 0.6 mm/day leads to greater amounts of bone tissue 'bridging' the left and right sides of the callus (Fig. 10). It is possible that excessive bone quantities in this area may hinder the process of distraction because a premature bone union can occur. Therefore a faster distraction rate of 1.2 mm/day is preferable in cases where there is an increased risk of bone union.

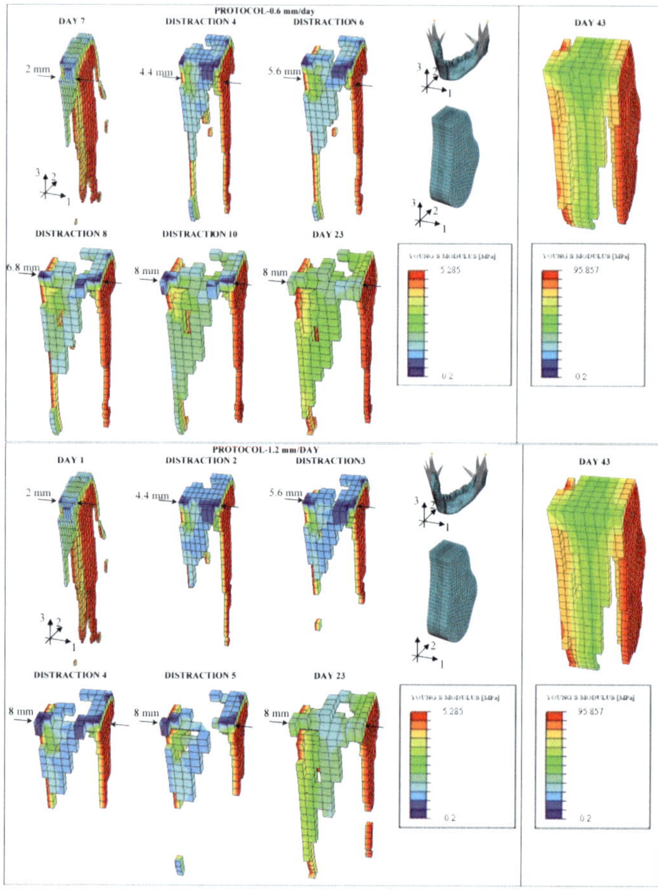

a)

b)

Fig. 10. Bone regeneration process for a distraction rate of (a) 0.6 mm/day and (b) 1.2 mm/day

4. Mechanobiology of fracture repair in vertebral bodies

Vertebral fractures commonly occur in elderly people with osteoporosis. For example, in the United States vertebral fractures account for nearly half of all osteoporotic fractures (Cummings et al., 2002). With age the structure of cancellous bone within vertebral bodies transforms from that characterized by predominately plate-like trabeculae to rod-like trabeculae. This change leads to an age-related decrease in trabecular bone mass (Amling et al., 1996). The reduced bone mass observed in vertebral bodies, particularly with osteoporosis, is generally accompanied by greater amounts of microcallus formations around injured trabeculae (Hansson and Roos, 1981). This weakening of the tissue means that spine fractures may occur after minimal trauma (Einhorn, 2005).

The objective of this study was to investigate if biophysical stimuli play a role in regulating the process of tissue differentiation and bone remodeling in a fractured vertebral body. Our hypothesis is that the mechano-regulation model for tissue differentiation proposed by Prendergast et al. (Prendergast et al., 1997) and that has previously been used to predict the time-course of fracture repair in long and flat bones (Lacroix and Prendergast, 2002, Boccaccio et al., 2007) can be used to predict trabecular bone healing in fractured vertebrae at the level of individual trabeculae.

To determine the magnitude of such stimuli at the level of individual trabeculae, a multi-scale finite element approach has been adopted. A macro-scale finite element model (Fig. 11) of the spinal segment L3-L4-L5, including a mild wedge fracture in the body of the L4 vertebra, is used to determine the boundary conditions acting on a micro-scale finite element model of a portion of fractured trabecular bone. The micro-scale model, in turn, is utilized to predict the local patterns of tissue differentiation within the fracture site and then how the equivalent mechanical properties of the macro-scale model change with time.

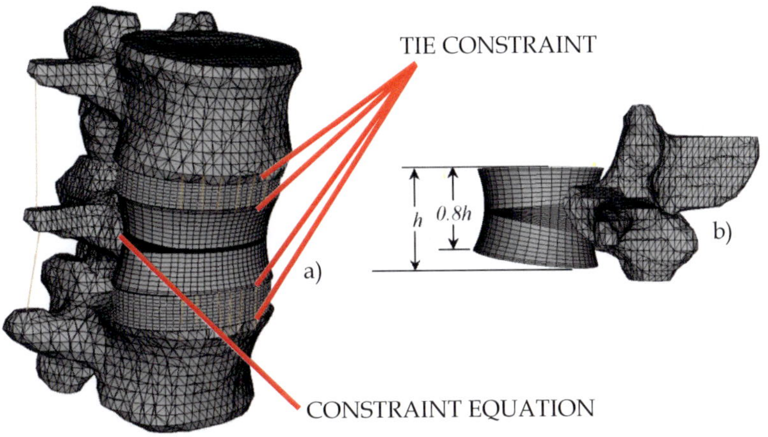

Fig. 11. (a) Finite element models of the spinal segment L3-L4-L5; (b) the body of fractured vertebra L4; its height decreases towards the anterior side.

The L3, L5 vertebrae and the posterior processes of the L4 were modelled as un-deformable rigid bodies. Deformable elements have been utilized to model the body of the L4 vertebra as well as the intervertebal discs. Between the intervertebral disc and the vertebral bodies a 'tie' constraint was applied (Fig. 11a). Constraint equations were used to attach the posterior processes to the body of the L4 vertebra (Fig. 11a). Each intervertebral disc includes the cartilagineous endplates, the nucleus polposus, the annulus fibrosus with the collagen fibres. The effects of the flavum, intertransverse, interspinous and supraspinous ligaments have been included in the model. Further details about the geometry of the intervertebral discs and the modelling of the ligaments are reported in Boccaccio et al. (Boccaccio et al., 2008c). The height of the fractured vertebra decreases by the 20% from the posterior processes towards the anterior side (Fig. 11 (b)). In the Genant grading (Genant et al., 1993), such a fracture is classified as a mild wedge fracture. The body of L4 includes the cortical shell of 0.5 mm thickness (Mizrahi et al., 1993), the cancellous bone and the fracture gap (Fig. 12(a-c)). The cancellous and the cortical bone have been modelled as biphasic poroelastic materials possessing transversely isotropic elastic properties. The distribution of the cancellous bone Young's modulus was assumed to be heterogeneous. An anisotropy ratio of 7/10, -i.e. the Young's modulus in the transversal plane is 7/10 the Young's modulus along the cranio-caudal direction-, was assumed (Eberlein et al., 2001). Further details about the spatial distribution of the Young's modulus of the cancellous bone are reported elsewhere (Boccaccio et al., 2008c).

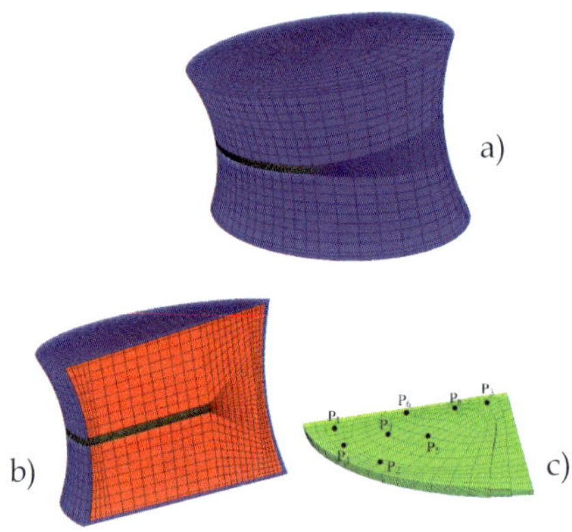

Fig. 12. The body of the fractured vertebra L4 includes the cortical shell (in blue, (a), (b)) the cancellous bone (in red, (b)) and the fracture gap (in green, (c)). The points P_1, P_2, …, P_8 within the fracture gap in correspondence of which the analysis of the fracture repair process was carried out are indicated.

The micro-scale model of the trabecular bone was similar in geometry to that used by Shefelbine et al. (Shefelbine et al., 2005) (Fig. 13). A diastasis of 0.5 mm was simulated, with the trabeculae bordering the gap idealized as prismatic domains 0.1 mm thick. The space between fractured trabeculae was hypothesized to be occupied by granulation tissue. Both, the trabecular bone and the granulation tissue were modelled as biphasic poroelastic materials.

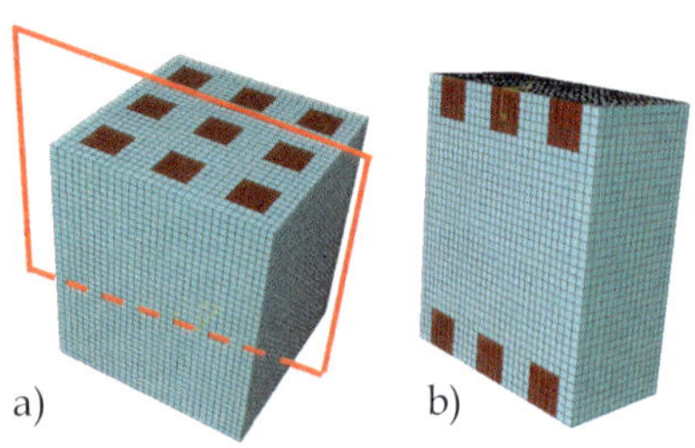

Fig. 13. Geometry (a) and section (b) of the micro-scale model. In red are represented the trabeculae spicules, in blue sky the granulation tissue.

Further details about the micro-scale finite element model of trabecular bone are reported in Boccaccio et al., (Boccaccio et al., 2011b).

A multi-scale approach was adopted. The equations describing tissue differentiation were implemented into an algorithm, a graphical summary of which is depicted in Fig. 14. The time period investigated corresponds to the first 100 days after the fracture event. The macro-scale model of the spinal segment was utilized to determine the elastic and poroelastic boundary conditions acting on eight different micro-scale models which were

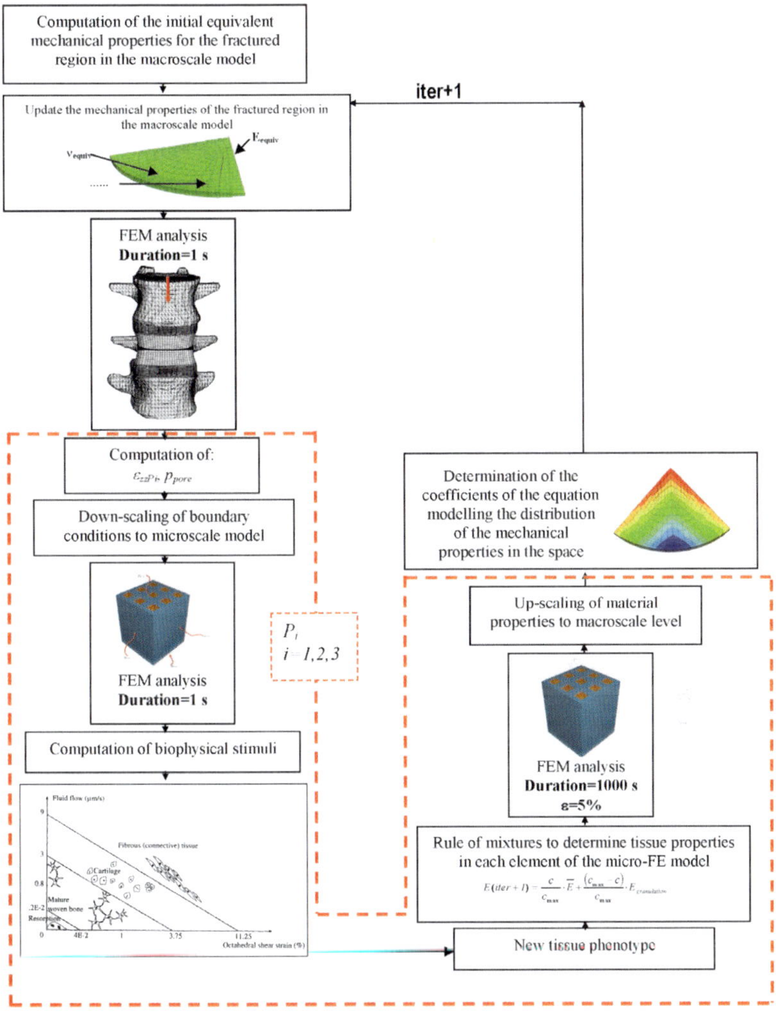

Fig. 14. Schematic of the algorithm utilized to model the fracture repair process in the L4 vertebra.

hypothesized to represent different regions in the fractured cancellous bone located in the neighbourhood of the points $P_1,\ldots,P_8$ (Fig. 12(c)). In order to evaluate the above mentioned boundary conditions, an axial compression of 1000 N -which is the typical load acting on the lumbar vertebrae of a 70 Kg subject in the erect standing position- was applied in the centre of mass of the L3 vertebra and ramped over a time period of 1 s (which can be considered the time in which a subject assumes the erect position). The nodes located on the inferior surface of the L5 vertebra have been clamped. To switch from the macro to the micro-scale model, proper localization rules have been utilized. The micro-scale model, in turn, served to predict the local patterns of the tissues differentiating during the fracture repair process. A compression test was simulated on the micro-scale model reproducing the same elastic and poroelastic boundary conditions as those determined from the macro-scale model. The results obtained from this finite element analysis were used to determine the biophysical stimulus acting in each element of the micro-scale model and then to implement the mechano-regulation model of Prendergast et al. (Prendergast et al., 1997). The change of the tissue phenotype leaded to a change of the equivalent mechanical properties possessed by the fracture gap of the macro-scale model. By adopting homogenization techniques the information obtained from the micro-scale model regarding the material properties was up-scaled to the macro-scale level. The new material properties were implemented into the macro-scale model and a new iteration initiated. Further details regarding the algorithm are reported in a previous study (Boccaccio et al., 2011b).

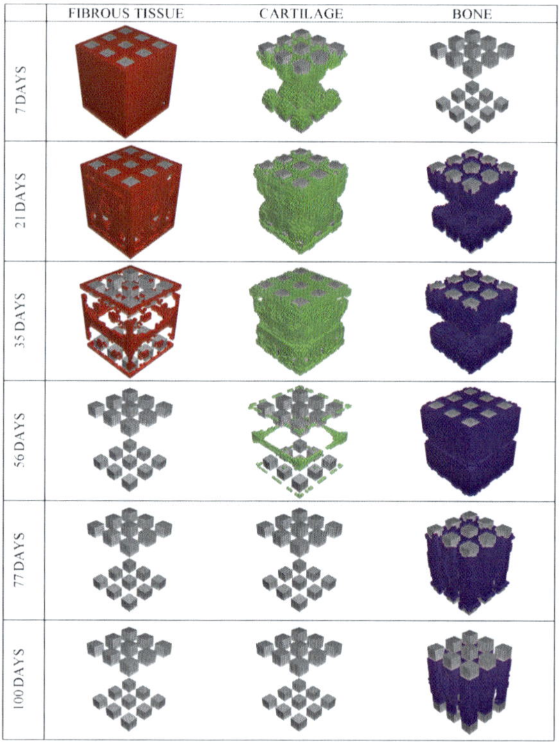

Fig. 15. Patterns of the tissues differentiating within the fractured vertebra during the fracture healing process.

The analyses carried out predicted that the space between the fractured trabeculae is mostly occupied by fibrous tissue in the first days after the fracture event (Fig. 15) During the first 30-35 days after the fracture event the amount of fibrous tissue decreases significantly and disappears completely after six weeks. Small amounts of cartilage appear during the first week, and approximately 40% of the space between the fractured trabeculae is occupied by cartilage after one month. This cartilaginous tissue is completely replaced by bone after two months (Fig. 15). Small amounts of bone are predicted after the first two weeks and after the second month the space is entirely occupied by bone. Bone deposition is predicted to initiate at the fractured trabecular ends. The bone remodeling process appears to start after the second month and reaches equilibrium at the end of the third month. The remodeled trabeculae are aligned with those bordering the fractured region (Fig. 15).
The spatial and temporal patterns of tissue differentiation predicted by this model are in general agreement with those observed experimentally. Diamond et al., (Diamond et al., 2007) describe 4 stages of fracture healing process in the vertebral body, with significant overlap between the various stages of healing. Chondrogenesis was evident in the second stage of the fracture healing process, which followed the initial granulation tissue stage. The appearance of cartilaginous tissue in the days following the fracture event is also predicted by the model (Fig. 15). This cartilaginous tissue is predicted to be gradually replaced by woven bone. The model then predicts a peak in bone formation (see 56th day, Fig. 15).
Hyperosteoidosis/Osteosclerosis (excessive formation of osteoid) is also observed experimentally at comparable time-points (Diamond et al., 2007). Finally remodeling of the cancellous bone architecture is predicted. Complete new trabeculae are predicted to form due to bridging of the microcallus between the remnant trabeculae, leading to restructuring of the bone architecture (Amling et al., 1996).

5. Discussion

In this Chapter the basic principles of mechanobiology are described as well as the principal theories and the main models utilized to simulate the cellular processes involved in fracture healing. Two examples have been illustrated that show how mechanobiology can be used to predict the patterns of tissue differentiation in a human mandible osteotomized and submitted to distraction osteogenesis as well the regrowth and the remodelling process of the cancellous bone in a fractured lumbar vertebra.
Different are the limitations of the above outlined mechano-regulation theories. The main criticism raised against the models of Pauwels (Pauwels, 1960), Carter and colleagues (Carter et al., 1988, Carter and Wong, 1988) and Claes and Heigele (Claes and Heigele, 1999) is that there are several reasons that interstitial fluid flow could be a more realistic mechanical variable for feedback information to the cells during tissue differentiation than hydrostatic pressure (Owan et a., 1997, Jacobs et al., 1998). The interfragmentary strain theory, although has the advantage of being simple to be used since interfragmentary movement can be easily monitored, presents the limitation that it models the fracture as a one dimensional entity thus ignoring the three dimensional complexity of the callus. The model of Prendergast et al. (Prendergast et al., 1997) although takes into account the interstitial fluid flow neglects osmotic effects and charged-density flows in the tissue (Mow et al., 1999). Several mechano-regulation algorithms proposed to control tissue differentiation during bone healing have been shown to accurately predict temporal and spatial tissue distributions during normal fracture healing. As these algorithms are different

in nature and biophysical parameters, it raises the question of which reflects the actual mechanobiological processes the best. Isaksson et al. (Isaksson et al., 2006), addressed this issue by corroborating the mechano-regulatory algorithms of Carter and colleagues (Carter et al., 1988, Carter and Wong, 1988), Claes and Heigele (Claes and Heigele, 1999, Claes et al., 1998) and Prendergast and coworkers (Prendergast et al., 1997), with more extensive in vivo bone healing data from animal experiments. They compared the patterns of tissue differentiation predicted by the different models and the patterns observed in vivo in an ovine tibia model. They concluded that none of the algorithms predicted patterns of healing entirely similar to those observed experimentally. However, patterns predicted by the algorithm based on deviatoric strain and fluid velocity (i.e. the model of Prendergast et al., (Prendergast et al., 1997)) was closest to experimental results.

Another important limitation for computational mechanobiology is represented by the fact that the mechano-regulatory algorithms include empirical constants, the values of which must be determined by comparison to a biological reality. For example, in the mechano-regulation rule developed by Prendergast et al. (Prendergast et al., 1997) the constants b and a (see equation (3)) do not have a specific physical meaning and can be determined by following the 'trial and error' method outlined in van der Melulen and Huiskes (van der Melulen and Huiskes, 2002): "Computational mechano-biologists hypothesize a potential rule and determine if the outcome of this hypothesis produces realistic tissue structures and morphologies, hence 'trial-and-error'. If the results correspond well, they might be an explanation for the mechanism being modelled. This method of research is common practice and productive in physics, less common in biology (Huiskes, 1995); although 'theoretical biology' is based on this type of approach". Certainly, physicists can use this approach (the computational gedanken experiment) because there are so few rules in physics and the predictions are amenable to exact quantitative testing. In biology the phenomena to be observed and analysed are much more complicated than in physics, so cut-and-try theoretical experimentation could not be really useful. Further research should be carried out on the efficiency and the correctness of this philosophy of biological research.

Concerning the mechano-regulation model of fracture repair in the body of the L4 vertebra, the most important limitation is that the implemented algorithm does not include a damaged tissue region that would allow tissue to fracture and new callus to form in regions experiencing high levels of biophysical stimulation (e.g. strain). Therefore this study has only considered the original injury event. In reality, histological analyses (Diamond et al., 2007) revealed that a typical feature of vertebral fractures is the overlap between the different tissues corresponding to the different temporal stages of the fracture healing process. This can be justified with the argument that in vertebral bodies the fracture stabilization that permits orderly repair in long bones is not possible due to repetitive injury.

As far as concerns the model of the human mandible osteotomized and distracted, the most important limitation is that after the first simulation the numerical predictions state that the callus consists of a mixture of bone, cartilage and fibrous tissue (Figures 8-9), where it might be more accurate to state that in the first few days after the osteotomy the callus consists of progenitor cells subjected to a stimulus that if maintained will result in these cells differentiating into either fibroblasts, chondrocytes or osteoblasts, depending on the magnitude of the stimulus. This may explain why histological findings (Loboa et al., 2005) from animal model studies differ from the initial model predictions as progenitor cells take time to differentiate and produce a tissue phenotype that is recognised by appropriate histological staining. For example, significant bone and soft tissue formation is predicted during the latency period which is not observed histologically. Explicitly including in the model the time taken for mineralization etc following differentiation of progenitor cells into osteoblasts may result in model predictions more comparable to *in vivo* findings. Another important limitation of the mechano-regulation model used to assess the bone regeneration process in a human mandible osteotomized and distracted as well as in a fractured vertebra is represented by the utilization of the exponential law. Such a law was introduced to account for the fact that mesenchymal cells not only require time to differentiate but, that differentiated cells require some time also for synthesising and remodelling new tissue. In reality, the exponential law should be utilized only to model the early stages of the fracture healing process; when this process is close to the end, saturation phenomena (e.g. the mineralization process) occur within the fracture callus and therefore, at this point, the exponential law should be replaced with another law that allows to better describe these conclusive processes. As a first approximation, we utilized the exponential law to model the early stages of the fracture healing (Boccaccio et al., 2011b) while, toward the end of the process, we replaced the exponential law with a linear constant law. Further research should be carried out on the mathematical function that better describes the entire process of fracture healing, both, in the early and in the final stages.

Many experiments on skeletal failure and repair have been performed in the last century aimed to determine the influence of biological, mechanical, hormonal factors on the healing process. Despite this effort, there are still many unanswered questions. This indicates the complexity of the biological problems and has stimulated the development of computational models that can analyze the influence of all factors and make predictions under different boundary and loading conditions. These models must also be validated with experimental analyses. However, in many cases the computational models cannot be validated directly because of the difficulties in performing some measurements in vivo. Despite this, indirect validations can be performed if the conclusions of the computer simulations are similar to the experimental or clinical results. Once the mechano-regulation model has been validated, it can be conveniently utilized to assess the regeneration process within the fracture site in the case in which different boundary and loading conditions act on it. For instance, the mechano-regulation model of fracture repair in vertebral bodies illustrated above can be used to predict the spatial and temporal patterns of repair during altered loading conditions, which may prove beneficial in developing rehabilitation regimes following vertebral fractures. Also, this same model can be utilized to evaluate how the patterns of tissue differentiation change if the fractured vertebra is supported with minimally invasive percutaneous fixation devices (Palmisani et al., 2009). Furthermore, the mechanobiological model of the human mandible osteotomized and distracted can be utilized to estimate how the bony tissue regeneration process within the fracture callus change for different mandibular distraction devices such as those analyzed in previous studies (Boccaccio et al., 2008d; Boccaccio et al., 2011c).

Future perspectives include the development of computer power. A more robust integration is required, in future, between biology, mechanics and materials science. This should lead to the development of mechano-regulation models that more accurately describe physiological processes such as fracture healing, tissue genesis etc. A very promising research area for mechanobiology is in the field of tissue engineering. Mechanobiology could be an efficient and cheap tool to determine optimal parameters governing scaffold performance. Future perspectives of numerical simulations of biomaterial scaffolds for tissue engineering rely also on the development of new methods to account for the multi-scale dimension of the problems. At the micro-scale level one can analyse cell/biomaterial interactions and how these interactions influence the tissue differentiation process, at the macro-scale level one can evaluate the 'average' boundary and loading conditions acting on the scaffold implanted in the specific anatomical site.

6. Conclusions

This Chapter presented the principal mechano-regulation theories recently developed to simulate the tissue differentiation and the main cellular processes involved in fracture healing. Two examples have then been given illustrating how a mechano-regulation algorithm - where the bone callus is modeled as a biphasic poroelastic material and the stimulus regulating tissue differentiation is hypothesized to be a function of the strain and fluid flow -, can be utilized to assess the bone regeneration process both, in a human mandible submitted to distraction osteogenesis and in a fractured lumbar vertebra. The principal limitations of mechanobiological algorithms as well as the future research lines in the field have been finally outlined.

7. References

Amling, M.; Pösl, M.; Ritzel, H.; Hahn, M.; Vogel, M.; Wening, V.J. & Delling, G. (1996). Architecture and distribution of cancellous bone yield vertebral fracture clues. A histomorphometric analysis of the complete spinal column from 40 autopsy specimens. *Archives of orthopaedic and trauma surgery*, Vol.115, No.,5, pp. 262-269; ISSN 1434-3916

Andreykiv, A.; Prendergast, P.J.; van Keulen, F.; Swieszkowski, W. & Rozing, P.M. (2005). Bone ingrowth simulation for a concept glenoid component design. Journal of Biomechanics,Vol.38, No.5, pp. 1023-1033, ISSN 1873-2380

Bailón-Plaza, A. & van der Meulen, M.C.H. (2001). A mathematical framework to study the effects of growth factor influences on fracture healing. *Journal of Theoretical Biology*, Vol.212, No.2, pp. 191-209, ISSN 1095-8541

Ballini, A.; De Frenza, G.; Cantore, S.; Papa, F.; Grano, M.; Mastrangelo, F.; Teté, S. & Grassi, F.R. (2007). In vitro stem cell cultures from human dental pulp and periodontal ligament: new prospects in dentistry. *International Journal of Immunopathology and Pharmacology*, Vol.20, No.1, pp. 9-16, ISSN 0394-6320

Ballini, A.; Capodiferro, S.; Cantore, S.; Crincoli, V.; Lajolo, C., De Frenza, G.; Favia, G. & Grassi, F.R. (2010). Dental pulp stem cells curriculum vitae. *Journal of Osteology and Biomaterials*, Vol.1, No.1, pp. 23-27, ISSN 2036-6795.

Barry, F.P. & Murphy, J.M. (2004). Mesenchymal stem cells: clinical applications and biological characterization. *International Journal of Biochemistry and Cell Biology*, Vol.36, No.4, pp568-584, ISSN 1878-5875

Baxter, M.A.; Wynn, R.F.; Jowitt, S.N.; Wraith, J.E.; Fairbairn, L.J. & Bellantuono, I. (2004). Study of telomere length reveals rapid aging of human marrow stromal cells following in vitro expansion. *Stem Cells*, Vol.22, No.5, pp. 675–682, ISSN 0250-6793

Boccaccio, A.; Lamberti, L.; Pappalettere, C.; Carano, A. & Cozzani, M. (2006). Mechanical behavior of an osteotomized mandible with distraction orthodontic devices. *Journal of Biomechanics*, Vol.39, No.15, pp. 2907-2918, ISSN 1528-8951

Boccaccio, A.; Pappalettere, C. & Kelly, D.J. (2007). The influence of expansion rates on mandibular distraction osteogenesis: a computational analysis. *Annals of Biomedical Engineering*, Vol.35, No.11, pp. 1940-1960, ISSN 1521-6047

Boccaccio, A.; Prendergast, P.J.; Pappalettere, C. & Kelly, D.J. (2008a). Tissue differentiation and bone regeneration in an osteotomized mandible: a computational analysis of the latency period. *Medical & Biological Engineering & Computing*, Vol.46, No.3, pp. 283-298, ISSN 1741-0444

Boccaccio, A.; Lamberti, L. & Pappalettere, C. (2008b). Effects of ageing on the latency period in mandibular distraction osteogenesis: a computational mechano-biological analysis. *Journal of Mechanics in Medicine and Biology*, Vol. 8, No.2, pp. 203-225, ISSN 0219-5194

Boccaccio, A.; Vena, P.; Gastaldi, D.; Franzoso, G.; Pietrabissa, R. & Pappalettere, C. (2008c). Finite Element Analysis in cancellous bone failure in the vertebral body of healthy and osteoporotic subjects. *Proceedings of the Institution of the Mechanical Engineers, Journal of Engineering in Medicine, Part H*, Vol.222, No.7, pp. 1023-1036, ISSN 0954-4119

Boccaccio, A.; Lamberti, L.; Pappalettere, C.; Cozzani, M. & Siciliani, G. (2008d). Comparison of different distraction orthodontic devices: a finite element study. *American Journal of Orthodontics and Dentofacial Orthopaedics*, Vol.134, No.2, pp. 260-269, ISSN 1097-6752

Boccaccio, A.; Ballini, A.; Pappalettere, C.; Tullo, D.; Cantore, S. & Desiate, A. (2011a). Finite Element Method (FEM), Mechanobiology and Biomimetic Scaffolds in Bone Tissue Engineering. *International Journal of Biological Sciences*, Vol.7, No.1, pp. 112-132, ISSN 1449-2288

Boccaccio, A.; Kelly, D.J. & Pappalettere, C. (2011b). A mechano-regulation model of fracture repair in vertebral bodies. *Journal of Orthopaedic Research*, Vol.29, No.3, pp. 433-443, ISSN 1554-527X

Boccaccio, A.; Cozzani, M. & Pappalettere, C. (2011c). Analysis of the performance of different orthodontic devices for mandibular symphyseal distraction osteogenesis. *European Journal of Orthodontics*, Vol. 33, No.2, pp. 113-120, ISSN 1460-2210

Brighton, C.T. & Hunt, R.M. (1991). Early histological and ultrastructural changes in medullary fracture callus. *Journal of Bone and Joint Surgery. American Volume*, Vol.73, No.6, pp.832-847, ISSN 1535-1386

Byrne, D.P.; Lacroix, D.; Planell, J.A.; Kelly, D.J. & Prendergast, P.J. (2007). Simulation of tissue differentiation in a scaffold as a function of porosity , Young's modulus and dissolution rate: application of mechanobiological models in tissue engineering. *Biomaterials*, Vol.28, No.36, pp. 5544-5554, ISSN 1878-5905

Byrne, D.P. (2008). Computational modelling of bone regeneration using a three dimensional lattice approach. PhD Thesis, Trinity College Dublin.

Carter, D.R.; Blenman, P.R. & Beaupré, G.S. (1988). Correlations between mechanical stress history and tissue differentiation in initial fracture healing. *Journal of Orthopaedic Research*, Vol.6, No.5, pp. 736–748, ISSN 1554-527X

Carter, D.R. & Wong, M. (1988). The role of mechanical loading histories in the development of diarthrodial Joints. *Journal of Orthopaedic Research*, Vol.6, No., pp. 804-816, ISSN 1554-527X

Carter, D. R.; Beaupré, G. S.; Giori, N. J. & Helms, J. A. (1998). Mechanobiology of skeletal regeneration. *Clinical Orthopaedics and Related Research* Vol.355, pp. S41-S55, ISSN 1528-1132

Checa, S., Prendergast, P.J. (2009). A mechanobiological model for tissue differentiation that includes angiogenesis: A lattice-based modeling approach. *Annals of Biomedical Engineering*, Vol.37, No., pp. 129-145, ISSN 1528-8951

Chen, J.; Sotome, S.; Wang, J.; Orii, H,; Uemura, T. & Shinomiya, K. (2005). Correlation of in vivo bone formation capability and in vitro differentiation of human bone marrow stromal cells. *Journal of medical and dental sciences*, Vol.52, No.1, pp. 27-34, ISSN 1342-8810

Chen, F.H.; Song, L.; Mauck, R.L.; Li, W.J. & Tuan, R.S. (2007). Mesenchymal stem cells, In: R. Lanza, R. Langer, J.P. Vacanti, (Ed.). *Principles of Tissue Engineering*. 3rd Edition. Elsevier/Academic Press ISBN 0-12-370615-7

Claes, L.E.; Heigele, C.A.; Neidlinger-Wilke, C.; Kaspar, D.; Seidl, W.; Margevicius, K.J. & Augat, P. (1998). Effects of mechanical factors on the fracture healing process. *Clinical Orthopaedics and Related Research,* Vol.355, pp. S132-S147, ISSN 1528-1132

Claes, L.E. & Heigele, C.A. (1999). Magnitudes of local stress and strain along bony surfaces predict the course and type of fracture healing. *Journal of Biomechanics*, Vol.32, No.3, pp. 255-266, ISSN 1528-8951

Conley, R. & Legan, H. (2003). Mandibular symphyseal distraction osteogenesis: diagnosis and treatment planning considerations. *Angle Orthodontics*, Vol.73, No.1, pp. 3-11, ISSN 1945-7103

Cummings, S. & Melton, Iii L.J. (2002). Epidemiology and outcomes of osteoporotic fractures. *Lancet*, Vol.359, No.9319, pp. 1761-1767, ISSN 1474-547X

Diamond, T.H.; Clark, W.A. & Kumar, S.V. (2007). Histomorphometric analysis of fracture healing cascade in acute osteoporotic vertebral body fractures. *Bone*, Vol.40, No. 3, pp. 775-780, ISSN 1873-2763

Doblaré, M.; García, J.M. & Gómez, M.J. (2004). Modelling bone tissue fracture and healing: a review. *Engineering Fracture Mechanics*, Vol.71, No.13-14, pp. 1809-1840, ISSN 0013-7944

Einhorn, T.A. (1998). The cell and molecular biology of fracture healing. *Clinical Orthopaedics and Related Research*, Suppl. 355, pp. S7–S21, ISSN 1528-1132

Einhorn, T.A. (2005). The science of fracture healing. *Journal of orthopaedic trauma*, Vol.19 (10 SUPPL.), pp. S4-S6, ISSN 1531-2291

Eberlein, R.; Holzapfel, G.A. & Schulze-Bauer, C.A.J. (2001). An anisotropic model for annulus tissue and enhanced finite element analyses of intact lumbar disc bodies. *Computer Methods in Biomechanics and Biomedical Engineering*, Vol.4, No.3, pp. 209-229, ISSN 1476-8259

Genant, H.K. ; Wu, C.Y. ; van Kuijk, C. & Nevitt, M.C. (1993). Vertebral fracture assesssment using a semi-quantitative technique. *Journal of bone and mineral research : the official journal of the American Society for Bone and Mineral Research*, Vol.8, No.9, pp. 1137-1148, ISSN 1523-4681

Geris,L.; Andreykiv, A.; Oosterwyck, H.V.; Sloten, J.V.; van Keulen, F.; Duyck, J. & Naert, I. (2004). Numerical simulation of tissue differentiation around loaded titanium implants in a bone chamber. *Journal of Biomechanics*, Vol.37, No.5, pp. 763-769, ISSN 1873-2380

Geris, L.; Gerisch, A.; Vander Sloten, J., Weiner, R. & Oosterwyck, H.V. (2008). Angiogenesis in bone fracture healing : A bioregulatory model. *Journal of Theoretical Biology*, Vol.251, No.1, pp.137-158, ISSN 1095-8541

Glowacki, J. (1998). Angiogenesis in fracture repair. *Clinical Orthopaedics and Related Research*, Suppl.355, pp. S82-S89, ISSN 1528-1132

Gòmez-Benito, M.J., Garcìa-Aznar, J.M., Kuiper, J.H. & Doblaré, M. (2005). Influence of fracture gap size on the pattern of long bone healing: a computational study. *Journal of Theoretical Biology*, Vol.235, No.1, pp. 105-119, ISSN 1095-8541

Hansson, T. & Roos, B. (1981). Microcalluses of the trabeculae in lumbar vertebrae and their relation to the bone mineral content. *Spine*, Vol.6, No.4, pp. 375-380, ISSN 1528-1159

Huiskes, R. (1993). Failed innovation in total hip-replacement - diagnosis and proposals for a cure. *Acta Orthopaedica Scandinavica* Vol.64, No.6, pp. 699–716, ISSN 0001-6470

Huiskes, R. (1995). The law of adaptive bone remodeling: a case for crying newton? In: Bone Structure and Remodeling, Odgaard, A.; Weinans, H. (eds.), 15-24, World Scientific Publishing, Singapore, ISBN 978-9810221904, River Edge, London.

Huiskes, R., van Driel, W.D., Prendergast, P.J. & Søballe, K. (1997). A biomechanical regulatory model for periprosthetic fibrous-tissue differentiation. *Journal of Materials Science. Materials in Medicine*, Vol.8, No.12, pp. 785–788, ISSN 1573-4838

Isaksson, H.; Donkellar, C.C. ; Huiskes, R. & Ito, K. (2006). Corroboration of mechanoregulatory algorithms for tissue differentiation during fracture healing: Comparison with in vivo results. *Journal of Orthopaedic Research*, Vol.24, No.5, pp. 898-907, ISSN 1554-527X

Jacobs, C.R. ; Yellowley, C.E. ; Davis, B.R.; Zhou, Z.; Cimbala, J.M.; & Donahue, H.J. (1998). Differential effect of steady versus oscillating flow on bone cells. *Journal of Biomechanics*, Vol.31, No.11, pp. 969–976, ISSN 1873-2380

Kelly, D.J. & Prendergast, P.J. (2005). Mechano-regulation of stem cell differentiation and tissue regeneration in osteochondral defects, *Journal of Biomechanics*,Vol.38, No.7, pp. 1413–1422, ISSN 1873-2380

Kelly, D.J. & Prendergast, P.J. (2006). Prediction of the optimal mechanical properties for a scaffold used in osteochondral defect repair. *Tissue Engineering*, Vol.12, No.9, pp. 2509-2519, ISSN 1557-8690

Lacroix, D.; Prendergast, P.J.; Li, G. & Marsh, D. (2002). Biomechanical model to simulate tissue differentiation and bone regeneration: application to fracture healing. *Medical & Biological Engineering & Computing*, Vol.40, No.1, pp. 14-21, ISSN 1741-0444

Lacroix, D. & Prendergast, P.J. (2002). A mechano-regulation model for tissue differentiation during fracture healing: analysis of gap size and loading. *Journal of Biomechanics*, Vol.35, No.9, pp. 1163-1171, ISSN 1873-2380

Lazar, F.C.; Klesper, B., Siessegger, M.; Zoeller, J.E. & Hidding, J. (2003). Modified distraction protocols in vertical distraction osteogenesis, *International Poster Journal Dental Oral Medicine*, Vol.5, Poster 185.

Loboa, E.G.; Fang, T.D.; Parker, D.W.; Warren, S.M.; Fong, K.D.; Longaker, M.T. & Carter, D.R. (2005). Mechanobiology of mandibular distraction osteogenesis: finite element analyses with a rat model. *Journal of Orthopaedic Research*, Vol.23, No.3, pp. 663-670, ISSN 1554-527X

Martin, I.; Wendt, D. & Heberer, M. (2004). The role of bioreactors in tissue engineering. *Trends in Biotechnology*, Vol.22, No.2, pp. 80–86, ISSN 1879-3096

Mattik, C.R.; Chadwick, S.M. & Morton, M.E. (2001). Mandibular advancement using an intra-oral osteogenic distraction technique: a report of three clinical cases. *Journal of Orthodontics*, Vol.28, No.2, pp. 105-114, ISSN 1465-3133

McKibbin, B. (1978) The biology of fracture healing in long bones. *Journal of Bone and Joint Surgery*, Vol.60, No.B2, pp. 150–162, ISSN 0301-620X

Mendes, S.C.; Tibbe, J.M.; Veenhof, M.; Bakker, K.; Both, S.; Platenburg, P.P.; Oner, F.C.; De Bruijn, J.D. & Van Blitterswijk, C.A. (2002). Bone tissue-engineered implants using human bone marrow stromal cells: effect of culture conditions and donor age. *Tissue Engineering*, Vol.8, No.6, pp. 911–920, ISSN 1557-8690

Meyer, U.; Kleinheinz, J. & Joos, U. (2004). Biomechanical and clinical implications of distraction osteogenesis in craniofacial surgery. *Journal of Cranio-Maxillofacial Surgery*, Vol.32, No.3, pp. 140-149, ISSN 1878-4119

McNamara, J.G. & Brudon, W.M. (1993). *Orthodontic and orthopaedic treatment in the mixed dentition*. Ann Arbor (MI): Needham Press; pp. 131-145.

van der Meulen, M.C.H. & Huiskes, R. (2002). Why mechanobiology? A survey article. *Journal of Biomechanics*, Vol.35, No.4, pp. 401-414, ISSN 1873-2380

Milan, J.L.; Planell, J.A. & Lacroix, D. (2009). Computational modelling of the mechanical environment of osteogenesis within a polylactic acid-calcium phosphate glass scaffold. *Biomaterials*, Vol.30, No.25, pp. 4219-4226, ISSN 1878-5905

Mizrahi, J.; Silve, M.J.; Keaveny, T.M.; Edwards, W.T. & Hayes, W.C. (1993). Finite-element stress analysis of the normal and osteoporotic lumbar vertebral body. *Spine*, Vol.18, No.14, pp. 2088-2096, ISSN 1528-1159

Moreo, P.; Garcìa-Aznar, J.M. & Doblaré, M. (2009a). Bone ingrowth on the surface of endosseous implants: Part 1: Mathematical model. *Journal of Theoretical Biology*, Vol.260, No.1, pp: 1-12, ISSN 1095-8541

Moreo, P.; Garcìa-Aznar, J.M. & Doblaré, M. (2009b). Bone ingrowth on the surface of endosseous implants: Part 2: Theoretical and numerical analysis. *Journal of Theoretical Biology*, Vol.260, No.1, pp: 13-26, ISSN 1095-8541

Mow, V.C.; Wang, C.C.-B. & Hung, C.T. (1999). The extracellular matrix, interstitial fluid and ions as a mechanical signal transducer in articular cartilage. *Osteoarthritis and Cartilage*, Vol.7, No.1, pp. 41-58, ISSN 1522-9653

Murray, J.D. (1989). *Mathematical Biology*. Springer-Verlag, ISBN 978-0-387-95223-9, Berlin, Germany.

Nagel, T. & Kelly, D.J. (2010). Mechano-regulation of mesenchymal stem cell differentiation and collagen organisation during skeletal tissue repair. *Biomechanics and Modelling in Mechanobiology*, Vol.9, No.3, pp. 359-372, ISSN 1617-7940

Olivares, A.; Marsal, E.; Planell, J.A. & Lacroix, D. (2009). Finite element study of scaffold architecture design and culture conditions for tissue engineering. *Biomaterials*, Vol.30, No.30, pp. 6142-6149, ISSN 1878-5905

Owan, I.; Burr, D.B.; Turner, C.H., Qiu, J.; Tu, Y.; Onyia, J.E. & Duncan, R.L. (1997). Mechanotransduction in bone: osteoblasts are more responsive to fluid forces than mechanical strain. *American Journal of Physiology*, Vol.273, No. 3 Pt 1, pp. C810-815, ISSN 0002-9513

Palmisani, M,; Gasbarrini, A.; Barbanti Brodano, G.; De Iure, F.; Cappuccio, M.; Boriani, L.; Amendola, L. & Boriani, S. (2009). Minimally invasive percutaneous fixation in the treatment of thoracic and lumbar spine fractures. *European Spine Journal* , Vol.18, No.1, pp. S71-S74, ISSN 1432-0932

Park, J.S.; Kim, H.Y.; Kim, H.W.; Chae, G.N.; Oh, H.T.; Park, J.Y.; Shim, H.; Seo, M.; Shin, E.Y.; Kim, E.G.; Park, S.C. & Kwak, S.J. (2005). Increased caveolin-1, a cause for the declined adipogenic potential of senescent human mesenchymal stem cells, *Mechanisms of ageing and development*, Vol.126, No.5, pp. 551–559, ISSN 1872-6216

Pauwels, F. (1960). Eine neue theorie über den einfluβ mechanischer reize auf die differenzierung der stützgewebe. *Z Anat Entwickl*, Vol.121, pp. 478-515. Translated as A new theory concerning the influence of mechanical stimuli on the differentiation of the supporting tissues. In: *Biomechanics of the Locomotor apparatus*, Maquet, P. & Furlong, R. (Eds), 375-407, Springer, ISBN 978-0387091310, Berlin, Germany

Pérez, M.A. & Prendergast, P.J. (2007). Random-walk models of cell dispersal included in mechanobiological simulations of tissue differentiation. *Journal of Biomechanics*, Vol.40, No., pp. 2244-2253, ISSN 1873-2380

Perren, S.M. Physical and biological aspects of fracture healing with special reference to internal fixation. (1979). *Clinical Orthopaedics and Related Research*, Vol.138, pp. 175–196, ISSN 1528-1132

Prendergast, P.J. & Huiskes, R. (1995). An investigation of Pauwels' mechanism of tissue differentiation. *Transactions of EORS*, Munich, Germany.

Prendergast, P.J.; Huiskes, R. & Søballe, K. (1997). Biophysical stimuli on cells during tissue differentiation at implant interfaces. *Journal of Biomechanics*, Vol.30, No.6, pp. 539–548, ISSN 1528-8951

Prendergast, P.J. (2006). Prosthesis fixation for orthopaedics In: *Encyclopaedia of Medical Devices and Instrumentation*, Webster J.E., (Ed.), 192-198, Wiley, ISBN 0471829366 New Jersey.

Prendergast, P.J.; Checa, S. & Lacroix, D. (2009). Computational Models of Tissue Differentiation. In *Computational modelling in Biomechanics*, De S.; Guilak, F. & Mofrad F., (Eds.), 353-372, Business Media: Springer Science, ISBN 978-90-4081-3575-2

Richardson, J.B.; Kenwright, J. & Cunningham, J.L. (1992). Fracture stiffness measurement in the assessment and management of tibial fractures. *Clinical Biomechanics*, Vol.7, pp. 75–79, ISSN 1879-1271

Sanz-Herrera, J.A.; García-Aznar, J.M. & Doblaré, M. (2009). On scaffold designing for bone regeneration: A computational multiscale approach. *Acta Biomaterialia*, Vol.5, No.1, pp. 219-229, ISSN 1878-7568

Schwartz-Dabney, C.L. & Dechow, P.C. (2003). Variations in cortical material properties throughout the human dentate mandible. *American Journal of Physical Anthropology*, Vol.120, No.3, pp. 252-277, ISSN 1096-8644

Shefelbine, S.J.; Augat, P.; Claes, L. & Simon, U. (2005). Trabecular bone fracture healing simulation with finite element analysis and fuzzy logic. *Journal of Biomechanics*,Vol.38, No.12, pp. 2440-2450, ISSN 1528-8951

Sherratt, J.A.; Martin, P. ; Murrayjd, J.D. & Lewis, J. (1992). Mathematical models of wound healing in embryonic and adult epidermis, *IMA Journal of Mathematics Applied in Medicine and Biology*, Vol.9, No.3, pp. 177-196, ISSN 0265-0746

Simmons, D.J. (1985). Fracture healing perspectives. *Clinical Orthopaedics and Related Research*, Vol.200, pp. 100-113, ISSN 1528-1132

2

Evolution of Locomotor Trends in Extinct Terrestrial Giants Affected by Body Mass

Valery B. Kokshenev[1] and Per Christiansen[2]
[1]*Departamento de Física, Universidade Federal de Minas Gerais, Belo Horizonte*
[2]*University of Aalborg, Department of Biotechnology, Chemistry, and Environmental Engineering, Sohngaardsholmsvej 57, DK-9000 Aalborg*
[1]*Brazil*
[2]*Denmark*

1. Introduction

It is generally accepted that bone morphology may be influenced by functional bone strains or stresses (McMahon, 1973, 1975a, b; Alexander, 1977; Bertram & Biewener 1990, 1992; Biewener, 1990; Christiansen, 1999, 2002a, b). However, the problem as to which specific mechanical characteristics are most relevant remains open (e.g., Rubin & Lanyon, 1984; Fritton et al., 2000; Biewener, 2000, 2005). Aiming to establish correlations between structural proportions and posture of mammalian limbs coping with body's locomotory functions, including support of mass in the gravitational field, scaling studies of limb long bones in terrestrial mammals have been subject to long standing debate and controversy (Biewener, 1982, 1983, 1989, 1990, 2000, 2005; Biewener et al., 1983; Biewener & Taylor, 1986; Selker & Carter, 1989; Bertram & Biewener, 1990, 1992; Christiansen, 1997, 1998, 1999, 2002a, b, 2007; Fariña et al., 1997; Carrano, 1998, 1999, 2001; Currey, 2003; Kokshenev, 2003; Kokshenev et al., 2003). The exploration of basic concepts of stability of ideal and non-ideal solid cylinders loaded in non-critical, transient and near critical mechanical regimes, mapped to arbitrary loaded curved limb long bones, resulted in a number of mechanical patterns of similarity in long bones adjusted to their design (Kokshenev, 2007). Established under fairly general assumptions, the proposed scaling rules (for peak longitudinal-bone and transverse-bone elastic forces and momenta, compressive and shear strains, corresponding to axial and non-axial bending and torsional components of tensorial stress) congruent with bone allometry explained the two basic patterns of functional stresses *in vivo* revealed in the limb bones of fast running terrestrial mammals by Rubin & Lanyon (1982, 1984).

The theoretically established patterns of bone design (Kokshenev, 2007) have been also tested (Kokshenev & Christiansen, 2010) by the surprisingly varied differential scaling of the limb long bones in Asian (*Elephas maximus*) and African (*Loxodonta africana*) elephants. These terrestrial giants have more upright limb bones to vertical, notably much more upright propodials (humerus and femur), which are held at a distinctly greater angle compared to the ground than is the case in other large, quadrupedal mammals. Studies of their locomotor mechanics have also indicated differences from other terrestrial mammals, in that fast locomotion is ambling with no suspended phase in the stride, but with duty factors exceeding 0.5 (Alexander et al., 1979; Hutchinson et al., 2006). The theoretical predictions by Kokshenev (2007) were compared with data from a phylogenetically wide sample of proboscideans from Christiansen (2007). Consequently, some salient features distinguishing limb postures characteristic of locomotion in proboscideans and mammals were established. The limb bone allometry in Asian elephants and the Elephantidae was shown to be congruent with adaptation to bending-torsion proportions of stress induced by muscular forces, likewise in other mammals, whereas limb bones in African elephants appear adapted for coping with the dominating axial compressive forces of gravity. Since the hindlimb bones in extant and most likely extinct elephants were shown to be more compliant than forelimb bones, the limb compliance gradient of limb locomotory function, contrasting in sign to other mammals, was shown to constitute a new important dynamic constraint preventing elephants from achieving a full-body aerial phase in fast gaits of locomotion.

Considering the athletism of non-avian dinosaurs and adopting the assumption of *dynamic similarity*, Alexander (1976) analyzed inferred bending stress in their limb bones, which led him to the hypothesis (Alexander, 1981, 1985a) that animals appear to be built with universal (equal bodyweight-independent) *limb safety factors* (bone strengths related to corresponding peak bone stresses). However, systematic studies of functional limb bone stress by Rubin & Lanyon (1982, 1984) clearly demonstrated that the dimensionless factor of limb safety may not be chosen as the determinant of dynamic similarity revealed across body mass through the speed and frequency in fast running bipeds and quadrupeds. Instead, a new kind of *dynamic strain similarity* (physically equivalent to dynamic stress similarity) observed in limb bones of walking, trotting, and galloping animals experimentally established by many researchers (Rubin & Lanyon, 1982, 1984; Rubin & Lanyon, 1982; Biewener et al., 1983; Biewener & Taylor, 1986) has been only recently understood in light of more general *mechanical elastic similarity* (Kokshenev, 2007). It has been in particular demonstrated that the consistency between the elastic strain similarity by Rubin & Lanyon (1982, 1984) and the *elastic static stress similarity* by McMahon (1975a) exists, since both are underlaid by the same patterns of elastic forces emerging in solids, that can be revealed if the external gravitational forces are substituted by predominating functional muscular forces (Kokshenev, 2003; Kokshenev et al., 2003). In this chapter, we try to establish a link between the mechanical elastic similarity in limb bones of different-sized animals (McMahon, 1973, 1975a, b; Rubin & Lanyon, 1982, 1984; Kokshenev, 2003, 2007) and the seminal dynamic similarity in locomotion of animals (Alexander, 1976, 1989; Alexander & Jayes, 1983), arising in turn from the more general mechanical similarity of uniform classical systems (Kokshenev, 2011a, b).

Following Schmidt-Neielsen (1984), it has been widely recognized that body mass is often a major locomotory factor scaling muscle force output establishing limits for body ability in animals (Alexander, 1985b; Hutchinson & Garcia, 2002; Biewener, 2005, Hutchinson et al., 2005; Marden, 2005), through their maximal speed (Garland, 1983; Jones & Lindstedt, 1993; Sellers & Manning, 2007) and maximal size (Hokkanen, 1986a; Biewener, 1989; Kokshenev, 2007). Reconstructing body mass and locomotion in extinct animals (Alexander, 1989, 1991, 1998, 2006; Fariña & Blanco, 1996; Fariña et al., 1997; Carrano, 1998; 2001; Carrano & Biewener, 1999; Farlow et al., 2000; Wilson & Carrano, 1999; Hutchinson & Gatesy, 2006, Sellers & Manning, 2007), the biomechanical modeling also includes their locomotor habits (e.g., Fariña, 1995; Paul & Christiansen, 2000; Christiansen & Paul 2001; Blanco & Jones, 2005; Fariña et al., 2005). The evolutionary history of dinosaurs and mammals provide evidence for convergent similarities of skeletal design (e.g., near parasagittal limb postures and hinge-like joints), locomotor kinematics (Alexander, 1991, 1998; Farlow et al., 2000; Carrano, 1998, 1999; 2001; Paul & Christiansen, 2000; Hutchinson et al., 2006), and biomechanics (see reviews by Hutchinson, 2006; and Alexander, 2006), as well as inferred physiology and growth rates (e.g., Ji et al., 1998; Horner et al., 1999; Rensberger & Watabe, 2000; Sander, 2000; Erickson, 2004; Padian et al., 2004). However, locomotor complexity cannot be captured in a simple model since the number of required parameters increases rapidly as a model becomes more complex (Hutchinson & Gatesy, 2006). One issue of great importance in biomechanics is therefore to more accurately employ generalizations following from dynamic similarity concepts suggested a few dimensionless universal (body mass independent) numbers (Alexander & Jayes, 1983; Gatesy & Biewener, 1991) or a few number of universal scaling (exponents in scaling) rules (Garland, 1983; Heglund & Taylor, 1988; Biewener, 1990; Farley et al.,1993; Bejan & Marden, 2006; Kokshenev, 2010), which potentially make a bridge between locomotory trends in large modern elephants, the largest extant, and the largest extinct proboscideans (e.g., Kokshenev & Christiansen, 2010). Although the experimental exploration of dynamic similarity determinants was repeatedly questioned, e.g., in the context of dimensionless body safety factors (Biewener, 1982, 1990, 2000, 2005) or Froude numbers (Hutchinson et al., 2006), the empirical studies of locomotor evolution in extinct animals (e.g., archosaurs reviewed by Hutchinson, 2006) evidence for that evolution in running and turning abilities in extinct giants, accomplished by transformations in poses and postures of animals, expose a certain kind of adaptive similarity driven by body mass. Developing here the application of dynamic stress similarity generally supported by some available dynamic data on reconstructed extinct giants, we demonstrate how the empirically established traits of locomotory evolution in extinct terrestrial giants can be explained as affected by maximal body mass through limb-bone adaptations.

2. Materials and methods

2.1 Materials

2.1.1 Maximal body mass

The principal sources of data on *maximal body masses* $M_{\max}^{(\exp)}$ inferred from remains of some of the largest non-avian dinosaurs and mammals are listed in Table 1. Other published data are cited at appropriate points.

2.1.2 Dynamic strain and stress similarities

The *in vivo* studies by Rubin & Lanyon (1982, 1984) on the individual-bone functional peak stress $\sigma_{bone}^{(peak)}(M, V)$, resulted from gauge implantation in the long limb bones, revealed the dynamic stress (or strain) similarity in animals of different body mass M running at a certain *speed* V. For the special studied case of biped and quadruped animals (from a turkey to an elephant) running at their *fastest speeds* $V_{\max}$, the corresponding pattern of dynamic stress similarity (shown below Table 2 in Rubin & Lanyon, 1984) can be read here as

$$\sigma_{bone}^{(\max)}(M, V_{\max}) - \sigma_{axial}^{(\exp)}(M) + \upsilon_{bend}^{(\exp)}(M). \tag{1}$$

The axial and bending components of the compressive *tibial* stress where scaled to body mass (ranged from 7.3 kg to 2500 kg) and analyzed by the least-squares liner regression method resulted in

$$\sigma_{axial}^{(\exp)}(M) = C_{axial}^{(\exp)} M^{-0.05}, \text{with } \sigma_{bend}^{(\exp)}(M) = C_{bend}^{(\exp)} M^{0.08}, \tag{2}$$

Taxon	Largest species	$M_{\max}^{(\exp)}$, kg	References	$\beta_{duty}^{(pred)}$
Dinosauria,Sauropoda,	*Argentinosaurus*	70000	Mazetta et al., 2004	> 0.5
Dinosauria, Sauropoda	*Supersaurus*	38000	Lovelace et al., 2007	> 0.5
Dinosauria, Sauropoda	*Giraffatitan*	38000	Taylor, 2009	> 0.5
Dinosauria, Theropoda	*Giganotosaurus*	9000	Mazetta et al., 2004	< 0.5
Dinosauria, Theropoda	*Tyrannosaurus*	8000	Mazetta et al., 2004	< 0.5
Dinosauria, Ornithopoda	*Shantungosaurus*	16000	Horner et al., 2004	< 0.5
Mammalia, Proboscidea	*Mammuthus trogontherii*	20000	Christiansen, 2004	≈ 0.5
Mammalia, Proboscidea	*Deinotherium giganteum*	18000	Christiansen, 2004	≈ 0.5
Mammalia, Perissodactyla	*Indricotherium*	19000	Fortelius & Kappe-lmann, 1993	< 0.5

Table 1. Some data on maximal body masses in terrestrial giants. The limb duty limb factor is provided as an expected characteristics indicating that animals could run with a suspended phase in the stride (with $\beta_{duty} < 0.5$) or would able to progress with a walking gait only (with $\beta_{duty} > 0.5$).

where

$$C_{axial}^{(\exp)} = 11MPa \cdot (kg)^{0.05} \text{ and } C_{bend}^{(\exp)} = 28MPa \cdot (kg)^{-0.08}. \qquad (3)$$

Testing the dynamic stress similarity hypothesis by Rubin & Lanyon (1984), the continuous-speed dynamic similarity between different-sized animals, moving in a certain *gait*, was studied by Biewener & Taylor (1986) through the gait-dependent individual-bone stress function $\sigma_{bone}^{(\max)}(M,V)$, also analyzed by Rubin & Lanyon (1982). Experimental studies of the peak stress measured in the midshaft of long bones in fast walking, moderately running (or trotting) animals, and fast running (or galloping) animals with smoothly changing speed, resulted in that $\sigma_{bone}^{(\max)}(M,V)$ is a linear piecewise function of speed, which domains are limited by the gait-dependent "speed-equivalent" points $V_{trans}^{(\max)}$, as suggested by Biewener & Taylor (1986).

When the allometric data from individual bones in running mammals are generalized to *effective limb bone* (e.g., Kokshenev, 2003), the corresponding peak functional stress is suggested here in the form

$$\sigma_{limb}^{(\max)}(M,V) = \sigma_{axial}^{(\max)}(M) + \sigma_{bend}^{(\max)}(M)\frac{V}{V_{trans}^{(\max)}}, \qquad (4)$$

where the *transient* speeds $V_{trans}^{(\max)}$ are characteristic points of the crossover-gait (walk-to-run) dynamic states or transient-mode (trot-to-gallop) dynamic states, discussed in the context of dynamic similarity theory (Kokshenev, 2011a, b). The reliably of the suggested gait-dependent pattern of dynamic stress similarity in an effective bone shown in Eq. (4) can be inferred from the *in vivo* compressive stress data exemplified by those from three walking, trotting, and galloping adult goats analyzed by Biewener & Taylor (1986, Figs. 2B and 4), which generally unify the experimental data from the radius and tibia in a goat with those in a dog (Rubin & Lanyon, 1982) and a horse (Rubin & Lanyon, 1982; Biewener et al., 1983).

2.1.3 Limb bone design

Aiming to make a bridge between limb bone design in extant and extinct animals listed in Table 1, for which systematic data on the bone length (L) and bone circumference (C) as

	Mammals			Proboscidea			Elephantidae		
Limb bones	N	$\lambda^{(\exp)}$	r	N	$\lambda^{(\exp)}$	r	N	$\lambda^{(\exp)}$	r
Humerus	189	0.7631	0.9738	16	*1.134*	0.831	7	0.912	0.990
Radius	189	0.7530	0.9957	10	*1.078*	0.878	6	0.813	0.853
Ulna	189	0.849	0.9600	14	0.929	0.866	6	0.727	0.888
Femur	189	0.8431	0.9763	14	0.802	0.816	7	0.747	0.966
Tibia	189	0.7641	0.9499	11	0.772	0.857	6	0.751	0.925
Limb bone	189	**0.795**	0.971	13	**0.943**	0.850	6	**0.790**	0.924

Table 2. Statistical data on the slenderness of individual and effective limb bones in animals reproduced from Table 1 in Kokshenev & Christiansen (2010). The mean slenderness exponents are presented by the slopes $\lambda^{(\exp)}$ derived in N species through the least-squares (LS) regression with the *correlation coefficient* r. The LS characterization of the effective limb bone corresponding to the overall-bone mean data is introduced as the standard mean of all data on five bones. The *bold numbers* are the data used below. The *italic numbers* indicate some the slope data contrasting to systematic mammalian data $\lambda^{(\exp)}_{(mam)} < 1$.

functions of body mass are not available, the effective limb bone for extinct species can be introduced through the statistical data on the *slenderness exponents* λ $(= dLog_{10}L/dLog_{10}C)$ obtained regardless of the body mass data. Some employed below examples of extinct Mammalia are listed in Table 2.

2.2 Theory

2.2.1 Stress similarity

In fast gaits of locomotion, all types of elastic strains (and thus stresses), including axial uniform compressive strains, non-uniform tensile strains and transverse non-uniform shear strains, are generally involved in the hindlimbs of terrestrial animals. Considering the cases of the fastest speed dynamic regimes discussed in Eq. (1), we employ the principle of superposition for the simple axial, and complex bending and shear-strain (torsional) elastic fields, resulted in the total compressive stress

$$\sigma^{(\max)}_{limb}(M, V_{\max}) = \alpha\sigma^{(\max)}_{axial} + \beta\sigma^{(\max)}_{bend} + \tau\sigma^{(\max)}_{tors}, \text{ with } \alpha + \beta + \tau = 1, \quad (5)$$

emerging in an effective limb bone. The peak stress appears as a combination of the partial functional axial, bending, and torsional stresses weighted respectively by relative probabilities α, β, and τ. These mass-independent probabilities play the role of indicators of the dynamic stress similarity, likewise the limb duty factors and swept angles discussed in the theory of dynamic similarity in animal locomotion (Kokshenev, 2011a, b).

Unlike the individual-bone data discussed in Eq. (1), we introduce an *effective mammalian limb bone* unifying six long bones (humerus, radius, ulna, femur, tibia, and fibula), through their geometric similarity determined by the bone-diameter and bone-length *allometric exponents*

$$d^{(\exp)}_{limb} = 0.36 \pm 0.02 \text{ and } l^{(\exp)}_{limb} = 0.28 \pm 0.02, \text{ with } \lambda^{(pred)}_{limb} = 0.78 \pm 0.02 \quad (6)$$

established (Kokshenev, 2007, Table 1) via the LRS data from mostly running extant mammals (79 species, 98 specimens, Table 2 in Christiansen, 1999). One can see that the data on *slenderness exponent* $\lambda_{limb}^{(pred)} = l_{limb}^{(exp)}/d_{limb}^{(exp)}$ shown in Eq. (6) match well those established from a wider spectrum of extant mammals (189 species, 612 specimens, see Table 3 below). The theory of stress similarity, arising from the more general mechanical elastic similarity, provides three patterns of elastic similarity functional stresses discussed in Eq. (5), namely,

$$\sigma_{func}^{(\max)}(M) = C_{func}^{(\max)} M^{\mu}, \tag{7}$$

establishing the stress similarity through the corresponding scaling exponents

$$\mu_{bend} = \mu_{tors} = d - l, \text{ with } d + l = \frac{2}{3}, \text{ and } \mu_{axial} = -\frac{2}{3}\mu_{bend}, \tag{8}$$

in limbs of adult, or large species of different-sized animals (Kokshenev, 2007, Fig. 2). Leaving for a while the scaling parameters $C_{func}^{(\max)}$ in Eq. (7), requiring a special consideration beyond the scaling theory, we stress that the bone-diameter d and the bone-length l scaling exponents are also external parameters of the dynamic similarity theory.

When the most simplest isometric similarity ($d_0^{(isom)} = l_0^{(isom)} = 1/3$) is adopted for the limb design, evidently excluding bone curvature effects in bone stress (e.g., Bertram & Biewener, 1992), the only one type of functional stress associated with the oversimplified *body support function* can be distinguished through the weight-independent isometrically universal stresses

$$\sigma_{bend}^{(isom)} \sim \sigma_{tors}^{(isom)} \sim \sigma_{axial}^{(isom)} \propto M^0, \tag{9}$$

straightforwardly following from Eqs. (7) and (8). In contrast, when the mammalian-limb realistic design discussed in Eq. (6) is adopted, the scaling rules for *stress similarity functions* determined by the scaling exponents

$$\mu_{bend}^{(pred)} = \mu_{tors}^{(pred)} = 0.08 \text{ and } \mu_{axial}^{(pred)} = -0.05 \tag{10}$$

become well theoretically observable through the axial-bone and bending-bone stress similarity discussed in Eq. (2). Thereby, it has been repeatedly demonstrated that the dynamic strain similarity experimentally established in limbs of fast running animals (Rubin & Lanyon, 1982, 1984) is grounded by the mechanical elastic similarity established for effective limb bones (Kokshenev, 2007). In other words, we have shown that the effective limb bone from running mammals shown in Eq. (6) is designed as adapted to the primary locomotory functions, presented by the *body mobility* and support functions patterned in Eq. (10).

The experimental data by Rubin & Lanyon (1982) for the axial and bending stress discussed in Eqs. (1) and (2) have been obtained at special experimental conditions of a special choice of the local-midshaft coordinate systems consequently excluding shear strains. In the context of the limb stress similarity suggested in Eqs. (5) and (7) these conditions are viewed as to be conventionally introduced by the two sets of stress indicators (α, β, τ) presented by $(1,0,0)$ and $(0,1,0)$, respectively. Restoring the torsional stress $\sigma_{tors}^{(\max)}$ in all stress-similarity equations through the corresponding scaling exponent in Eq. (10), we also adopt in Eq. (5) the scaling factors

$$C_{bend}^{(\max)} = C_{tors}^{(\max)} = C_{mobil}^{(exp)} = 27MPa \cdot (kg)^{-0.08} \text{ and } C_{axial}^{(\max)} = C_{supp}^{(exp)} = 11MPa \cdot (kg)^{0.05}. \tag{11}$$

When compared with Eq. (3), the experimental data $C_{supp}^{(exp)}$ for the body support function is adopted without change, whereas the data for the body mobility function $C_{mobil}^{(exp)}$ is slightly modified by the statistical analysis extended by *in vitro* data on the tibial failure in torsion (Kokshenev, 2007, Fig. 1).

2.2.2 Critical body mass

Taking into consideration that instead of the axial-bone stress the bending and torsional functional stresses limit the body mobility of animals involved in strenuous activity, the upper limit of body mass, or the *critical body mass* $M_{\max}^{(crit)}$, follows from the relevant functional-stress constraint

$$\sigma_{mobil}^{(\max)}(M) = C_{mobil}^{(exp)} M^{0.08} = s_{mobil}^{(\max)} \left(\frac{M}{M_{\max}^{(crit)}} \right)^{0.08}, \text{ providing } M_{\max}^{(crit)} = \left(\frac{s_{mobil}^{(\max)}}{C_{mobil}^{(exp)}} \right)^{\frac{1}{0.08}}, \quad (12)$$

introduced on the basis of Eqs. (5) and (10). Here $s_{mobil}^{(\max)}$ is the strength of the bone subjected to complex bending-torsion loading and $C_{mobil}^{(exp)}$ is shown in Eq. (11).

The *in vitro* data on the mean individual-bone strength $s_{funct}^{(mean)}$ are known for a compact long bones damaged under pure axial compression, i.e., $s_{axial}^{(mean)} \approx 200\ MPa$ employed by Alexander (1981) and Biewener (1990), pure bending and torsion, i.e., $s_{bend}^{(mean)} \approx 51\ MPa$ and $s_{tors}^{(mean)} \approx 60\ MPa$ reported by Taylor et al. (2003). Given that generally the ± 10 % domain is adopted for the statistically established mean bone strengths, the maximal amplitude data

$$s_{bend}^{(\max)} = 56.1\ MPa,\ s_{tors}^{(\max)} = 66\ MPa, \text{ and } s_{axial}^{(\max)} = 220\ MPa \quad (13)$$

result in limiting estimates for the critical masses (Kokshenev, 2007)

$$M_{bend}^{(crit)} = \left(\frac{s_{bend}^{(\max)}}{C_{bend}^{(\max)}} \right)^{\frac{1}{0.08}} = 9.3\ tons \text{ and } M_{tors}^{(crit)} = \left(\frac{s_{tors}^{(\max)}}{C_{tors}^{(\max)}} \right)^{\frac{1}{0.08}} = 71\ tons. \quad (14)$$

These two critical body masses determine two kinds of similarity patterns of well distinct *body postures* in giants, whose body mobility is supposedly limited by critical pure bending and pure torsional stresses emerging in their limbs at maximal speeds of critical locomotion. Using empirical data in Table 1, the patterns of *most erect posture* and *most sprawling posture* in giants, may be respectively presented by the obligate biped *Giganotosaurus*, likely capable for relatively fast running and the largest terrestrial quadruped *Argentinosaurus*, an animal so huge that a true run would likely have severely injured the limb bones via critical torsional stresses. Indeed, sauropod anatomy speaks vehemently against anything other than a walk gait anyway.

2.2.3 Body safety

Bearing in mind that the limb safety during strenuous activity of terrestrial animals establishes the risk level of skeleton damage (Alexander, 1981; Biewener, 1982, 1989, 1990), a generalized body-skeleton *safety function* $S_{body}(M,V)$ based on the additivity of functional stresses $\sigma_{funct}^{(\max)}(M,V)$ could be suggested as

$$S_{body}(M,V) = \left(\sum_{functions} \frac{\sigma_{funct}^{(\max)}(M,V)}{s_{funct}^{(\max)}} \right)^{-1}. \quad (15)$$

The dynamic stress similarity experimentally and theoretically represented in, respectively, Eqs. (1), (4), (11) and (5), (7), (8), suggests the following piecewise functional form, namely

$$S_{body}^{-1}(M,V) = \frac{\alpha}{s_{axial}^{(\max)}} C_{supp}^{(\exp)} M^{\mu_{axial}} + \left(\frac{\beta}{s_{bend}^{(\max)}} + \frac{\tau}{s_{tors}^{(\max)}} \right) C_{mobil}^{(\exp)} M^{\mu_{bend}} \frac{V}{V_{\max}}, \text{ with } S_{body} \geq 2, \quad (16)$$

for the body safety function activated in slow (walk) and fast (walk and run) gaits of animals moving within a certain speed domain limited by $V_{\max}$. The shown domain (analyzed in Figs. 1 and 3 in Kokshenev, 2007) conventionally establishes a condition for realization of the mechanically equilibrated, *non-critical* dynamic similarity states in slow and moderately fast gaits of locomotion, as exemplified by the non-critical axial stress (Kokshenev, 2007, Table 2, Eq. (2)).

Coming back to the problem of the maximal mass of terrestrial giants mentioned in the Introduction, a question arises whether the body support function may establish the critical body mass $M_{body}^{(crit)}$ determined by critical-point condition $S_{body}^{(crit)}(M_{body}^{(crit)}, V_{\max}) = 1$, which in fact violate the domain of validation shown in Eq. (16)? Searching for the answer, let analyze the relevant model solution $M_{body}^{(crit)}(\alpha,\beta,\tau)$ provided by

$$\frac{\alpha}{s_{axial}^{(\max)}} C_{supp}^{(\exp)} M_{body}^{\mu_{axial}} + \left(\frac{\beta}{s_{bend}^{(\max)}} + \frac{\tau}{s_{tors}^{(\max)}} \right) C_{mobil}^{(\exp)} M_{body}^{\mu_{bend}} = 1, \text{ with } \alpha + \beta + \tau = 1, \quad (17)$$

following from Eq. (16). In Eq. (14), the two particular solutions $M_{body}^{(crit)}(0,1,0) = 9.3$ *tons* and $M_{body}^{(crit)}(0,0,1) = 71$ *tons* were discussed as critical masses attributed, respectively, to the largest theropod and the largest sauropod, obtained in the effective limb-bone approximation (shown in Eqs. (10) and (11)). One can see that the obtained limiting masses introduce the validation domain for the *body mobility function* in giants, namely

$$S_{mobil}(M,V) = \left(\frac{M_{\max}^{(crit)}}{M} \right)^{\mu_{bend}} \frac{V_{\max}}{V}, \text{ with } S_{mobil} \geq 1. \quad (18)$$

The critical mass discussed in Eq. (12) is now specified by

$$M_{\max}^{(crit)}(\beta) = \left(\frac{C_{mobil}^{(\exp)-1} s_{bend}^{(\max)} s_{tors}^{(\max)}}{\beta s_{tors}^{(\max)} + \tau s_{bend}^{(\max)}} \right)^{\mu_{bend}^{-1}}, \text{ with } \tau = 1 - \beta, \quad (19)$$

as follows from Eq. (16) taken at the critical condition $S^{(crit)}_{mobil}(M, V_{\max}) = 1$, with $\alpha = 0$.
The domain shown in Eq. (18) for the body mobility function conventionally indicates the condition for realization of the near-critical transient states of continuous dynamic similarity, associated with locally equilibrated universal transformations of near-critical compressive strains into non-critical global shear strains, eventually decreasing the resulted compressive bone stress (Kokshenev, 2007).

3. Results

Several aspects concerning the problem of evolution of locomotory trends in extinct animals are discussed in view of generalizations suggested by the dynamic stress similarity approach.

3.1 Critical mass

In order to establish the role of competing axial, bending, and torsional stresses in the problem of the maximal mass of terrestrial giants, we analyze the domains of observation of the corresponding probabilities α, β, and τ through Eq. (17) where the critical mass $M^{(crit)}_{body}(\alpha, \beta, \tau)$ is associated with maximal body mass $M^{(\exp)}_{\max}$ known for the largest giants (Table 1). Since in most cases of bone specimens for extinct species the allometric exponents d and l are not available, we employ statistical data on the slenderness exponent $\lambda^{(\exp)}$ for the effective limb bone (Table 2). Instead of Eq. (10), the theoretical predictions for the scaling exponents in Eq. (17) are estimated through

$$\mu^{(pred)}_{axial} = -\frac{4}{9}\frac{1-\lambda}{1+\lambda} \text{ and } \mu^{(pred)}_{bend} = \mu^{(pred)}_{tors} = \frac{2}{3}\frac{1-\lambda}{1+\lambda} \tag{20}$$

established with the help of the definitive equation for the exponent $\lambda = l/d$ excluding d and l from those shown in Eq. (8). Allowing the whole domains for all kinds of stresses to be exploited by giants during near-critical locomotion, e.g., for bending stress $0 \le \beta \le 1$, hereafter designated as [0;1], the resulted observable domains are shown in Table 3.
Fig. 1 illustrates the analysis in Table 3 indicating domains of exploration of the axial, bending and torsional stresses by limb bones in the largest mammalian species running or walking at the critical condition $S^{(crit)}_{body} = 1$. The semi-qualitative analysis[1] indicates that neither maximal critical mass nor maximal near-critical mass of terrestrial giants is affected by axial stress. In other words, instead of body safety function lying beyond the critical locomotion domain, as shown in Eq. (16), the body mobility function establishes the critical behavior (see Fig. 2) determined by the critical mass

$$M^{(crit)}_{mobil}(\beta) = \left[\frac{137.1}{(1-\beta)56.1 + \beta 66}\right]^{\frac{1}{0.08}}, \text{ with } 0 \le \beta \le 1, \tag{21}$$

represented from Eq. (19) in the mammalian limb-bone approximation discussed in Eq. (6).

$$M^{(crit)}_{mobil}(\beta) = \left[\frac{137.1}{(1-\beta)56.1 + \beta 66}\right]^{\frac{1}{0.08}}, \text{ with } 0 \le \beta \le 1, \tag{22}$$

[1] The provided analysis is treated as semi-qualitative since, unlike the scaling exponents (Table 3), the data on the scaling factors, discussed in Eq. (10), are still taken in the mammalian-limb approximation.

Largest giants in	N, n	$\lambda^{(\exp)}$	$\mu^{(pred)}_{axial}$	$\mu^{(pred)}_{bend}$	$M^{(\exp)}_{\max}, kg$	α	τ	β
Mammals	$N = 189$	0.795	-0.051	0.076	20000	[0; 0.03]	[0.85; 0]	[0.15; 0.97]
Proboscidean	$N = 13$	0.943	-0.013	0.020	20000	*n.e.s.*	[1; 0.95]	[0.95; 1]
Elephantidae	$N = 6$	0.790	-0.520	0.078	20000	*n.e.s.*	[1; 0.30]	[0.40; 1]
Asian elephant	$n = 106$	0.851	-0.036	0.054	8000	*n.e.s.*	[1; 0.35]	[0.45; 1]
African elephant	$n = 56$	0.648	-0.094	0.141	10000	[0.35; 0.45]	[0.65; 0]	[0; 0.55]

Table 3. Maximal body mass and limb bone design determine the stress-similarity domains through the corresponding stress indicators. The domains of the axial (α), bending (β), and torsion (τ) stresses explored by the body safety function (shown in squared brackets) are obtained through Eq. (17) where the scaling exponents $\mu^{(pred)}_{axial}$ and $\mu^{(pred)}_{bend} = \mu^{(pred)}_{tors}$ are estimated through Eq. (20). The data on the critical mass $M^{(\exp)}_{\max}$ for *Mammuthus trogontherii* is used for the largest taxon in both Mammalia, Proboscidea, and Elephantidae (Table 1). The largest masses for extant Asian (*Elephas maximus*) and African (*Loxodonta africana*) elephants are for exceptionally large bulls (Wood, 1976; Nowak, 1991; McFarlan, 1992; Blashford-Snell & Lenska, 1996). The LS regression data on the slenderness exponents $\lambda^{(\exp)}$ of long bones from N species are taken from Table 2 and from n specimens for elephants are taken from Table 2 in Kokshenev & Christiansen (2010). *Notation*: *n.e.s.* - not employing stress.

Dynamic conditions	Optimum speed		Maximum power		Near critical regime	
Locomotory muscle type	slow	fast	slow	fast	slow	fast
Contraction frequency	L_m^{-1}	$L_m^{-1/2}$	$L_m^{-3/2}$	L_m^{-1}	L_m^{-2}	$L_m^{-3/2}$
Contraction velocity	L_m^{0}	$L_m^{1/2}$	$L_m^{-1/2}$	L_m^{0}	L_m^{-1}	$L_m^{-1/2}$

Table 4. Dynamic characterization of the slow and fast striated muscles (of resting length L_m) contracting at optimum-speed (maximum-efficiency), maximum-speed (maximum-power), and near critical (low-safety) dynamic conditions (reproduced from Table 4 in Kokshenev, 2009).

represented from Eq. (19) in the mammalian limb-bone approximation discussed in Eq. (6). In Fig. 3 we extend the analysis of locomotory trends in Fig. 2 to other large giants, modeled by near critical safety factors lying in narrow domain $1.0 < S_{mobil} \leq 1.1$, corresponding to the 10% domain established for the mean bone strengths, as discussed in Eq. (13).

3.2 Froude numbers

Modeling the animal locomotion by contractions of locomotory muscles activated at natural frequencies, the data on optimal speeds $V^{(\exp)}_{opt} \sim M^{1/6}$ of bipeds (Gatesy& Biewener, 1991) and quadrupeds (Heglund & Taylor, 1988) running in fast locomotor modes can be explained by activation of the fast locomotor muscles of length, linearly scaling with *limb length* (or hip height) $L^{(isom)}_b \sim M^{1/3}$ (Kokshenev, 2009, 2010) presented in the isometric-similarity approximation discussed in Eq. (9). Modeling the low-safety locomotion of large giants by critical-velocity muscle contractions (see Table 4), let us adopt the scaling relations $V^{(\mathrm{mod})}_{walk} \sim L_b^{-1}$ and $V^{(\mathrm{mod})}_{run} \propto L_b^{-1/2}$ for critically walking or running giants moving due to activation of slow and fast limb muscles, respectively.

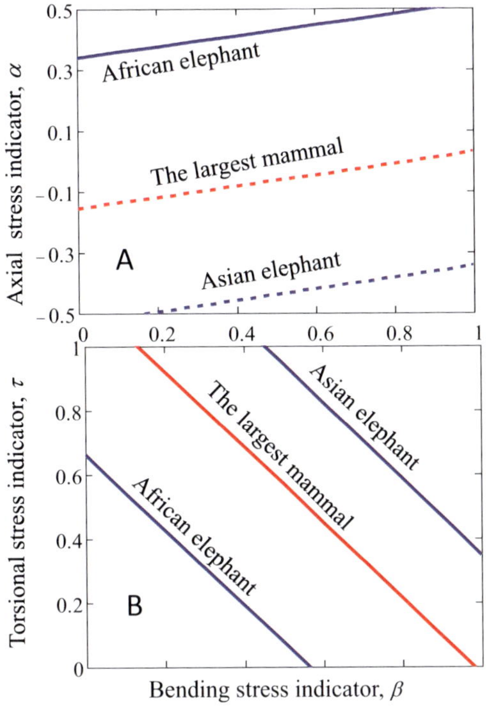

Fig. 1. The comparative role of limb adaptation in the largest mammal and elephant (extinct species) through the elastic reaction to muscle loading forces (via turning-bending stress, Fig. 1A) and ground-reaction forces (mostly via axial stress, Fig. 1B). The *solid* and *dashed lines* correspond to employing and non-employing domains (Table 3).

Choosing the *model* critical-state *Froude number* ($Fr^{(mod)}_{critic} = V^2_{crit}/gL_b$, where g is the gravitational field) as a relative squared-speed characteristics of animal locomotion (Alexander & Jayes, 1983; Gatesy& Biewener, 1991), one obtains the scaling relations $Fr^{(mod)}_{walk} \sim L_b^{-3}$ and $Fr^{(mod)}_{run} \sim L_b^{-2}$, adopted for model Froude numbers in the simplest isometric geometry approximation $L_b^{(isom)} \sim L_m^{(isom)} \sim M^{1/3}_{\max}(\beta)$. Hence, one obtaines the critical-mass scaling rules $Fr^{(mod)}_{walk} \sim M^{-1}_{\max}(\beta)$ and $Fr^{(mod)}_{run} \sim M^{-2/3}_{\max}(\beta)$ distinguishing dynamic similarities in a walk and a run gaits in giants, moving in the near critical mobility regime. When the walk-to-run continuous transition, *in vivo* established for modern elephants by Hutchinson et al. (2006) at Froude numbers $Fr^{(exp)}_{w-r} \approx 1$ and duty factors $\beta^{(exp)}_{duty} \approx 0.5$ is mapped onto the walk-to-run crossover in evolution of trends in extinct largest giants indicated by transient bending-torsion stress similarity at $\beta = 0.5$, the model similarity scaling equations for near critical level of walking and running quadrupedal giants are suggested as

$$Fr^{(quadr)}_{walk} = 24.7M^{-1}_{\max}(\beta) \text{ and } Fr^{(quadr)}_{run} = 8.48M^{-2/3}_{\max}(\beta), \tag{23}$$

(here critical mass is taken in *tons*) with the help of Eq.(22).

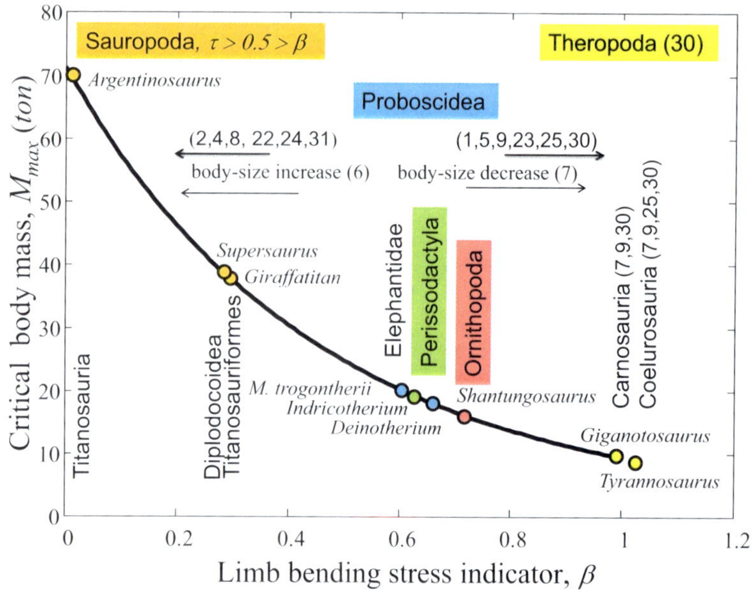

Fig. 2. Analysis of locomotor evolution of the largest terrestrial giants scaled by the limb bending parameter. The *solid line* is critical mass drawn by Eq. (22). The *points* correspond to giants in Table 1. The *arrows* indicate the biomechanical trends described by competitive empirically revealed traits (Hutchinson, 2006, Table 1): (1), more erect posture; (2), less erect posture; (4), quadrupedalism; (5), striding bipedalism; (6), body-size increase; (7), body-size decrease; (8), more upright pose; (9), more crouched pose; (22), poor bipedal running ability; (23), good bipedal running ability; (24), poor turning ability; (25); improved turning ability; (30), more cursorial limb proportions; (31), less cursorial limb proportions.

3.3 Turning and bending mobilities

Being remarkably similar, both limb-bone longitudinal bending elastic force F_{bend} and transverse torsion force F_{tors} scale with body mass as M^{3d-l}, within the domain of similar dynamic states including transient near-critical states (Kokshenev, 2007, Eq. (17), Table 2). The force scaling equations, taken in the mammalian limb-bone approximation, i.e., with $3d - l = 1.20$, are completed by the scaling factors approximated by muscle-reaction forces from the largest 6-*ton Tyrannosaurus* modeled by Hutchinson et al. (2007).[2] Treating the total force exerted by leg muscles over the center of body mass as the vectorial sum of vertical and horizontal forces, resulted in the total muscle force output, the corresponding skeletal body reaction force, limiting body mobility is found as the root mean square of the corresponding elastic forces emerging in the effective limb bones, i.e., $F_{mobil}^{(mod)} = (F_{bend}^{(mod)2} + F_{tors}^{(mod)2})^{1/2}$. When extrapolated to other largest extinct giants, the relative forces provide the model estimates,

[2] Specifically, for the case of F_{tors} we employ the data (Hutchinson et al., 2007, Table 6, Model 3) on maximal (medial and lateral) rotation muscle moments and moment arms of turning force exerted about center of mass of the trunk. The case of $F_{bend}^{(mod)}$ is adjusted with the maximal vertical ground reaction force that the limb could support (Hutchinson et al., 2007, Table 9, Model 23).

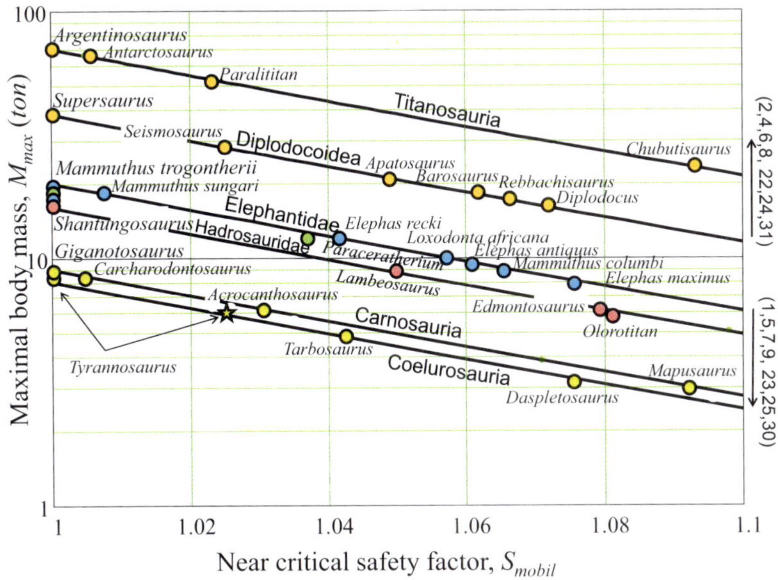

Fig. 3. Maximal body masses for terrestrial giants modeled by the near-critical locomotor behavior. *Solid lines* are drawn by Eq.(18) taken at maximal stride speeds. The *points* are data from Table 1 and other available sources. The star corresponds to 6-*ton* modeled *Tyrannosaurus* (Hutchinson et al., 2007; Sellers & Manning, 2007).

namely

$$\frac{F_{tors}^{(mod)}}{Mg} = 0.87 \cdot M^{-0.20}, \quad \frac{F_{bend}^{(mod)}}{Mg} = 1.89 \cdot M^{-0.20}, \quad \frac{F_{mobil}^{(mod)}}{Mg} = 2.08 \cdot M^{-0.20}, \text{ with } S_{mobil} \geq 1, \tag{24}$$

discussed in Fig. 5.

4. Discussion

Our study develops Alexander's hypothesis on that the locomotor dynamic similarity in non-avian dinosaurs can be inferred from the bending stress in their limbs (Alexander, 1976). We have demonstrated how the knowledge on elastic stress (or strain) similarity reliably established in limbs of different-sized running mammals may provide rationalizations of locomotory trials empirically suggested for extinct terrestrial giants. Allowing the generalized mammalian limb bone to be arbitrary loaded, the body functions of giants of different taxa subjected to cyclic loading during locomotor activity are viewed in terms of a few dynamic similarity patters provided by elastic theory of solids. Our theoretical study suggests that even though the dynamic similarity is underlaid by a certain set of *elastic force patterns*, there are several ways in which they may be realized and thus described.

The elastic patterns of forces emerging in the effective mammalian limb bone loaded in distinct (globally equilibrated non-critical stationary states and near-critical transient states

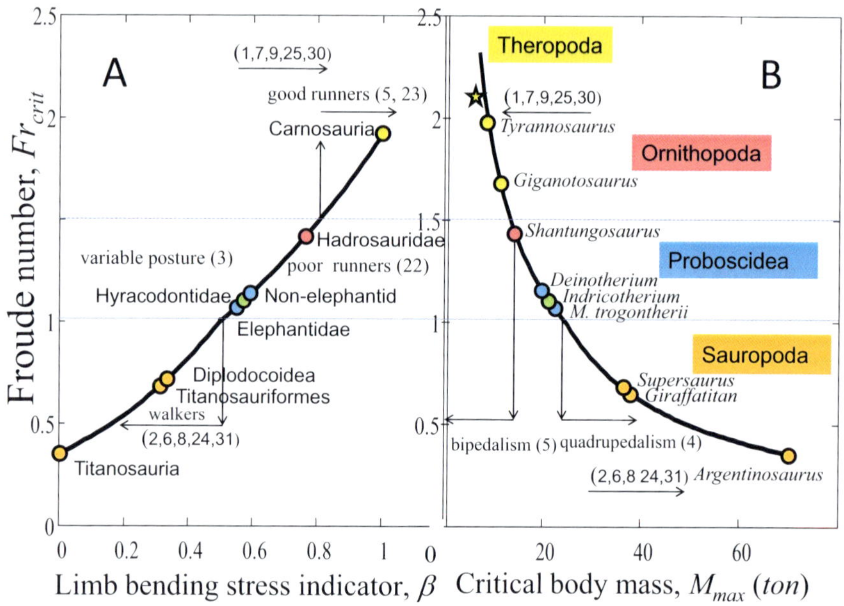

Fig. 4. Froude numbers expected from the largest terrestrial giants during near-critical locomotion. The *solid curves* are drawn through Eqs. (23) and Eq. (22); The *points* (Table 1) and notations for taxa and traits correspond to those in Fig. 1. The *star* shows the experimental data $Fr_{run}^{(exp)} = 2.1$ for the fast running 6-*ton Tyrannosaurus* modeled by Sellers & Manning (2007).

of) dynamic similarity regimes (Kokshenev, 2007) have been revealed earlier through the bone design observed in different-sized animals through the allometric data on linear bone dimensions (Kokshenev et al., 2003; Kokshenev, 2007) and slenderness (Kokshenev, 2003; Kokshenev & Christiansen, 2010). All theoretical studies of the data were critically discussed within the context of McMahon's pioneering criteria of elastic similarity (McMahon, 1973, 1975a, b). The observation of elastic force patterns through the locomotory functions evaluated on the basis of available data on the maximal masses of extinct giants is one of the objectives of the presented approach. The critical-state similarity regime is treated as theoretically established if the observable characteristics are shown to be driven by one of the predominating critical-force patterns.

Even though animals are built from the same bone tissue and muscle tissue materials, the safety factors of limbs in running animals are not universally equal (Kokshenev, 2007, Fig. 3), as was suggested by earlier estimates (Alexander, 1981, 1985a) of the isolated dynamic stress states and systematical observations of limb safety factors (Biewener, 1982, 1983, 1989, 1990, 2000, 2005). On the other hand, in non-critical dynamic regimes of locomotion the body safety function discussed in Eq. (16) could also conventionally be observed, either theoretically or experimentally, as "almost" universal. The first kind of observations could be made through

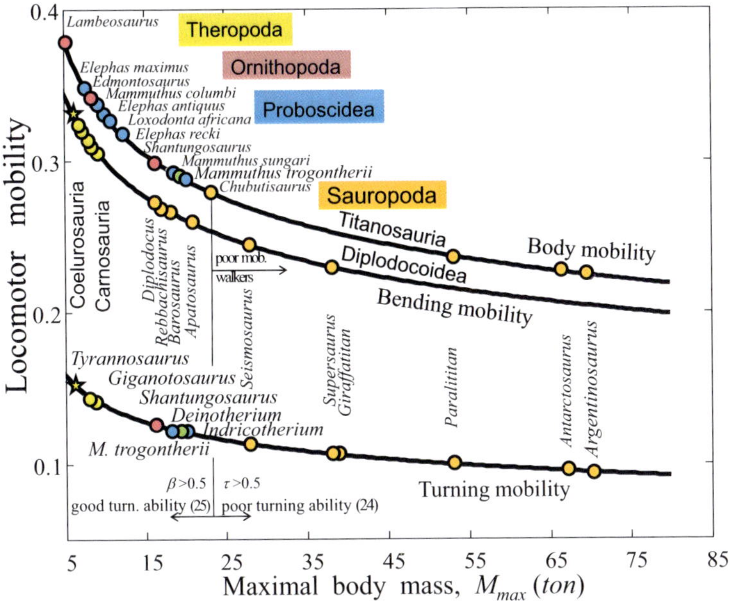

Fig. 5. Locomotor mobilities expected for extinct giants. The curves for relative limb bone elastic forces are drawn via Eq. (24) and notations correspond to Figs. 2 and 4. The *stars* are the data on 3D *Tyrannosaurus* experimentally modeled by Hutchinson et al. (2007).

the corresponding oversimplified bending stress estimated under assumption of the almost isometric mammalian bones, as shown in Eq. (9). In this case we have ignored small by finite scaling bone-mass effects (Prange et al., 1979), which significance in limb bone allometry has previously been discussed (Kokshenev et al., 2003) and statistically evaluated (Kokshenev, 2007). In the second case, the desirable observation of the seemingly universal functional limb stress implies that the safety factor domain reliably established in running mammals as lying between 2 and 4 should indicate almost invariable safety function approximated by the number 3 ± 1. In the current research, the dynamic similarity features in giants moving in near-critical dynamic regimes are revealed through the stress-similarity indicators of the underlying patterns of axial, bending and torsional elastic forces. As is common in dynamic similarity theories, the patterns of scaling rules and related dimensionless numbers (Kokshenev, 2011a) or functions (Kokshenev, 2011b) determine the conditions of observation of dynamic similarity states.

Our recent study of similarities and dissimilarities in locomotory trends of extant and extinct proboscideans, indicated by the slenderness characteristics of design of the effective limb bones (Kokshenev & Christiansen, 2010), has revealed new features of their locomotory functions. The Asian elephants (*E. maximus*) are dynamically similar to the family Elephantidae and have been found to be distinct from the African elephants (*L. africana*). Moreover, the Elephantidae as group including both kinds of extant elephants, clearly exposed a negative limb duty gradient (with respect to other mammals, Fig. 6) in the body mobility function, closely related to the proximal-distal gradient (Biewener et al., 2006) in body ability function. Qualitatively, the hind-to-fore gradient in limb locomotor activity

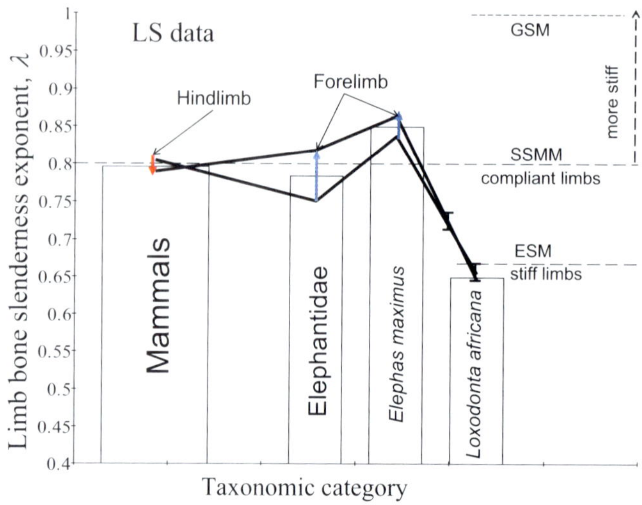

Fig. 6. The observation of elastic similarity across different taxa via bone slenderness exponents (Table 2) for the effective forelimb bone (humerus, radius, and ulna) and hindlimb bone (femur and tibia). The *arrows* indicate deviations in the trends of adaptation of forelimb and hindlimb bones associated with gradients in the corresponding mechanical functions. The *bar* shows statistical error. *Notations*: GSM and ESM indicate the predictions of the geometric similarity model and elastic similarity model of McMahon (1973, 1975a); SSMM indicates the static stress similarity model (McMahon, 1975a, SSM) modified by muscle forces (Kokshenev, 2003). For further details, see Fig. 4 in Kokshenev & Christiansen (2010).

caused by the difference in bone proportions of hind and fore limbs (Fig. 6, mammals) explains the differing *postures* in mammals as group as well as elephants (Kokshenev & Christiansen, 2010, Fig. 5). The negative gradient of limb functions for the Elephantidae (including the extant species, but mainly comprising of extinct species) suggests a trend for forelimbs to be designed more isometrically, and also for the forelimbs of *E. maximus* to be mechanically stiffer than the hindlimbs. The newly established dynamic constraint, contrasting in sign to that of other mammals and mechanically extending the hindlimb ground contact duration, explains why elephants are prevented from achieving a full-body aerial phase during fast gaits of locomotion.

The design remarkably observed (Table 6) for the effective limb bone in the African elephant (5 limb bones, 56 specimens, Table 3) is surprisingly similar to that established in adult ungulates (5 limb bones, 118 specimens, McMahon, 1975b) mostly from the family Bovidae (see also analysis by Selker & Carter, 1989). The distinct from other effective bones, say, *pillar-type limb bone*, is statistically established via the slenderness exponent $\lambda^{(\exp)} \approx \lambda_0^{(ESM)} = 2/3$ predicted by the elastic similarity model (ESM, Fig. 6). The pillar-like limb bone pattern underlaid by the *critical buckling force* (McMahon, 1973, 1975a) is well distinguished from the mammalian-type limb bone, determined experimentally in Eq. (6) and predicted by SSMM through $\lambda_0^{(SSMM)} = 7/9$ (Kokshenev & Christiansen, 2010, footnote 1). The buckling force was introduced in the theory of elasticity of solids by Euler as the critical axial elastic force provoking critical bending deformations under loading conditions of the absence of non-axial external forces (e.g., Kokshenev et al., 2003; Kokshenev, 2003). McMahon therefore proposed that terrestrial animals would optimize their skeleton support function so that were similarly in danger of elastic mechanical failure by buckling under gravity (e.g., Christiansen, 1999). The corresponding to buckling mechanism loading, the simplest model for terrestrial giants, as an animal standing on one leg and subjected to increasing with weight gravitational force, was proposed by Hokkanen (1986a). Although it has been clearly demonstrated that the maximal body mass of terrestrial giants is not limited by axial critical forces, associated with buckling mechanism of damage of naturally curved bones (e.g., Currey, 1967; Hokkanen, 1986a, b; Selker & Carter, 1989), the corresponding scaling pattern of the Euler's force (e.g., Kokshenev et al., 2003, Eq. (1)) emerging under aforesaid dynamic conditions may survive and even predominate at loads far from critical. Moreover, as one may infer from the reliable observation of the effective pillar-type bone, the pattern of critical buckling force most likely controls the limb elastic stress of animals, in which limb muscles function as to resist non-axial external forces, through the proximal-distal functional gradients, evolutionary resulting in the limb bone design mostly adapted to the axial-bone peak loading. Hence, when one considers competitive patterns of functional elastic stresses in a certain effective bone of unknown design, as discussed on general basis in Eq. (5), equally with the term of non-critical axial stress $\sigma_{axial}^{(\max)}$, which negative allometry ($\mu_{axial} < 0$) was predicted by $\sigma_{axial}^{(pred)} \propto M^{2/3-2d}$ (Kokshenev, 2007, Eq. (5), Table 3), one should not exclude the possibility of axial stress predicted as $\sigma_{axial}^{(ESM)} \propto M^{2(d-l)}$ (Kokshenev et al. 2003, Eq. (4)) underlying the pattern of pillar-type bones.

Following the ESM (Fig. 6), the individual limb bones in *L. africana* are mostly influenced by gravitational and ground reaction forces, generating buckling-type dynamic elastic stress of the peak amplitude $\sigma_{axial}^{(ESM)}$. This finding is supported by our study of the competing functional axial, bending and torsional stresses occurring in the limbs of the largest extinct giants at similar critical states modeled by the maximal body masses of Asian and African elephants, Elephantidae, and mammals as whole (Table 3, Fig. 1). Unlike the case of Asian elephants and running mammals, the axial predominating stress becomes observable through the maximal body mass of African elephants (Fig. 1A). As follows from Fig. 6, more reliable observation of the stress similarity in African elephants, as well as bovids (McMahon, 1975b), might be obtained when the scaling exponents $\mu_{axial}^{(pred)} = -0.05$ and $\mu_{bend}^{(pred)} = 0.08$ in Eq. (16) are substituted by $\mu_{0axial}^{(ESM)} = 1/4$ and $\mu_{0bend}^{(ESM)} = 1/8$, predicted by McMahon's elastic similarity model. Since the exponent for critical axial stress is expected to be twice as high as that for critical bending stress, we have thereby shown that in near-critical dynamic regimes the buckling force effects appear to dominate over bending-torsional force effects. Since the effective pillar-type limb bones, scaled to body mass as $\lambda_0^{(ESM)} = 2/3$, are not ideal long cylinders, the critical (yield-state) bending strains (Kokshenev et al., 2003; Eq. (4)) dynamically transform into transient-state pure bending elastic strains (Kokshenev, 2007; Eq. (15)), as has been explained earlier by Currey (1967).

The analysis of elastic peak forces developed in ideal solid cylinders indicated that various conditions of application of external loads affect solely scaling factors, leaving unchanged scaling exponents determining elastic force patterns (e.g., Kokshenev et al., 2003, Eq. (1)) employed above in rationalization of the functional stress in Eq. (5) when applied to extinct animals. Unlike ideal cylinders, the individual long skeletal bones are mostly curved along the longitudinal axis in all but the largest extant mammals (Bertram & Biewener, 1988, 1992), and even in the largest, elephant-sized theropod dinosaurs (e.g., Farlow et al., 1995; Christiansen, 1998). Hence, external loads produce a complex non-axial compression in long bones, causing different components (axial and non-axial) of reactive (elastic) bending and torsional stresses. Moreover, since the bone cross section is also not an ideal circle, near maximal bending stress can be avoided via the transient non-critical dynamic regimes by deviation of the bone from the sagittal plane, thereby decreasing bending stress through torsional stress (Kokshenev, 2007). Switching from bending deformation to out-off-plane torsion, such a mechanism reduces the risk of limb damage, naturally increasing bone safety factors. In this study, the stress in the non-uniformly loaded limbs of animals is modeled by an arbitrary composition of axial, bending, and torsional stresses, as shown in Eq. (5).

Unlike the case of the ESM underlaid by Euler's force, no explicit bending force pattern for McMahon's static stress similarity model (SSM, McMahon, 1975a) was established. Instead, in the *in vitro* experimental studies of long bone strength the *critical transverse-bone force* has been discussed as the *perpendicular* bending force that a bone can withstand without breaking (e.g., Hokkanen, 1986b, Eq. (11)) under either three-point or cantilever loading (Selker & Carter, 1989; Eq. (4)). In spite of that it was widely adopted that most fractures in limbs of living animals are due to longitudinal-bone and transverse-bone torsional forces (e.g., Carter et al., 1980; Rubin & Lanyon, 1982; Biewener et al., 1983; Biewener & Taylor, 1986; Selker & Carter, 1989) such generalizations resulting in transverse-bending, longitudinal-bending, and transverse-torsional elastic force patterns unified by the SSM have recently been established and tested (Kokshenev, 2007, Eq. (17) and Table 3). In this study, we have repeatedly demonstrated in Eq. (10) that the dynamic elastic stress similarity patterns (Kokshenev, 2007, Eq. (15)) can be observed through the effective (mammalian) limb bone design, which appears to be common to both extant and extinct large animals (Fig. 6). It is well established that the peak muscle contractions involved in locomotion are primarily responsible for bending and torsional stresses in bones (Carter et al., 1980; Biewener, 1982). Consequently, the definitive scaling equations of the SSM of long bones (McMahon, 1975a), completely ignoring predominating muscular forces, required a modification as indicated by the bone stress index (Selker & Carter, 1989; Table 2). When experimentally indicated modifications have been provided through the gravitational forces substituted by external bending and torsional muscle's forces, the *modified* McMahon's model (SSMM) had turned to be reliable, i.e., observable through the bone allometry data from extant mammals (Kokshenev et al., 2003, Fig. 1, dashed area 2; Kokshenev, 2003, Fig. 2) and extinct animals (Fig. 6, SSMM). According to the SSMM, in the Elephantidae and in particular in *E. maximus*, the external bone off-axial muscular forces, causing a complex bending-torsion elastic bone stress during fast locomotion, provide a relatively high level of limb compliance conducted by the limb bones. These qualitative SSMM predictions are well supported by the analysis illustrated in Fig. 1B. Asian elephants are involved in torsional effects with the probability ($0.35 \leq \tau \leq 1$) that on average is twice as high as that ($0 \leq \tau \leq 0.65$) of the largest extant African elephants (Table 3). Relatively large domains of exploration of bending-torsional stress, completely excluding the axial stress domain common to mammals, Proboscideans and Elephantidae (Table 3). These distinct dynamically features of limb bone functions accomplished by different predominating critical stresses result in distinct bone designs, as illustrated by the running-mammal and pillar-like effective limb bones.

In Fig. 2, the maximal masses of some extinct giants, from the largest theropod (9-*ton Giganotosaurus* and 8-*ton Tyrannosaurus*) to the largest sauropod (70-*ton Argentinosaurus*), are scaled by the bending stress set up in the limbs of animals moving at critically low limb safety factors. Our analysis, indicating probabilities of bending (β) and torsional (τ) limb stresses as seen in various maximal body masses, is expected to establish a bridge between body size traits 6 and 7 and other biomechanical traits established for dinosaurs and reviewed by Hutchinson (2006). The anatomical data from bipedal (trait 5) theropods (long legs, long tibia relative to femur, long metatarsus, and very large limb muscles) suggest that they had well developed anatomical adaptations for running modes, as shown through the expected duty factor in Table 1. These generally agree with the observation in Fig. 2 of Sauropoda in, say, *run-mode domain* $\beta > 0.5 > \tau$ (we recall that $\tau = 1 - \beta$) indicated by limbs adapted for peak bending effects rather than peak torsional effects. Anatomy leaves no doubt whatsoever that all sauropods (trait 4) were capable of progression with a walking gait only, which generally determines the *walk-mode* domain $\tau > 0.5 > \beta$. The established trends linked to locomotor characterization of the limbs of giants, developing with body mass (trait 6) are supported by changes in competing biomechanical traits: from striding bipedalism (trait 5), related to good bipedal running ability (trait 23) to quadrupedalism (trait 4) through decreasing bipedal running ability (22). Likewise, the trend of changes in posture, pose, and limb proportions with body mass (varying from corresponding traits 1, 9, and 30 to traits 2, 8, and 31) could also be elucidated through the limb stress indicators.[3] A crossover between giants found in run-mode and walk-mode domains during the evolution of competitive locomotory traits is indicated by the transient indicators $\tau \approx \beta \approx 0.5$, corresponding approximately to the Elephantidae (Fig. 2), whose limbs are expected to be biomechanically adapted to the transient (walk-to-run) dynamic similarity states.

In Fig. 3, the analysis of locomotor traits from Fig. 2 for the largest extinct giants is extended to smaller giants, belonging to the same anatomical type and large-scale taxon (e.g., family, order). When the critical (and near-critical) body mass criterion of the similarity in evolution of locomotory trends is adopted, the largest representatives of the taxa Titanosauria, Diplodocoidea, Titanosauriformes, Elephantidae, non-elephantid, proboscideans (a paraphyletic group of morphologically comparable taxa), Perissodactyla, Hadrosauridae, Carnosauria, and Coelurosauria are treated as *locomotory patterns of similarity* presented by biomechanically similar animals having limbs adaptively designed to explore the bending and torsion stresses in the strict narrow domains indicated (Fig. 2) by the corresponding probabilities β and τ. For example, the dynamic similarity pattern of *Mammuthus trogontherii* (Fig. 2) is now extended by the Elephantidae, including the largest extant 10-*ton* African and 8-*ton* Asian elephants (Fig. 3). Being analyzed by the body safety function in Eq. (16), where $\tau \neq 1 - \beta$, these two compared elephants also differ in the *mean stress indicators* $\tau_{African}^{(mean)} \approx \beta_{African}^{(mean)} < 0.5$, for African elephant, and $\tau_{Asian}^{(mean)} \approx \beta_{Asian}^{(mean)} > 0.5$, for Asian elephant (Table 3, Fig. 1B). These different limb bone traits imply that even though both elephants generally fall into the transient walk-to-run evolutionary domain indicated by $\tau_{eleph}^{(mean)} \approx \beta_{eleph}^{(mean)}$, Asian elephants, showing $\beta_{Asian}^{(mean)} > 0.5$, reminiscent of running mammals rather than walking animals. In contrast, African elephants fall into the domain of walkers indicated by $\beta_{African}^{(mean)} < 0.5$.

[3] In this context, the set of traits (6, 8, 31) suggested for the Carnosauria by Hutchinson et al. (2006) should be likely substituted by the set (7, 9, 30), if this group is indeed characteristic of the non-avian Theropoda as whole.

The top-speed dynamic regimes, broadly related to maximal body mobility, should not be expected for large animals (Garland, 1983; Christiansen, 2002b) especially if they move at near critical conditions. Within the framework of the current approach to critical locomotion, the top speed of the fastest land mammal, the cheetah (Sharp, 1997), conventionally separating small and large fast-running animals (Jones & Lindstedt, 1993) and possibly determining a crossover in mammalian scaling trends of the appendicular skeleton (Christiansen, 1999), corresponds to the non-critical domain of body safety function discussed in Eq. (16) and the data $S_{mobil} = 3/2$ (Kokshenev, 2007) for the body mobility function discussed in Eq. (18).

The non-critical linear dynamic similarity as seen in optimal locomotion by stride speeds $V_{opt}^{(\mathrm{mod})} \sim M^{1/6}$and natural frequencies $T_{opt}^{(\mathrm{exp})-1} \sim M^{1/6}$ in running bipeds (Gatesy & Biewener, 1991) and trotting and galloping quadrupeds (Heglund & Taylor, 1988; Farley et al., 1993) can be explained by the optimal-speed regime of muscle activation shown in Table 4. As such, dynamic similarity was shown (Kokshenev, 2009, 2010, 2011a) to be determined by minimum mechanical muscle action controlled during contractions by the condition of *linear* dynamic-length changes with muscle length L_m (Table 4). The non-critical *bilinear* dynamic regime (maximum-power regime, Table 4) was proven to be responsible for muscle design adaptation to the primary locomotory functions (Kokshenev, 2008), whereas the higher non-linear regime of contraction of fast and slow muscles is associated here with near critical loading dynamic conditions ($1 < S_{mobil} \leq 1.1$, Fig. 3) resulting in model speeds $V_{walk}^{(\mathrm{mod})} \sim M_{max}^{-1/3}$ and $V_{run}^{(\mathrm{mod})} \sim M_{max}^{-1/6}$, which follow from Table 4. When the near critical regime speeds are compared with maximal speeds (limited by 2 m/s for large quadrupedal sauropods and by 4 m/s for bipedal dinosaurs) obtained by Tulborn (1990) using graphs of relative stride length against Froude number (Alexander, 1976), the estimates $V_{walk}^{(\mathrm{mod})} = 8.3M_{max}^{-1/3}$ and $V_{run}^{(\mathrm{mod})} = 8.1M_{max}^{-1/6}$ (masses are taken in *tons*) for the relatively slow-walking *Argentinosaurus* and slow-running *Giganotosaurus* (Table 1) are suggested. However, these estimates do not corroborate the idea of a continuos-speed evolution in gaits during a crossover from striding bipedalism (trait 5) to quadrupedalism (trait 4), as generally expected near the crossover-gait duty factor of around one half (Table 1) at a transient critical mass of around 25 *tons* (Fig. 2). Indeed, the estimates suggested for speeds within the scenario of a one-step continuous transition are not consistent, since they do not match when taken at the transient critical mass. We therefore propose a *two-step scenario* for evolution of locomotory functions: from (i) good bipedal running ability (trait 23), via (ii) decreasing bipedal running ability (trait 22), to (iii) quadrupedalism (trait 4).

Instead of speeds, the study of locomotor dynamic similarity in different-sized animals through Froude numbers is more appropriate (Alexander, 1976; Alexander & Jayes, 1983, Gatesy & Biewener, 1991). Most mammals appear to change their gait from walking to running discontinuously (abruptly) at a duty factor close to one half and Froude numbers below one (Ahlborn & Blake, 2002; Alexander & Jayes, 1983, Gatesy & Biewener, 1991). Extant elephants, however, exhibit a *continuous* walk-to-run transition at magnitudes $Fr_{w\text{-}r}^{(\mathrm{exp})} \approx 1$ (Hutchinson et al., 2006; for comparative analysis of quadrupeds see Kokshenev, 2011b, Fig. 1). Mapping this transient-state similarity point onto the transient critical mass discussed in the context of similarity in locomotor evolution in extinct giants, Eq. (23) describes the crossover from striding bipedalism (trait 5) to quadrupedalism (trait 4). Then, when introducing the two-step evolution scenario via locomotor traits 23→ 22→ 24 (Fig. 4) in the run-mode domain ($0.5 < \beta \leq 1$), we determine two locomotory patterns: (i) *good runners* capable of showing relatively high numbers $Fr_{run}^{(mod)} > 1.5$, since they have limbs mostly subjected to and, thus, adapted to near-critical bending stress of the domain, say, $0.8 \lesssim \beta < 1$, and (ii) *poor runners* attributed to Froude numbers lying in the transient-state domain $1 < Fr_{w\text{-}r}^{(mod)} \leq 1.5$ and using moderate bending and moderate torsional stress indicated by $0.5 < \beta \lesssim 0.8$. The walk-mode domain ($0 < \beta \leq 0.5$) establishes the locomotory pattern of (iii) *walkers*, for which $Fr_{walk}^{(mod)} \leq 1$ is generally expected. The suggested scenario of evolution in giants of gait-dependent *Froude function* $Fr(M)$ is found to be in good agreement with the data $Fr_{Tyrus}^{(exp)} = 2.10$ (shown by star in Fig. 4B) for the experimentally modeled 6-*ton* *Tyrannosaurus* showing relatively high running speed 8 m/s (Sellers & Manning, 2007). One may also expect that more reliable estimates for critical speeds discussed above could be derived from the predicted Froude numbers (Fig. 4B) by re-scaling method.

It generally follows from Fig. 4 that with increasing body mass the evolution of locomotory patterns from *good runners* through *poor runners* to *walkers* is controlled by decreasing bending stress and increasing torsional elastic stress in the limbs. Based on the corresponding indicators β and τ, we are broadly able to characterize the accompanied evolution in postures and limb proportions, changing in striding running bipeds from (i) erect posture (trait 1) and more cursorial limbs (trait 30) to (iii) sprawling, or less erect posture (trait 2) and less cursorial limb proportions (trait 31), attributed to quadrupeds. The intermediate biped-to-quadruped locomotory evolution indicated by near equal proportions of moderate bending and torsional stress in limbs, may roughly be approached by elephantid and non-elephantid proboscideans, having rather short and compact bodies and fairly long limbs; these animals were undoubtedly not fast running with a suspended phase and therefore are found (Fig. 4) to be poor runners (trait 22). The largest land animal, *Argentinosaurus*, certainly could not run at all, but grouping in the walk-mode domain, it may be broadly regarded as having been a good walker.

While locomotor ability is provided by the relative body force output, body mobility is generally associated with the corresponding reaction-body elastic force, provided in most part by limb bone elastic forces. The evolution of body mobility, resulting from turning and bending limb mobilities, moderately decreasing with body mass (Fig. 5), is concomitant with a suggested evolution from striding bipedalism (trait 5) to quadrupedalism (trait 4). The walking and running mobilities are distinguished through the walk-mode and run-mode domains of the bone-stress similarity indicators. The animals considered by Hutchinson (2006) to possess good running abilities (trait 23) as well as improved turning abilities (trait 25) are presented (Figs. 4 and 5) by a single pattern of good runners, which relatively high mobility is due to bending effects exceeding torsional effects in the limb bones. The animals characterized by poor turning ability (trait 24) and poor bending ability are treated as walkers constrained by relatively high-level torsional elastic stress developed in long bones.

As can be inferred from Fig. 5, smaller quadrupedal giants from the Proboscidea, poorly running elephants at relatively high safety factors, may expose the same body mobility as the slow running largest bipedal giants of the Theropoda, operating close to critical levels. The body mobility of extinct elephants, moving at near critical levels, e.g., presented by *Deinotherium giganteum* (Fig. 5), is one-fourth of that of running African and Asiatic elephants (Kokshenev, 2011b, Fig. 2).

5. Conclusion

We hope to have shown how a simple theoretical treatment of the similarities in the peak functional stress reliably established for the effective mammalian limb bone may provide new generalizations in the evolution with body mass of locomotory trends in extinct terrestrial giants, accompanied by evolution in postures and limb proportions affected by maximal body mass through limb-bone adaptations to primary locomotor body functions.

6. Acknowledgments

One of the authors (V.B.K.) acknowledges financial support by the national agency FAPEMIG.

7. References

Ahlborn, B.K. & Blake, R.W. (2002). Walking and running at resonance, *Zoology* 105:165–174.

Alexander,R.McN. (1976). Estimates of speeds of dinosaurs, *Nature* 261: 129-130.

Alexander, R. McN. (1977). Allometry of the limbs of antelopes (Bovidae), *Journal of Zoology* 183: 125-146.

Alexander, R.McN. (1981). Factors of safety in the structure of animals, *Science Progress Oxford* 67: 109–130.

Alexander, R. McN. (1985a). Mechanisms of posture and gait of some large dinosaurs, *Zoological Journal of Linnean Society* 83:1-25.

Alexander, R. McN. (1985b). The maximum forces exerted by animals, *Journal of Experimental Biology* 115: 231-238.

Alexander, RMcN. (1989). Optimization and gaits in the locomotion of vertebrates, *Physiological Review* 69: 1199-1227.

Alexander, R.McN. (1991). Doubts and assumptions on dinosaurs mechanics, *Interdisciplinary Scientific Review* 16: 175-1981.

Alexander, R. McN. (1998). All-time giants: The largest animals and their problems, *Paleontology* 41: 1231-1245.

Alexander, R.McN. (2006). Dinosaur biomechanics, *Proceedings of Royal Society B*, 273: 1949-1855.

Alexander, R.McN. & Jayes, A.S. (1983). A dynamic similarity hypothesis for the gaits of quadrupedal mammals, *Journal of Zoology* (London)201: 135-152.

Barriel, V., Thuet, E. & Tassy, P. (1999). Molecular phylogeny of Elephantidae. Extreme divergence of the extant forest African elephant, *Comptes Rendus de L'Academie des Sciences* (Ser. III) 322: 447 454.

Bertram, J.E.A. & Biewener, A.A. (1988). Bone curvature: Sacrificing strength for load predictability? *Journal of Theoretical Biology* 131: 75-92.

Bertram, J.E.A. & Biewener, A.A. (1990). Differential scaling of the long bones in the terrestrial Carnivora and other mammals, *Journal of Morphology* 204: 157-169.

Bertram, J.E.A. & Biewener, A.A. (1992). Allometry and curvature in the long bones of quadrupedal mammals. *Journal of Zoology* 226: 455-467.

Biewener, A.A. (1982). Bone strength in small mammals and bipedal birds: do safety factors change with body size? *Journal of Experimental Biology* 98: 289-301.

Biewener, A.A. (1983). Allometry of quadrupedal locomotion: the scaling of duty factor, bone curvature, and limb orientation to body size, *Journal of Experimental Biology* 105: 147-171.

Biewener, AA. (1989). Mammalian terrestrial locomotion and size. Mechanical design principles define limits, *Bioscience* 3: 776-783.

Biewener, A.A. (1990). Biomechanics of mammalian terrestrial locomotion, *Science* 250: 1097-1103.

Biewener, A.A. (2000). Scaling of terrestrial support: differing solutions to mechanical constraints of size, *in Scaling in Biology* of editors Brown, J. H. and West, G. B., Oxford University Press, Oxford, pp. 51-66.

Biewener, A.A. (2005). Biomechanical consequences of scaling, *Journal of Experimental Biology* 208: 1665-1676.

Biewener, A.A., Thomason, J. & Lanyon, L.E. (1983). Mechanics of locomotion and jumping in the forelimb the of the horse *(Equus): in vivo* stress developed in the radius and metacarpus *Journal of Zoology* 201: 67-82.

Biewener, A. & Taylor, C.R. (1986). Bone strain: a determinant of gait and speed?, *Journal of Experimental Biology* 1235: 383-400.

Blanco, R.E. & Jones, W.W. (2005). Terror birds on the run: A mechanical model to estimate its maximum running speed, *Proceedings of the Royal Society of London* 272: 1769-1773.

Blashford-Snell J. & Lenska, R. (1996). Mammoth hunt, *in Search for the Giant Eephants of Bardia*, Harper-Collins, London.

Carrano, M.T. (1998). Locomotion in non-avian dinosaurs: integrating data from hindlimb kinematics, in vivo strains, and bone morphology, *Paleobiology* 24: 450–469.

Carrano, M.T. (1999). What, if anything, is a cursor? Categories versus continua for determining locomotor habit in mammals and dinosaurs, *Journal of Zoology* 247: 29-42.

Carter, D.R., Smith, D.J., Spengler, D.M., Daly, C.H. & Frankel, V.H. (1980). Measurements and analysis on *in vivo* bone strains on the canine radius and ulna, *Journal of Biomechanics* 13: 27-38.

Carrano, M.T. (2001). Implications of limb bone scaling, curvature and eccentricity in mammals and non-avian dinosaurs, *Journal of Zoology* 254: 41–55.

Carrano, M.T. & Biewener, A.A. (1999). Experimental alteration of limb posture in the chicken (Gallus gallus) and its bearing on the use of birds as analogs for dinosaur locomotion, *Journal of Morphology* 240: 237-249.

Christiansen, P. (1997). Locomotion in sauropod dinosaurs, *GAIA* 14: 45-75.

Christiansen, P. (1998). Strength indicator values of theropod long bones, with comments on limb proportions and cursorial potential, *GAIA* 15: 241-255.

Christiansen, P. (1999). Scaling of the limb long bones to body mass in terrestrial mammals, *Journal of Morphology* 239: 167-190.

Christiansen, P. (2002a). Mass allometry of the appendicular skeleton in terrestrial mammals, *Journal of Morphology* 251: 195-209.

Christiansen, P. (2002b). Locomotion in terrestrial mammals: the influence of body mass, limb length and bone proportions on speed, *Zoological Journal of the Linnean Society* 136: 685-714.

Christiansen, P. (2004). Body size in proboscideans, with notes on elephant metabolism, *Zoological Journal of the Linnean Society* 140: 523-549.

Christiansen, P. (2007). Long-bone geometry in columnar-limbed animals: allometry of the proboscidean appendicular skeleton, *Zoological Journal of the Linnean Society* 149: 423-436.

Christiansen, P. & Paul, G.S. (2001). Limb bone scaling, limb proportions, and bone strength in neoceratopsian dinosaurs, *GAIA* 16: 13-29.

Currey, J.D. (1967). The failure of exoskeletons and endoskeletons, *Journal of Morphology* 123: 1-16.

Currey, J.D. (2003). The many adaptations of bone, *Journal of Biomechanics* 36: 1487-1495.

Erickson, G.M., Makovicky, P.J., Currie, P.J., Norell, M.A.,Yerby, S.A. & Brochu, C.A. (2004): Gigantism and comparative life-history parameters of tyrannosaurid dinosaurs, *Nature* 430: 772-775.

Fariña, R.A. (1995). Limb bone strength and habits in large glyptodonts, *Lethaia* 28: 189-196.

Fariña, R.A., Blanco, R.E. & Christiansen, P. (2005). Swerving as the escape strategy of *Macrauchenia patachonica* Owen (Mammalia; Litopterna), *AMEGHINIANA* (Review of Association of Paleontologists in Argentina) 42: 751-760.

Fariña, R.A. & Blanco, R.E. (1996). Megatherium, the stabber, *Proceedings of the Royal Society of London* (Series B) 263: 1725-1729.

Fariña, R.A., Vizcaino, S.F. & Blanco, R.E. (1997). Scaling of the indicator of athletic capability in fossil and extant land tetrapods, *Journal of Theoretical Biology* 185: 441-446.

Farley, J.R., Glasheen, J. & McMahon, T. A. (1993). Running springs: speed and animal size, *Journal of Experimental Biology* 185: 71-86.

Farlow, J.O., Smith, M.B. & Robinson, J.M. (1995). Body mass, bone "strength indicator", and cursorial potential of *Tyrannosaurus rex*, *Journal of Vertebrate Paleontology* 15: 713-725.

Fortelius, M. & Kappelman, J. (1993). The largest land mammal ever imagined,*Zoological Journal of the Linnean Society* 107 (1): 85-101.

Fritton, S.P., McLeod, K.J. & Rubin, C.T., (2000). Quantifying the strain history of bone: spatial uniformity and self-similarity of low magnitude strains, *Journal of Biomechanics* 33: 317–325.

Gambaryan, P.P. (1974). *How Mammals Run*. John Wiley & Sons, New York.

Garland, T. (1983). The relation between maximal running speed and body mass in terrestrial mammals, *Journal of Zoology* 199: 157–170.

Gatesy, S.M. & Biewener, A.A. (1991). Bipedal locomotion: effects of speed, size and limb posture in birds and humans, *Journal of Zoology* 224: 127–147.

Gatesy, S.M., Holtz, Jr.T.R., Hutchinson, J.R., & Robinson, J.M. (2000). Theropod locomotion, *American Zoology* 40: 640–663.

Heglund, N.C., McMahon, T.A. & Taylor, C.R. (1974). Scaling stride frequency and gait to animal size: mice to horses *Science* 186: 1112-1113.

Heglund, N.C. & Cavagna, G.A. (1985). Efficiency of vertebrate locomotory muscles, *Journal of Experimental Biology* 115: 283-292.

Heglund, N.C. & Taylor, C.R. (1988). Speed, stride, frequency and energy cost per stride: how do they change with body mass and gait?, *Journal of Experimental Biology* 138: 301-318.

Hokkanen, J.E.I. (1986a). The size of the largest land animal, *Journal of Theoretical Biology* 118: 491-499.

Hokkanen, J.E.I. (1986b). Notes concerning elastic similarity, *Journal of Theoretical Biology* 120: 499-4501.

Horner, J.R., Ricqles, A.J. de & Padian, K. (1999). Long bone histology of the hadrosaurid dinosaur Maiasaura peeblesorum: Growth dynamics and physiology based on an ontogenetic series of skeletal elements, *Journal of Vertebrate Paleontology* 20: 115-129.

Horner, J.R., Weishampel, D.B. & Forster, C. A. (2004). Hadrosauridae, *in The Dinosauria*, editors Weishampel, D.B., Dodson, P. and Osmólska, H. Berkeley, University of California Press. pp. 438–463.

Howell, A.B. (1944). *Speed in Animals. Their Specialization for Running and Leaping*. University of Chicago Press, Chicago.

Hutchinson, J.R., 2006. The evolution of locomotion in archosaurs, *Comptes Rendus Palevol* 5: 519-530.

Hutchinson, J.R. & Garcia, M. (2002). Tyrannosaurus was not a fast runner, *Nature* 415: 1018 -1021.

Hutchinson, J.R. & Gatesy, S.M. (2006). Beyond the bones, *Nature* 440: 292-294.

Hutchinson, J.R., Anderson, F.C., Blemker, S.S. & Delp, S.L. (2005). Analysis of hindlimb muscle moment arms in Tyrannosaurus rex using a three-dimensional musculoskeletal computer model: implications for stance, gait, and speed, *Paleobiology* 31: 676–701.

Hutchinson, J.R., Schwerda, D., Famini, D.J., Dale, R.H.I., Fischer, M.S. & Kram, R. (2006). The locomotor kinematics of Asian and African elephants: changes with speed and size, *Journal of Experimental Biology* 209: 3812-3827.

Hutchinson, J.R, Ng-Thow-Hing, V. & Anderson, F.A. (2007). A 3D interactive method for estimating body segmental parameters in animals: Application to the turning and running performance of *Tyrannosaurus rex*, *Journal of Theoretical Biology* 246: 660–680.

Ji, Q., Currie, P.J., Norell, M.A. & Ji, S.-A. (1998). Two feathered dinosaurs from northeastern China, *Nature* 393: 753-761.

Jones, J.H. & Lindstedt, S.L. (1993). Limits to maximal performance, *Annual Review Physiology* 55: 547-569.

Kokshenev, V.B. (2003). Observation of mammalian similarity through allometric scaling laws, *Physica A* 322: 491-505.

Kokshenev, V.B. (2007). New insights into long-bone biomechanics: Are limb safety factors invariable across mammalian species?, *Journal of Biomechanics* 40: 2911–2918.

Kokshenev, V.B. (2008). A force-similarity model of the activated muscle is able to predict primary locomotor functions, *Journal of Biomechanics* 41: 912–915.

Kokshenev, V.B. (2009). Scaling functional patterns of skeletal and cardiac muscles: New non-linear elasticity approach, *arXiv:0909.1444v1*.

Kokshenev, V.B. (2010). Key principle of the efficient running, swimming, and flying, *Europhysics Letters* 90: 48005.

Kokshenev, V.B. (2011a). Physical insights into dynamic similarity in animal locomotion. I. Theoretical principles and concepts, In: *Theoretical Biomechanics*, Vaclav Klika (ed.), pp. 267-284, ISBN 978-953-307-851-9

Kokshenev, V.B. (2011b). Physical insights into dynamic similarity in animal locomotion. II. Observation of continuous similarity states, In: *Theoretical Biomechanics*, Vaclav Klika (ed.), pp. 285-302, ISBN 978-953-307-851-9

Kokshenev, V.B., Silva, J.K.L. & Garcia, G.J.M. (2003). Long-bone allometry of terrestrial mammals and the geometric-shape and elastic-force constraints of bone evolution, *Journal of Theoretical Biology* 224: 551-555.

Kokshenev, V.B. & Christiansen P. (2010). Salient features in locomotion of proboscideans revealed via the differential scaling of limb long bones, *Biological Journal of Linnean Society* 100: 16-29.

Lovelace, D. M., Hartman, S. A. & Wahl, W. R. (2007). Morphology of a specimen of Supersaurus (Dinosauria, Sauropoda) from the Morrison Formation of Wyoming, and a re-evaluation of diplodocid phylogen, *Arquivos do Museu Nacional* 65: 527–544

Marden, J.H. (2005). Scaling of maximum net force output by motors used for locomotion, *Journal of Experimental Biology* 208: 1653-1664.

Mazetta, G.V., Christiansen, P. & Fariña, R.A. (2004). Giants and Bizarres: Body Size of Some Southern South American Cretaceous, Dinosaurs. *Historical Biology* 16: 71-83.

McFarlan, D. (1992). *The Guinness book of records*. Guinness Publ. Ltd, Enfield, Middlesex.
McMahon, T.A. (1973). Size and shape in biology, *Science* 179: 1201-1204.
McMahon, T.A. (1975a). Using body size to understand the structural design of animals: quadrupedal locomotion, *Journal of Applied Physiology* 39: 619-627.
McMahon, T.A. (1975b). Allometry and biomechanics: limb bones in adult ungulates, *American Naturalist* 109: 547-563.
Nowak, R. (1991). *Walker's mammals of the World*. Johns Hopkins University Press, Baltimore.
Padian, K., Horner, J.R. & Ricqles A. de (2004). Growth in small dinosaurs and pterosaurs: The evolution of archosaurian growth strategies, *Journal of Vertebrate Paleontology* 24: 555-571.
Paul, G.S. & Christiansen, P. (2000). Forelimb posture in neoceratopsian dinosaurs: implications for gait and locomotion, *Paleobiology* 26: 450-465.
Prange, H.D., Anderson, J.F. & Rahn, H. (1979). Scaling of skeletal mass to body mass in birds and mammals, *American Naturalist* 113: 103-122.
Rensberger, J.M. & Watabe, M. (2000). Fine structure of bone in dinosaurs, birds and mammals, *Nature* 406: 619-622.
Rubin, C.T. & Lanyon, L.E., (1982). Limb mechanics as a function of speed and gait: a study of functional stains in the radius and tibia of horse and dog. *Journal of Experimental Biology*: 101 187–211.
Rubin, C.T. & Lanyon, L.E. (1984). Dynamic strain similarity in vertebrates; an alternative to allometric limb bone scaling, *Journal of Theoretical Biology* 107: 321-327.
Sander, M.P. (2000). Longbone histology of the Tendaguru sauropods: Implications for growth and biology, *Paleobiology* 26: 466-488.
Selker, F. & Carter, D.R. (1989). Scaling of long bone fracture strength with animal mass. *Journal of Biomechanics* 22: 1175-1183.
Schmidt-Neielsen, K. (1984). *Scaling: Why Is Animal Size So Important?* Cambridge University Press, Cambridge.
Sharp, N.C.C. (1997). Timed running speed of a cheetah (*Acinonyx jubatus*), *Journal of Zoology* 241: 493-494.
Sellers, W.I. & Manning, P.L. (2007). Estimating dinosaur maximum running speeds using evolutionary robotics, *Proceedings of Royal Society B* 274: 2711-2716.
Taylor, M.P. (2009). A Re-evaluation of Brachiosaurus altithorax Riggs 1903 (Dinosauria, Sauropoda) and its generic separation from Giraffatitan brancai (Janensh 1914), *Journal of Vertebrate Paleontology* 29: 787-806
Taylor, D., O'Reilly, P., Vallet, L. & Lee, T.C. (2003). The fatigue strength of compact bone in torsion, *Journal of Biomechanics* 36: 1103-1109.
Tulborn, R.A. (1990). *Dinosaur Tracks*. Chapman and Hall, London.
Wilson, J.A. & Carrano, M.T. (1999). Titanosaurs and the origin of 'wide-gauge' trackways: a biomechanical and systematic perspective on sauropod locomotion, *Paleobiology* 25: 252–267.
Wood, G.L. (1976). *The Guinness Book of Animal Facts and Feats*. Guinness Superlatives Ltd, Enfield, Middlesex.

3

Mechanical Properties of Living Cells and Tissues Related to Thermodynamics, Experiments and Quantitative Morphology – A Review

Miroslav Holeček, Petra Kochová and Zbyněk Tonar
Department of Mechanics, Faculty of Applied Sciences
University of West Bohemia, Pilsen
Department of Histology and Embryology, Faculty of Medicine in Pilsen
Charles University in Prague, Pilsen
Czech Republic

1. Introduction

Physics and living matter

Although Galileo Galilei laid down the fundamentals for a mathematical description of natural processes, a long time passed before living organisms became a focus in physics. Given the high-spirited concept from René Descartes, living organisms were considered subject to the same universal laws as all objects. However, this approach did not provide scientists with an apparatus for systematically describing the physics of living matter. Isaac Newton's examination of physical reality was based on analysis of the forces that cause movement of objects. Although he developed a very efficient and fruitful mathematical apparatus, living organisms appeared as "black boxes" therein. Terms such as "trajectory" and "force" became highly problematic when attempting to describe such phenomena as the growth, assembly, and physical activities of complex biological systems. These problems became apparent during the 20th century with advances in thermodynamics, molecular physics, computer simulations, and highly sophisticated experimental and imaging methods.

From the perspective of physics, living cells are considered physical systems, i.e., material structures composed of atoms and molecules governed by the laws of physics. A living cell becomes material with certain rheological properties. Its molecular structure is described using terms from macromolecular chemistry, polymer physics, statistical mechanics, and thermodynamics. Most of the biological attributes for living matter are reduced or neglected on purpose, as they are typically undefined using these physical methods. However, even physicists must reflect the enormous complexity of biological systems. When considering a living cell as a "material", we cannot ignore that the phenomena, such as the "material", is able to move spontaneously, and cells can migrate through pores and avoid barriers while simultaneously changing their shape as well as their viscoelastic and rheological properties. Moreover, these physical objects of interest are growing and multiplying in number, and they can even undergo cell death (e.g., apoptosis). Therefore, physicists must be careful when interpreting results from highly idealized models. This is an issue especially when confronting models with real experiments, as living systems typically do not behave as passive objects during an experiment. They are able to actively respond to the experimental conditions by changing their mechanical properties.

2. Thermodynamics of living structures

By publishing his "Reflections on the Motive Power of Fire" (Carnot, 1824), Sadi Carnot provided not only a theory and description useful for machine and design engineers, but he also laid the foundations for the second law of thermodynamics. At first, this theory was unnoticed as a universal natural law that cannot be simply deduced from physics based on Newtonian mechanics. This led Rudolf Clausius to become one of the founders of a new discipline: thermodynamics. Thermodynamics was based on physical quantities that were unknown until then, i.e., internal energy (U) and entropy (S). Both of these quantities contribute to the Helmoltz *free energy*, F ($F=U-TS$), where T is the absolute thermodynamic temperature. Free energy is a consideration for systems interchanging heat with the surrounding matter, which is exactly the case for living cells and tissues in organisms.
Let us consider a sample material at a resting state without any unbalanced forces between the system and adjacent systems and in a state of thermodynamic equilibrium with its surroundings. The macroscopic conditions in such a system may be described using a set of working parameters ($\mathbf{A}^{(0)}$). These parameters can be set by mechanical, electrical, or magnetic actions, thus characterizing, for example, the shape or volume of the sample, its surface, and electrical polarization. Let us consider a change in these parameters caused by an external action, where surrounding the system is a heat reservoir at a steady temperature. The work done by these external forces (W) depends on the structure of that material and realization of such a change. As long as the change is *reversible*, W equals the free energy difference between the initial and the final state $\Delta F=F(\mathbf{A})-F(\mathbf{A}^{(0)})$. According to the second law of thermodynamics, relationship (1) applies to *any* process:

$$W \geq \Delta F . \tag{1}$$

The relationship between free energy and the parameters **A** is extremely important when describing our sample materials. Obviously, it is a measure of the *minimum amount of work* required to change the parameters of the material. However, the condition of reversibility is non-trivial. Changing the macroscopic configuration of most materials inevitably leads to a number of irreversible processes, such as the initiation and propagation of lattice defects in polycrystalline materials. In living tissues, it is logical to assume that certain processes are reversible, as tissues are clearly able to change their configuration across a broad range without any irreversible structural changes. However, the processes must be performed slowly to eliminate the effects from viscosity.
Free energy appears to be a key quantity in characterizing the rheological properties of living cells and tissues. When applying the laws of physics to living systems, it is a great challenge to describe the relationship between free energy and the working and structural parameters of the living system. However, both U and TS contribute to free energy, i.e., free energy is determined by energetic and entropic factors. This renders the task extremely difficult, which can be demonstrated using the biopolymer networks responsible for most

mechanical properties in tissues. These networks are *semiflexible*, i.e., the persistence length (l_p) is comparable to the typical distance between adjacent nodes (the contour length, L_C); see Fig. 1.

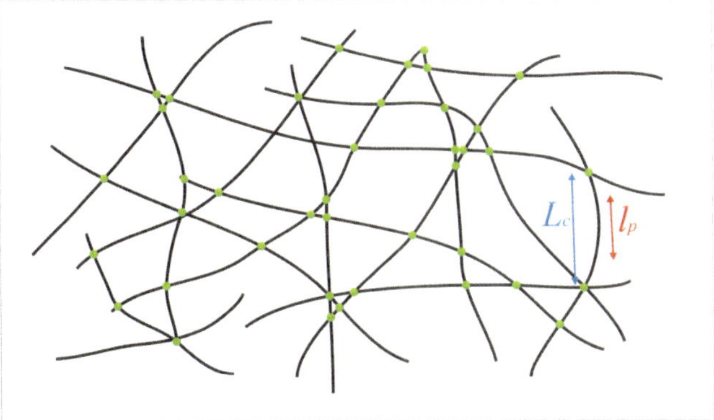

Fig. 1. Schematic for a network of semiflexible cytoskeleton biopolymer chains responsible for biomechanical properties in cells. The relationship between the persistence length (l_p) and contour length (L_C) is shown. For persistence length, correlations in the tangent direction are lost. The contour length of the chain is the distance between two nodes, measured as the mean length of the chain at the maximum physical extension.

Semiflexible networks typical in rubber-like materials have $l_p << L_C$; therefore, the elasticity is determined mainly by the entropic factors. The number of possible configurations for the fibers is reduced by stretching, and entropy is a log function for the number of these configurations. Nevertheless, analysis of biopolymer networks is a much more complex issue that solved in the most prestigious journals. According to Storm et al. (2005), the energy of a biological chain can be modeled as follows:

$$U = \int_0^{L_c} \left\{ \frac{\kappa}{2} |u''|^2 + \frac{f}{2} |u'|^2 \right\} dz , \tag{2}$$

where z is the projected coordinate along the end-to-end vector, κ is the bending stiffness related to persistence length via $\kappa = k_B T\, l_p$ (k_B is the Boltzmann constant), f is the applied force, and $u(z)$ describes deviation of the filament from its straight conformation. In small deformations, the entropic factor dominates, as the polymer chains can still embody a number of potential conformations. At higher deformations, the energetic factor prevails, which results in *strain-stiffening* (Onck et al., 2005), and the stress grows rapidly with increasing strain. However, other issues arise at higher deformations, such as the loss of fiber stability, and, therefore, more corrections could be necessary (Chadhuri et al., 2007). Strain-stiffening is typical for biological materials (Fung, 1993; De Santis et al., 2004; Kochova et al., 2008) and has several interesting consequences.

The validation of these theoretical models seems to be successful, especially with experimental data characterizing artificial biopolymer networks created *in vitro* and separate from other biopolymers (e.g., collagen network, vimentin filaments, and fibrillar actin microfilaments). However, the *in vivo* experiments performed in living cells remain a problem, even for simple cell cultures, where cells are separate and free from the context of the entire tissue. The main issue is that the cells, which are supposed to be the object of the experiment, are remodeling during the experiment, thus altering its conditions. This raises a fundamental paradox: how can we measure the mechanical behavior of living cells if they react to our measurement tools (Bao & Suresh, 2003)?

Another issue is that living structures, unlike artificial biopolymers, behave as open systems, far from thermodynamic equilibrium. The cells require a constant influx of energy and behave as dissipative systems. For the application of non-equilibrium thermodynamics as devised by Onsager and Prigogine for cell membrane transport, see e.g., Dickel (1984). Biopolymer networks *in vivo* are in a non-equilibrium state, which results in the presence of a permanent mechanical *prestress*, not caused by any external force. The elastic behavior of these networks is non-linear (Fig. 2). Due to prestress, the material is more stiff, which has been demonstrated in experiments on actin cytoskeletal microfilaments (Gardel et al., 2006). While the elastic module for *in vitro* actin networks reaches 0. 1 Pa, the moduli in living cells were 10,000 times higher. Although this difference is also caused by the presence of additional networks, it can be concluded that prestress increases stiffness in living cells by at least 10 times. Prestress is based in part on active forces generated by molecular motors (such as within the contractile apparatus of muscle cells, see Fig. 3). Other chemical energy-driven phenomena might take part in prestress, such as ion pumps regulating cell volume and intracellular osmotic pressure.

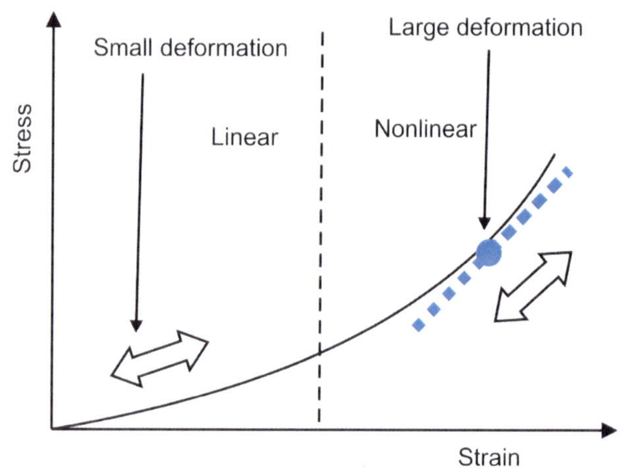

Fig. 2. Graphical interpretation of the stress-strain relationship describing the nonlinear strain-stiffening effect, which is characteristic of higher deformations in biological materials. For an explanation, see the text in this section related to modeling the energy, stiffness, and forces acting on a biopolymer chain (Storm et al., 2005; Chadhuri et al., 2007).

3. The living cell as a physical system

The cell is the basic functional and morphological unit in living organisms (Alberts et al., 2002). The typical cell size is 10-20 μm, and the shape can be spheroidal, ellipsoidal, fusiform, polyhedric, or squamous. Cells are either free units or are surrounded by other cells and an extracellular matrix within tissue. There are two types of cells: prokaryotic

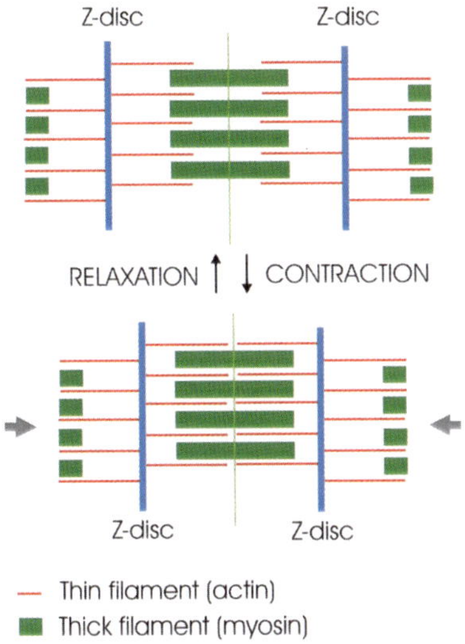

Fig. 3. Arrangement of myofibrils within contracted and relaxed sarcomeric muscle cells and fibers. The schematic illustrates the information in the paragraph on prestress generated by molecular motors and proteins associated with actin microfilaments (Gardel et al., 2006).

(bacteria) and eukaryotic (containing the cell nucleus and other membrane-bound compartments). Because of the plasma membrane (all cells) and even the cell wall (bacteria, plants, fungi, algae), the cell is an autonomous thermodynamic unit. The plasma membrane serves as an interface between intracellular and extracellular space. However, it does not insulate the cell from the extracellular environment. Rather, it is a selectively permeable barrier that hosts membrane transport systems. It is also involved in cell adhesion, cell signaling, ion conductivity, anchoring the cytoskeleton, attaching the extracellular matrix, maintaining cell volume, and the electric membrane potential. Maintaining stable and constant conditions within the cell, i.e., cell homeostasis, entails multiple dynamic equilibrium adjustments and regulatory mechanisms, which require approximately 30-70% of the energy available to the cell.

The intracellular space is compartmentalized by a number of membrane structures, while the space among them is filled with a colloidal liquid, the cytoplasm. In addition to the organelles and various inclusions, the intracellular space is reinforced by a scaffold, the cytoskeleton. This provides the cell with structure and shape. Cytoskeletal elements interact with cellular organelles and membranes. The cytoskeleton is also involved in cell motility, intracellular transport, cell division, and other processes.

From the physics point of view, the cell can be regarded as a structure comprised of heterogeneous materials, which correspond to the cytoskeleton, nucleus and other compartments. These constituents are considered continuous bodies with various material characteristics. Each of these materials is a viscoelastic continuum with a high degree of anisotropy and non-linear behavior. This approach is used to perform computational simulations of experiments performed with real cells using variety of techniques (e.g., atomic force microscopy as well as twisting, compressing, and pulling the cells, see Fig. 4-5). Describing the cellular structures as a sum of mechanical continua is useful only in tasks with dimensions exceeding the level of intracellular changes (Vaziri & Gopinath, 2008). Models based on the interaction of multiple physical phases can simulate interactions between the cytosol and solid objects using constitutive laws that describe the flow of fluid through a porous medium, such as Darcy's law (Rohan & Cimrman, 2010). Such multiphase models are applicable when analyzing experiments based on the interaction of liquid and solid phases, such as micropipette aspiration experiments (Fig. 4C, see also Mofrad & Kamm, 2006).

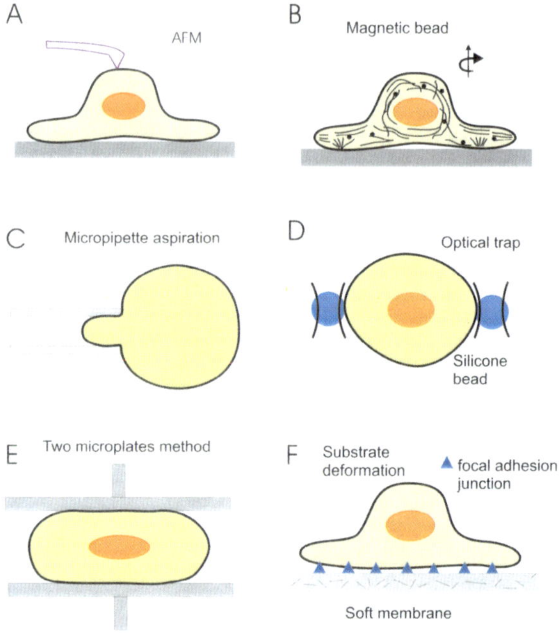

Fig. 4. Schematics of experimental methods currently used for measuring mechanical properties at the cellular level. These include atomic force microscopy (A), magnetic twisting and pulling cytometry (B), micropipette aspiration (C), optical particle trapping and optical tweezers (D), the two microplates method (E), and traction force microscopy (F).

However, for a better understanding of the cell as a physical system, more structures must be employed in our models. Probably the most important is the cytoskeleton (Fig. 6, see also Boal, 2002). The three main types of cytoskeletal filaments present in eukaryotic cells are microfilaments, intermediate filaments, and microtubules (Alberts et al., 2002). In prokaryotic cells, several types of structural and functional homologs of these cytoskeletal filaments were found (Carballido-López & Errington, 2003).

The *actin filaments* are the thinnest in the cytoskeleton at only 7 nm in diameter and are referred to as microfilaments. They are composed of linear actin polymers and are capable of generating force by elongation and shrinking at the ends. They also act as tracks for the movement of myosin molecules that attach to the microfilament, sliding along them. Actin microfilaments can be found both in the cortical and the deep cytoplasm. They are involved in cell motility, phagocytosis, cell division, and the transmission of force between the extracellular and intracellular structures. Several actin-binding proteins (e.g., α-actinin) contribute to actin cross-linking, thus modulating its *in vivo* mechanical properties. Unlike artificial microfilaments, *in vivo* actin is stiffer from prestress.

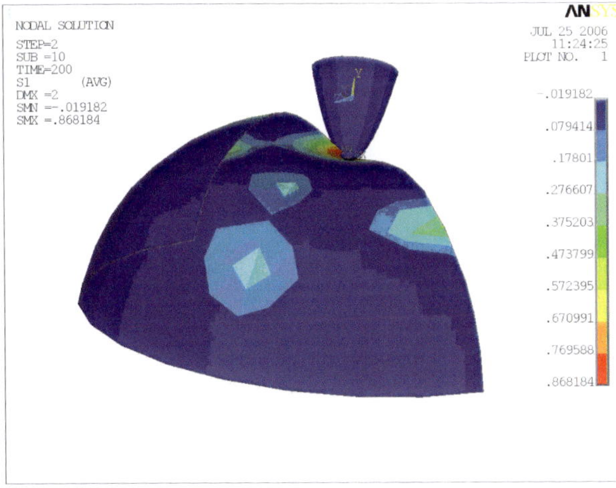

Fig. 5. Distribution of principal stress in the plasma membrane of a cell during a simulation of the indentation test. The figure demonstrates simulations by considering cellular compartments as viscoelastic mechanical continua with variable material properties (with kind permission of Dr. J. Burša, according to Burša & Fuis, 2009).

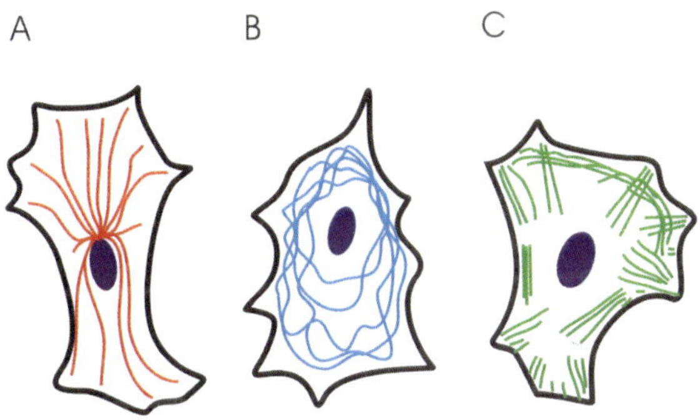

Fig. 6. Schematics for three different distribution patterns of cytoskeletal filaments. (A) Microtubules *(red)* are hollow cylindrical filaments with a diameter of 25 nm, radiating from the cell nucleus. Microtubules are organized by the microtubule organizing centers (centrioles and basal bodies). They are capable of growing and shrinking to generate force. They can be used by motor proteins that support the movement of organelles and other cellular factors along the microtubules. (B) The intermediate filaments *(blue)* have an average diameter of 10 nm, and they are mostly cytoplasmic (except the nuclear filaments known as lamins). These filaments are deformable proteins that can be stretched to several times their initial length. Such a large deformation is possible due to their hierarchical structure (Qin et al., 2009). (C) The actin microfilaments *(green)* are the thinnest cytoskeletal filaments (7 nm in diameter). They are assembled in highly versatile bundles and networks, they can be cross-linked and they resist both tensile and compressive forces. They are distributed both in the cortical cytoplasm and throughout the entire cell. They are able to generate force by either elongating or depolymerizing, and they work as part of the actomyosin molecular motor (Alberts et al., 2002).

The *intermediate filaments*, approximately 10 nm in diameter, are more stable than actin filaments. Like actin filaments, they help maintain the cell-shape by resisting tensional forces. Therefore, the cells are able to resist a tension of 10^2-10^5 Pa (Bao & Suresh, 2003). Intermediate filaments organize the internal structure of the cell and anchor the organelles.
Microtubules are rigid, hollow cylinders approximately 25 nm in diameter, and are polymers of the protein tubulin. They exhibit a highly dynamic behavior as they polymerize and depolymerize. They are commonly organized by the centrosome, play role in the intracellular transport of organelles and vesicles, and construct the cilia, flagella, and mitotic spindles. They resist compression, and thus, in *tensegrity models* (tensional integrity, Stamenovic, 2006), they are considered rigid bars (rods). These rigid microtubules are interconnected by prestressed, extensible microfilaments (cables) (Fig. 7). These models are used to explain cellular tension and complex interactions between stiffness and prestress, thus describing even viscoelastic properties (Canadas et al., 2002). Tensegrity models may be combined with continuum models. However, they are highly sensitive to the spatial arrangement of the cables and rods.

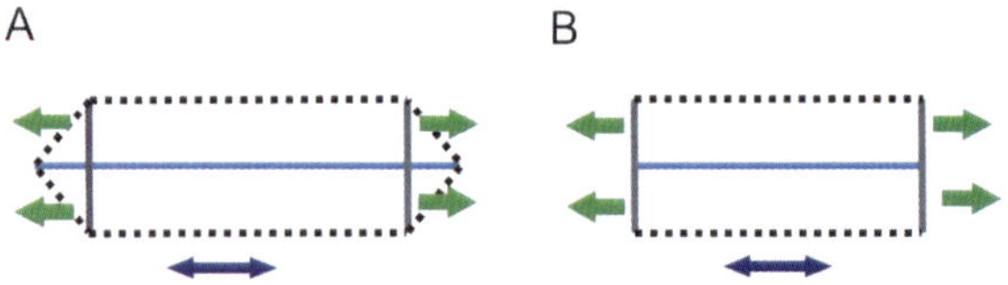

Fig. 7. A combination of rigid bars (rods, full lines) and viscoelastic fibers (cables, dotted lines) illustrate the tensegrities (Stamenovic, 2006) in models based on the balance between tension and compression in linear cytoskeleton components. In a steady state (A), the oblique cables are prestressed so that they can carry the tensile force, balanced by compression of the rigid rods (B). This approach may be used to demonstrate the non-trivial explanation of prestressed behavior in intracellular biopolymer networks.

As demonstrated by the tensegrity models, whenever physics aims to describe cell mechanics, it tends to choose a remarkable phenomenon, which becomes the basis for physical analysis. The cell has been considered a either mixture of polymer networks, a prestressed construction created from rods and fibers, or a multiphase continuum. Each of these strategies can explain certain features of cell behavior and may be used for planning and describing various experiments. Still, there is a demand for more general models, often inspired by non-trivial physical approaches. An interesting model is based on the similarity between cell behavior and the rheology of colloidal materials.

4. Biological cells and soft glassy materials

Despite the obvious presence of cytoskeletal semiflexible networks within the cells, physical description of these networks does not explain their complex behavior. The *in vivo* networks are not passive. On the contrary, the cell is a living structure; the networks undergo constant remodeling, and the activity of the molecular motors change over time. Despite the molecular level of these adaptive processes, their outcome is global and even macroscopic, i.e., at the level of the entire cell or tissue. Therefore, the next task is to describe the physical global effects from these molecular processes.

Recent advances in the rheology of soft glassy materials are at least a partial response to this problem (Fabry et al., 2001; Bursac et al., 2005; Deng et al., 2006). An experimental description of the frequency dependence for the complex modulus of the cell *G(f)* via magnetic cytometry (Fig. 4B) showed that the complex modulus of the cell consists of an elastic modulus G' and a loss of this modulus iG'', i.e., $G = G' + iG''$. These measurements were transformed into traditional elastic and loss moduli using a geometric factor, α, that depends on cell shape and thickness. For frequency dependence of the complex modulus for a semiflexible polymer network (e.g., fibrillar *in vitro* actin), *G* is either independent from the frequency (at lower frequencies) or is related (for higher frequencies) as follows:

$$G \sim f^{3/4}. \tag{3}$$

Equation (3) complies with the theory of entropic elasticity. At higher frequencies, the heat-driven bending fluctuations of the semiflexible fibers contribute to the complex modulus. This relationship (3) has also been measured for cell cytoskeletons *in vivo*. However, there should be a considerable contribution from prestress *in vivo*, generating higher stiffness in the cytoskeletal network. Because of prestress, the energetic component should prevail over the entropic contribution (represented by the ¾ index in Equation (3)). Another discrepancy was found at lower frequencies. Unlike *in vitro* networks, the real cytoskeleton has a frequency dependence even at lower frequencies:

$$G \sim f^{\alpha}, \tag{4}$$

where α varies between 0.1-0.3. Such behavior no longer complies with semiflexible polymer networks. Instead, it corresponds to special materials referred to as *soft glassy materials* (Sollich, 1998). These material represent various foams, emulsions, slurries and colloidal systems. These "glassy materials" share features of structural disorder and metastability. Local elements in this material are either too large, or they are trapped by their neighbors. Therefore, they cannot rapidly reach heat-induced equilibrium, and their rearrangement via thermal activation, referred to as *aging,* is rather slow. However, this rearrangement can be facilitated by external energy (Fig. 8). The behavior depends on mesoscopic elements, which are regions small enough for a macroscopic piece of material to contain them in a large number, thus providing a description of its behavior as an average over elements. They are also large enough such that deformations at the scale of a single element can be described using an elastic strain variable (Sollich, 1998).

The application of these experiments and conceptual tools to the cytoskeleton provides evidence for a non-equilibrium cytoskeletal state. Prestress corresponds to the "densities" of colloidal particles trapped within the glassy system, causing the metastability. The ATP (adenosine triphosphate)-driven molecular motors (e.g., myosin, dynein, kinesin) and cytoskeleton-associated proteins rearrange the network *in vivo,* thus modifying the local non-equilibria within the cytoskeletal configuration. As a result, the macroscopic behavior of the cytoskeleton is observed (Fabry et al., 2001). The value of α is the central characteristic for the entire process. When α=1, the material is a fluid, and when α=0, the material is solid. As soft glassy materials, the cells may be near the *glass transition*. Upon activating the contractile apparatus, α (Equation 4) decreases to zero, which corresponds to the glassy transition. In contrast, the loosening and relaxing the cytoskeleton leads to an increase in α. The "glassy dynamics" appear at frequencies of 10^2 Hz, which is the transition frequency between the characteristics described by Equation (3) and (4). In other words, describing the cell in terms of soft glassy rheology is useful for processes at a scale of approximately 0.01 s. However, this is exactly the time scale for many cellular events, such as cell motility, movement of kinocilia, and phagocytosis, among others. (Deng et al., 2006).

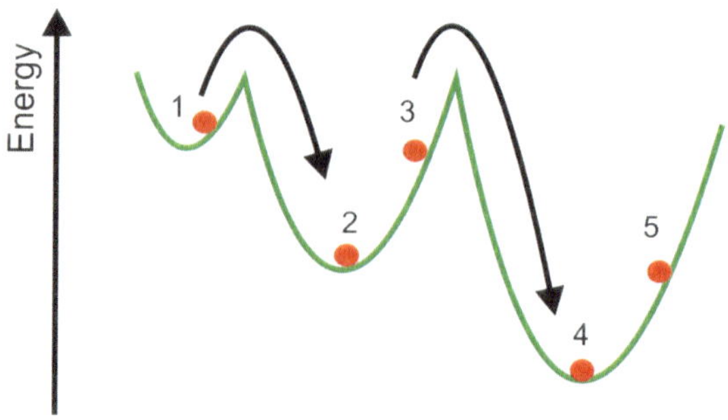

Fig. 8. Schematic illustrating the soft glassy rheology model of the cytoskeleton. The natural reorganization and dynamics for intracellular biopolymers can be modeled as a series of transitions (red positions labeled 1-5) between a fluid and solid state.

It is noteworthy that when applying soft glassy rheology to cell behavior, the physical approach is far from a "naive reductionism". There are no simulations at the molecular level. Conversely, the molecular processes remain in the background, varying only as a typical response to the stimulating frequencies. However, the "global" parameter, α, appears to be more important, as it characterizes the condition of the cytoskeleton and its typical response. The individual molecular mechanisms likely contribute to changes in α, thus affecting the global cellular response. Even the definition and experimental identification of such a parameter must be appreciated.

5. Cells and "intelligent materials"

In multicellular organisms, the cells are arranged in tissues, which usually compose organs. The cells are interconnected with cell-to-cell junctions that involve both plasma membranes and the intercellular matrix. The extracellular matrix consists of fibers and a ground "amorphous" substance. The prevailing matrix fibers in vertebrates are the collagen, elastin, and reticular fibers. The ground substance is constructed mainly of glycoproteins and glycosaminoglycans. In some tissues, the cells prevail, while other types of tissue are formed mainly by the matrix. Quantitative analysis of the tissue requires either a combination of microscopy and image processing or, preferably, unbiased *stereological methods* (Howard & Reed, 2005). The tissue can be characterized using volume fractions of the constituents (Fig. 9A), a description of the degree of anisotropy of the cells, the spatial orientation of the matrix fibers, cell clustering, the fiber length density, the microstructure surface area (Fig. 9B), and the numerical density of the objects in three dimensions, among others. Volumes, surfaces, lengths, numbers, and other microstructural characteristics can be estimated using stereological methods (Howard & Reed, 2005), which apply various geometrical principles for fair sampling of histological sections (Gundersen & Jensen, 1987). Stereology is based on methods related to the three-dimensional measurements available on the sections. A typical example includes the point-interception method, which estimates the area by counting the intersections between a randomly placed test grid and the objects of interest. The total number of points intersecting with the objects of interest is then multiplied by the reference area corresponding to each point. This is the reason stereology is also known as "stochastic geometry".

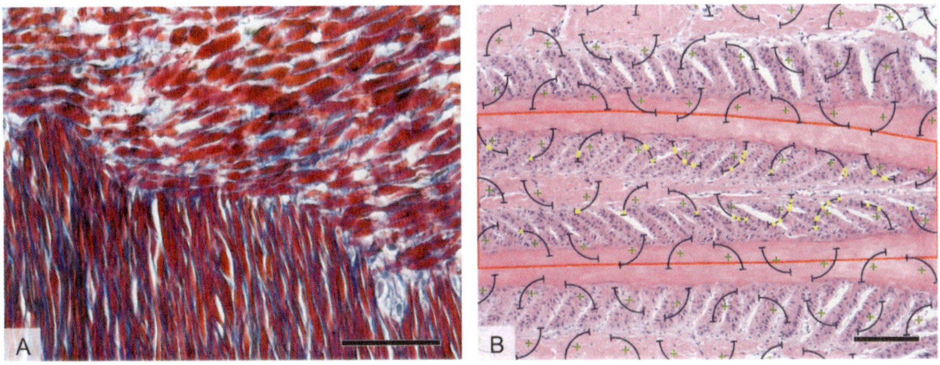

Fig. 9. Micrographs of composite biological tissues undergoing quantitative histological analysis. To elucidate how the principal constituents in biological tissues contribute to the mechanical behavior of macroscopic biological samples, either the volume fractions or surface densities of the tissue compartments must be assessed, preferably using unbiased point-interception stereological methods. (A) Smooth muscle *(red)* within the amphibian intestine is arranged in two perpendicular systems. The volume fractions from the active component (smooth muscle, stained *red*) and passive matrix (collagen fibers, *blue*) can be quantified. (B) A section through a junction for two types of tissues at the border between the dermis and epidermis of an equine hoof. Repeating epithelial lamellae interdigitate with the collagenous connective tissue of the dermis. The lamellar surface area can be estimated by counting the intersections *(yellow)* between the lamellae and a linear stereological system (circular arcs, *black*). The *red* borders delimit the reference space that corresponds to a single primary lamella, thus, the lamellar surface can be related to a volume unit of the tissue via the surface density of the junction. Mallory trichrome stain (A) and hematoxylin-eosin stain (B). Scale bars 50 μm (A), 100 μm (B).

In biological tissues, the cells are interconnected with the matrix fibers. The most abundant are collagen fibers. In fact, the hierarchical organization of collagen is complicated. Bundles of collagen fibers are constructed from fibrils, which consist of microfibrils, made from protofibrils that are overlapping trihelices of tropocollagen. In small deformations, the collagen fibers have a wavy appearance, and, unlike elastin fibers, they almost never contribute to the stress-strain behavior (Fig. 10, region I).

With increasing deformation (Fig. 10, region II), the collagen fibers become stretched and contribute to the total elastic modulus of the tissue. Further deformation (Fig. 10, region III) is characterized by fully stretched collagen fibers, which lead to sample stiffening. When increased stress reaches the ultimate strength of the tissue (region IV), microcracks are initiated and propagate through the tissue (Fig. 11). According to the arrangement of the collagen fibers, different tissues have different extensibility under uniaxial loading. For example, the mesentery of the peritoneal cavity can be distented by 100-200%, while ureters, arteries and veins can extend by approximately 60%; in addition, the cardiac muscle and tendons can extend to 15% and 2-5% of their initial length, respectively (Viidik, 1979; Ahlfors et Billiar, 2007). Therefore, we must consider that biological tissues have a complex microstructure and a non-linear, non-Hookean stress-strain response. Even under physiological conditions, they are subjected to large deformations.

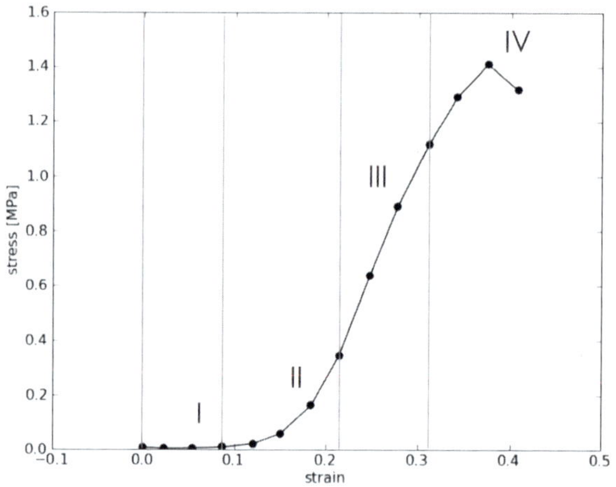

Fig. 10. An illustration of the non-linear stress-strain relationship for connective tissue exposed to a uniaxial tensile test. Region I represents the linear region for small deformations, region II is characterized by tissue stiffening, region III is the linear region for large deformations, while, at the end of region IV, the rupture is initialized.

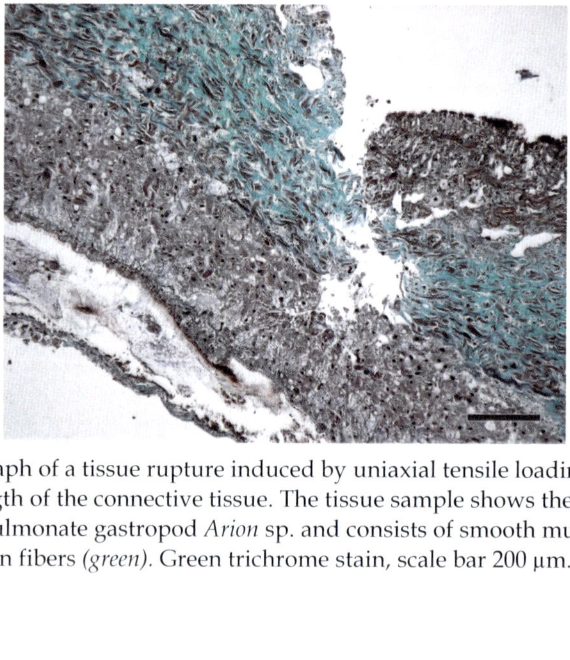

Fig. 11. A micrograph of a tissue rupture induced by uniaxial tensile loading that exceeds the ultimate strength of the connective tissue. The tissue sample shows the pedal integument of a pulmonate gastropod *Arion* sp. and consists of smooth muscle *(reddish to brown)* and collagen fibers *(green)*. Green trichrome stain, scale bar 200 μm.

From the perspective of rheology, the tissues can be considered viscoelastic materials, and therefore, they have properties such as stress relaxation, creep, and hysteresis. These parameters are identified using mechanical experiments, while preserving experimental conditions close to the *in vivo* state. The viscous properties result from biopolymers and the presence of intracellular and extracellular fluid. The intracellular fluid corresponds to approximately 40% of the tissue weight, while the extracellular fluid composes approximately 20% of the tissue weight. Deformation of the tissue is accompanied by redistribution of the fluid; however, the fluid renders the tissues incompressible.

Materials that can adapt to their environment and those that, more modestly, can alter their properties as required by their users are referred to as "intelligent". This is observed, for example, in the muscle tissue, which can change the microscopic contractility of the cytoskeletal filaments, causing either macroscopic peristalsis of the intestine, blood vessel vasoconstriction or blood vessel vasodilatation.

Let us consider a possible physical description for these mechanisms, enabling the number of *N* cells to modulate the mechanical behavior of the entire tissue. The free energy of a cell $F_{cell}(\mathbf{A}_C,\alpha)$ is determined by a set of working parameters $\mathbf{A}_C$ (describing the cell geometry) and a set of intrinsic parameters α (governed by the cell itself, e.g., the activity of molecular motors and degree of polymerization of the actin network, etc.). Now let us define the free energy of the extracellular matrix F_{ECM}, which is determined by the working parameters $\mathbf{A}$ of the sample and the values for all cells present within the sample $\mathbf{A}_c^i$, $i = 1,\ldots,N$. These values define the geometry of the cells and, therefore, the geometry of the matrix. At the level of the entire tissue sample, the working parameters for individual cells are considered free variables, as they are not controlled from "outside" of the cells; rather, they are set by the cells to minimize the free energy of the entire system:

$$\Delta F = \min_{\mathbf{A}_c^i}\left\{\Delta F_{\mathrm{ECM}}(\ldots,\mathbf{A}_c^j,\ldots) + \sum \Delta F_{\mathrm{cell}}(\mathbf{A}_c^i,\alpha_i)\right\}. \tag{5}$$

As the cells are much softer than the matrix, the consequence of Equation (5) is that the geometry of a cell is adapted to minimize deformation of the matrix, i.e., the cells will be deformed rather than the matrix. The contribution of the free energy is small; therefore, should the deformation mainly involve the cells, the intracellular processes would not be able to change the free energy of the entire tissue, i.e., they would not be able to alter the mechanical properties of the entire tissue.

In addition, the shape of the cells should not be deformed without limits, i.e., the values for parameters $\mathbf{A}_c^i$ are limited. It is well-known that most animal cells tend to maintain their shape and volume using a variety of compensating mechanisms related to homeostasis and constant intracellular osmotic pressure (Pollard & Earnshaw, 2004). Therefore, constant volume is another factor limiting the shape of the cell. Maintaining constant cell volume is an efficient way to enable additional intrinsic mechanisms to alter the tissue stiffness. This can be demonstrated using a model structure constructed of elastic balloons (or balls) interconnected with linear springs (Fig. 12); the balls represent the cells, and the springs are analogous to the tissue matrix. Similar to living tissues, this material is incompressible as a whole (the space inside and among the balls is filled with fluid). Let us study orthogonal deformations of this material, which can be described as changes in individual dimensions $\Delta x_{i0} \to \Delta x_i$, i = 1,2,3, while $\beta_i \equiv \Delta x_i/\Delta x_{i0}$ is the relative deformation in the i-th direction (the incompressibility of the material can be expressed as $\beta_1\beta_2\beta_3 = 1$). Change in the internal energy during deformation is determined by deformations of the springs and balls. For compressible balls (i.e., their wall is permeable to the fluid), the ratio between deformations of the balls and springs could be optimized in all three directions independently from each other. If the balls are much softer than the springs, an external mechanical loading in the system causes a deformation of the balls only such that the overall stiffness of the material is close to the balls' stiffness. Should the balls' wall become impermeable, such optimization would be impossible. Changes in the free energy during deformation within a system made of incompressible balls ΔF would be much higher than the change in free energy for a system containing compressible balls ΔF_0:

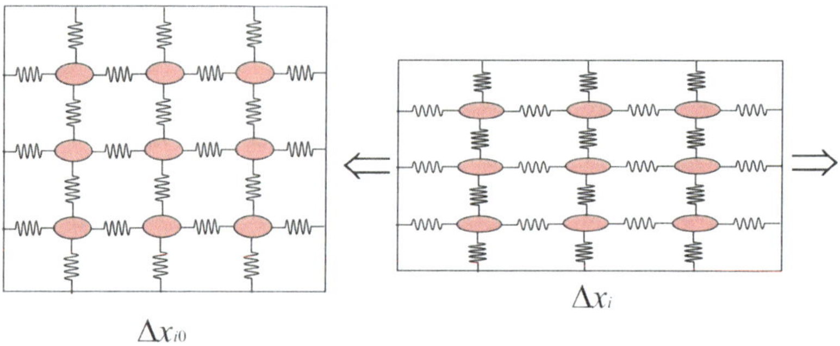

Fig. 12. An illustrative explanation of a two-dimensional model formed by flexible balls connected with linear springs (according to Holeček & Moravcová, 2006). Due to the incompressibility of the system as a whole, the total volume for the tissue model is constant. However, an external force may deform both the balls and springs, while the maximum deformation occurs in the balls, as this deformation requires less energy. For compressible balls, the material becomes extremely soft and deformation occurs almost entirely in the balls. This approach appears to be useful for modeling non-trivial modulation of macroscopic mechanical behavior of tissues (or even entire organs) by setting the properties of various cell types and intercellular fibers or junctions.

$$\begin{aligned} \Delta F &= \Delta F_0 + \Delta F', \\ \Delta F' &>> \Delta F_0. \end{aligned} \tag{6}$$

While the free energy ΔF_0 corresponds to linear elastic material, the free energy ΔF corresponds to non-linear material. This is caused by the optimization process described by Equation (5), which describes a system with non-linear relationships (Holeček & Moravcová, 2006). The involvement of the balls is determined by physical and geometric parameters describing the inner structure of the material. The more behavior of the material that is controlled by the balls entirely, the nearer the product of $\beta_1^{eff}\beta^{eff}{}_2\beta^{eff}{}_3$ to 1, where β_i^{eff} describes an efficient relative deformation in the i-th direction:

$$\beta_i^{\mathrm{eff}} = \frac{1+\delta_i}{1+k_i}\left(\frac{\Delta x_i}{\Delta x_{i0}} - 1\right) + 1 \cdot \tag{7}$$

δ_i is the ratio of the distance between the balls to the diameter of the ball in the i-th direction (in a non-deformed condition, thus corresponding to the ratio of initial spring lengths and the initial ball diameters), and k_i is a ratio between the ball stiffness and the stiffness of the spring in the i-th direction. In any part of the material, provided that

$$\beta_1^{\text{eff}} \beta_2^{\text{eff}} \beta_3^{\text{eff}} = 1, \tag{8}$$

the geometric and mechanical parameters are optimized such that even with incompressible balls, the material behaves as if the balls were compressible, i.e., deformation of the material relies on deformation of the balls only. Under the condition described by Equation (8), the local inner energy $\Delta F'=0$ (Fig. 13). However, even a small change in either δ_i or k_i will impair Equation (8). Further deformation of the entire material also depends extensively on deformation of the springs, which are much stiffer than the balls. This leads to an increase in inner energy ΔF, necessary for local deformation. Equation (8), therefore, indicates the presence of a local minimum for deformation energy among the intrinsic material parameters at a given external deformation.

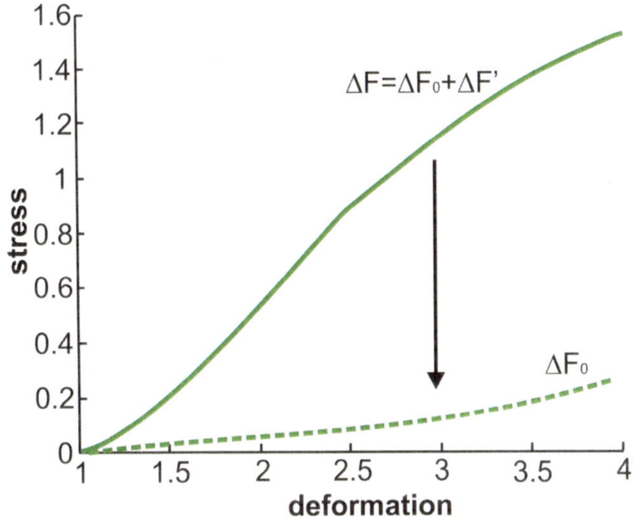

Fig. 13. Numerical simulation of free energy for a model constructed from balls and reinforced with springs *(full line)*. For high deformability of the balls, the energy of the material drops to a minimum and the stress-strain characteristics of the material are illustrated with a *dashed* line. Along this minimum, it is possible to change the stiffness of the material in an efficient manner. This simulation demonstrates the considerable number of macroscopic mechanical characteristics in biological tissues that result from the properties of its microscopic constituents.

Nevertheless, do the living cells really use this principle? Taking the interaction between the actin and myosin myofilaments as an example, it is obvious that the sliding of the myosin heads along the actin microfilaments corresponds to changes in the initial lengths of the springs. Using these intrinsic processes driven by chemical energy, the cell changes the geometric parameters δ_i, thereby setting $\beta_1^{eff} \beta^{eff}{}_2 \beta^{eff}{}_3$ close to 1. Indirect evidence for such a structural optimization is demonstrated by comparing the efficiencies of the smooth and skeletal muscle. Both muscle cell types share the same intrinsic mechanisms for the sliding myofilaments, i.e., altering the overlap between the actin and myosin filaments. However, the ultrastructural organization of the contractile apparatus (i.e., the geometric properties of the system) varies. In skeletal muscle, the contractile apparatus is arranged as periodical sarcomeres. In smooth muscle cells, the actin and myosin chains stretch across the cytoplasm, and spatial reorganization of the contractile machinery optimizes force development during contraction. The smooth muscle cell can be shortened to 2/3 its initial length, while contraction in a skeletal muscle fiber is limited to approximately 1/4. According to the experiments performed, the skeletal muscle requires 10-300 times the chemical energy (ATP) to achieve the same isometric contractile force compared with smooth muscle (Mofrad & Kamm, 2006). In smooth muscle cells, each isometric contraction is accompanied by a lower number of interactions between actin and myosin (each of these interactions is compensated with the ATP), which more efficiently maintains muscular tone. The drawback of this adaptation is that the onset of contraction is much slower in smooth than skeletal muscle.

6. Conclusion

Modeling the mechanical behavior of living cells and tissues is one of the biggest challenges in biomechanics. The models should comprise the properties of the cytoskeleton, plasma membrane, cell-to-cell junctions, as well as fibrillar and amorphous extracellular matrix. The macroscopic mechanical parameters of tissues can be identified much easier than microscopic parameters; therefore, the models serve as translators between macroscopic and microscopic phenomena. We reviewed several current approaches used in various branches of biophysics to devise non-trivial models of biological tissues.

Beginning with thermodynamics, which led us to study the free-energy dependence of microscopic parameters for living tissues, we continued with special mechanical properties of living cells (Bao & Suresh, 2003) and the important role of prestress in the cytoskeleton. We mentioned the tensegrity models (Stamenovic, 2006) and the approach in which the biological cell is regarded as a soft glassy material (Sollich, 1998). Active adaptations of intracellular structures require a physical description of such cytoskeletal remodeling (Bursac et al., 2005). We then discussed the problems with description and experimental identification of properties in living tissues and used an example to outline a purely mechanical explanation for the way that smooth muscle cells efficiently control the mechanical behavior of the entire tissue. We discussed the current methods for quantitative microscopic analysis of biological samples using stereological methods (Howard & Reed, 2005). We also outlined the importance of simple physical models in understanding the important features of biological structure functions (e.g., Holeček & Moravcová, 2006). To enhance this review's availability to a broad audience, a number of illustrations accompanied the text.

We conclude that the mechanical properties of biological cells and tissues depend on their underlying complex microstructure. At the tissue level of organization, computer simulations based on a stochastic interpretation of real morphology allow us to pursue the effects from stiffness and elasticity of both the cytoskeleton and extracellular matrix on the mechanical behavior of entire organs. Despite the limitations in our knowledge and methods, physical models of cell mechanics offer powerful tools for researching the structural principles governing living matter.

7. Acknowledgment

The study was supported by the Grant Agency of Czech Republic under Project No. 106/09/0734 and Ministry of Education, Youth and Sports of the Czech Republic under Project No. MSM4977751303

8. References

Ahlfors, J. E. W. ; Billiar, K L. (2007). Biomechanical and biochemical characteristics of a human fibroblast-produced and remodeled matrix. *Biomaterials*, Vol. 28, pp. 2183-2191, ISSN 0142-9612.

Alberts, B. ; Johnson, A. ; Lewis, J. ; Raff, M. ; Roberts, K. ; Walter, P. (2002). *Molecular Biology of The Cell,* (4th edition), Garland Science, ISBN 978-0815332183, New York.

Bao, G. ; Suresh, S. (2003). Cell and molecular mechanics of biological materials. *Nature Materials*, Vol. 2, pp. 715-725, ISSN 1476-1122.

Boal, D. (2002). *Mechanics of the Cell,* Cambridge University Press, ISBN 978-0521796811, Cambridge.

Burša, J. ; Fuis, V. (2009). Finite element simulation of mechanical tests of individual cells. *IFMBE Proceedings,* Vol. 25, pp. 16-19, ISSN 1680-0737.

Bursac, P. ; Lenormand, G. ; Fabry, B. ; Oliver, M. ; Weitz, D.A. ; Viasnoff, V. ; Butler, J.P. ; Fredberg, J. J. (2005). Cytoskeletal remodelling and slow dynamics in the living cell. *Nature Materials*, Vol. 4, pp. 557-561, ISSN 1476-1122.

Canadas, P. ; Laurent, V.M. ; Oddou, C. ; Isabey, D. ; Wendling, S. (2002). A cellular tensegrity model to analyze the structural viscoelasticity of the cytoskeleton. *Journal of Theoretical Biology,* Vol. 218, pp. 155-173, ISSN 0040-5809.

Carballido-López, R. ; Errington, J. (2003). A dynamic bacterial cytoskeleton. *Trends in Cell Biology,* Vol. 13, pp. 577-583, ISSN 0962-8924.

Carnot, S. (1824). Réflexions sur la puissance motrice du feu et sur les machines propres à développer cette puissance. Bachelier, Paris.

Chadhuri, O.; Parekh, S.H.; Fletcher, D.A. (2007): Reversible stress softening of actin networks. *Nature,* Vol. 445, pp. 295-298, ISSN 0028-0836.

De Santis, R. ; Sarracino, F. ; Mollica, F. ; Netti, P.A. ; Ambrosio, L. ; Nicolais, L. (2004). Continuous fibre reinforced polymers as connective tissue replacement. *Composites Science and Technology,* Vol 64, pp. 861-871, ISSN 0266-3538.

Deng, L. ; Trepat, X. ; Butler, J.P. ; Millet, E. ; Morgan, K.G. ; Weitz, D.A. ; Fredberg, J. J. (2006). Fast and slow dynamics of the cytoskeleton. *Nature Materials,* Vol. 5, pp. 636-640, ISSN 1476-1122.

Dickel, G. (1984). The variational principles of Onsager and Prigogine in membrane transport. *Faraday Discussions of the Chemical Society,* Vol. 77, pp. 157-168, ISSN 0301-7249.

Fabry, B. ; Maksym, G.N., Butler, J.P; Glogauer, M.; Navajas, D.; Fredberg, J.J. (2001). Scaling the microrheology of living cells. *Physical Review Letters,* Vol. 87, pp. 148102-1-148102-4, ISSN 0031-9007.

Fung, Y.C. (1993): *Biomechanics. Mechanical Properties of Living Tissues.* Springer-Verlag, ISBN 03-879-7947-6, New York.

Gardel, M.L. ; Nakamura, F. ; Hartwig, J.H. ; Crocker, J.C. ; Stossel, T.P. ; Weitz, D.A. (2006). Prestressed F-actin networks cross-linked by hinged filamins replicate mechanical properties of cells. *Proceedings of the National Academy of Sciences,* Vol. 103, pp. 1762-1767. ISSN 1091-6490.

Gundersen, H.J.G. ; Jensen, E.B. (1987). The efficiency of systematic sampling in stereology and its prediction. *Journal of Microscopy,* Vol. 147, pp. 229-263, ISSN 0022-2720.

Holeček, M.; Moravcová F. (2006). Hyperelastic model of a material which microstructure is formed by "balls and springs". *International Journal of Solid and Structures,* Vol. 43, pp. 7393-7406, ISSN 0020-7683.

Howard, C.V.; Reed, M.G. (2005). *Unbiased Stereology: Three Dimensional Measurement in Microscopy,* (2nd edition), Garland Science/BIOS Scientific, ISBN 978-1859960899, New York.

Kochova P.; Tonar, Z.; Matejka, V.M.; Sviglerova, J.; Stengl, M.; Kuncova, J. (2008). Morphology and mechanical properties of the subrenal aorta in normotensive and hypertensive rats. *Biomedical papers of the Faculty of Medicine of Palacký University, Olomouc, Czech Republic,* Vol. 152, pp. 239-245, ISSN 1213-8118.

Mofrad, M.R.K.; Kamm, R.D. (2006). *Cytoskeletal Mechanics. Models and Measurements in Cell Mechanics,* Cambridge University Press, ISBN 978-0521846370, New York.

Onck, P.R.; Koeman, T.; van Dillen, T.; van der Giessen, E. (2005). Alternative explanation of stiffening in cross-linked semiflexible networks. *Physical Review Letters,* Vol. 95, pp. 178102-1-178102-4, ISSN 0031-9007.

Pollard, T.D.; Earnshaw, W.C. (2004). *Cell Biology.* W.B. Saunders Company, ISBN 0-7216-3360-9, Philadelphia.

Qin, Z.; Kreplak, L.; Buehler, M.J.; Schnur, J.M. (2009). Hierarchical Structure Controls Nanomechanical Properties of Vimentin Intermediate Filaments. *PLoS ONE,* Vol. 4, p. e7294, ISSN 1932-6203.

Rohan, E.; Cimrman, R. (2010). Two-scale modeling of tissue perfusion problem using homogenization of dual porous media. *International Journal for Multiscale Computational Engineering,* Vol. 8, pp. 81–102, ISSN 1543-1649.

Sollich, P. (1998). Rheological constitutive equation for model of soft glassy materials. *Physical Review E,* Vol. 58, pp. 738-759, ISSN 1539-3755.

Stamenovič, D. (2006). Models of cytoskeletal mechanics based on tensegrity. In: *Cytoskeletal Mechanics,* Mofrad, M.R.K.; Kamm, R.D. (Eds), pp. 103-128, Cambridge University Press, ISBN 978-0521846370, New York.

Storm, C.; Pastore, J.J.; MacKintosh, F. C.; Lubensky, T.C.; Janmey, P.A. (2005). Nonlinear elasticity in biological gels. *Nature,* Vol. 435, pp. 191-194, ISSN 0028-0836.

Vaziri, A.; Gopinath, A. (2008). Cell and biomolecular mechanics in silico. *Nature Materials,* Vol. 7, pp. 15-23, ISSN 1476-1122.

Viidik, A. (1979). Biomechanical behavior of soft connective tissues, In: Akkas N. (Ed) *Progress in Biomechanics,* pp. 75-113, Springer and Sijthoff & Nordhoff´, ISBN 978-9028604797, New York.

Part 2

Biomechanical Modelling

4

Biomechanical Computer Models

K. Engel[1], R. Herpers[2] and U. Hartmann[3]
[1]*German Sport University Cologne*
[2]*Bonn-Rhine-Sieg University of Applied Sciences*
[3]*University of Applied Sciences Koblenz*
Germany

1. Introduction

In the past decade computer models have become very popular in the field of biomechanics due to exponentially increasing computer power. Biomechanical computer models can roughly be subdivided into two groups: multi-body models and numerical models. The theoretical aspects of both modelling strategies will be introduced. However, the focus of this chapter lies on demonstrating the power and versatility of computer models in the field of biomechanics by presenting sophisticated finite element models of human body parts. Special attention is paid to explain the setup of individual models using medical scan data. In order to reach the goal of individualising the model a chain of tools including medical imaging, image acquisition and processing, mesh generation, material modelling and finite element simulation -possibly on parallel computer architectures- becomes necessary. The basic concepts of these tools are described and application results are presented. The chapter ends with a short outlook into the future of computer biomechanics.

The field of biomechanics suffers from one very severe restriction; in general it is not possible for ethical reasons to measure forces and pressure inside the human body. Thus, typical measurement technology in biomechanics works on the interface between body and environment. Force platforms dynamically quantify reaction forces when a person is walking or running across the sensor, electromyography (EMG) monitors action potentials of contracting muscles with electrodes attached to the human skin. The information provided by the measurement technology is very important to investigate the mechanics of movements, but is not sufficient to answer questions like:

- How can we optimise movements (e.g. in sports or rehabilitation) in order to minimise the loads on the joints? How can we better understand mechanisms of injury and thus improve prevention? These questions are related to the human body.
- How do we have to design the equipment to optimally suit the patient's or the athlete's requirements in terms of mechanical behaviour? These questions are related to the medical or technical equipment. This optimisation process has three aspects:
    - Ineffective and destructive loading has to be minimised (e.g. by damping through innovative cushions in the shoe sole or improved orthotic devices).
    - Body protection has to be maximised (e.g. through better design of cyclists' helmets or the interior of automobiles).

- The patient's outcome and the athlete's output have to be maximised (e.g. by a novel concept for the design a prosthesis or the aerodynamics of a bob sleigh).

The only possible way to answer the questions related to the human body is to set up mechanical models of the human body or at least of human body parts. The setup of a biomechanical model is the only possibility to gain insight into the mechanical behaviour of the inner human body. Thus, modelling has become extremely popular because it -to some extent- heals the fundamental dilemma of biomechanics that has been described at the beginning of the chapter. Therefore, a software tool chain for the automatic generation of *individual* anatomical structures is presented in this book chapter. The setup of models representing medical or sports equipment is also an important task in computational biomechanics. Here, computer analyses are applied to better understand the mechanics of equipment during exercise. Despite the success of modelling techniques in the field of biomechanics, measurement technology still plays an important role: the information provided by the measurements is either input for a model (e.g. reaction forces acting on the foot) or used to validate the model (e.g. comparing the simulation results with EMG data). Thus, it is almost trivial to mention that models are of no scientific use without validation. When looking at the progress being made in the field of biomechanical modelling one can observe two major directions of development:

- Multi body systems (MBS) have been set up yielding important results in prevention and sports (Gruber et al.,1998; Blajer & Czaplicki, 2001; Wojtyra, 2003).
- Numerical models using finite elements (FEM) or computational fluid dynamics (CFD) have been successfully applied to a variety of biomechanical problems such as improving injury prevention (Penrose & Hose, 1998), ameliorating the design of equipment (Dabnichki & Avital, 2006) and for optimising movement techniques (Wangerin et al., 2007).

Both types of models have their advantages and disadvantages: numerical models enable the computation of the whole body's deformation, whereas multi-body models only provide forces at a limited number of body points. But, the price to pay for taking into account the body's deformation is a much higher demand in terms of computer power for the finite element method. This fact partially explains why sometimes parallel computers enter the stage in order to arrive at accurate FE results. Meanwhile, software packages are available that enable the user to use both methods, MBS and FEM simultaneously. The remainder of this text is organised as follows: the next chapter deals with the basic concept of multi body models to then discuss one MBS model in detail. The subsequent chapter gives a short introduction to the finite element method, describes a software tool chain to set up FE models of human body parts starting from medical image data. Chapter 4 provides insight into two example applications. Finally, a short outlook into the future of computer modelling in the field of biomechanics is given.

2. Multi body systems in biomechanics

Within the last two decades multi body models have frequently been applied to solve biomechanical problems (see Figure 1). Some selected MB applications are for instance simulations for impact analysis (Gruber et al.,1998), investigations of the trampoline jumping (Blajer & Czaplicki, 2001), studies about walking and running (Wojtyra, 2003) or the discussion of forces encountered in bicycle sports (Wangerin et al., 2007). Multi body systems can be used in two different ways: as forward or as inverse models. Here, we focus on forward models. The physical forces and moments (e.g. gravitation and external forces, see Figure 2) are the given quantities. Together with geometric data (e.g. length of body segment) and mechanical parameters (e.g. moments of inertia J, centre of mass) the resulting body movement can be computed. The movement is fully described by the laws of Newtonian dynamics that is mathematically described by the following equations.

$$\mathbf{F} = m\,\mathbf{a} \tag{1}$$

$$\mathbf{M} = J\,\boldsymbol{\alpha} \tag{2}$$

In general, **F**, **a**, **M** and $\boldsymbol{\alpha}$ are three-dimensional vectors denoting force, linear acceleration, moments and angular acceleration respectively. The mass m is a scalar and the moment of inertia J is in general a tensor represented by a 3x3 matrix. To be able to solve the underlying differential equations a kinematical chain of simple geometric entities (e.g. an ellipsoid representing the thigh) has to be set up (see Figures 1 and 2). In order to arrive at the quantities of interest (e.g. the load in the hip joint while landing) segment after segment has to be processed. The segments are linked by joints whose degrees of freedom are defined according to those of the anatomical articulations. The rigid body motion (i.e. translation and rotation) of the current segment (e.g. the foot) can be calculated when the external forces (e.g. measured by a force platform) and the body weight of the segment are given. The mechanical influence of the next segment in the chain (e.g. the shank) on the current segment is represented by a reaction force. These reaction forces are most interesting as they give a measure of the load present in the joint during sports exercise. The reaction force determined for one segment is then input (only switching the sign) for the calculation of the rigid body motion of the next segment. After having processed all body segments the complete dynamics for the motion of interest is computable if a time integration scheme is applied. Figure 2 shows the results of such a computation for different kinds of landing after a jump. The reaction forces in the hip joint are depicted for a soft landing (with the use of the body damping system) and a very hard landing (with the body kept stiff). The analysis shows that peak force in the hip joint is more than doubled for the hard landing. The forward model has to be validated against experimental data. Here, the measurement of the landing phase for the different types of landing are monitored and subsequently compared with the body reaction forces calculated with the multi-body model. The simulation results are in good accordance with the experimental data. Another example application of MB models in the field of sports is briefly presented in Figure 3. A back flip jump has been investigated with three different analysis tools. The last row shows the results of a forward solution using a multi-body model of the human body. The computed motion almost perfectly matches the real body movement that is captured by a high-speed camera depicted in the second row. The first row shows the typical result of a motion analysis.

3. The finite element method

3.1 A short history

The finite element method (FEM) is a very popular tool in the field of (fluid)-mechanical and electrical engineering to solve partial differential equations (PDEs) on a computer. The first application of the FEM in biomechanics was presented in 1972. FEM was used to build a model of the human femur for orthopaedic applications (Brekelmans et al., 1972). The authors

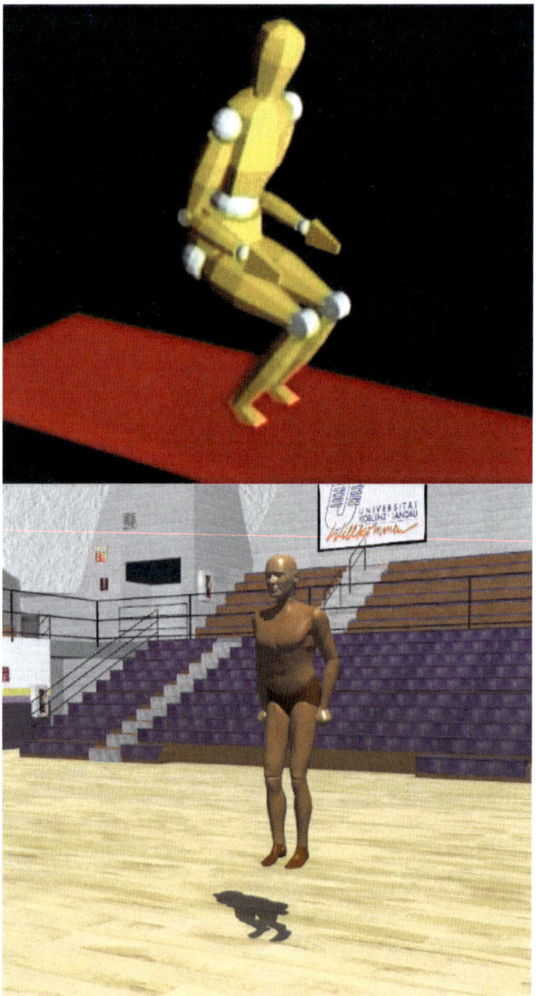

Fig. 1. Multi-body models in different visualisations.

set up a two-dimensional isotropic model with roughly 1000 triangular elements and investigated different loading conditions for the human leg. Due to increasing computer power it soon became possible to realise three-dimensional models enabling an improved representation of the complex anatomy of human body parts. Huiskes and Chao, 1983 gave an overview of the first decade of Finite Element modelling in the field of orthopaedic biomechanics. In the last three decades the number of FE models grew exponentially and the application areas cover a large variety of biomechanical problems. Currently, FE models are widely used in research and industry. The application spectrum ranges from trauma to sports-medical biomechanics. This is not only explained by the rapidly increasing availability of fast computers (today with multi-core processors) but also by the advent of efficient algorithms exploiting the advantages of parallel hardware architectures.

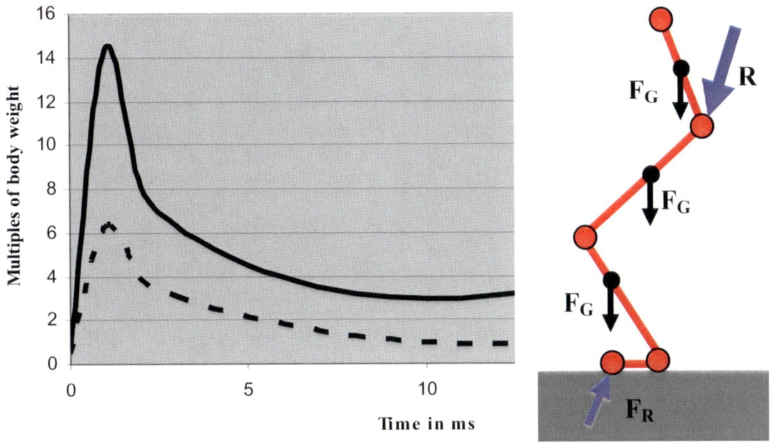

Fig. 2. Link segment model of the human leg and calculated forces in the hip joint for different kinds of landing (dotted line=soft landing, straight line =hard landing).

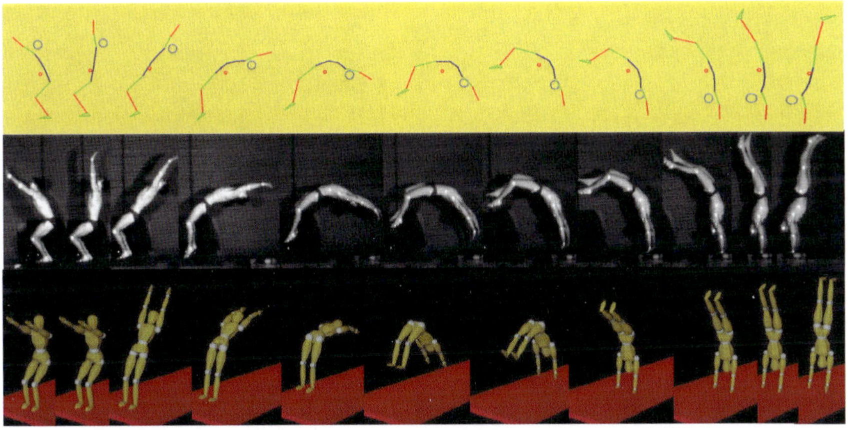

Fig. 3. The analysis of a back flip by motion analysis, high speed video and multi body models.

3.2 The basic concept of the finite element method

The basic idea of FEM is quite simple: let us assume that a physical problem that can be described by a partial differential equation which is defined on a complex geometry (e.g. the human head or knee). Due to the complex geometry an analytical (i.e. a mathematically correct) solution is impossible. Perfect mathematical solutions can only be determined if the system under consideration has a simple geometry (e.g. a sphere or an ellipsoid). At this point FEM enters the stage: the idea is to approximate the complex geometry by a multitude of simple geometric entities (e.g. triangular, tetrahedral or hexahedral elements). Each element is then individually processed. Within an element adequate functions (so-called basis functions) are chosen that are used to interpolate the *unknown* function. The general procedure of FEM is summarised in six steps:

a. Generation of a discrete representation of the object of interest.

The mesh generation step is crucial for the rest of the analysis as the spatial resolution and the element quality to a large extent affect the robustness and the accuracy of the simulation result. In order to achieve high accuracy in a physically interesting region (e.g. the area of large deformation in an impact scenario) a mesh refinement in such regions of special interest is indicated. Mesh refinement means to increase the number of elements and likewise the number of mesh nodes (in the simplest case nodes can be regarded as the corner points of an element). Thus, FE meshes can have millions of mesh nodes. The result of 3D mechanical FE study is the displacement function of the nodes (i.e. the body's deformation) in three dimensions of space.

b. Defining the physical behaviour

In order to set up a realistic model the physical behaviour of the object has to be integrated. At this stage two important decisions have to be made. An appropriate material model (e.g. elastic or viscoelastic behaviour) has to be chosen and the boundary conditions (e.g. fixed or free) have to be selected. The simulation results are very sensitive to these settings. Human soft tissue can be modelled in the simplest case by assuming linear elastic behaviour. Here, two mechanical parameters (Young's modulus and Poisson's ratio) suffice. However, the results provided by such a simple model might not be satisfactory.

c. Setup of the stiffness matrix

For each finite element a stiffness matrix has to be set up. A prerequisite for this step is the choice of adequate interpolation or basis functions within an element. Depending on the number of nodes of the element (e.g. a tetrahedral element can be defined to have four nodes on each of its corners or ten if nodes on the connecting lines are added) the interpolation functions are chosen to be linear or quadratic. Increasing the polynomial order improves the accuracy of the simulation results, but the price to pay is a higher demand in terms of computer resources. The element stiffness matrices are then summed up (taking into account the element connectivity) to form the global stiffness matrix K that represents the complete system. If a transient or dynamic FE analysis is desired a mass matrix M and a damping matrix D have to be assembled to describe the inertial and the damping behaviour of the system respectively.

d. Numerical solution of the problem

After the system matrices M, D and K have been assembled a numerical equation solver is started to calculate the vector of nodal displacements U of the body when an external force defined by a force F is applied. The simplest FE analysis is the computation of the new static equilibrium for a body under load. The equation system to solve is then given by

$$\mathbf{KU} = \mathbf{F}. \tag{3}$$

Sometimes it is of great interest for the developer what the eigenfrequencies ω of an object are and how the corresponding eigenmodes U look like. Then the eigenvalue equation system looks like

$$\mathbf{KU} = \omega^2 \mathbf{MU} \tag{4}$$

In general, only a few of the eigenmodes U are of interest. To solve the above equation system sophisticated software is needed. For a dynamical analysis the velocities and accelerations of the mesh nodes are calculated as well. The integration scheme is then solving the following system of linear equations.

$$\mathbf{M}\ddot{\mathbf{U}}(t) + \mathbf{D}\dot{\mathbf{U}}(t) + \mathbf{K}\mathbf{U}(t) = 0 \tag{5}$$

The purpose of the next chapter is to give a detailed description of the workflow for creating finite element models of human body parts starting with medical image acquisition.

4. FE Applications in biomechanics

4.1 A high resolution model for impact studies

In principle, accurate FE calculations can be carried out on personal computers. However, very complex simulations are candidates for the use of high performance computing. In particular, applications stemming from the field of biomechanics can profit from the use of parallel computers (Hartmann et al., 2001). The complex geometry of anatomical structures often requires a very high spatial resolution of the model leading to possibly huge demand of computer power. In Figure 4 an automatic tool chain to generate *individual* models of human body parts is presented that takes advantage of the application of parallel computers. The software environment has been tested for impact analyses on the human head. It includes the complete chain of tools necessary for the geometric model generation from medical scan data (segmentation, mesh generation and mesh manipulation), computer simulation and visualisation. The software tools are public domain and are available on the web (Berti,2010).

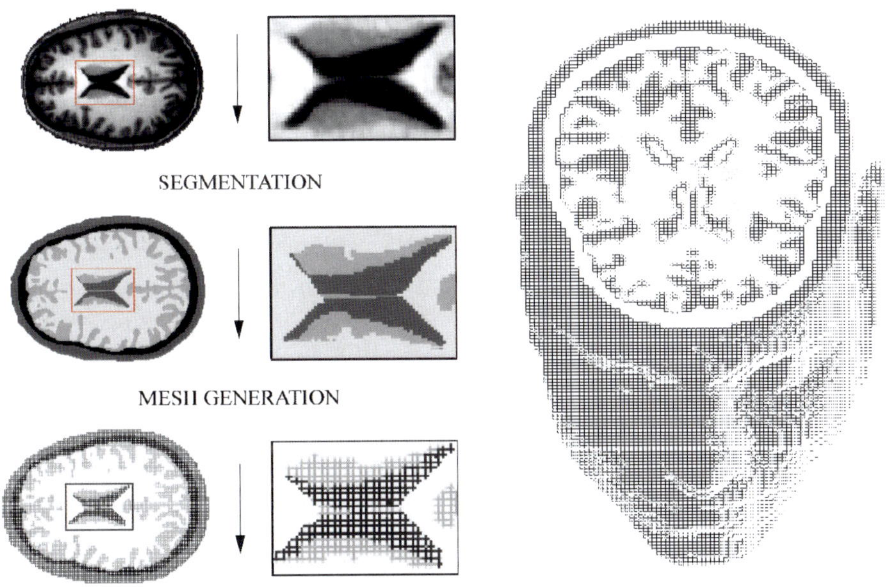

Fig. 4. From medical scan data to finite elements.

The first step is the identification of anatomical structures of interest in a 3D voxel dataset derived from medical scan data (CT or MRI). After this image processing step follows the geometric modelling of the structures identified in the previous step. The important difference to standard engineering problems is the lack of continuum geometry. The starting point is a discrete voxel dataset with a typical resolution of 1 mm or less. The chosen algorithm to generate a discrete representation of the object suitable for FE simulations is based on an octree data structure. It allows the fast generation of very large tetrahedral and hexahedral meshes. The scan data provide information about geometry only. The computer model is not complete without initial and boundary conditions and reliable information about material behaviour. The FE code for solving the underlying PDE is fully parallel and runs on a Linux cluster with distributed memory architecture. This enables the calculation of millions of unknowns.

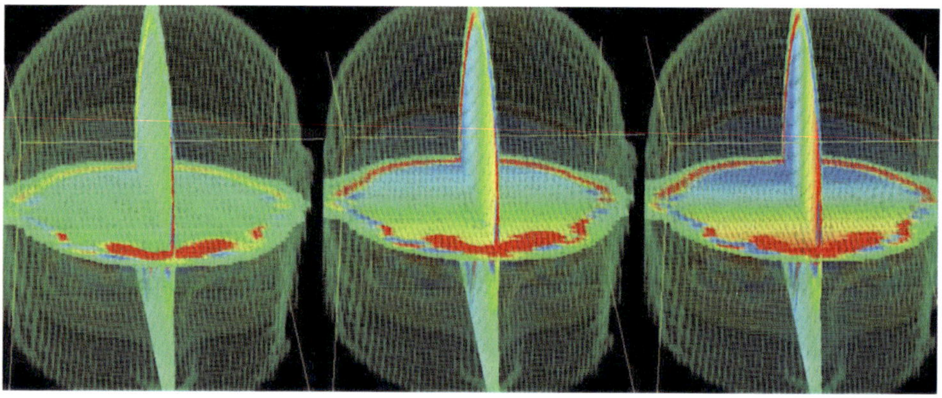

Fig. 5. Evolution of a pressure wave in the brain after frontal impact.

Figure 5 shows an example of a high-resolution impact analysis based on the above described tool chain. This analysis investigated the mechanics of the *coup-contrecoup*, a phenomenon that is well known in neurology. After a heavy (often deadly) impact to the forehead the neurologist observes a brain contusion at the frontal brain and surprisingly enough a second contusion at the occipital brain lobe. The calculation that provides an FE solution for equation (5) shows that there are two distinct regions of pressure developing in the brain. In the frontal region an area of increased pressure is spreading out whilst on the opposite side an area of low pressure is starting to grow. Low and high-pressure zones are related to an increased risk of brain damage. Thus, the simulation confirms the clinical findings. Furthermore, the results have been validated against crash experiments proving the reliability of the FE model (Hartmann & Kruggel, 1998). However, for many applications the use of parallel computers is not necessary. But the pre-processing becomes much more sophisticated because the number of finite elements has to be controlled during the meshing process. Mesh regions of high physical interest have to be refined whereas other mesh areas might show a lower spatial resolution. This explains the demand for commercial meshing and simulation tools. In the following chapter a very complex model of the human knee joint is described. The model is developed on a typical desktop PC making use of commercial software.

4.2 A model for contact analysis in the tibio-femoral joint

4.2.1 Introduction

Due to the complex anatomy and the high loading the knee joint is one of the most frequently injured joints of the human body. In addition to injuries like ruptures of the ligaments caused by accidents, chronic diseases as osteoarthritis affect a high amount of the population. Caused by the estimated demographic progression an increase of total knee joint replacements will be observed in the near future. FE models help to understand the behaviour of the structures of the human knee joint under dynamic loading. The strain on the cartilage and the load distribution effects of the menisci can show how the load is transferred through the different anatomical parts. Another line of application is the investigation of the mechanics of the main ligaments of the knee joint. The anterior and posterior cruciate ligaments (ACL, PCL) and the medial and lateral collateral ligaments (MCL, PCL) play an important role in stabilising the knee joint during daily activities and restrain the joint motion in nearly all degrees of freedom. The understanding of the combined role of the knee joint structures in stabilising and restraining the motion of the joint is fundamental for diagnostic procedures (Blankevoort & Huiskes, 1991). This knowledge can help to develop interventions such as training strategies or surgical procedures for the prevention of a knee joint disease. Also an optimization of orthopaedic devices is possible by the use of FE simulations. Even though many studies have been done, the kinematic and kinetic behaviour of the human knee joint is still not fully understood. Furthermore, the complex injury mechanisms and the development of degenerative joint injuries need additional research. Experimental studies often cannot satisfy this demand due to several limitations like for instance their high costs, the difficult measuring situation and the fact that the experiments can hardly be reproduced. As shown at the beginning of this section accurate FE models have proven to be a good alternative in determining knee joint mechanics. In order to get reliable and accurate results a good segmentation of the anatomical structures is highly important. Other quality influencing parameters are the mesh resolution and the choice of the finite elements. Most of the commercial meshing software products offer the possibility to create surface or volume meshes. The quality of the models has become much better within the last decade because of the high-performance computer chips that enable more complex and detailed models with smaller elements. In order to get an idea of the improvement of FE modelling related to biomechanics of the knee joint we will briefly describe some interesting models developed in the last twenty years.

A three dimensional model of the human knee joint was presented by Blankevoort et al., 1991, to investigate the articular contact of femur and tibia. The paper gave a good mathematical description of the modelling process and the material properties for the different structures. A more detailed model with 798 eight-node solid elements for the cartilage and the menisci, 1212 truss elements for the reinforcing of the solid elements was built to simulate the compression of the knee joint. Only 39 uniaxial elements represented the ligaments (Bendjaballah et al., 1995). Two years later the same authors restructured the model to study the biomechanical influence of varus-valgus (Bendjaballah et al., 1997) followed by an analysis of the tibio-femoral joint in axial rotation (Jilani et al., 1997). These studies are good examples for the advantages of FE models. After a detailed geometry reconstruction and a reliable validation process a lot of biomechanical problems can be explored with only few variations of the same model saving time and money. The availability of commercial software tools and faster multi-core computers lead to an increased number of models and application fields such as prosthesis development (Godest et al., 2002; Soncini et al., 2002).

4.2.2 Image acquisition

The reconstruction process of the individual geometry of the investigated object is based on medical image data obtained by Computed Tomography (CT) or Magnetic Resonance Imaging (MRI). Both methods create two-dimensional images with a predefined slice thickness and slice distance of a specified region. A set of these slices is called image stack and represents a three-dimensional recording of the knee joint. The advantage of using MRI is the possibility to visualise muscles and ligaments in addition to the bony structures whereas CT gives a better representation of the bony structures. It is obvious that the choice of the imaging procedure is depending on the specific research question.

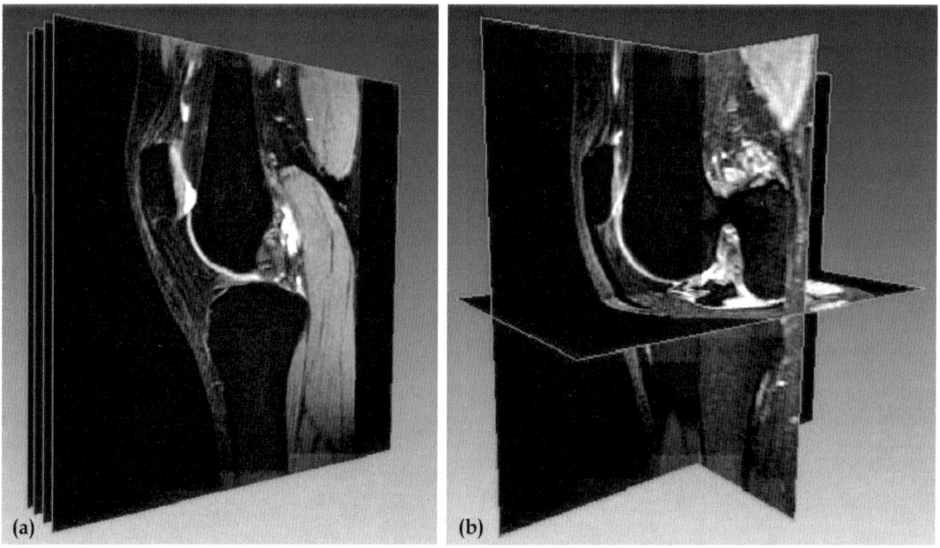

Fig. 6. Image stack of the knee joint from MRI, b) different orientations of the images

In the study presented it is important to have a nearly full representation of the knee joint including the articulating bones (femur, tibia and patella) and also the stabilizing ligaments and the meniscus. The images of a healthy female knee joint are taken in a Philips Gyroscan Intera MRI with a field intensity of 1.0 Tesla.

We use the software Amira (Version 4.0, Mercury Systems) for the data visualisation and segmentation. The program offers the option to apply several image processing tools such as filters for a better differentiation of the structural edges resulting in a more accurate segmentation. In order to get a first and fast overview of the joint geometry a volume rendering depending on the grey values can be done. From a clinical point of view the deviations of the grey values within a structure can show possible pathological changes (for example in the cartilage or the bones).

4.2.3 Segmentation process

The segmentation of the images is done to define anatomical structures in the three-dimensional image stack. This image processing is an important step in the workflow and crucial for the quality of the simulation results. Segmentation can be done with respect to different kinds of concepts; but the output remains the same. A range of grey values characterise the different structures in an image. Different automatic segmentation principles are based on pixel grey values, region or edge detection. These can be used for images in which the anatomical structures show a huge difference in the grey values. For images of the knee joint obtained by MRI a full automatic segmentation is *not* possible due to the fact that the differences of grey values are not high enough. Therefore it is recommended to use a semi-automatic segmentation, which starts with one of the automatic segmentation principles for detection of large connected areas. After this pre- segmentation an interactive improvement of the segmentation by hand leads to a clearly defined differentiation of the structures. A short overview of the numerous automatic methods and the workflow of the process will be shown in the following. The threshold operation is one of the best-known automatic detection procedures. It belongs to the pixel-based procedures, is fast but not very accurate for homogeneous images. It is often used for fast overview segmentations, if no detailed information is necessary. The algorithm compares each pixel grey value with a user-defined threshold; the pixel is assigned to the structure if the pixel value is in the range of the threshold. The application on the whole image is called global thresholding which can often lead to an excluding of pixels that belong to the same structure. Better results can be obtained by using a local thresholding, where the image is separated into different areas with varying thresholds. As mentioned in the beginning it is not sensible enough to detect small changes in an image, but can be applied on regions with nearly the same grey values like the bones.

Another method to identify different regions in an image is based on edge detection. The principle of operation can be compared to the threshold method. Instead of defining a specific value the algorithm checks for grey value changes in an image by comparing two neighbouring pixels. Is there a clear difference of their grey values a part of the edge is detected and two structures are found. The combining of all grey values differences provides a line between the detected parts and all pixels of one region are then merged. In the field of image processing the Sobel-operator, the Laplace-operator or the gradient search are well known filters to find edges in an image. The detected edges have to be combined by special edge tracing algorithms. Like with the threshold method the edge detection algorithm is often not sensitive enough for a satisfying segmentation, so that a manual improvement is applied.

Figure 7 illustrates the mentioned problems occurring with the automatic segmentation algorithms. As a simple example a pure automatic segmentation of the femur is shown on the left (a). It can be seen that it was not possible to define the threshold such that only the bony parts are detected. The expected edge is not straight-lined; in regions with similar grey values protuberances can be found and the inner part is not completely detected. Without a manual correction of the border it is not possible to detect a clear defined region by only defining a threshold.

Therefore different tools are available to mark areas, which are incorrectly detected or omitted. After the whole structure is marked it is added to the specified part.

In this example the automatic detection can be applied to all 100 slices at the same time, but this also increases the number of errors because the grey values of a specified structure differ from image to image in the image stack. For the above-mentioned reasons it is only applicable for the large bony structures. The soft tissues like the meniscus or the ligaments cannot be detected automatically. The homogeneous grey value parts of the soft tissue in the middle of the knee joint and the partly thin cartilage are completely manually segmented with a live wire procedure. In total 11 structures in the 100 slices are segmented. This is needed in the following meshing procedure and for the subsequent calculations of the FE solver. An example of one segmented slice is shown in Figure 8.

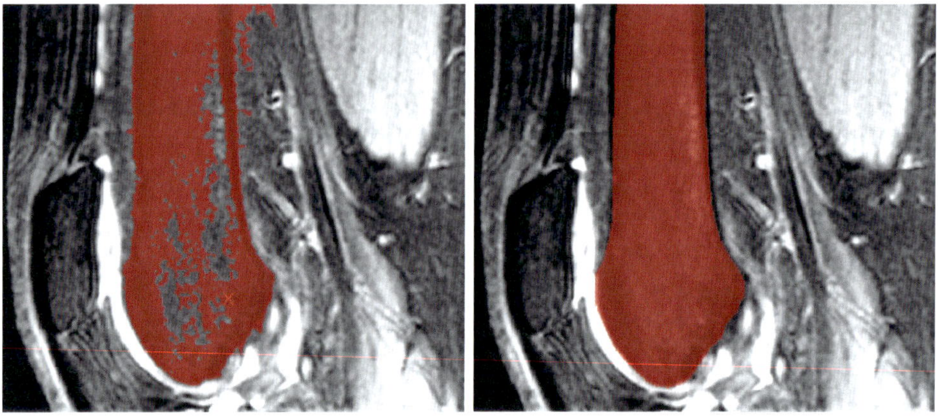

Fig. 7. a) Automatic segmentation of the femur with protuberances, b) segmented femur after improvement

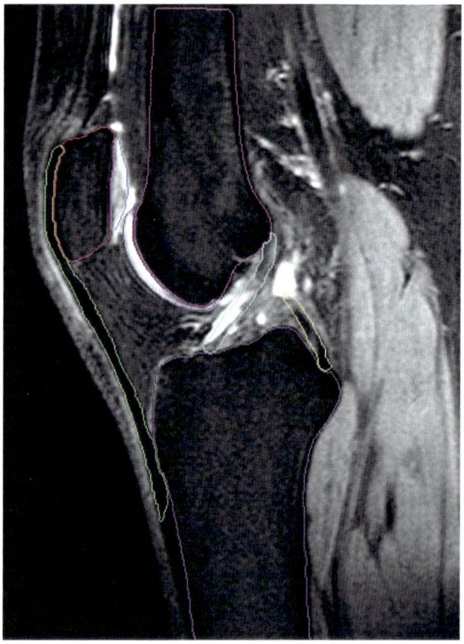

Fig. 8. Fully segmented slice of the knee joint.

Due to the image acquisition procedure a specified slice thickness and distance is given causing errors in the reconstruction process. The gap between each slice does not provide any information about the shape of the anatomic structures. This leads to stairs in the 3D reconstruction in areas where the alteration of the structures is smaller then the slice distance. It is obvious that these stairs adulterate not only the design but also the simulation results. Therefore it is mandatory to make the stairs as small as possible by interpolating the segmented structures and smoothing the surface, before the meshing begins.

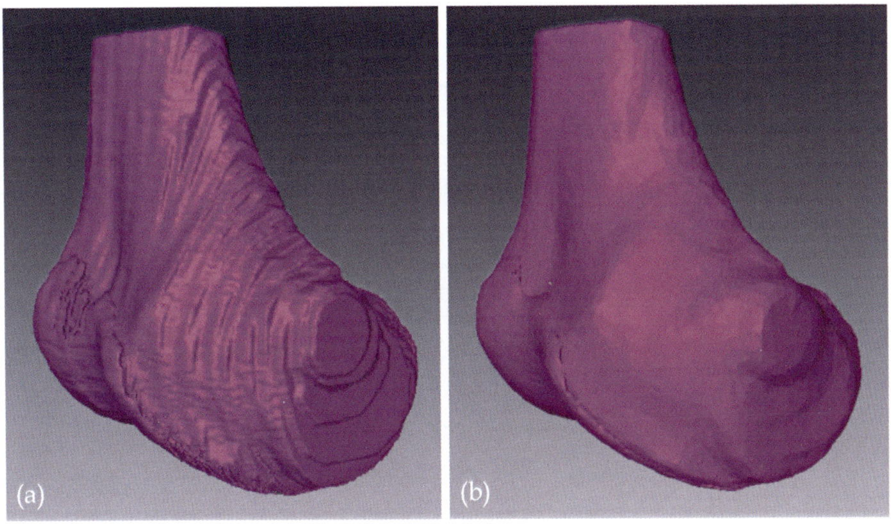

Fig. 9. a) Reconstructed femur with existing stairs due to the slice distance, b) surface of the femur after the interpolation and smoothing process

In the interpolation process imaginary points, calculated with the existing points of the segmentation are included between two slices thus minimising the effect of the stairs. This can either be done by a linear or a cubic interpolation. Following the interpolation step the surface is reconstructed from the segmented structures. This is a pre-processing step before the real meshing procedure where the surface will be divided into the small tetrahedral elements. Directly after the meshing process a smoothing filter is applied. A comparison between the femur condyles after the surface generation with existing stairs and after the interpolation and smoothing is shown in Figure 9.

4.2.4 Meshing of the segmented images

The reconstructed three-dimensional surface of the anatomic structures is transformed into a surface mesh consisting of triangles using a Marching Cube algorithm before an Advancing Front algorithm constructs the volume mesh. For the surface triangulation Amira uses a modified type of the Marching Cube algorithm developed by Lorensen and Cline [20]. The algorithm assumes a lattice model of a volumetric dataset with a specific value at each intercept point of the lattice. The space is subdivided into a constant grid consisting of cubes, where each cube has eight pixels and eight grey values from two successive slices. Four pixels belong to a slice. In the case that the vertices of a cube's edge are lying on different sides of the isosurface, it is given that this edge is cut by the surface. The detected intersection points of the cube and the isosurface are combined so that a polygon and a triangle are created. Theoretically there are 256 different possible combinations given how the cut goes through the surface. Due to symmetries these can be reduced to 14 classes. The summary of all polygons leads to the 3D reconstruction of the surface. This surface is used to create a volumetric mesh using the above-mentioned Advancing Front algorithm. With this it is possible to create elements and nodes at the same time. The edge is set by nodes, which are divided into connections lines. The length of such a line is depending on the specified size of the elements and results in a closed polygon, the "advancing front". Along this front the elements are created, which should go into the inner part of the area to be meshed. An update of this front includes only the connection lines, which are needed for subsequent construction of the mesh. This method is properly suited for complex geometries with inner edges because the boundary of the area is done first. Both algorithms are often used in commercial meshing software and described in detail by Nigel et al., 1999.

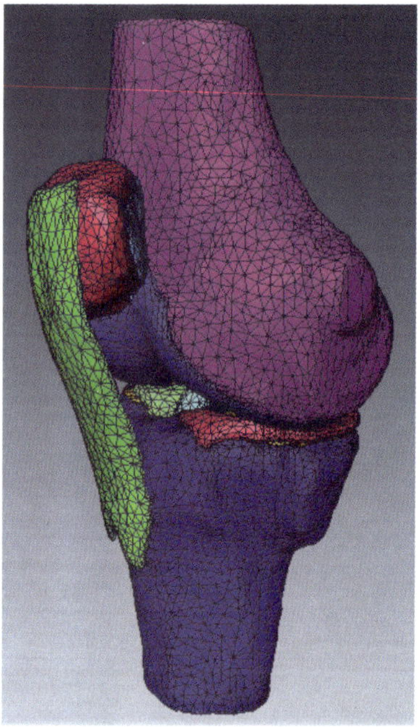

Fig. 10. Mesh of the human knee joint consisting of tetrahedral elements.

Before starting the surface generation the minimal edge length of the triangles and the choice for a first smoothing of the surface have to be set. The result is a closed surface mesh with rather small elements, which leads to a high amount of nodes and elements. The more elements exist, the better is the reconstruction of the surface but also the computation times increases extremely. Therefore it is recommended to reduce the amount of elements using the simplification editor. The positions of the elements are recalculated, so that the same surface is constructed using fewer elements. The meshing procedure is highly important for the whole FE analysis as the quality of the mesh influences the robustness and the accuracy of the results. It is obvious that a compromise between size and amount of elements and the computation time has to be found. After the simplification step the mesh is smoothed to eliminate the mentioned stairs in case they still exist. During this second smoothing the edge points of the elements are moved. For the calculation of the new position, the middle point of the neighbour elements is determined, and the point to be moved is shifted into the new direction. This is done for all elements, which do not have a uniform changeover from one element to another. Is the form of the mesh satisfying and close to the original structures, its quality has to be determined through several tests. If the mesh quality is not satisfactory, an additional smoothing can be helpful. Checking the dihedral angle, the orientation and the aspect ratio of the elements provides a good measure of the mesh quality. These tests should be done consecutively, as well as the intersection and closeness test. If a problem or a bad triangle is found, the element is highlighted and can be improved using the editor by shifting, subdividing or drawing. If no problems are present the generation of the volume mesh can be started. Based on the surface the mesh of the inner volume is constructed. The described tests for the surface should also be done for the volume mesh. For special regions of interest, e.g. the meniscus or the articulating surfaces of femur and tibia, a refinement of the mesh is taken into account. The existing elements are bisected, so that a finer and smoother structure is achieved. This increases not only the number of nodes and elements but also the quality of the results of the simulation. The complete mesh of the 3D reconstruction of the human knee joint is shown in Figure 10.

4.2.5 Implementation of the model

Madymo (Mathematic dynamic modelling, Version 6.3, Tass–safe, Netherlands) is used for the FE analyses based on the meshes depicted in Figure 10. Madymo enables a combination of a multi-body and finite element parts. Models are built in a kinematic chain where the rigid multi-body elements are connected by joints. The mesh obtained by Amira is attached to those bodies thus ensuring that a prescribed joint motion results in a movement of the bones. The several steps of the implementation in Madymo are described in the following.

After having chosen a reference frame three bodies are defined; one for the femur, one for the tibia and one for the patella. To each of these bodies, the elements and nodes belonging to the specified bony structure are assigned. The described x, y and z coordinates of the nodes, the part numbers and the elements for each part, which were exported from Amira, are imported in two different tables. The part numbers are crucial for the assignment to the bodies and for the differentiation of the material properties. Free joints, which have three translational and three rotational degrees of freedom are used for the connection of the bodies. To guarantee a realistic kinematic and kinetic behaviour of the model, the physical properties like the moment of inertia and the mass with its centre are essential. The determination of these parameters is a complex physical procedure and individual for each subject. For this reasons it is common to take values from literature, which were gained, in cross-sectional studies. The inertial characteristics of several human segments can be found in Zatsiorsky, 2002.

The material properties are important for a realistic model and essential for the stress calculation. In the material sciences there are different typical laws known to describe a material's behaviour with mathematical formulae. Such mathematical material models are also used in finite element simulations to compute the resulting stress from the displacement field of the nodes. The properties of a biological material are always an approximation because they vary due to different influencing factors like age or training. For this reason simplifications in expressing the material laws are often made. The isotropic elastic material is one of the easiest to describe because only two parameters are needed. Elastic means that a force-loaded material returns completely to its initial shape after it is unloaded. Isotropic indicates, the loading direction is of no matter, so there is no distinct direction. The describing parameters for an isotropic elastic material are Young's modulus **E** (in Mega Pascal, MPa) and the Poisson ratio **ν** (without a unit). When expecting small strains, it is common to use these two parameters for the material description because of the low computation costs. Other biomechanical models use a hyperelastic material law for the description, due to the fact, that the results obtained by a linearised model are not applicable for finite strain calculations.

The response of biological soft tissues of the human body is often time or load dependent. This means, that these viscoelastic materials show creep or relaxation effects. Applying a constant force to a material produces a lengthening. Creeping is given if a material shows an enlarging displacement in addition to the normal response to the outer force. Relaxation of a material stands for the reduction of the inner stresses if a constant force is applied. For the human knee joint the different material responses mentioned above are used to specify the biological tissues. All properties are taken from the literature. The femur, the tibia and the patella are assumed to be rigid with a density of 1000 kg/m^3. For the cartilage of the bones viscoelastic behaviour was neglected due to a short loading time. Therefore the assumption of a linear elastic and isotropic material was made and a Young's modulus of $E = 5$ MPa and a Poisson ratio of $\nu = 0.46$ were chosen (Li et al., 2001). The menisci are hydrated tissues. They are modelled as linear elastic for the same reason that holds true for the cartilage but with a much higher Young's modulus of $E = 59$ MPa and a Poisson ratio of $\nu = 0.49$ (LeRoux & Setton, 2002). The ligament properties are defined by a stress strain function (Lee & Hyman, 2002).

The articulating surfaces of the human knee joint show a complex geometry with curved shapes in all directions. Due to this fact it is important to have a look on the contact modelling that will influence the computed strains. During a movement of the femur, the menisci and the cartilage parts of the bones are in contact with each other. Therefore a contact definition for each contact pair is defined, the result of a contact between two surfaces is a deformation of at least one of these. Also a self-contact of one structure is possible. Three algorithms are well known for the description of a finite element contact: Node-to surface, point-to surface and surface-to surface.

In the node-to surface contact the nodes of structure 1 are in contact to the surface of the elements of structure 2. The time consuming tracking of contacts between nodes and the surface is simplified with special search strategies. For a three-node element, all nodes can have contact to the elements of the penetrated surface. If elements have an additional point in the middle of the element, the point-to-surface method should be used, which also looks for other points that can apply forces due to penetration. The surface-to-surface method is mainly used for the contact between rigid bodies with a special penetration characteristic and for heavily curved shapes.

The first step is to make a decision, which part is *Master* and which one is *Slave*. For the case that the mesh has different element sizes due to a refinement of a structure, the finer mesh should be chosen as *Slave*. Is this not the case the surface with the more curved shape should be the *Slave*. In this model, the surface-to-surface method is chosen, because of the curved

shapes of the femur and the menisci. The gap can either be set as a function or is defined by program. The contact edge search algorithm can find additional contacts, which could be lost in presence of the curved shapes. The penalty method is used for the calculation of contact forces, with a damping coefficient of 0.05 and a variable FE time step, given that the contact force is dependent on the time step, to keep the simulation stable.
For the kinematic boundary conditions a simple knee bending is used for the prescribed motion, which is obtained in a three-dimensional movement analysis using retro reflective markers and infrared cameras (Vicon Nexus, Vicon Motion System, Oxford, UK). The calculated joint angles in three directions are given as an angle vs. time function. The kinetic boundary conditions are applied by a gravity function which includes the mass of the investigated subject.

4.2.6 First results

The goal of the simulation is the calculation of the contact forces and stresses in three directions as well as the resultants. A distribution of the forces and stresses acting on the articulating surfaces is shown with a specified colour bar referring to the calculated values. The results provide a better understanding of the transduction of applied outer forces in the inner structures of the human knee joint. In addition different scenarios like meniscal tears or ligament ruptures can easily be simulated and the biomechanical effects on the joint investigated. The influence of joint alignment like a varus or valgus condition is of great interest in these simulations. In Figure 11 the results of the knee bending simulation under body weight condition are shown. The menisci and the cruciate ligaments are removed for a better illustration of the forces on the articulating cartilage. The distribution shows a peak in the direct contact area and a decrease from the middle to the border.

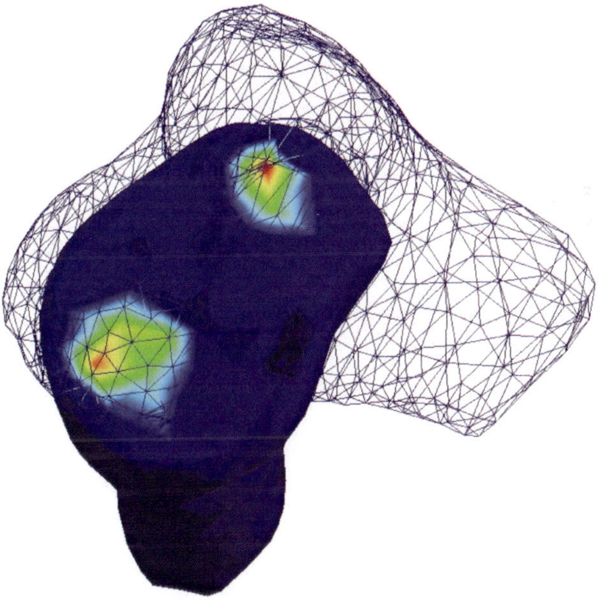

Fig. 11. Calculated contact forces of the simulation of a knee bending.

Having the option to prescribe motion enables the determination of the influence on the motion of the inner structures, like shifting of the menisci or the stretching of the ligaments. Using simulated muscle forces as input for the simulation the resulting locomotion and the acting forces on the articulating surfaces can be studied.

5. Conclusion

The increasing availability of computational resources will lead to more detailed and complex models of the human body. In the future, efforts like the Virtual Physiological Human (Coveney, 2010) will provide a framework for developing and coupling biomechanical and bioelectric models of different scales and body parts. The term Virtual Physiological Human (VPH) indicates a shared resource formed by a federation of disparate but integrated computer models of the mechanical, physical, and biochemical functions of living human body in both physiological and pathological conditions. VPH models will be both descriptive and predictive. They comprise

- large collections of anatomical, physiological, and pathological data stored in digital format,
- predictive simulations developed from these collections,
- services aimed to support the researchers in the creation and maintenance of these models and
- services aimed to empower clinical, industrial and societal users in the use of the VPH resource.

The Virtual Physiological Human is a methodological and technological framework that once established, will enable collaborative investigation of the human body as a single complex system. VPH is not 'the supermodel' that will explain all possible aspects of human physiology or pathology. It is away to share observations, to derive predictive hypotheses from them, and to integrate them into a constantly improving understanding of human physiology/pathology, by regarding it as an integrated system.

6. Acknowledgements

The authors would like to thank Prof. Dr. Karin Gruber (University of Koblenz, Germany) for providing valuable input related to MB models and motion analysis. Many thanks go as well to J. Seybold (University of Stuttgart) for making available his computer studies on the reaction forces for soft and hard landing. Special thanks go to Dr. Torsten Hans (University of Tübingen, Germany) for the visualisation of the jumping gymnast.

7. References

Bendjaballah, M., Shirazi-Adl, A. & Zukor, D. (1995) Biomechanics of the human knee joint in comparison reconstruction, mesh generation and finite element analysis. *The Knee* 2 , pp. 69-79

Bendjaballah, M., Shirazi-Adl, A. & Zukor, D. (1997). Finite element analysis of human knee joint in varus-valgus, *Clinical Biomechanics* 12 (3), pp. 139-148

Berti, G. (Nov 2010). Open Source Software for Medical Simulation, 04/12/2011, Available from http://www.rheinahrcampus.de/~hartmann/

Blajer, W. & Czaplicki, A. (2001). Modelling and inverse simulation of somersaults on the trampoline. *Journal of Biomechanics* 34, pp. 1619-1629

Blankevoort, L. & Huiskes, R. (1991). Ligament-bone interaction in a three-dimensional model of the knee. *Journal of Biomechanical Engineering* 113 (3), pp. 263-269

Blankevoort, L., Kuiper, J. H., Huiskes, R. & Grootenboer, H. J. (1991) Articular contact in a three-dimensional model of the knee. *Journal of Biomechanics* 24 (11), pp. 1019-1031

Brekelmans, W., Poort, H. & Slooff, T. (1972). A new method to analyse the mechanical behaviour of skeletal parts. *Acta orthopaedica Scandinavica*, 43(5), pp. 301-317

Coveney P. (2010) Virtual Physiological Human Network of Excellence, 04/09/2011, Available from http://www.vph-noe.eu/

Dabnichki, P. & Avital, E. (2006). Influence of the position of crewmembers on aerodynamics performance of two-man bobsleigh. *Journal of Biomechanics* 39(15) , pp. 2733-2742

Godest, A., Beaugonin, M., Haug, E., Taylor, M., & Gregson, P. (2002). Simulation of a knee joint replacement during a gait cycle using explicit finite element analysis. *Journal of Biomechanics* 35 (2), 267-275

Gruber, K., Ruder, H., Denoth, J. & Schneider, K. (1998). A comparative study of impact dynamics: wobbling mass model versus rigid body models. *Journal of Biomechanics* 31, pp. 439-444

Hartmann, U. & Kruggel, F. (1998). Transient Analysis of the Biomechanics of the Human Head with a High-Resolution 3D Finite Element Model. *Computer Methods in Biomechanics and Biomedical Engineering* 2(1), pp. 49-64

Hartmann, U., Kruggel, F., Hierl, T., Lonsdale, G. & Kloeppel, R. (2001) Skull mechanics simulations with the prototype SimBio environment. *In: Proceedings of the M.I.T. Conference on Computational Solid and Fluid Mechanics* Boston May 2001

Huiskes, R. & Chao, E. (1983). A survey of finite element analysis in orthopaedic biomechanics: the first decade. *Journal of Biomechanics* 16 (6), pp. 385-409

Jilani, A., Shirazi-Adl, A. & Bendjaballah, M. (1997). Biomechanics of human tibio-femoral joint in axial rotation. *The Knee* 4, pp. 203-213

Lee, M., & Hyman, W. (2002). Modeling of failure mode in knee ligaments depending on the strain rate. *BMC musculoskeletal disorders* 3, 3, pp.

LeRoux, M. A., Setton. L. A. (2002). Experimental and biphasic FEM determinations of the material properties and hydraulic perme- ability of the meniscus in tension. *ASME Journal of Biomechanical Engineering* 124, pp. 315-321

Li, G., Lopez, O., Rubash, H. (2001). Variability of a three-dimensional finite element model constructed using magnetic resonance images of a knee for joint contact stress analysis. *ASME Journal of Biomechanical Engineering* 123, pp. 341-346

Lorensen, W. & Cline, H. (1987) Marching Cubes: A high resolution 3D surface reconstruction algorithm. *Computer Graphics*, 21 (4), pp 163-169

Penrose, J.M.T. & Hose, D.R. (1998). Finite Element Impact Analysis of a Flexible Cricket Bat for Design Optimisation. In: The Engineering of Sport - Design and Development, S. Haake (ed.), pp. 531-539, Blackwell Science Ltd.

Soncini, M., Redaelli, A., & Montevecchi, F., (2002). FE Dynamic Analysis Of A Knee Joint Prosthesis During The Walking Cycle. *Proceeding of 2003 Summer Bioengineering Conference*, Key Biscayne, Florida, June 2003

Wangerin, M., Schmitt, S., Stapelfeldt, B. & Gollhofer, A. (2007). Inverse Dynamics in Cycling Performance, Proceedings in Physics: Advances in Medical Engineering, Springer-Verlag: Berlin and New York, Remagen, September 2007

Weatherill N.P., Soni, B.K. & Thompson, J.F. (1999). *Handbook of grid generation*, CRC press, 978-0-8493-2687-5

Wojtyra, M. (2003). Multibody Simulation Model of Human Walking, *Mechanics Based Design of Structures and Machines*, 31(2), pp. 357-379,

Zatsiorsky, V. M. (2002). *Kinetics of Human Motion* . Human Kinetics, USA, 978-0-7360-3778-5

5

Biomechanics and Modeling of Skeletal Soft Tissues

Rami K. Korhonen[1] and Simo Saarakkala[2,3]
[1]*Department of Applied Physics, University of Eastern Finland, Kuopio*
[2]*Department of Medical Technology, University of Oulu, Oulu*
[3]*Department of Diagnostic Radiology*
University of Oulu and Oulu University Hospital, Oulu
Finland

1. Introduction

1.1 Articular cartilage

Articular cartilage is a specialized connective tissue that covers the ends of the bones in the diarthrodial joints. The thickness of human articular cartilage is typically between 1-6 mm. The main functions of articular cartilage are to dissipate and distribute contact stresses during joint loading, and to provide almost frictionless articulation in diarthrodial joints. In order to accomplish these demanding tasks, articular cartilage has unique mechanical properties. The tissue is a biphasic material with an anisotropic and nonlinear mechanical behaviour.

Articular cartilage is composed of two distinct phases. Fluid phase of the cartilage tissue consists of interstitial water and mobile ions. The water phase constitutes 68-85 % of the cartilage total weight and is an important determinant of the biomechanical properties of the tissue. Solid phase (or solid matrix) of the cartilage tissue consists mainly of collagen fibrils and negatively charged proteoglycans. The cell density is relatively small - in human adult tissue only ~2% of the total cartilage volume is occupied by the chondrocytes. Collagen molecules constitute 60-80% of the cartilage dry weight or approximately 10-20% of the wet weight. The collagen molecules assemble to form small fibrils and larger fibers that vary in organization and dimensions as a function of cartilage depth. The diameter of collagen fibers is approximately 20 nm in the superficial zone and 70-120 nm in the deep zone, and it varies between different collagen types. The collagen fibrils of the cartilage tissue consist mainly of type II collagen, although small amounts of other collagen types can be also found in cartilage, e.g. collagen type VI is common form in the vicinity of cells (pericellular matrix). In addition to the collagen fibrils, proteoglycan macromolecules constitute 20-40% of the cartilage dry weight or approximately 5-10% of the wet weight. The proteoglycan aggrecan is composed of a protein core and numerous glycosaminoglycan (GAG) chains attached to the core. Many aggrecan molecules are further bound to a single hyaluronan chain to form a proteoglycan aggregate.

The basic structure of the articular cartilage can be divided into four zones based on the arrangement of collagen fibril network (Benninghoff, 1925): 1) *Superficial zone*: here the chondrocytes are flattened and aligned parallel to the cartilage surface. The collagen fibrils are relatively thin and run parallel to each other. The proteoglycan content is at its lowest and the water content is at its highest. 2) *Middle zone*: here the collagen fibrils have a larger diameter and they are oriented randomly. The cell density and water content is lower and proteoglycan content is higher than in the superficial zone. 3) *Deep zone*: here the diameter of the collagen fibrils is at its largest, and the collagen fibrils are oriented perpendicular to the articular surface. The cell density and water content are at their lowest, the proteoglycan content at its highest but the collagen content is variable. 4) *Calcified cartilage*: this thin layer is located between the deep zone and the subchondral bone and it joins the cartilage tissue to the subchondral bone. Here the chondrocytes usually express a hypertrophic phenotype.

It is nowadays widely accepted that collagen fibrils are primarily responsible for the cartilage tensile stiffness and the dynamic compressive stiffness. In contrast, proteoglycans are primarily responsible for the equilibrium properties during compression, and fluid contributes to the dynamic and time-dependent properties of the tissue. For more comprehensive description of structure-function relationships of cartilage, the reader may consult *e.g.* the book by Mow et al. (2005).

1.2 Meniscus

Meniscus is a wedge-shaped fibrocartilaginous structure between femoral and tibial articular cartilage surfaces inside the knee joint capsule. The function of the meniscus is to bear and dissipate loads, provide stability to the knee joint, and protect articular cartilage from excessive loads by functioning as a shock absorber. Similarly as in articular cartilage, meniscus has complex mechanical properties in order to accomplish these tasks.

Meniscus has also biphasic composition. Such as in cartilage, fluid phase of the meniscus consists of interstitial water and mobile ions. The water phase constitutes 60-70% of the meniscus total weight and is similarly important determinant of the biomechanical properties of the tissue. Solid phase of the meniscus consists of highly organized collagen fibril network, negatively charged proteoglycans and meniscal cells (fibrochondrocytes). Collagen molecules constitute 15-25 % of the meniscus wet weight. In contrast with articular cartilage, the collagen fibrils of meniscus consist mainly of type I collagen, *i.e.* also found in skin and bone tissues, although smaller amounts of types II, III, V, and VI can be also found in meniscus (McDevitt&Webber, 1990). Furthermore, meniscus contains significantly less proteoglycan than articular cartilage, only 1-2% of the wet weight.

The basic structure of meniscus can be divided into different layers based on the arrangement of the collagen fibril network. Since the meniscus is located between femoral and tibial articular surfaces, it has two surface layers both in top and bottom. Below surface layers are intermediate layers and in the center of the meniscus is the central layer. At the femoral surface layer the collagen fibrils are relatively thick and run parallel to each other and the femoral surface. In contrast, at the tibial surface layer the collagen fibrils are oriented randomly. At inner layers, the arrangement of collagen fibrils is more variable. The central layer can be further divided into four zones in the axial plane: anterior and posterior parts of the central layer exhibit relatively parallelly organized collagen fibrils, middle part of the central layer exhibits irregular organization medially, wheras organization changes more regular and circular-shaped at the lateral side. For a more comprehensive and graphical description of structure and organization of collagen fibril network in the different layers of meniscus, the reader is recommended to consult the study of human meniscus structure by Cui&Min (2007).

Similarly as in cartilage, the collagen fibrils are mainly responsible for the tensile properties of meniscus and proteoglycans contribute strongly to the equilibrium response. Fluid has a significant role in carrying impact and dynamic loads. For more information of the general anatomical and functional properties of the meniscus, the reader may consult *e.g.* the review by Messner&Gao (1998).

1.3 Ligaments and tendons

Ligaments and tendons are soft tissues connecting bones to bones or bones to muscles, respectively. Their primary functions are to stabilize joints and transmit the loads, hold the joints together, guide the trajectory of bones, and control the joint motion area. Ligaments and tendons are also biphasic tissues having fluid and solid phases similarly as in articular cartilage and meniscus. Therefore, they also possess highly viscoelastic mechanical properties.

The fluid phase constitutes 60-70% of the total weight of ligaments and tendons. Solid phase consists of highly organized longitudinal collagen fibril network (over 15 % of the wet weight), elastin network, and proteoglycans. Similarly than in meniscus, the collagen fibrils of ligaments and tendons consist mainly of type I collagen. Since ligaments and tendons have so tightly packed and organized long collagen fibril network they have extremely high tensile strength and nonlinear stress-strain behavior.

For more information of the anatomical and functional properties of the ligaments and tendons, the reader may consult *e.g.* the book chapter by Woo et al. (2005).

	Collagen (wet weight)	**Proteoglycan (wet weight)**	**Fluid (wet weight)**	**Young's modulus**
Articular cartilage	10-20% (type II)	5-10%	68-85%	~0.5 MPa (compression)
Meniscus	15-25% (type I)	1-2%	60-70%	~0.1 MPa (compression)
Ligament	20-30% (type I)	less than in cartilage	60-70%	>100 MPa (tension)
Tendon	more than in ligament (type I)	less than in ligament	60-70%	>1000 MPa (tension)

Table 1. Main compositional parameters and elastic properties of articular cartilage, meniscus, ligaments and tendons.

2. Experimental mechanical characterization of skeletal soft tissues

2.1 Introduction

When skeletal soft tissues are mechanically tested, one can apply either force or deformation to it and then follow the other parameter. For example, constant or changing force may be applied to a tissue and consequent change in the deformation is followed. Similarly, the change in force can be followed when constant or changing deformation is applied. Important parameter to describe the behavior of tissues under loading is strain (ε), defined as follows:

$$\epsilon = \frac{\Delta l}{l_0} \tag{2.1}$$

where Δl is the change in thickness/length of a tissue sample, and l_0 is the original thickness/length. The normalization with the original thickness/length ensures that the deformation is comparable between tissue samples with different thickness or length. It is important to note that, according to the definition, the strain is a unitless quantity.
Second important parameter in biomechanical testing is stress (σ), which is defined as:

$$\sigma = \frac{F}{A_0} \tag{2.2}$$

where F is the force applied to tissue, and A_0 is the original cross-sectional area in which the force is acting. Again here, the normalization with the cross-sectional area ensures that the load is comparable between different cross-sectional areas. The unit of stress is Pa, and the definition of stress is fundamentally the same as for pressure.
When both stress (σ) and strain (ε) are defined as above, mechanical behavior/properties of different skeletal soft tissues can be compared regardless of the size and shape of the samples. If the relation between stress and strain is assumed linear, one obtains the Hooke's linear model for solids from which the stiffness (elastic modulus) of the tissue can be calculated (see section 3.2).
When the compressive or tensile stress is applied to, say, excised soft tissue sample, consequent strain occurs in the direction of the loading. However, when the strain occurs in one direction in a three-dimensional soft tissue sample, there is always corresponding strain in the perpendicular direction. For example, when a soft tissue sample is stretched in one direction it typically simultaneously compresses in perpendicular direction changing its shape. The change of shape is the third important parameter in biomechanical testing. It is quantified with the parameter called the Poisson's ratio (ν), defined as follows:

$$\nu = -\frac{\varepsilon_{lat}}{\varepsilon} \tag{2.3}$$

where ε is the strain in loading direction and ε_{lat} is the corresponding strain in horizontal direction. The Poisson's ratio is the intrinsic parameter of a tissue, and it is unique for different materials. For example, an isotropic elastic material, e.g. rubber, has the Poisson's ratio of 0.5 in compression which means that the volume of the material does not change during mechanical loading. Since the major component of all human soft tissues is interstitial water, mechanical loading causes water to flow out of the tissue. Finally, after the complete relaxation, i.e. in equilibrium state, no fluid flow or pressure gradients exist in a tissue and, consequently, the entire stress is carried by the solid matrix. Because of this time-dependent viscoelastic nature, all human soft tissues have typically lower Poisson's ratios in compression than elastic materials, being in the range of 0.0 - 0.4 in

compression (Jurvelin et al., 1997; Korhonen et al., 2002a; Sweigart et al., 2004). On the other hand, Poisson's ratios in tension, shown for anisotropic materials, can be even more than 1 (Hewitt et al., 2001; Elliott et al., 2002).
It is also possible to apply load or deformation to a soft tissue sample parallel to the surface. This requires fixed contact between the tester and the surface of the sample. Then, so called shear strain (γ) is defined as follows:

$$\gamma = \frac{\Delta l_{shear}}{l_0} \tag{2.4}$$

where Δl_{shear} is the deformation of a surface point parallel to the surface, and l_0 is the sample thickness (perpendicular to the surface). Similarly, shear stress (τ) is defined as follows:

$$\tau = \frac{F_{shear}}{A_0} \tag{2.5}$$

where F_{shear} is the force applied parallel to the surface, and A_0 is the cross-sectional area of the contact between the tester and the surface of the sample.

2.2 Mechanical testing geometries

Mechanical testing geometries for soft tissues can be divided into compression, tension, bending and torsion. We will now consider only compression and tension since they are the most relevant geometries for skeletal soft tissues.
Compression testing is widely used especially for determination of mechanical properties of articular cartilage and meniscus. This is a relevant choice since also in vivo, e.g. during normal walking cycle, articular cartilage and meniscus experiences external compressive forces. When the tissue is mechanically tested in compression, three different measurement configurations can be used: unconfined compression, confined compression and indentation. In unconfined compression, a soft tissue sample is compressed between two smooth metallic plates to a predefined stress or strain. This geometry allows interstitial fluid flow out of the tissue only in the lateral direction (Fig. 1). In confined compression, a soft tissue sample is placed in a sealed chamber and, subsequently, compressed with a porous filter (Fig. 1). In this geometry the interstitial fluid can only flow axially through the tissue surface into the filter. In indentation geometry, a soft tissue is compressed with a cylindrical, typically plane-ended or spherical-ended indenter (Fig. 1). In this geometry, fluid flow outside the indenter-tissue contact point is possible in both the lateral and axial directions. It should be emphasized that the indentation is the only compressive geometry which is not limited into the laboratory use. Since indentation testing does not require a preparation of separate tissue samples it can be also performed in vivo. For example, stiffness of femoral articular cartilage has been measured during arthroscopy in vivo (Vasara et al., 2005).
Tensile testing is widely used especially for determination of mechanical properties of ligaments and tendons, while it is less used for the characterization of cartilage and meniscus properties. Again, this is a relevant choice for these tissues since they exhibit mainly tensile stresses in vivo. In tensile testing, a soft tissue sample is fixed with two ends, e.g. by using metallic clamps, and the sample is then streched to a predefined stress or strain.

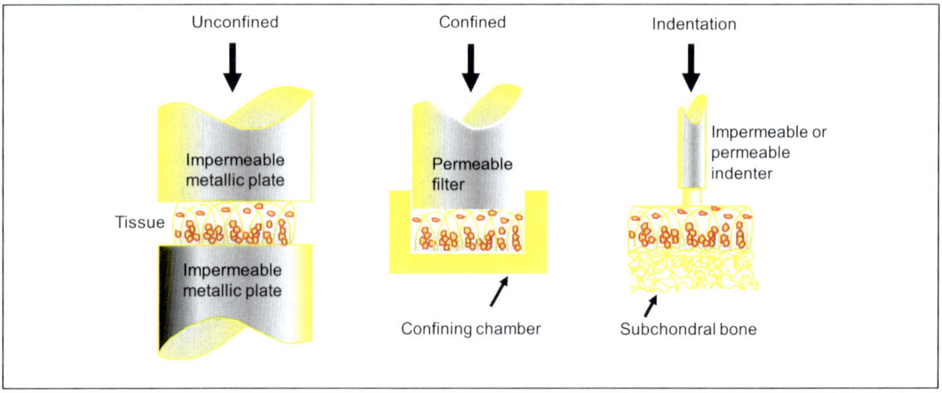

Fig. 1. Unconfined, confined and indentation loading geometries for testing of mechanical properties of articular cartilage.

2.3 Destructive and nondestructive testing protocols

In all experimental mechanical testing geometries it is possible to conduct both destructive and non-destructive testing. In non-destructive protocol tissue is tested with small strains or loads and all the changes induced to the tissue are reversible. In contrast, destructive protocol involves larger strains or loads inducing non-reversible changes to a tissue.

Most common non-destructive testing protocols are called creep and stress-relaxation. These tests can be conducted both in compression and tension geometries. In creep test, constant compressive or tensile stress is applied to a tissue and corresponding strain is followed as a function of time (Fig. 2). In stress-relaxation test, predefined compressive or tensile strain is applied and corresponding stress is followed as a function of time (Fig. 2). All biphasic and viscoelastic soft tissues exhibit first the relaxation phase in both testing protocols, and finally when the tissue reaches its equilibrium state, no fluid flow or pressure gradients exist. Consequently, after the relaxation phase, strain (in creep test) or stress (in stress-relaxation test) stabilizes at the constant level, and then the entire load is carried by the solid matrix of a tissue.

Destructive testing is typically conducted for skeletal soft tissues only in tension geometry. Then it is common to follow the tissue mechanical behaviour from the stress-strain curve. At the beginning phase of tension test of skeletal soft tissue, one can observe so called toe region (Fig. 3). In this region, the relation between stress and strain is nonlinear and the slope is increasing with increased loading. The reason for the increasing slope is the straightening of the wavy-like collagen fibrils. After the collagen fibrils are completely straightened begins the elastic region (Fig. 3). In this region, the stress and strain are linearly related and the slope of the curve is called the Young's modulus of tissue. In the elastic range, all changes of a tissue are still reversible, i.e. if the stress is removed tissue returns to the original strain. All non-destructive tests, such as creep and stress-relaxation tests mentioned above, should be conducted in this elastic region. It should be also noted that in human skeletal soft tissues the loading rate affects the slope of the elastic range, i.e. higher loading rate results to steeper slope and higher Young's modulus value.

When the stress is further increased from the elastic region, the slope of the curve changes and the plastic region begins. This is called the yield point (Fig. 3). After the yield point tissue begins to experience destructive changes, e.g. microfractures in the collagen fibril network. In the plastic region irreversible changes have occurred in a tissue and it does not return to the original strain although the stress would be completely removed. The yield point is one typical parameter reported for soft tissues under destructive testing.

After the plastic region, the sudden failure of the tissue occurs and stress disappears (Fig. 3). The location of the breakdown is called the failure point, which is one typical parameter reported for soft tissues under destructive tensile testing.

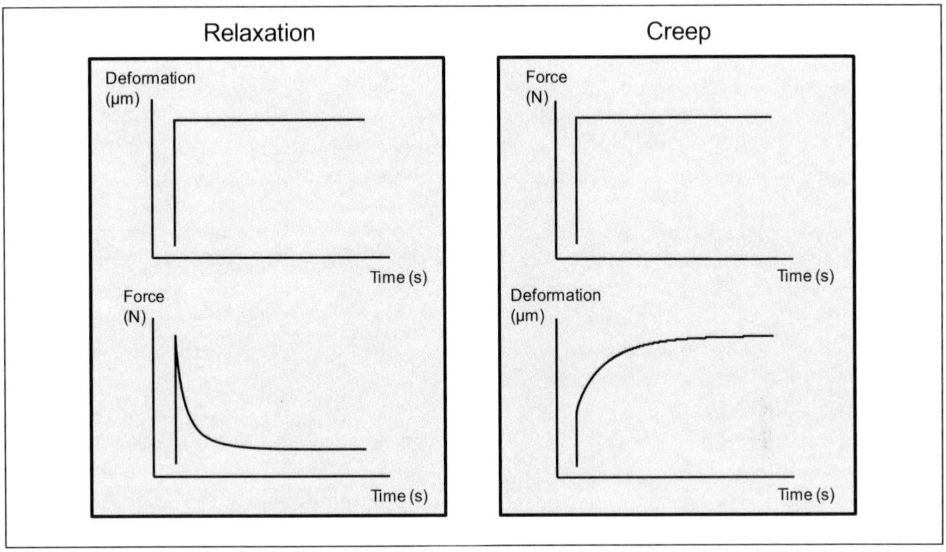

Fig. 2. Stress-relaxation (left) and creep (right) testing protocols.

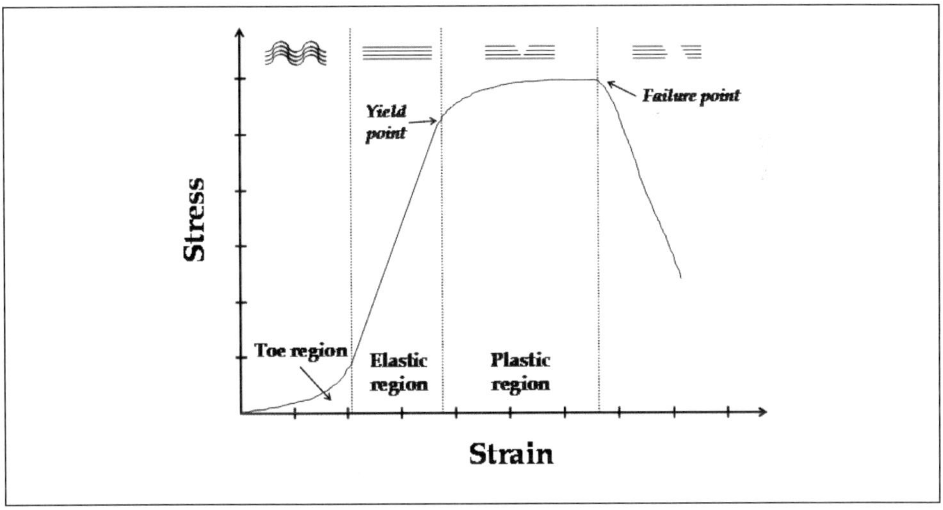

Fig. 3. Typical stress-strain curve for destructive tensile testing of skeletal soft tissues. Collagen fibril straightening and failure, related to different regions of the stress-strain curve, are also schematically shown.

3. Biomechanical modeling of skeletal soft tissues

3.1 Introduction

In this section, we will present the development of computational models applied for the characterization of biomechanical properties of cartilage, meniscus, ligaments and tendons. We will start from traditional linearly elastic models that can be applied for the characterization of static or dynamic properties of tissues by a simple Hookean relation. As the linear elastic model is only applicable for small strains, we will also introduce hyperelastic models that can be applied for nonlinear problems in larger strains.

Second, we will show traditional solid viscoelastic models, i.e. Maxwell, Voigt and Kelvin models. We will show the basic equations of these models. Then, we will take fluid into account in the model and present a biphasic, poroelastic model. We will present biphasic models with isotropic and anisotropic solid matrixes, improving the prediction of experimentally found mechanical behavior of fluid-saturated soft tissues.

Finally, we will present the fibril reinforced biphasic model of cartilage. In this model, the solid matrix is divided into fibrillar and non-fibrillar parts. We will also present different forms of nonlinearities formulated especially for the collagen fibers and the swelling properties due to the fixed charge density of proteoglycans. At the end of the section, we will summarize the application of the presented constitutive models for cartilage, menisci, ligaments and tendons.

3.2 Linear elastic model

The most traditional and simplest mechanical model for skeletal soft tissues is Hooke's linear elastic model for solid materials. This model assumes the linear relation between stress and strain, corresponding to a spring fixed from one end and compressed or strecthed from the other. Hooke's model can be presented as follows:

$$\sigma = E\epsilon, \tag{3.1}$$

where σ is stress, ε is strain, and E is the elastic (Young's) modulus: This model is easy to apply for various testing geometries and protocols, and consequently stiffness of a tested soft tissue can be expressed by the Young's modulus. However, it should be realized that this simple model is limited to one-dimensional geometry and it assumes tissue as elastic and isotropic material. Hooke's law can be generalized to three-dimensional geometry and then also the Poisson's ratio (ν) is needed to describe the mechanical behaviour of the tested soft tissue (see section 3.5.1). Obviously, this is still not adequate for viscoelastic and anisotropic skeletal soft tissues.

Hooke's law can be further generalized for an anisotropic elastic material, when it can be expressed as a matrix form:

$$[\sigma] = [C][\epsilon], \tag{3.2}$$

where $[\sigma]$ is the stress tensor, $[\varepsilon]$ is the strain tensor, and $[C]$ is the stiffness matrix. In order to completely characterize the mechanical behaviour of anisotropic and elastic tissue, altogether 21 stiffness components are needed in $[C]$. For the material with mutually perpendicular planes of elastic symmetry, i.e. orthotropic material, nine elastic constants are needed in $[C]$. Furthermore, if one assumes the same mechanical properties in one plane (e.g. in x–y plane) and different properties in the direction normal to this plane (e.g. z-axis), five independent elastic constants are needed in $[C]$ and the material is referred as transversely isotropic (see section 3.5.2).

Even though one could determine all required stiffness components for an anisotropic elastic material, the mechanical behaviour of skeletal soft tissues still cannot be described by this linear model. In general, the linear elastic model can be applied for skeletal soft tissues when strains are small and the stress-strain relationship can be assumed linear. However, many soft tissues experience large strains in vivo. Furthermore, time-dependent behaviour (due to viscoelasticity) and different mechanical responses in compression and tension, both typical to skeletal soft tissues, cannot be described with this simple model. Therefore, more sophisticated models are needed for the mechanical characterization of skeletal soft tissues.

3.3 Hyperelastic model

Many biological tissues experience large deformations and then the stress-strain relationship becomes nonlinear. These materials are called hyperelastic materials. There are several hyperelastic material models developed, e.g. Neo-Hookean, Arruda-Boyce, Mooney-Rivlin, Ogden models. We will present here one of these models (Neo-Hookean model) that has been typically applied for many biological soft tissues.
The Neo-Hookean material model uses a general strain energy potential for finite strains:

$$U = C_1(\bar{I}_1 - 3) + \frac{1}{D_1}(J_{el} - 1)^2, \tag{3.3}$$

where C_1 and D_1 are material parameters, J_{el} is the elastic volume ratio and $\bar{I}_1$ is the first deviatoric strain invariant defined as:

$$\bar{I}_1 = \bar{\lambda}_1^{\,2} + \bar{\lambda}_2^{\,2} + \bar{\lambda}_3^{\,2}, \tag{3.4}$$

where $\bar{\lambda}_i = J^{-\frac{1}{3}}\lambda_i$ are the deviatoric stretches, J is is the total volume ratio, and λ_i are the principal stretches. The material parameters are given by:

$$C_1 = \frac{G_0}{2}, \quad D_1 = \frac{3(1-2\nu)}{G_0(1+\nu)} \tag{3.5}$$

where G_0 is the initial shear modulus and v is the Poisson's ratio. For linear elastic materials, the shear modulus can be expressed with the Young's modulus ($E = 2G_0(1+\nu)$).

3.4 Viscoelastic models

There are three typical viscoelastic solid materials that have been applied for biological soft tissues; Maxwell, Voigt and Kelvin (Standard linear solid) (Fig. 4). In contrast to the elastic or hyperelastic materials, these models have a time-dependent component that enables the modelling of creep, stress-relaxation and hysteresis.
The solid voscoelastic models are composed of elastic and viscous components. The elastic component is that shown in eq. 3.1, while the viscous component (dashpot) is velocity dependent as:

$$F = \eta\frac{dx}{dt} \tag{3.6}$$

where η is the damping coefficient, F is force and x is deformation/elongation. F and x can also be replaced with stress (σ) and strain (ε). In the Maxwell model, both the spring and dashpot experience the same force, while their deformation and velocity are different. The total velocity becomes:

$$\frac{dx}{dt} = \frac{1}{\mu}\frac{dF}{dt} + \frac{F}{\eta} \tag{3.7}$$

In the Voigt model, the forces of the spring and dashpot elements are different, but their deformation is the same. Thus, the total force is the sum of forces acting on the spring and dashpot:

$$F = \mu x + \eta \frac{dx}{dt} \tag{3.8}$$

In the Kelvin model, the combination of two springs and one dashpot complicates the equation of motion. The same principles as with the Maxwell and Voigt models can be applied, i.e. the elements that are side by side, undergo the same deformation but different force, while those that are arranged consecutively, experience the same force but different deformation. Subsequently, it can be proven that the equation of motion becomes:

$$F + \tau_\epsilon \frac{dF}{dt} = E_R\left(x + \tau_\sigma \frac{dx}{dt}\right) \tag{3.9}$$

where

$$\tau_\epsilon = \frac{\eta_1}{\mu_1}, \tau_\sigma = \frac{\eta_1}{\mu_0}\left(1 + \frac{\mu_0}{\mu_1}\right), E_R = \mu_0. \tag{3.10}$$

There are several textbooks that derive creep and stress-relaxation equations of the aforementioned viscoelastic models. See for instance Fung (2004).

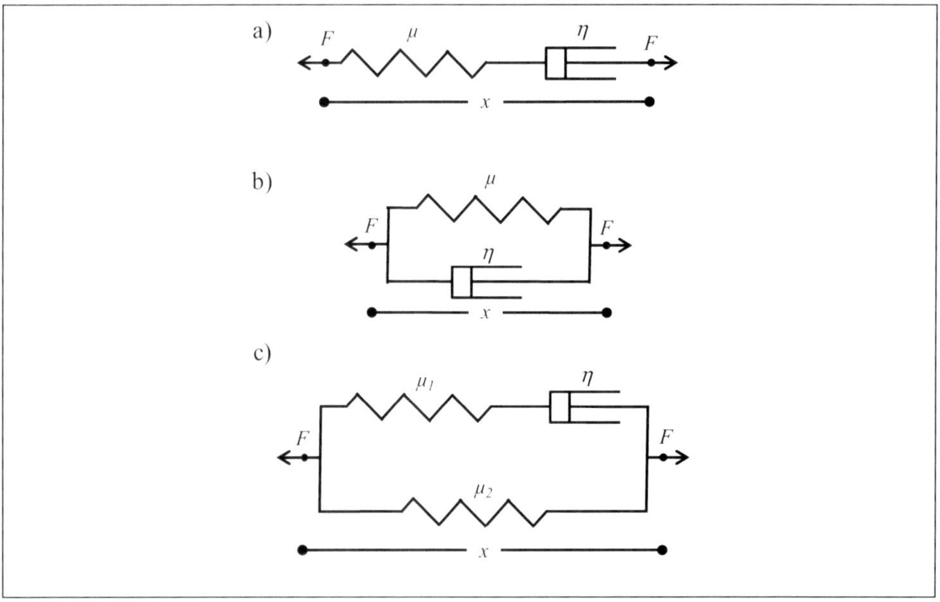

Fig. 4. Solid viscoelastic models: a) Maxwell, b) Voigt, c) Kelvin. F=force, μ=spring constant, η=damping coefficient, x=distance.

3.5 Biphasic, poroelastic model

The biphasic model is the most traditional model of articular cartilage and other fluid-saturated tissue which takes the interstitial fluid movement into account (Mow et al., 1980). In the biphasic theory, the solid matrix and fluid are assumed to be intrinsically incompressible and nondissipative. The only dissipative factor is the fluid flow in the tissue. The constitutive equations, i.e, the stress-strain relations for the solid, fluid and entire tissue are given by:

$$\boldsymbol{\sigma}_s = -\phi_s p\boldsymbol{I} + \boldsymbol{\sigma}_E, \tag{3.11}$$

$$\boldsymbol{\sigma}_f = -\phi_f p\boldsymbol{I}, \tag{3.12}$$

$$\boldsymbol{\sigma}_t = \boldsymbol{\sigma}_s + \boldsymbol{\sigma}_f = -p\boldsymbol{I} + \boldsymbol{\sigma}_E, \tag{3.13}$$

where $\boldsymbol{\sigma}_s$, $\boldsymbol{\sigma}_f$ and $\boldsymbol{\sigma}_t$ are solid, fluid and total stress tensors, respectively, ϕ_s and ϕ_f are volume fractions for the solid and fluid, respectively, p is the fluid pressure, $\boldsymbol{I}$ is the unit tensor and $\boldsymbol{\sigma}_E$ is the effective solid stress tensor.

For the biphasic material with linearly elastic Hookean solid matrix (see eqs. 3.1 and 3.2), the effective solid stress can be written as follows:

$$\boldsymbol{\sigma}_E = \boldsymbol{C}\boldsymbol{\epsilon}, \tag{3.14}$$

where $\boldsymbol{C}$ is the stiffness matrix and $\boldsymbol{\epsilon}$ is the elastic strain tensor. The effective solid stress tensor alone resists the deformation at equilibrium, when the fluid flow has ceased.

With both solid and fluid phases considered intrinsically incompressible and homogenous, the balance of mass (continuity equation) is given by:

$$\nabla \cdot (\phi_s \boldsymbol{v}_s + \phi_f \boldsymbol{v}_f) = \boldsymbol{0}, \tag{3.15}$$

where $\boldsymbol{v}_s$and $\boldsymbol{v}_f$ are velocity vectors of the solid and fluid phases. Neglecting inertia effects (acceleration = 0), the momentum equations for the solid and fluid phases are:

$$\nabla \cdot \boldsymbol{\sigma}_\alpha + \boldsymbol{\pi}_\alpha = \boldsymbol{0}, \tag{3.16}$$

$$\boldsymbol{\pi}_s = -\boldsymbol{\pi}_f = \frac{\phi_f^2}{k}(\boldsymbol{v}_f - \boldsymbol{v}_s) \tag{3.17}$$

$$\nabla \cdot \boldsymbol{\sigma}_t = \boldsymbol{0}, \tag{3.18}$$

where permeability k is related to the diffusive drag coefficient K by:

$$k = \frac{\phi_f^2}{K}. \tag{3.19}$$

The permeability k can be defined to be dependent on the porosity and void ratio, i.e. ratio of fluid to solid content, according to the following equation:

$$k = k_0 \left(\frac{1+e}{1+e_0}\right)^M, \tag{3.20}$$

where k_0 is the initial permeability, e_0 and e are initial and current void ratios, and M is a positive constant. The void ratio or fluid fraction has also been modeled in a depth-dependent manner, e.g,

$$\phi_f = 0.80 - 0.10\text{z}, \tag{3.21}$$

where z is the tissue depth (0: cartilage surface, 1:cartilage-bone interface).

3.5.1 Isotropic model

The elastic parameters of the biphasic poroelastic tissue can be obtained from the equation 3.14. The simplest form of linear elasticity is the isotropic case. The stress-strain relationship becomes:

$$\boldsymbol{\sigma_E} = \frac{E}{(1+\nu)(1-2\nu)} \begin{bmatrix} 1-\nu & \nu & \nu & 0 & 0 & 0 \\ \nu & 1-\nu & \nu & 0 & 0 & 0 \\ \nu & \nu & 1-\nu & 0 & 0 & 0 \\ 0 & 0 & 0 & 1-2\nu & 0 & 0 \\ 0 & 0 & 0 & 0 & 1-2\nu & 0 \\ 0 & 0 & 0 & 0 & 0 & 1-2\nu \end{bmatrix} \boldsymbol{\epsilon}. \tag{3.22}$$

Subsequently, the isotropic biphasic or poroelastic model consists of three material parameters: elastic parameters (Young's modulus (E), Poisson's ratio (ν)) and permeability (k, eq. 3.19)).

The biphasic isotropic material is equivalent to the elastic isotropic material at equilibrium and under dynamic loading. In these representations, it is assumed that at equilibrium all fluid flow has ceased and that the instantaneous response ($t \to 0$) of the biphasic tissue corresponds to that of an incompressible elastic material (ν = 0.5). These elastic isotropic models are useful if one wishes to obtain simple material parameters for the tissue. However, a more detailed description of the complex mechanical properties of skeletal soft tissues can only be obtained by using more sophisticated models.

3.5.2 Transversely isotropic model

In the transversely isotropic material, the mechanical parameters depend on the three mutually orthogonal directions. However, the properties are considered isotropic in the x-y plane. Then, the stiffness matrix relates the stress and strain tensors as follows:

$$\boldsymbol{\sigma_E} = \begin{bmatrix} \frac{1-\nu_{pz}\nu_{zp}}{E_pE_z\Delta} & \frac{\nu_p+\nu_{zp}\nu_{pz}}{E_pE_z\Delta} & \frac{\nu_{zp}+\nu_p\nu_{zp}}{E_pE_z\Delta} & 0 & 0 & 0 \\ \frac{\nu_p+\nu_{pz}\nu_{zp}}{E_zE_p\Delta} & \frac{1-\nu_{zp}\nu_{pz}}{E_zE_p\Delta} & \frac{\nu_{zp}+\nu_{zp}\nu_p}{E_zE_p\Delta} & 0 & 0 & 0 \\ \frac{\nu_{pz}+\nu_p\nu_{pz}}{E_p^2\Delta} & \frac{\nu_{pz}(1+\nu_p)}{E_p^2\Delta} & \frac{1-\nu_p^2}{E_p^2\Delta} & 0 & 0 & 0 \\ 0 & 0 & 0 & 2G_{zp} & 0 & 0 \\ 0 & 0 & 0 & 0 & 2G_{zp} & 0 \\ 0 & 0 & 0 & 0 & 0 & \frac{E_p}{1+\nu_p} \end{bmatrix} \boldsymbol{\epsilon}, \tag{3.23}$$

where

$$\Delta = \frac{(1 + \nu_p)(1 - \nu_p - 2\nu_{pz}\nu_{zp})}{E_p^2 E_z}. \tag{3.24}$$

The total number of transversely isotropic biphasic poroelastic parameters can now be written in terms of the Young's modulus and Poisson's ratio in the transverse plane, i.e. parallel to the articular surface (E_p and ν_p), out-of-plane Young's modulus and Poisson's ratio (E_{pz} and ν_{pz}), out-of-plane shear modulus (G_{zp}), and permeability (k, eq. 3.19).
Under an instantaneous loading ($t \to 0$), when fluid is entrapped in the tissue, the transversely isotropic biphasic or poroelastic material behaves like an incompressible elastic material (Garcia et al., 2000; Korhonen et al., 2002b), similarly as in the case of the isotropic model. The elastic parameters are then:

$$E_{pz}, E_p, \nu_{pz} = 0.5, \nu_p = 1 - 0.5\frac{E_p}{E_{pz}}, G_{zp}. \tag{3.25}$$

Similarly at equilibrium, when the fluid flow has ceased and only the solid matrix resists the compression, the material can be assumed to be elastic with the five independent material parameters in eq. 3.23.

3.5.3 Fibril reinforced model

In the fibril reinforced biphasic model, the fibril network (collagen network), in addition to the isotropic biphasic matrix, contributes to the mechanical response of tissues under loading (Korhonen et al. 2003). Thus, the total stress becomes:

$$\boldsymbol{\sigma}_t = \boldsymbol{\sigma}_{nf} + \boldsymbol{\sigma}_{fibril} - p\boldsymbol{I}, \tag{3.26}$$

where $\boldsymbol{\sigma}_{nf}$ and $\boldsymbol{\sigma}_{fibril}$ are nonfibrillar and fibril network stresses, respectively. The isotropic biphasic nonfibrillar matrix has been modeled as Hookean or Neo-Hookean materials with Darcy's law for the fluid flow (sections 3.2 and 3.3). The material parameters for the nonfibrillar part are the Young's modulus (E_m), Poisson's ratio (ν_m) and permeability (k). The fibril network properties are controlled by the Young's modulus of the fibril network (E_f). Elastic properties of the fibril network have been characterized with a nonlinear relation:

$$E_f = E_f^0 + E_f^\epsilon \epsilon_f, \text{for } \epsilon_f > 0, \tag{3.27}$$

$$E_f = 0, \text{for } \epsilon_f \leq 0, \tag{3.28}$$

where E_f^0 is the initial fibril network modulus, E_f^ϵ is the strain-dependent fibril network modulus, and ϵ_f is the fibril strain. The significant difference between the fibril reinforced and transversely isotropic poroelastic model is that the fibrils in the fibril reinforced model resist only tension, whereas E_p in the transversely isotropic model is the same for both compression and tension.
The collagen fibril stresses (σ_f) have also been modeled as viscoelastic:

$$\sigma_f = -\frac{\eta}{2\sqrt{(\sigma_f - E_f^0\varepsilon_f)E_f^\varepsilon}}\dot{\sigma_f} + E_f^0\varepsilon_f + \left(\frac{\eta E_f^0}{2\sqrt{(\sigma_f - E_f^0\varepsilon_f)E_f^\varepsilon}} + \eta\right)\dot{\varepsilon_f}, \text{for } \varepsilon_f > 0, \tag{3.29}$$

$$\sigma_f = 0, \text{for } \varepsilon_f \leq 0,$$

where η is the viscoelastic damping coefficient, and $\dot{\varepsilon}$ and $\dot{\sigma}$ are the stress- and strain-rates, respectively.

The fibrillar part has also been modeled with primary and secondary fibrils (Wilson et al., 2004). The primary fibrils represent the collagens detected with polarized light microscopy (Arokoski et al., 1996; Korhonen et al., 2002b), which cause a depth-dependent tensile modulus for the tissue. The fibrils are oriented vertically in the deep zone, curve in the middle zone, and reach a parallel orientation with the articular surface in the superficial zone (Benninghoff, 1925). Two parameters are needed to describe the fibril orientation: thickness of the superficial zone (d_{vec}) and bending radius of the collagen fibrils in the middle zone (r_{vec}). The secondary fibrils mimic the less organized collagen network which are observed in scanning electron microscopy (Kaab et al., 2003). The stresses for primary and secondary fibrils can be formulated as:

$$\sigma_{f,p} = \rho_z C \sigma_f, \tag{3.30}$$

$$\sigma_{f,s} = \rho_z \sigma_f, \tag{3.31}$$

where ρ_z represents the depth dependent fibril density, and C is the density ratio of primary and secondary fibrils. The stress of the fibril network is then determined as the sum of the stresses in each individual fibril ($\sigma_{f,all}^{i}$),

$$\sigma_f = \sum_{i=1}^{totf} \sigma_{f,all}^{i}. \tag{3.32}$$

3.5.4 Other models of skeletal soft tissues

There are also other models of biological soft tissues than those presented above. The conewise linear elastic model is able to characterize compression-tension nonlinearity of the tissues (Soltz&Ateshian, 2000). The poroviscoelastic model includes both fluid flow dependent and fluid flow independent viscoelasticities (DiSilvestro&Suh, 2001). The triphasic model includes ion flow (Lai et al., 1991) and it is equivalent to the biphasic swelling model at equilibrium (Wilson et al., 2005a). In the biphasic fibril reinforced swelling model, after inclusion of osmotic swelling and chemical expansion, the total stress becomes:

$$\boldsymbol{\sigma}_t = \boldsymbol{\sigma}_{nf} + \boldsymbol{\sigma}_{fibril} - \Delta\pi \boldsymbol{I} - T_c \boldsymbol{I} - \mu_f \boldsymbol{I}, \tag{3.33}$$

where $\Delta\pi$ is the osmotic pressure gradient, T_c is the chemical expansion stress, and $\mu_f = p - \Delta\pi$ is the chemical potential of fluid (Huyghe&Janssen, 1997; Wilson et al., 2005a; Wilson et al., 2005b; Korhonen et al., 2008). The osmotic pressure gradient is caused by the difference in ion concentration of the cartilage and that of the surrounding fluid (Huyghe&Janssen, 1997; Wilson et al., 2005a; Wilson et al., 2005b). It is also referred to as the Donnan swelling pressure gradient. The chemical expansion stress comes from the repulsion between negative charges in the solid matrix (Lai et al., 1991; Wilson et al., 2005a; Wilson et al., 2005b). Swelling of the tissue is resisted by the collagen network, inducing pre-stresses in the collagen fibrils. This model has been applied specifically for cartilage since its swelling properties due to the fixed charge density have a significant role for the deformation behavior of the tissue, especially under static loading. For the implementation of swelling properties, the fixed charge density can be taken from experimental measurements (Maroudas, 1968; Chen et al., 2001).

Other anisotropic and nonlinear representation have also been presented for biological soft tissues. Specifically the collagen fibrils and their nonlinear stress-strain tensile behavior has been presented as follows:

$$P_1 = E_1(e^{k_1 \varepsilon_f} - 1), \tag{3.34}$$

$$P_2 = E_2(e^{k_2 \varepsilon_e} - 1), \tag{3.35}$$

$$P_f = P_1 + P_2, \tag{3.36}$$

where P_f is the first Piola-Kirchhoff fibril stress, ε_f is the total fibril strain, ε_e is the strain of the spring μ_1 (Fig. 3c), and E_1, E_2, k_1 and k_2 are constants (Wilson et al., 2006; Julkunen et al., 2008). Tensile stress-stretch relationship for collagen fibrils has also been presented in the following form

$$\lambda \frac{\partial F_2}{\partial \lambda} = \begin{cases} 0, & \lambda < 1, \\ C_3\left(e^{C_4(\lambda-1)} - 1\right) & 1 < \lambda < \lambda^*, \\ C_5\lambda + C_6 & \lambda > \lambda^*, \end{cases} \tag{3.37}$$

where

$$C_6 = C_3\left(e^{C_4(\lambda^*-1)} - 1\right) - C_5\lambda^*. \tag{3.38}$$

In these equations, F_2 is the strain energy function for the collagen fibers, usually in conjunction with the hyperelastic model, such as Neo-Hookean (eq. 3.3), λ is fiber stretch, λ^* is the stretch where collagen fibers are straightened, and C_3, C_4, C_5 and C_6 are material constants (Pena et al., 2006; Zhang et al., 2008).

3.6 Models applied for skeletal soft tissues

Articular cartilage has been modelled using almost all the above mentioned models (Mow et al., 1980; Lai et al., 1991; Li et al., 1999; Garcia et al., 2000; Guilak&Mow, 2000; Soltz&Ateshian, 2000; DiSilvestro&Suh, 2001; Korhonen et al., 2003; Laasanen et al., 2003; Wilson et al., 2004; Julkunen et al., 2007). The choice of the material model has been mainly based on the study purpose and loading protocol. Recently, however, the fibril reinforced material description has been applied by many researchers and it is probably the most realistic approach for cartilage (Li et al., 1999; Li et al., 2000; Korhonen et al., 2003; Wilson et al., 2004; Wilson et al., 2005b; Julkunen et al., 2007; Korhonen et al., 2008; Julkunen et al., 2009). It should also be noted that in articular cartilage negative fixed charges create tissue swelling pressure and is very important for the mechanical behaviour of the tissue. Thus, tissue swelling model or triphasic approaches are important phenomena. Meniscus, ligaments and tendons have only a small amount of fixed charges and swelling mechanisms have thus been neglected in the models.

Meniscus has been typically modelled as isotropic or transversely isotropic material (Spilker et al., 1992; Meakin et al., 2003; Sweigart et al., 2004; Guess et al., 2010). Poroelastic properties have also been included in meniscus models. Typical models for ligaments and tendons have been transversely isotropic nonlinear with hyperelastic behaviour (Pena et al.,

2006; Zhang et al., 2008). Also viscoelastic solid models (Thornton et al., 1997) and poroelastic models have been applied for ligaments (Atkinson et al., 1997). However, the fluid-flow dependent viscoeasticity may not be that important in ligaments and tendons because they experience mainly tensile forces under physiological loading and it has been suggested that fluid has only a minor role in contributing to soft tissue response in tension (Li et al., 2005). Furthermore, viscoelastic models with anisotropic nonlinear stress-strain behaviour have been developed to capture the strain rate dependent nonlinearity of ligaments and tendons (Pioletti et al., 1998; Limbert&Middleton, 2006).

3.7 Optimization of material parameters

The optimization of material parameters of the model can be done by typically minimizing the mean squared error (MSE), root mean squared error (RMSE) or mean absolute error (MAE) between the simulated and experimental force curves (Fig. 5). This can be done for instance using a multidimensional unconstrained nonlinear minimization routine (fminsearch) available in Matlab (Mathworks Inc., Natick, MA, USA). The optimization should be first tested with different initial values of the material parameters, and the optimized parameter values should be always the same, independent on the initial guess. Then one of the equations for MSE, RMSE and MAE,

$$MSE = \frac{1}{n}\sum_{j=1}^{n}\left(F_{model,j} - F_{exp,j}\right)^2, \tag{3.39}$$

$$RMSE = \frac{1}{n}\sum_{j=1}^{n}\sqrt{(F_{model,j} - F_{exp,j})^2}, \tag{3.40}$$

$$MAE = \frac{1}{n}\sum_{j=1}^{n}\left|F_{model,j} - F_{exp,j}\right|, \tag{3.41}$$

where $F_{model,j}$ is the model output and $F_{exp,j}$ is the experimental result at any time point (j), can be applied. The optimizations have also been conducted using normalized MSE, RMSE and MAE, i.e. by dividing equations 3.39-3.41 with $F_{exp,j}$ at each time point.

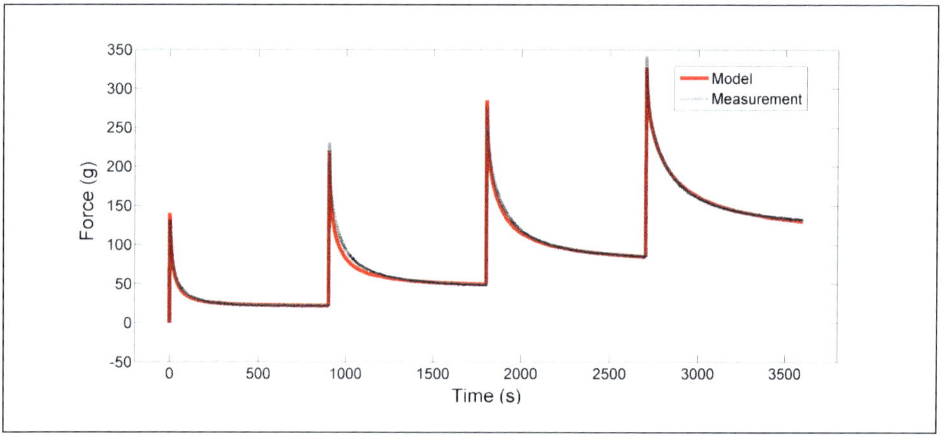

Fig. 5. A typical stress-relaxation measurement of articular cartilage and corresponding optimized model fit using a fibril reinforced poroviscoelastic model.

4. References

Arokoski, J. P., Hyttinen, M. M., Lapveteläinen, T., Takacs, P., Kosztaczky, B., Modis, L., Kovanen, V., Helminen, H., (1996). Decreased birefringence of the superficial zone collagen network in the canine knee (stifle) articular cartilage after long distance running training, detected by quantitative polarised light microscopy. *Ann Rheum Dis* 55, 253-264.

Atkinson, T. S., Haut, R. C., Altiero, N. J., (1997). A poroelastic model that predicts some phenomenological responses of ligaments and tendons. *J Biomech Eng* 119, 400-405.

Benninghoff, A., (1925). Form und bau der gelenkknorpel in ihren beziehungen zur function. *Zeitschrift fur Zellforschung* 2, 783-862.

Chen, A. C., Bae, W. C., Schinagl, R. M., Sah, R. L., (2001). Depth- and strain-dependent mechanical and electromechanical properties of full-thickness bovine articular cartilage in confined compression. *J Biomech* 34, 1-12.

Cui, J. H., Min, B. H., (2007). Collagenous fibril texture of the discoid lateral meniscus. *Arthroscopy* 23, 635-641.

DiSilvestro, M. R., Suh, J. K., (2001). A cross-validation of the biphasic poroviscoelastic model of articular cartilage in unconfined compression, indentation, and confined compression. *J Biomech* 34, 519-525.

Elliott, D. M., Narmoneva, D. A., Setton, L. A., (2002). Direct measurement of the Poisson's ratio of human patella cartilage in tension. *J Biomech Eng* 124, 223-228.

Fung, Y. C., (2004). Biomechanics-Mechanical properties of living tissues, second edition. Springer, New York.

Garcia, J. J., Altiero, N. J., Haut, R. C., (2000). Estimation of in situ elastic properties of biphasic cartilage based on a transversely isotropic hypo-elastic model. *J Biomech Eng* 122, 1-8.

Guess, T. M., Thiagarajan, G., Kia, M., Mishra, M., (2010). A subject specific multibody model of the knee with menisci. *Med Eng Phys* 32, 505-515.

Guilak, F., Mow, V. C., (2000). The mechanical environment of the chondrocyte: a biphasic finite element model of cell-matrix interactions in articular cartilage. *J Biomech* 33, 1663-1673.

Hewitt, J., Guilak, F., Glisson, R., Vail, T. P., (2001). Regional material properties of human hip joint capsule ligaments. *J Orthop Res* 19, 359-364.

Huyghe, J. M., Janssen, J. D., (1997). Quadriphasic theory of swelling incompressible porous media. *Int J Eng Sci* 35, 793-802.

Julkunen, P., Kiviranta, P., Wilson, W., Jurvelin, J. S., Korhonen, R. K., (2007). Characterization of articular cartilage by combining microscopic analysis with a fibril-reinforced finite element model. *J Biomech* 40, 1862-1870.

Julkunen, P., Wilson, W., Jurvelin, J. S., Korhonen, R. K., (2009). Composition of the pericellular matrix modulates the deformation behaviour of chondrocytes in articular cartilage under static loading. *Med Biol Eng Comput* 47, 1281-1290.

Julkunen, P., Wilson, W., Jurvelin, J. S., Rieppo, J., Qu, C. J., Lammi, M. J., Korhonen, R. K., (2008). Stress-relaxation of human patellar articular cartilage in unconfined compression: prediction of mechanical response by tissue composition and structure. *J Biomech* 41, 1978-1986.

Jurvelin, J. S., Buschmann, M. D., Hunziker, E. B., (1997). Optical and mechanical determination of Poisson's ratio of adult bovine humeral articular cartilage. *J Biomech* 30, 235-241.

Kaab, M. J., Richards, R. G., Ito, K., ap Gwynn, I., Notzli, H. P., (2003). Deformation of chondrocytes in articular cartilage under compressive load: a morphological study. *Cells Tissues Organs* 175, 133-139.

Korhonen, R. K., Julkunen, P., Wilson, W., Herzog, W., (2008). Importance of collagen orientation and depth-dependent fixed charge densities of cartilage on mechanical behavior of chondrocytes. *J Biomech Eng* 130, 021003.

Korhonen, R. K., Laasanen, M. S., Toyras, J., Lappalainen, R., Helminen, H. J., Jurvelin, J. S., (2003). Fibril reinforced poroelastic model predicts specifically mechanical behavior of normal, proteoglycan depleted and collagen degraded articular cartilage. *J Biomech* 36, 1373-1379.

Korhonen, R. K., Laasanen, M. S., Töyräs, J., Helminen, H. J., Jurvelin, J. S., (2002a). Comparison of the equilibrium response of articular cartilage in unconfined compression, confined compression and indentation. *J Biomech* 35, 903-909.

Korhonen, R. K., Wong, M., Arokoski, J., Lindgren, R., Helminen, H. J., Hunziker, E. B., Jurvelin, J. S., (2002b). Importance of the superficial tissue layer for the indentation stiffness of articular cartilage. *Med Eng Phys* 24, 99-108.

Laasanen, M. S., Toyras, J., Korhonen, R. K., Rieppo, J., Saarakkala, S., Nieminen, M. T., Hirvonen, J., Jurvelin, J. S., (2003). Biomechanical properties of knee articular cartilage. *Biorheology* 40, 133-140.

Lai, W. M., Hou, J. S., Mow, V. C., (1991). A triphasic theory for the swelling and deformation behaviors of articular cartilage. *J Biomech Eng* 113, 245-258.

Li, L. P., Buschmann, M. D., Shirazi-Adl, A., (2000). A fibril reinforced nonhomogeneous poroelastic model for articular cartilage: inhomogeneous response in unconfined compression. *J Biomech* 33, 1533-1541.

Li, L. P., Herzog, W., Korhonen, R. K., Jurvelin, J. S., (2005). The role of viscoelasticity of collagen fibers in articular cartilage: axial tension versus compression. *Med Eng Phys* 27, 51-57.

Li, L. P., Soulhat, J., Buschmann, M. D., Shirazi-Adl, A., (1999). Nonlinear analysis of cartilage in unconfined ramp compression using a fibril reinforced poroelastic model. *Clin Biomech* 14, 673-682.

Limbert, G., Middleton, J., (2006). A constitutive model of the posterior cruciate ligament. *Med Eng Phys* 28, 99-113.

Maroudas, A., (1968). Physicochemical properties of cartilage in the light of ion exchange theory. *Biophys J* 8, 575-595.

McDevitt, C. A., Webber, R. J., (1990). The ultrastructure and biochemistry of meniscal cartilage. *Clin Orthop*, 8-18.

Meakin, J. R., Shrive, N. G., Frank, C. B., Hart, D. A., (2003). Finite element analysis of the meniscus: the influence of geometry and material properties on its behaviour. *Knee* 10, 33-41.

Messner, K., Gao, J., (1998). The menisci of the knee joint. Anatomical and functional characteristics, and a rationale for clinical treatment. *J Anat* 193, 161-178.

Mow, V. C., Gu, W. Y., Chen, F. H., (2005). Structure and function of articular cartilage and meniscus. In: Mow, V. C., Huiskes, R. (Eds.), *Basic Orthopaedic Biomechanics and Mechano-biology*. Lippincott Williams & Wilkins, Philadelphia, pp. 181-258.

Mow, V. C., Kuei, S. C., Lai, W. M., Armstrong, C. G., (1980). Biphasic creep and stress relaxation of articular cartilage in compression: Theory and experiments. *J Biomech Eng* 102, 73-84.

Pena, E., Calvo, B., Martinez, M. A., Doblare, M., (2006). A three-dimensional finite element analysis of the combined behavior of ligaments and menisci in the healthy human knee joint. *J Biomech* 39, 1686-1701.

Pioletti, D. P., Rakotomanana, L. R., Benvenuti, J. F., Leyvraz, P. F., (1998). Viscoelastic constitutive law in large deformations: application to human knee ligaments and tendons. *J Biomech* 31, 753-757.

Soltz, M. A., Ateshian, G. A., (2000). A Conewise Linear Elasticity mixture model for the analysis of tension- compression nonlinearity in articular cartilage. *J Biomech Eng* 122, 576-586.

Spilker, R. L., Donzelli, P. S., Mow, V. C., (1992). A transversely isotropic biphasic finite element model of the meniscus. *J Biomech* 25, 1027-1045.

Sweigart, M. A., Zhu, C. F., Burt, D. M., DeHoll, P. D., Agrawal, C. M., Clanton, T. O., Athanasiou, K. A., (2004). Intraspecies and interspecies comparison of the compressive properties of the medial meniscus. *Ann Biomed Eng* 32, 1569-1579.

Thornton, G. M., Oliynyk, A., Frank, C. B., Shrive, N. G., (1997). Ligament creep cannot be predicted from stress relaxation at low stress: a biomechanical study of the rabbit medial collateral ligament. *J Orthop Res* 15, 652-656.

Vasara, A. I., Jurvelin, J. S., Peterson, L., Kiviranta, I., (2005). Arthroscopic cartilage indentation and cartilage lesions of anterior cruciate ligament-deficient knees. *Am J Sports Med* 33, 408-414.

Wilson, W., Huyghe, J. M., van Donkelaar, C. C., (2006). A composition-based cartilage model for the assessment of compositional changes during cartilage damage and adaptation. *Osteoarthritis Cartilage* 14, 554-560.

Wilson, W., van Donkelaar, C. C., Huyghe, J. M., (2005a). A comparison between mechano-electrochemical and biphasic swelling theories for soft hydrated tissues. *J Biomech Eng* 127, 158-165.

Wilson, W., van Donkelaar, C. C., van Rietbergen, B., Huiskes, R., (2005b). A fibril-reinforced poroviscoelastic swelling model for articular cartilage. *J Biomech* 38, 1195-1204.

Wilson, W., van Donkelaar, C. C., van Rietbergen, B., Ito, K., Huiskes, R., (2004). Stresses in the local collagen network of articular cartilage: a poroviscoelastic fibril-reinforced finite element study. *J Biomech* 37, 357-366.

Woo, S. L., Lee, T. Q., Abramowitch, S. D., Gilbert, T. W., (2005). Structure and function of ligaments and tendons. In: Mow, V. C., Huiskes, R. (Eds.), *Basic Orthopaedic Biomechanics and Mechano-biology*. Lippincott Williams & Wilkins, Philadelphia, pp. 301-342.

Zhang, X., Jiang, G., Wu, C., Woo, S. L., (2008). A subject-specific finite element model of the anterior cruciate ligament. In *30th Annual International Conference of the IEEE Engineering in Medicine & Biology Society*. Vancouver, British Columbia, Canada, August 20-24, pp. 891-894.

6

Functional Data Analysis for Biomechanics

Elizabeth Crane, David Childers, Geoffrey Gerstner and Edward Rothman
University of Michigan
U.S.A

1. Introduction

The application of nonlinear tools and advanced statistical methods is becoming more prevalent in biomechanical analyses. In a traditional biomechanics laboratory with motion analysis equipment, large amounts of kinematic data can be collected relatively easily. However, a significant gap exists between all the data that are collected and the data that are actually analyzed. Because movements occur over a period of time, whether seconds or minutes, each movement is represented by a continuous series of kinematic data (e.g., 60 or 120 observations per second). Using standard analytic methods, the continuous data associated with each movement are often reduced to a single discrete number. This reduction to a single summary value, such as a peak flexion, extension, or range of motion, excludes potentially valuable information. Reducing a curve representing hip motion during gait to a single range of motion value, for example, precludes the analysis of the entire movement pattern or the timing of the movement. A handful of investigations have recognized this limitation and have begun using functions to maintain the shape and timing of the movement in the analysis.

The primary purpose of this chapter is to introduce an emerging collection of statistical methods called Functional Data Analysis (FDA). FDA is distinct from traditional analytic methods because how data changes continuously over time can be assessed. Therefore, information in continuous signals can be retained, such as changes in joint angles or in landmark positions during a movement task. FDA can be used for both exploratory and hypothesis driven analyses with traditional multivariate statistical methods that have been modified for functional predictor and response variables. Although representing motion data as a set of functions is not new to biomechanics analyses (Chester & Wrigley, 2008; Deluzio & Astephen, 2007; Landry et al., 2007; Lee et al., 2009; Sadeghi et al., 2002; 2000), statistical methods developed specifically for analyzing these functions have not been available. More recently, FDA methods have been used within biomechanics to study mastication (Crane et al., 2010), back pain (Page et al., 2006), as well as age, gender, and speed effects on walking (Røislien et al., 2009). Given the interest in and need for treating motion data as functions, it is important that methods for analyzing a set a functions using emerging statistical methods are brought to the attention of those in the biomechanics community.

Although several excellent references exist for Functional Data Analysis (Ramsay, 2000; Ramsay et al., 2009; Ramsay & Silverman, 2002; 2005) there are important issues for biomechanists to be aware of when implementing this set of statistical tools. Therefore, the aims of this chapter are to provide an overview of the steps associated with FDA, to focus on issues related to aligning curves from cyclical data, to discuss specific statistical techniques, and finally to provide an example of how to implement the techniques introduced in the chapter.

2. Overview of basic FDA procedures

There are four primary procedures in FDA: transforming data into functions, smoothing functions, registering functions, and analysis. The purpose of this section is to provide a conceptual introduction to each of these procedures. Open source tools are available for performing the procedures described in this chapter using R statistical software (R Development Core Team, 2010) along with the freely available *fda* library (Ramsay et al., 2010).

2.1 Transforming data into functions

The first step in FDA is transforming the captured time series data into functions. For cyclical behaviors such as locomotion or mastication, it is common to begin by dividing a long sequence of motion data captured during walking or chewing into individual cycles (Fig. 1).

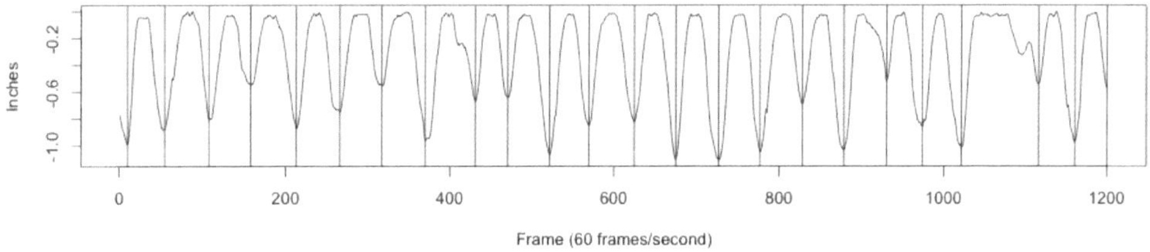

Fig. 1. Displacement data representing a time series of chewing kinematics captured using an optoelectronic motion capture system.

Each cycle is then transformed into a function. Therefore, if one cycle was represented by n observations, by transforming those data points into a function, the behavior can now be considered a single functional observation (Fig. 2).
In Functional Data Analysis, functions are represented as a linear combination of a set of basis functions (see Equation 1).

$$f(t) = \sum_{k=1}^{K} c_k \phi_k(t) \tag{1}$$

One of the first decisions that must be made is the type of basis system to use to represent the data. Typical selections are Fourier and spline basis systems, but others such as polynomials or wavelets can also be used. A Fourier basis system is typically used for periodic data, while splines (in particular b-splines) are used for non-periodic data. For K basis functions, there will be K corresponding coefficients. As the number of basis functions used to model the behavior increases, complexity also increases. While increasing the number of basis functions can produce an excellent fit to the data, the complexity of the function increases computational time for certain procedures and can increase the analytical complexity and interpretation.
An important advantage of transforming discrete data into functions is the ease with which derivatives can be computed and assessed, a common task in biomechanical analyses (Fig. 3). Two points should be given consideration when transforming data into functions if derivatives are going to be used. First, end point error can be amplified in derivatives (see

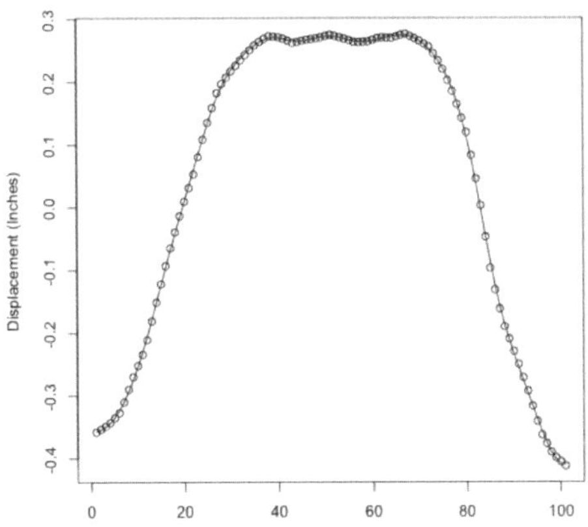

Fig. 2. A single chewing cycle. Dots indicate the recorded observations while the line represents the function that was fit to the observed data.

Section 2.2 for one possible solution to this issue). Second, wild fluctuations in the data can be amplified as a result of the basis system selected.

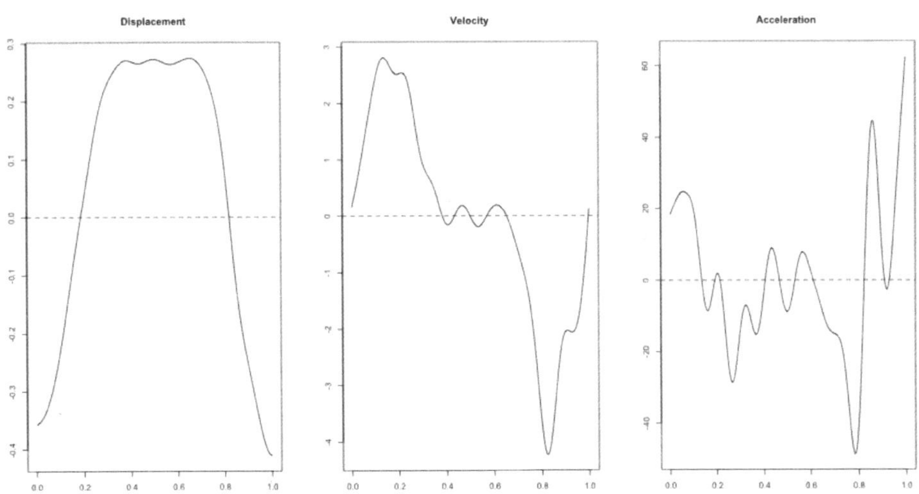

Fig. 3. Functions representing displacement, velocity, and acceleration for a single chewing cycle.

2.2 Smoothing

Functions can be smoothed by minimizing the number of basis functions and using regression analysis or by using a roughness penalty approach. Regression splines use a least squares estimation process. The advantage of regression splines is their simplicity. However, the use of a large number K of basis functions relative to the number of data points in the curve tends to overfit the data. Conversely, using a small number of regression splines risks losing localized functional features. Further, regression splines can produce end-point error in derivative estimates. Thus, regression splines can work well when simplicity is important, but have limitations for more complex cases.

An alternative to using regression splines to smooth the data is an approach that smoothes the data using a roughness penalty. With this approach it is common to have one basis function for each observation in the curve. Because this curve may contain noise, which can be especially amplified in derivatives, a measure of function complexity is penalized to impose smoothness. Unlike regression splines, the roughness penalty approach uses a large number of basis functions without overfitting or sigularity problems. Figure 4 illustrates the same curve fit with each type of smoothing.

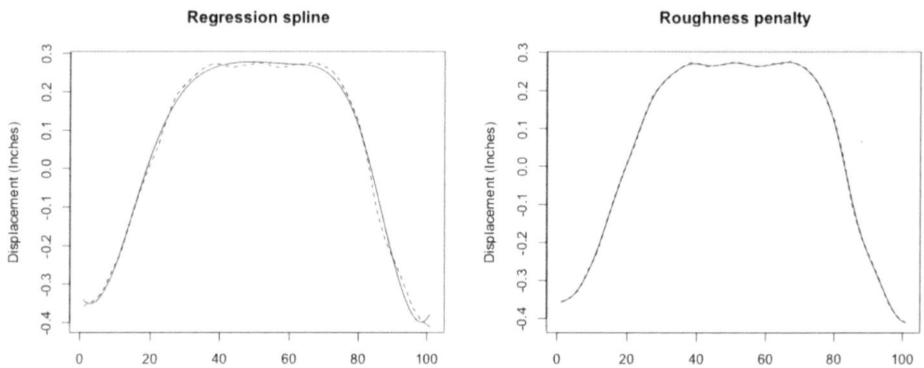

Fig. 4. The left plot overlays raw data (dashed line) from a chewing cycle with a function (solid line) fit to the data using a regression spline. The right plot overlays the same raw data (dashed line) with a function (solid line) fit to the data using a roughness penalty approach.

For further discussion and computational details related to smoothing see Ramsay et al. (2009). Briefly, the roughness of a curve f is typically measured as the integrated squared second derivative (Equation 2).

$$\mathrm{ROUGH}(f) = \int [D^2 f(t)]^2 \mathrm{d}t \tag{2}$$

In Equation 2, $[D^2 f(t)]^2$ is a measure of roughness of function f at value time t. The idea is that when a function contains noise, the noise is amplified in the second derivative. Therefore, the square of the second derivative will be large where noise is present in the curve. To create the smooth curve, a multiple of the roughness penalty is applied to the error sum of squares and a smoothing parameter λ is used to specify the degree of penalty. As λ approaches 0, the fit of the function to the observations improves.

Whether data are filtered using more traditional methods, such as digital filters, or are smoothed using regression splines or a roughness penalty approach, it is important to note that each of these smoothing techniques has the potential to impact the location of specific and biologically relevant points in the curve (Fig. 5). While this may seem obvious, it is important to understand the possible sources of noise introduced by the measurement technique as well as how the data smoothing method modified the curve to reduce the noise. We note that different techniques can produce different results that may affect interpretation of the behavior and analysis. This is illustrated below with a chewing cycle. Within a cycle, there are four biologically relevant phases and, therefore, three transition points between phases. The four phases, in order shown in Figure 5, are fast close (FC), slow close (SC), slow open (SO), and fast open (FO). When two different smoothing techniques are applied to the same curve prior to identifying the location of the transition points between these phases, it is clear how the smoothing technique can substantially change the location of these points.

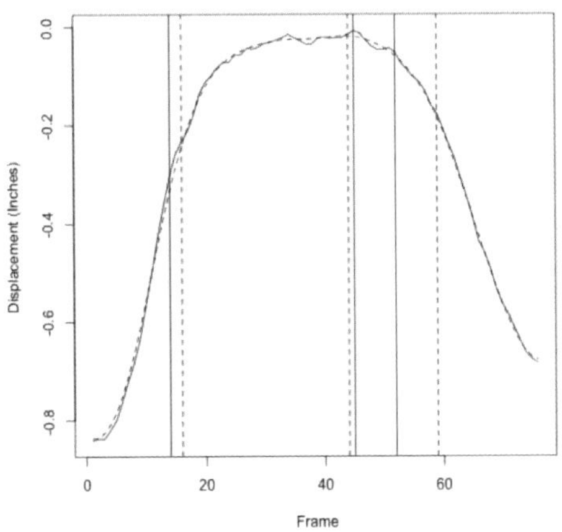

Fig. 5. From left to right are the FC-SC, maximum close, and SO-FO transitions. Dashed lines represent the location of transitions identified after regression spline smoothing and solid lines represent the location of transitions identified after roughness penalty smoothing.

2.3 Registering functions - Curve alignment

An important curve that many biomechanists generate is a mean curve to represent a specific behavior. It is well known that when a curve contains both phase and amplitude variation, they can not be easily compared and an average curve does not accurately represent the true behavior (Fig. 6). Therefore, the purpose of curve alignment is to reduce phase variability while preserving the curves shape and amplitude. A common method for aligning curves used in biomechanics applications is a linear time normalization procedure. An analogous procedure exists in Function Data Analysis called registration. Curves can be registered using a continuous method or by using landmarks. Both approaches use time warping functions, which align curves to minimize phase variation. Two curves are perfectly aligned if they differ only in amplitude. If f_1 and f_2 are perfectly aligned, then the plot of $f_1(t)$ versus $f_2(t)$ will yield a straight line. Continuous registration uses an iterative numerical approach to choose time warping functions that maximize the proportionality of all the functional observations. The algorithm begins by aligning each individual curve in the set of curves to the group average curve. Once the new set of aligned curves is generated, a new average curve is calculated and the set of aligned curves are aligned again to the new average curve. See Ramsay & Silverman (2005) for further details.

Landmark registration is in many ways a simpler form of registering a set of curves. A landmark is defined as a point that is identifiable in every curve. This may be a minima, maxima, or zero crossing. Landmark registration aligns all specified landmarks by transforming time for each curve so that the landmarks occur in the same location. A common procedure for landmark registration is to first identify the location of the landmark of interest for each individual curve. Next, an average of these landmarks is calculated. Finally, time is transformed for each curve such that the identified landmark occurs at the average location. Although landmark registration is computationally less intensive than continuous registration, there is an upfront data processing cost to identifying the location of the landmark(s) for each individual curve.

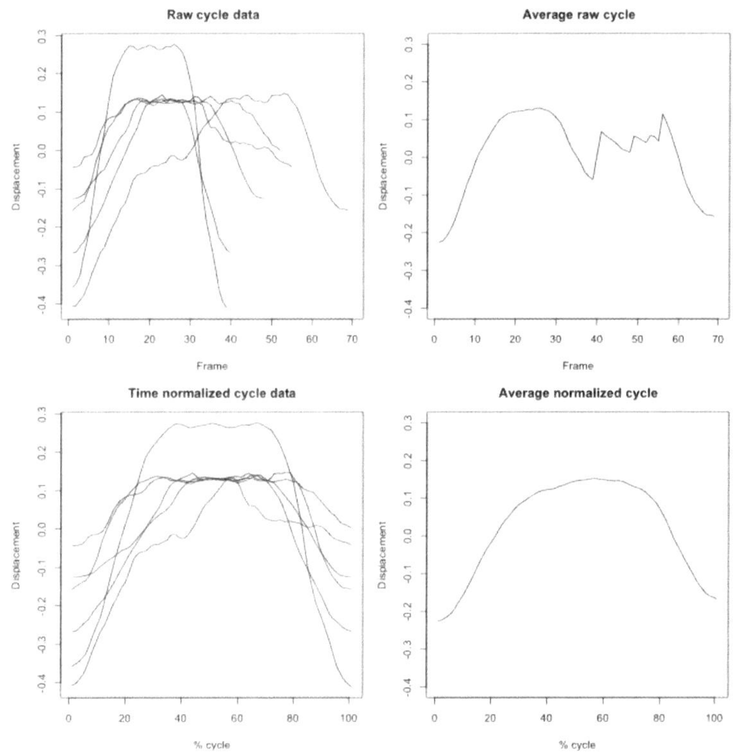

Fig. 6. A set of five curves illustrating the effect of curve alignment. Without alignment the average curve does not provide an accurate representation of the behavior.

Whether continuous registration or landmark registration is used, the outcomes include a new set of aligned curves as well as time warping functions. The time warping functions contain information about how phase was adjusted. A unique time warping function is associated with each individual curve. Figure 7 shows the warping functions associated with each of the registered curves.

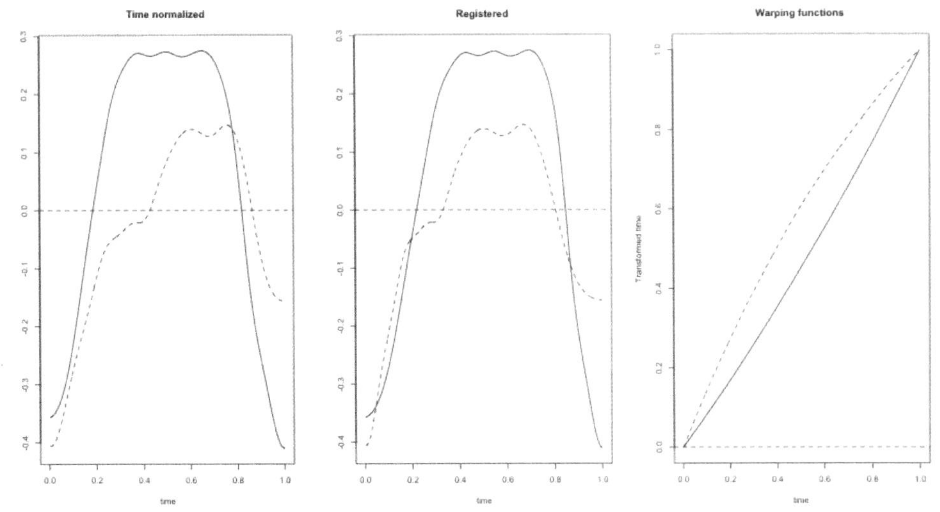

Fig. 7. This figure shows the warping functions associated with each of the registered curves.

2.4 Statistical tests

An important advantage of treating the behavior as a function rather than n discrete data points is that the data do not have to be reduced to a single number to be analyzed. For example, it is common to identify peak flexion or extension or range of motion for analysis using traditional multivariate statistical methods. However, reducing the data into one or two descriptive statistics, such as an average, maxima, or minima, eliminates a large amount of valuable information that cannot be summarized with one number. In traditional multivariate statistics, high correlation among predictor variables causes unstable results. Because the points of a curve in a time series are highly correlated, putting all of the points representing the curve into a multivariate analysis could result in severe collinearity. By using FDA and representing each curve as a function, it is possible to use a functional analogue of traditional methods without the problem of collinearity. An example is provided in Section 4.

3. Important considerations for curve registration

3.1 What makes a curve suitable for registration?

One advantage of FDA is that position variables, as well as their time derivatives, are all possibilities that can be considered for use in registration. However, there are characteristics associated with curves that improve registration. The presence or absence of these characteristics can suggest whether position or derivative variables should be used. The main consideration is that curves with characteristic features such as maxima, minima, or inflection points result in a set of registered curves with less phase variability compared to registering a set of curves without one or more of these features, particularly during continuous registration.

The issue of having a peak or inflection point that can be used for registration purposes is an important one. Take, for example, position data representing a chewing cycle. The chewing cycle can be defined two different ways, from maximum open to maximum open or maximum close to maximum close (Fig. 8). Defining the cycle from maximum close to maximum close produces a curve without characteristic features needed for registration. It is important to consider that position data may not always have characteristic features that are needed for registration, yet using position data is sometimes important for a particular analysis. The absence of a characteristic feature can be ameliorated in cyclical position data by two possible methods. First, one can consider dividing cycles using a different start and end event that may adjust the cycle to include a clearly defined maxima, minima, or zero crossing within the cycle. Second, a derivate of the position curves can be estimated and these derivative curves can be aligned. Once the derivative curves are aligned, the resulting time transformation information associated with each curve can be used to register the position curves. To illustrate the difference the selection of start and end events can make in the shape of the curve, Figure 8 is an example of a cycle that begins and ends with the teeth together (i.e., maximum close). Maximum opening represents the characteristics feature that can be used for registration. Therefore, a clearly defined minima is present in the displacement data. This curve can be compared to a chewing cycle that begins and ends with maximum open (see Fig. 2)

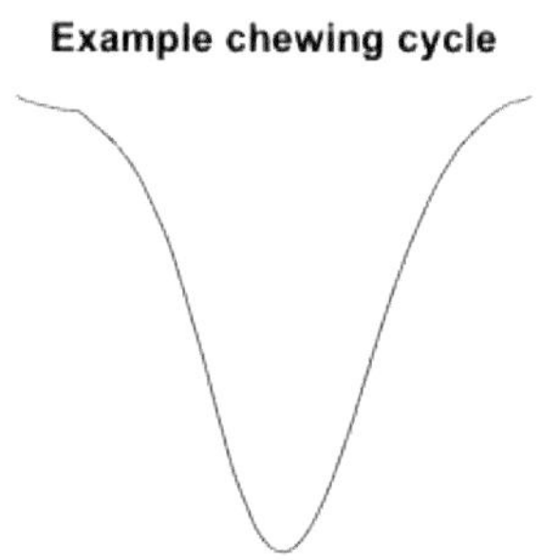

Fig. 8. Example chewing cycle define from maximum close to maximum close.

3.2 Is time normalization necessary?

As previously discussed, when curve alignment is required prior to an analysis, there are three registration methods from which to select: linear time normalization, continuous registration, and landmark registration. However, an issue occurs when working with cyclical data that require time normalization prior to continuous or landmark registration. That is, a prerequisite of the FDA registration procedures is that all curves have the same time interval. Three methods can be considered for achieving this prerequisite when cycles have variable durations.

The first method is a procedure used by Page et al. (2006) for creating a common time interval across all cycles. Their procedure recommends completing the raw data with a suitable number of pairs so that the trial with the longest duration becomes the duration for all trials. While this will work for single movements, such as the sit-to-stand movement presented in the Page et al. (2006) analysis, it does not work for cyclical data. When cycles are padded at the end to create a common time interval, artifacts are created in the data that create two problems precluding the generalization of results. First, artifacts in cyclical data change the interpretation of the actual behavior. For example, when individual chewing cycles are extended so that each cycle has the same duration, chewing is characterized as having an unusually long phase at the end of the cycle where the teeth are together (i.e., closed gape). Figure 9 illustrates a raw, unaltered cycle, the corresponding time-normalized cycle, and the cycle that has been padded at the end using Page et al. (2006) method. The problem that occurs is that the phase at the end is artificial, since it has only been added to extend the duration of the cycle. The consequence to this solution is that statistical analyses, such as functional principal component analysis or functional analysis of variance, will provide inaccurate results because data were inappropriately added to cycles, thereby changing the behavioral pattern of the movement. Therefore, the outcome of these types of typical FDA analyses will provide inaccurate results. Thus, although completing raw data may be suitable for discrete tasks, the interpretation of the behavior will be affected and incorrect if this method is applied to cyclical data.

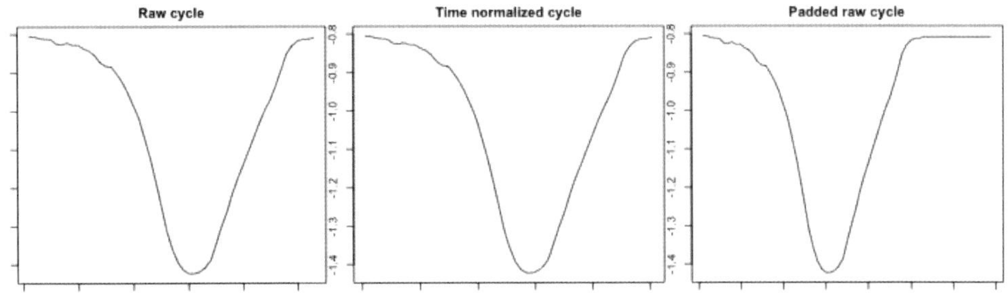

Fig. 9. Illustration of the outcome of creating a common time interval by completing the raw data with a suitable number of pairs. The new curve does not provide an accurate representation of the behavior.

As an alternative, padding cycles by evenly distributing missing values could be a potential solution. However, Figure 10 illustrates that the problem remains with the missing value method.

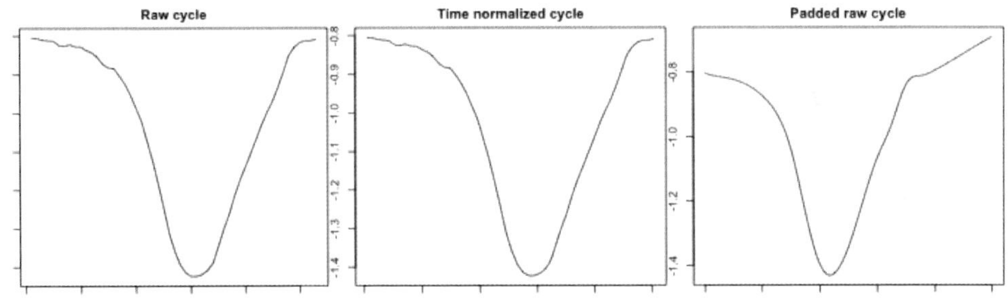

Fig. 10. Illustration of the outcome of creating a common time interval by padding the raw cycles by evenly distributing missing values. The new curve does not provide an accurate representation of the behavior.

Because a common time interval is required for FDA analyses, it is important to assess whether registration procedures are necessary after standard time normalization has been applied to the data. Crane et al. (2010) found that registration after time normalization may not always be necessary. They concluded that when obtaining an average curve was the purpose of registration, the additional alignment did not affect the interpretation of the behavior enough to warrant the additional data manipulation. So when might registration be useful? When specific functional data analyses, such as those discussed in Section 4, will be used, Crane et al. (2010) found that decreases in inter-subject variability within homogenous groups indicate registration may be justified. Because of this, when functional data analyses are used, registration improves the likelihood of finding significant differences between two or more populations, if they indeed exist.

4. Specific functional data analyses

This section discusses how the linear model, one of the classic methods of data analysis, can be extended to functional biomechanical data. We illustrate the ideas in this section using a subset of data collected as part of a study by Gross et al. (In Press) that contains knee angles during a gait cycle and height normalized walking speed for 60 trials.

4.1 Classical linear model

In the classical linear model, a response variable Y is modeled as a linear combination of predictor variables X and a random distrubance term ϵ.

$$Y = \beta_0 + \sum_{j=1}^{p} \beta_j X_j + \epsilon \tag{3}$$

We can think of β_j as the effect of X_j on the expected value of Y. Common goals of a linear model include

1. Estimating the β_j
2. Creating confidence intervals for β_j
3. Testing the hypothesis $H_0 : \beta_j = 0$

4.2 Functional linear model example

Figure 11 displays the knee angle throughout a gait cycle for one of the 60 trials. Time is normalized so that the start and end of the gait cycle are 0 and 1, respectively. Notice that peak flexion occurs at time ≈ 0.7.

Suppose we wish to investigate whether peak flexion (denoted X) can predict a scalar outcome such as walking speed (normalized velocity) Y. The method of least-squares can be used to fit a model of the form $\hat{Y} = \hat{\beta}_0 + \hat{\beta}_1 X$, where

1. $\hat{Y}$ is predicted value of Y
2. X is peak flexion
3. $\hat{\beta}_0$ is the intercept, and
4. $\hat{\beta}_1$ is the estimated effect of angle on Y

The results of the fitted linear model on the $n = 60$ trials are presented in Table 1. Note that there is no significant linear relationship between peak knee flexion and Y ($p = 0.73$)

The analysis above, however, only selects a single feature of the gait cycle (peak flexion) as a predictor of Y. An entire gait cycle contains much more information than just the maximum, and perhaps angles other than the absolute maximum can predict Y. With 100 time-normalized angle measurements on each of 60 trials, we *could* make use of all the information in a multiple regression by fitting a model of the form

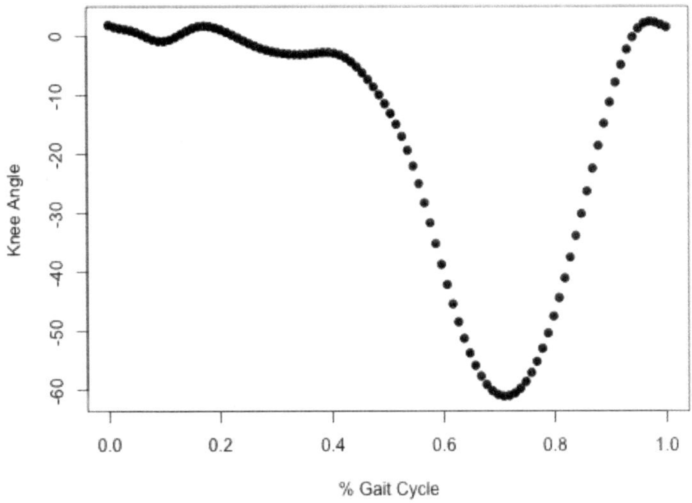

Fig. 11. Example of knee angle data from a gait cycle.

	Estimate	Std. Error	t	p-val
$\hat{\beta}_0$	0.55	.55	1.00	0.33
$\hat{\beta}_1$	-0.01	0.01	-0.34	0.73

Table 1. Y versus peak knee flexion

$$Y_i = \beta_0 + \sum_{j=1}^{100} \beta_j f_i(t_j) + \epsilon_i \tag{4}$$

- $i = 1, \ldots, 60$ indexes the trial
- t_j (j = 1, ... ,100) indexes the times during the cycle when gait is measured
- $f_i(t_j)$ denotes the knee angle for trial i at time t_j
- β_j is the effect of knee angle at time t_j on Y

This multiple regression model uses each angle measurement rather than just the angle at peak flexion. However, there are serious problems with this proposed model.

1. With 101 parameters (including the intercept) and only 60 trials, there is not enough data to reliably estimate a model of this complexity.
2. There would likely be a strong correlation between knee angles at nearby time points, causing instability in estimated effects.

The functional nature of knee angle is apparent in Figure 11. By considering the data as a sample of observations from a smooth underlying curve, we will be able to use all of the information without resorting to the problematic multiple regression model. Before fitting a functional linear model, we must first fit a smooth curve to the data in Figure 11. We do this using b-spline basis functions. To avoid overfitting, a roughness penalty is imposed on the curvature of the fitted function. The smooth fits for 3 trials are displayed in Figure 12.

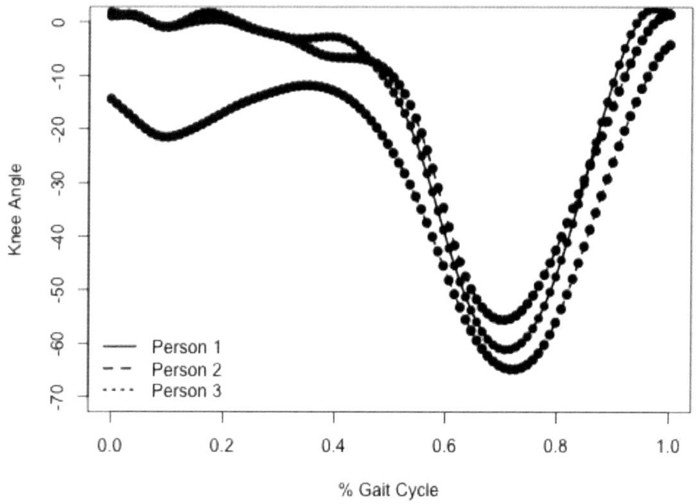

Fig. 12. Functions fit to three trials.

After estimating knee angle versus time functions for all 60 trials, we can replace the discrete angle measurements $f(t_1), ..., f(t_{100})$ with a continuous angle function $f(t)$. With this continuous function, we can write the form of the **functional** linear model:

$$y_i = \beta_0 + \int \beta(t) f_i(t) dt + \epsilon_i \tag{5}$$

In the functional linear model, $\beta(t)$ is a coefficient function whose values capture the effect of knee angle at time t on walking speed. The details of how the functional linear model is estimated are beyond the scope of this text (see Ramsay et al. (2009) for more details). The results, however, describe the power of the functional linear model. Figure 13 shows how knee angle affects Y at various points in the gait cycle. Recall that the results from the ordinary linear regression of Y versus maximum angle showed no relationship. This is consistent with Figure 13 which shows $\beta(t)$ close to 0 near the times of peak flexion (typically occurring between 0.71 and 0.73). Both the functional model and the ordinary linear model show no substantial relationship between Y and knee angle in this range of the gait cycle. The functional linear model does indicate that knee angle between .31 and .46, .55 and .64, as well as .85 and .95 seem to have an association with Y. When the confidence bands for the coefficient function are entirely above 0, this indicates that individuals with greater extension at these stages tend to also have an increased gait velocity Y. When the confidence bands for the coefficient are entirely below 0, this indicates that individuals with greater flexion at these stages tend to have a decreased velocity.

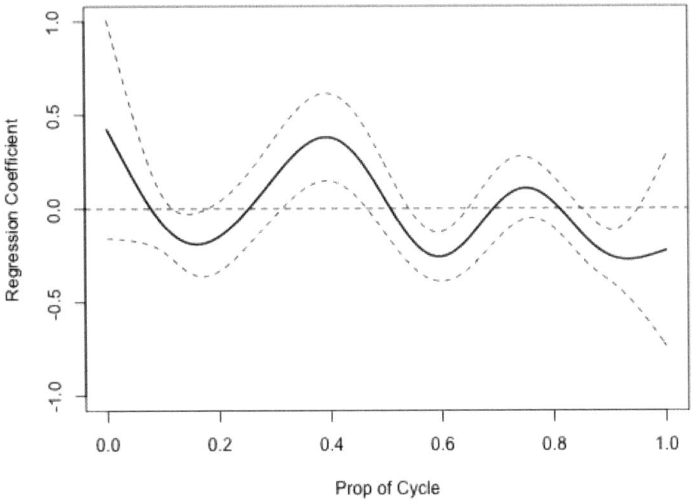

Fig. 13. Regression coefficient associated with the functional linear model. Dashed lines represent the 95% confidence interval. When this interval does not include zero there is a significant relationship between knee angle and Y.

4.3 Other functional data analyses

This section illustrates how the functional linear model reveals a more complete picture of a relationship than analysis of features (such as maxima). Our example involves a scalar outcome, but methodology exists for functional outcomes as well. Various other classic statistical methods also have functional analogues, including Analysis of Variance, Canonical Correlations, and Principal Components.

5. Implementation

The following code can be implemented in R (R Development Core Team, 2010) , an open source statistical software package. Once R is installed, the fda library (Ramsay et al., 2010) as well as the CraneLib will need to be installed. The fda library contains the functions that perform the procedures discussed in this chapter. The CraneLib contains the example data needed to run the following example.

```
library(fda)
library(CraneLib)
matplot(dataset)

knots=c(0,.2,.4,.6,.8,1)
mybasis <- create.bspline.basis(rangeval=c(0, 1), nbasis=NULL,
    norder=4, breaks=knots,
```

```
dropind=NULL, quadvals=NULL, values=NULL, names="bspl")
myfd <- Data2fd(dataset,argvals=seq(0, 1, len = 101),
    basisobj=mybasis)

plot(myfd)
plot(myfd[1]) # plots the first function
plot(myfd[1:3]) # plots the first three functions

samples <- seq(0,1, length=101)
par(mfrow=c(1,1), pty="m")
plotfit.fd(dataset, samples, myfd)

lambda <- 1e-12
norder <- 6
samples <- seq(0,1, length=101)
nbasis <- length(samples) + norder-2
mybasis <- create.bspline.basis(c(0,1), nbasis, norder, samples)
myfdPar <- fdPar(mybasis, 4, lambda)
myfd <- smooth.basis(samples, dataset, myfdPar)$fd

plot(myfd)
plot(myfd[1]) # plots the first function
plot(myfd[1:3]) # plots the first three functions

par(mfrow=c(1,1), pty="m")
plotfit.fd(dataset, samples, myfd)

FirstDeriv <- deriv.fd(myfd, 1)
plot(FirstDeriv)

DerivMat <- eval.fd(samples, FirstDeriv)
DerivMat[,1]

lambda <- 1
nbasis <- myfd$basis$nbasis
ntrials <- dim(dataset)[2]
y0fd <- mean.fd(myfd)
yfd <- myfd
y0vec <- eval.fd(samples, y0fd)
yvec <- eval.fd(samples, yfd)
coef0 <- matrix(0, nrow=nbasis, ncol=ntrials)
Wfd0 <- fd(coef0, mybasis)
WfdPar <- fdPar(Wfd0, 2, lambda)
reglist <- register.fd(y0fd, yfd, WfdPar, iterlim = 10, dbglev = 1)

names(reglist)
plot(reglist$regfd)
```

```
plot(reglist$warpfd)

origMean <- mean.fd(myfd)
regMean <- mean.fd(reglist$regfd)

plot(origMean)
lines(regMean, col=2)
```

6. Conclusions

Functional Data Analysis is an important analytical method that can be used for exploratory and hypothesis driven analyses. A primary advantage to FDA is the ability to assess continuous data that change over time without having to reduce the signal into discrete variables. However, there are some important issues for biomechanists to be aware of when implementing this set of statistical tools. Therefore, this chapter provided an overview of the steps associated with FDA, focused on issues related to aligning curves from cyclical data, discussed specific statistical analytical techniques, and finally provided an example using sample code in R.

7. References

Chester, V. L. & Wrigley, A. T. (2008). The identification of age-related differences in kinetic gait parameters using principal component analysis, *Clinical Biomechanics* 23(2): 212–220.

Crane, E. A., Cassidy, R. B., Rothman, E. D. & Gerstner, G. E. (2010). Effect of registration on cyclical kinematic data, *Journal of Biomechanics* 43(12): 2444–2447. doi:10.1016/j.jbiomech.2010.04.024.

Deluzio, K. J. & Astephen, J. L. (2007). Biomechanical features of gait waveform data associated with knee osteoarthritis: An application of principal component analysis, *Gait & Posture* 25(1): 86–93.

Gross, M. M., Crane, E. A. & Fredrickson, B. (In Press). Effort-shape and kinematic assessment of bodily expression of emotion during gait, *Human Movement Science* . doi:10.1016/j.humov.2011.05.001.

Landry, S. C., McKean, K. A., Hubley-Kozey, C. L., Stanish, W. D. & Deluzio, K. J. (2007). Knee biomechanics of moderate oa patients measured during gait at a self-selected and fast walking speed, *Journal of Biomechanics* 40(8): 1754–1761.

Lee, M., Roan, M. & Smith, B. (2009). An application of principal component analysis for lower body kinematics between loaded and unloaded walking, *Journal of Biomechanics* 42(14): 2226–2230.

Page, A., Ayala, G., LeÛn, M. T., Peydro, M. F. & Prat, J. M. (2006). Normalizing temporal patterns to analyze sit-to-stand movements by using registration of functional data, *Journal of Biomechanics* 39(13): 2526–2534.

R Development Core Team (2010). *R: A Language and Environment for Statistical Computing*, R Foundation for Statistical Computing, Vienna, Austria. ISBN 3-900051-07-0. URL: *http://www.R-project.org/*

Ramsay, J. O. (2000). Functional components of variaion in handwriting, *Journal of the American Statistical Association* 95(449): 9.

Ramsay, J. O., Hooker, G. & Graves, S. (2009). *Functional Data Analysis with R and MATLAB*, Use R!, Spinger, New York.

Ramsay, J. O. & Silverman, B. W. (2002). *Applied functional data analysis: methods and case studies*, Springer series in statistics, Springer, New York.

Ramsay, J. O. & Silverman, B. W. (2005). *Functional data analysis*, Springer series in statistics, 2 edn, Springer, New York.

Ramsay, J. O., Wickham, H., Graves, S. & Hooker, G. (2010). *fda: Functional Data Analysis*. R package version 2.2.5.
URL: *http://CRAN.R-project.org/package=fda*

Røislien, J., Skare, O., Gustavsen, M., Broch, N. L., Rennie, L. & Opheim, A. (2009). Simultaneous estimation of effects of gender, age and walking speed on kinematic gait data, *Gait & Posture* 30(4): 441–445.

Sadeghi, H., Allard, P., Barbier, F., Sadeghi, S., Hinse, S., Perrault, R. & Labelle, H. (2002). Main functional roles of knee flexors/extensors in able-bodied gait using principal component analysis (i), *The Knee* 9(1): 47–53.

Sadeghi, H., Prince, F., Sadeghi, S. & Labelle, H. (2000). Principal component analysis of the power developed in the flexion/extension muscles of the hip in able-bodied gait, *Medical Engineering & Physics* 22(10): 703–710.

7

Biomechanical Models of Endodontic Restorations

Antonio Pérez-González, Carmen González-Lluch, Joaquín L. Sancho-Bru, Pablo J. Rodríguez-Cervantes and José L. Iserte-Vilar
Universitat Jaume I
Spain

1. Introduction

Endodontic treatment is one of the most widely used techniques in present-day odontology owing to the tendency to save teeth whenever possible. In endodontic therapy, the injured pulp of a tooth (located in the interior of the tooth and containing nerves and other vital tissues) is cleaned out and then the space is disinfected and subsequently filled with restorative material. This process is commonly known as root canal treatment. The devitalised tooth resulting from endodontics, has a different stiffness and resistance as compared to the original tooth and is less resistant as a consequence of the loss of tooth structure (Walton & Torabinejad, 2002). The use of intraradicular posts has extended as a technique to restore teeth that have lost a considerable amount of coronal tooth structure. After removing the pulp, the intraradicular post is introduced into the devitalised root. The post helps to support the final restoration and join it to the root (Christensen, 1998). Fig. 1a shows the typical structure of a tooth endodontically restored with a post. The post is inserted into the devitalised root canal, which has previously been obturated at its apical end with a biocompatible polymer called gutta-percha. Cement is used to bond the post to the root canal and a core is placed over the remaining dentine and the post. Finally, an artificial crown is used to achieve an external appearance that is similar to that of the original tooth. Nowadays most of the posts are prefabricated in a range of different materials and designs (Scotti & Ferrari, 2004). However, before prefabricated post became generalised, cast post and cores were used as a single metal alloy unit (Fig. 1b). Cast post-core systems take longer to make and involve an intermediate laboratory stage in which the retention system is created, which makes the whole process more costly. In comparison, prefabricated posts do not need this intermediate stage, which means that the whole restoration process can be performed in a single visit and is obviously easier and cheaper for the patient (Christensen, 1998). Nonetheless, the adaptation of the prefabricated posts to the root canal may be less accurate (Chan et al., 1993).

As the endodontically restored tooth is composed of materials that are different to those of natural teeth, it is expected to have a different biomechanical response under oral loads. The deformation of the system under flexural, compressive or tension forces could be different and so its mechanical strength under static or fatigue loads. Ideally, it seems interesting that the biomechanical behaviour of the restored system should preferably resemble that of the original tooth as much as possible in order to avoid failure of the repaired tooth or its antagonists or adjacent teeth. Nevertheless, this is only an ideal for endodontic therapy and actual restored teeth would differ from this ideal depending on the geometry of the remaining tooth structure, the material and geometry of the components used in the restoration and the technique used by the dentist.

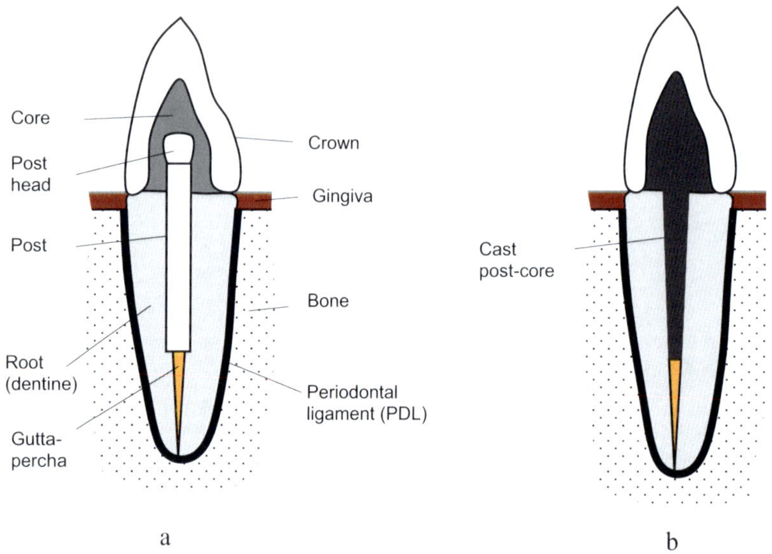

Fig. 1. Endodontic restoration with prefabricated post (a) and cast post-core (b)

The interest in performing an in-depth analysis of the mechanical response of restored teeth becomes apparent from the above considerations and in last few decades a considerable amount of research has been devoted to this objective. Some works have compared this mechanical response with that of natural teeth and others have studied the effect of using different procedures or components for the restoration in order to obtain conclusions about which is preferable for clinical use. The conclusions from these investigations have contributed to the advance of the restorative techniques in Endodontics, that have allowed achieving higher survival rates.

With regard to the methodology used in this field of research, three main lines are distinguished: *in vitro* experimentation, retrospective clinical studies and studies with numerical biomechanical models. The first usually covers the effects of the specific parameters (material, post design, post length or post diameter) on the resistance or the retention of the restoration (Fokkinga et al., 2005; Gallo et al., 2002; Pereira et al., 2006). The majority of these works are static experiments and very few studies have been carried out under cyclic loading or fatigue (Isidor et al., 1999; Sahafi et al., 2005). Retrospective studies are less common given that they require longer times to be performed, often years, and they are based on the study of failures in restorations performed on real patients (Fox et al., 2004; Nothdurft & Pospiech, 2006; Torbjorner et al., 1995). Although working conditions are the current oral dynamic conditions in these studies, the results may be conditioned by loss of control over parameters that are beyond the scope of what is being studied owing to the variability that exists from one patient to another. Finally, the number of studies based on numerical biomechanical models has considerably increased considerably in recent years (Barjau-Escribano et al., 2006; Boschian Pest et al., 2006; Genovese et al., 2005; Pegoretti et al., 2002). These biomechanical models mainly use the finite element analysis (FEA) technique to obtain a numerical representation of the real system and to compute mechanical stresses and strains under simulated loads. In FEA, the system to be studied is divided into a set of small discrete elements (finite elements, FE) defined by a limited number of nodes. A simplified constitutive equation for the finite elements is defined to represent their mechanical response, as a relationship between nodal loads and nodal displacements, and is expressed as the stiffness matrix of the element. By forcing the nodes shared by adjacent elements to have the same displacements, the element stiffness matrices of the elements are combined to give the global stiffness matrix. Nodal displacements can be solved by imposing boundary conditions on this problem, i.e. applied loads and forced displacements and, subsequently, the strains and stresses are then calculated from them. As the size of the finite elements decreases (thus increasing the number of elements), the accuracy of the method increases, but at the same time the computational cost also increases significantly.

The use of FEA for studying the restored tooth has some advantages with respect to the other alternatives cited above. Its main advantage is that it allows a highly controlled analysis of one or several specific parameters on a single tooth model. This results in a better comprehension of either the individual effect or that combined with different parameters. Moreover, numerical analysis with biomechanical models is faster and cheaper than *in vitro* experimentation and eliminates the ethical implications related with the collection of real tooth specimens for *in vitro* experiments or invasive *in vivo* measurements. In contrast, FEA also has some drawbacks namely, the clinical application of their results is conditioned by the accuracy of the model and its previous validation based on experimental data.

In this chapter, a comprehensive review of the state of the art of biomechanical models of endodontic restorations is presented. First, we describe a review of the evolution of these models throughout their brief history. Then, the different aspects related to the definition of the model are analysed with reference to the way they were treated in previous models in the literature. Finally, we provide an overview of the main conclusions reached in previous studies using biomechanical models about the effect of the different parameters involved in the endodontic restoration. Lastly, we present possible lines for future research that can be pursued in this field in order to obtain more comprehensive and accurate models.

2. Historical overview of biomechanical models for simulating endodontic restorations

FEA was developed in the fifties of the last century in the aircraft industry and was not used in dentistry until the seventies. One of the first works on the subject was the doctoral dissertation of Farah, at the University of Michigan, in 1972, which dealt with the simulation of molar restoration using photoelasticity and FEA. Some later works were presented by this research group in following years (Craig & Farah, 1977; Farah et al., 1973; Farah & Craig, 1974). Other pioneering works in those years were presented by Thresher and Saito (Thresher & Saito, 1973) and Selna et al.(Selna et al., 1975). These first works were two-dimensional and were conducted with programs developed by the researchers themselves. Later, the advances in computer resources and in commercial software for FEA extended the use of different commercial programs, allowing more accurate and predictive three-dimensional models to be developed (Asmussen et al., 2005; Barjau-Escribano et al., 2006;

Boschian Pest et al., 2006; Ferrari et al., 2008; Genovese et al., 2005; Gonzalez-Lluch et al., 2009b; Maceri et al., 2009; Rodríguez-Cervantes et al., 2007; Sorrentino et al., 2007).
The number of publications dealing with FE simulation in endodontics has increased exponentially in recent years. For example, in 2011 a manual search in the SCOPUS database in 2011 for papers containing simultaneously the terms *finite element* and *endodontic* within journals on the subjects of Engineering and Medicine and Dentistry found 14 papers until 2000, 31 papers from 2000 to 2009 and 11 papers in the short period including 2010 and first two months of 2011.
The number of elements in the mesh has an influence on the number of degrees of freedom considered in the FE model. Using a mesh with a smaller element size is equivalent to increasing the number of elements and nodes of the model and consequently in the number of degrees of freedom of the problem. This number of degrees of freedom has also increased exponentially in recent years, as shown in Fig. 2.

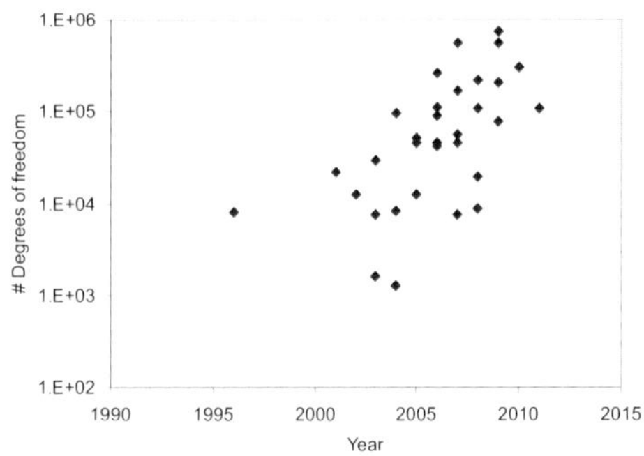

Fig. 2. Number of degrees of freedom of FE models in different works from the literature.

Most of the studies about endodontic restorations using FEA have dealt with incisor teeth, followed by premolars, molars and canines. In the majority of those works, the teeth were analysed under masticatory loads, although other load types, such as bruxism or accidental loads, were also simulated. The development of computers and simulation software has allowed more detailed models. Although an increasing number of studies consider all the components of the restored tooth in the model, other studies still simplify the model by eliminating some of the components. Sometimes the final crown is not included for the sake of simplification (Rodríguez-Cervantes et al., 2007), while in other cases the periodontal ligament (PDL), the luting cement, or both, are left out to simplify the model (Adanir & Belli, 2007; Asmussen et al., 2005; Hsu et al., 2009; Yaman et al., 2004; Zarone et al., 2006).
To date, most of the FE models have been linear and static. In linear static models, the stress-strain curve representing the material behaviour has a constant slope and the materials undergo deformation below their proportional limit. However, in some realistic situations this analysis is not accurate. Wakabayashi et al. (Wakabayashi et al., 2008) cited three main causes of non-linearity: (1) material non-linearities, like the response of the PDL, (2) the changing interrelation of objects, as when loads introduce contacts between components, and (3) geometric nonlinearities, as a consequence of large deformations in some components. In recent years, some works have introduced non-linear FE models as a better way to represent the response of endodontic restorations (Sorrentino et al., 2009; Uddanwadiker et al., 2007). On

the other hand, masticatory loads are variable, implying that the restoration is subject to fatigue, but very few fatigue simulations are found in the literature up until now (Huysmans & Van der Varst, 1993). The authors have recently presented a study on fatigue simulation of a whole endodontic restoration (Sancho-Bru et al., 2009).

3. Biomechanical model definition

The validity of the conclusions reached from biomechanical models of the endodontic restoration will depend on the accuracy with which these models can represent the real system. A number of different factors related to the definition of the model conditions the quality of the results obtained from FEA, namely the accuracy of the geometric representation of the system, the components included in the model, the quality of the discretisation and the constitutive equations for finite elements, the material properties, or the boundary conditions. Moreover, processing and interpreting the results is a challenging task that can compromise accuracy of the conclusions from FEA. All these questions are reviewed in this section.

3.1 Geometric model

The first step in the generation of an FE model is to obtain a geometrical representation of the real system. Some models use a simplified representation of the geometrical shape of the tooth, using elliptical paraboloids or similar shapes to represent the root (Asmussen et al., 2005; Bourauel et al., 2000; Holmes et al., 1996) or cylindrical blocks to represent the alveolar bone (Barjau-Escribano et al., 2006; Holmes et al., 1996; Mezzomo et al., 2011). Other researchers have tried to represent the real geometry better by using anatomical data (Adanir & Belli, 2007; Lanza et al., 2005), X-ray images (Maceri et al., 2007) or CT data (Magne, 2007; Tajima et al., 2009). Authors using two-dimensional data sometimes make use of appropriate algorithms to obtain a three-dimensional model (Maceri et al., 2007). With advances in CAD software and 3D scanning methods, most of the recent works obtain the external geometry of a real representative tooth or a plaster model using 3D digitising scanners (Ausiello et al., 2001; Ferrari et al., 2008; Ichim et al., 2006) and import it into a 3D CAD software application. The geometrical representation of the different components of the restoration is obtained later in CAD using Boolean algebra. The authors recently used this procedure (Gonzalez-Lluch et al., 2009b) to obtain a realistic geometrical model of a maxillary central incisor, which is shown, in a sagittal section, in Fig. 3.

3.2 Components in the model

The natural tooth is the reference for comparing the biomechanical behaviour of an endodontic restoration. Several works in the literature have modelled the natural tooth (Dejak et al., 2003; Middleton et al., 1996; Zarone et al., 2006). Most of modelled natural teeth included enamel, dentine, cortical and cancellous bone, pulp and ligament (Middleton et al., 1996; Rees & Jacobsen, 1997). Some of them did not include the ligament (Zarone et al., 2006). These studies used the model of the natural tooth to compare the calculated biomechanical response with the experimental results (Rees & Jacobsen, 1997), to evaluate the behaviour of a restored tooth against a natural tooth (Davy et al., 1981; Maceri et al., 2009; Soares et al., 2008b; Zarone et al., 2006) or both (Ferrari et al., 2008). Cementum is not considered in most of the models, due to its reduced thickness, although a recent work (Ren et al., 2010) has reported the importance of the cemento-dentinal junction and cementum in stress distribution in the root and the ligament.

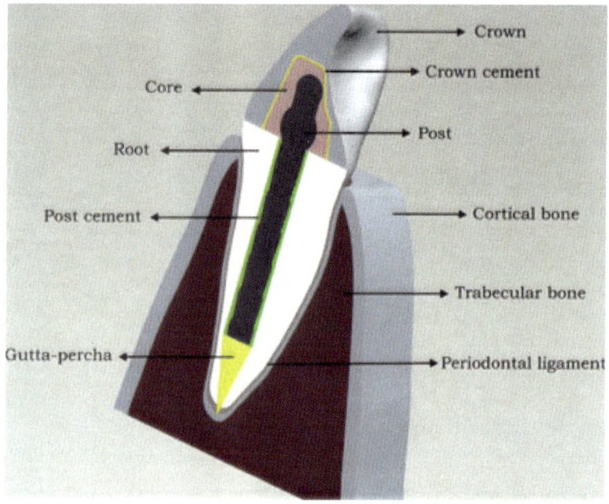

Fig. 3. Sagittal section of an endodontically restored maxillary central incisor

Previous works simulating post-core endodontic restorations have not always included all the actual components of the restoration. Some works assumed that bone deformation is negligible and did not include this component in the model (Boschian Pest et al., 2006; Davy et al., 1981; Maceri et al., 2009). Not all models in the literature include the bone. When included, sometimes it is modelled with uniform properties (Imanishi et al., 2003; Nakamura et al., 2006), although most of the models consider the cancellous bone and a layer of cortical bone near the bone surface (Asmussen et al., 2005; Gonzalez-Lluch et al., 2009b).

Thin structures, such as the PDL and cement are not always considered in the FE models. In natural teeth, the PDL thickness is approximately between 0.125 mm and 0.375 mm (Rees & Jacobsen, 1997). This range is covered in different biomechanical models (Asmussen et al., 2005; Boschian Pest et al., 2006; Ferrari et al., 2008; Ichim et al., 2006; Soares et al., 2010). However, some works did not include the ligament (Yaman et al., 1998; Zarone et al., 2006), despite it has been reported that stress distribution is affected to an important degree by this omission (Davy et al., 1981) or even by a geometrically simplified representation (Toms & Eberhardt, 2003). When cement layers are considered in the biomechanical model, they are usually represented with a constant small thickness (Asmussen et al., 2005; Maceri et al., 2009; Okamoto et al., 2008; Schmitter et al., 2010). However, some works simplify the model by obviating the cement in the interface between the core and the crown (Gonzalez-Lluch et al., 2009b; Lanza et al., 2005) or even in the interface between the post and the root (Adanir & Belli, 2007; Hsu et al., 2009).

Several types of endodontic posts can be found in the literature (Christensen, 1998; Fernandes et al., 2003). Originally, cast post-core systems were used as a single metal alloy unit. Subsequently, prefabricated posts made out of stainless steel, titanium or precious metals were used, while more recently prefabricated fibre posts were introduced. All these post types have been studied with FE models.

Some earlier laboratory studies maintain that preparing a ferrule might improve the resistance of post-core system (Assif & Gorfil, 1994; Aykent et al., 2006; Ichim et al., 2006; Tan et al., 2005; Zhi-Yue & Yu-Xing, 2003). Accordingly, many works in the literature prepared a ferrule of varying heights in the biomechanical model: 2 mm (Mezzomo et al.,

2011; Uddanwadiker et al., 2007), 2.5 mm (Coelho et al., 2009) , 1 mm (Toksavul et al., 2006). Ichim et al. (Ichim et al., 2006) prepared biomechanical models without a ferrule and with a ferrule of different heights (0.5, 1.0, 1.5, 2 mm) to study its effect on the strength of the restoration.

3.3 Mesh definition

Mesh definition is a key point in FEA. The mechanical behaviour of a continuous domain with an infinite number of degrees of freedom is approximated in the model with the simplified mechanical response of a set of discrete finite elements with a limited number of degrees of freedom. This process occurs when a mesh of finite elements is defined for the original system. The accuracy of the results is highly dependent on the characteristics of this mesh. A coarse mesh will produce results in a short computation time, but the accuracy of these results will be compromised. A finer mesh may improve the validity of the results but with the cost of a higher processing time. A coarse mesh is affected by two main sources of error: firstly, an error is introduced in representing the boundaries of the real geometry; and secondly, the mechanical response of the continuous material in each finite element is represented by a simplified polynomial function, which is only an approximation of the actual response. In biomechanical applications, such as dentistry, the geometry of the real system is highly irregular, so the mesh density should be enough to obtain a good geometrical representation.

Generation of a good mesh of FE for a restored tooth is always a challenge. The complicated shape of the tooth makes it difficult to produce a mesh manually. Moreover, some elements of a dental restoration present dimensions that are quite different from one another. For example, the luting cement used to bond the post to the root, or the PDL, have a thickness of a fraction of a millimetre, which is much smaller than the post dimensions, although its total length would be of several millimetres. To obtain a good mesh, a small element size has to be used in this thinner component, but such a size cannot be maintained for all the components, because, otherwise, the number of degrees of freedom would increase to a limit beyond the capacity of the computer or the computation time would increase excessively. A good meshing strategy should increase mesh density in areas where a greater expected stress gradient is expected or with thinner components, and increase the size of the elements in other parts of the model. Two different basic strategies can be used to improve finite element results from a first tentative model, namely the h-method or the p-method (Zienkiewicz & Taylor, 1989). In the h-method, the mesh is refined using elements of a smaller size, whereas in the p-method, the size of the elements is maintained but the order of the interpolation function is increased. A mixed strategy that combines both options can also be used. Most of the works in the literature about endodontic simulation use finite elements with linear or quadratic interpolation and refine the mesh using smaller elements to improve the representation, so the h-method is prevalent.

The first FE models used two-dimensional finite elements to represent the tooth and endodontic restoration (Craig & Farah, 1977; Davy et al., 1981), assuming the axisymmetric or plane strain hypothesis. In these planar models triangular or quadrangular elements with three or four nodes, respectively, are used to mesh the system. The size of the finite elements in these first models was relatively large owing to the limitations in computer resources. Davy et al. (Davy et al., 1981) used quadrangular elements for an incisor and tested different meshes to decide on the mesh density by comparing displacements of selected nodes. Finally the finer mesh tested was selected, with elements of about 1 mm in the coronal-apical direction and with a dimension close to 0.3 mm in the lingual-vestibular direction in the cervical area. Middleton et al. (Middleton et al., 1996) used quadrangular elements with eight nodes to study the effect of the PDL in bone modelling. Although the mesh used for tooth and bone was relatively coarse, the ligament was modelled with a much finer mesh, as it was the part of interest in that particular study. More recently, Pegoretti et al. (Pegoretti et al., 2002) also used plain strain two-dimensional elements and modelled the endodontic restoration using about 4000 quadrilateral elements of four nodes. The mesh presented in that work employed elements with an aspect ratio close to one and smaller elements were used near the cement and for the ligament. The aspect ratio for a finite element is the ratio of the longest to the shortest side of the element and should be as close to one as possible in order to minimise possible inaccuracies in the model. In other recent two-dimensional model, convergence tests were used to recommend the element size of 0.1 mm (Coelho et al., 2009). These planar FE models are simplifications of the real system and hence limited. Although they can be explained by the computer limitations in the last few decades, they are no longer justified nowadays. Some authors present pseudo three-dimensional models to represent the tooth (Adanir & Belli, 2007; Li et al., 2006). They obtain a planar representation of the geometry from a sagittal section of the tooth and then a solid from an extrusion normal to this planar model, using a fictitious small thickness. This approach is doubtful because it is as assuming a planar stress hypothesis, which is difficult to justify with the geometry of the real tooth. Similarly, an assumption of planar strain or axisymmetry is difficult to justify if a three-dimensional model can be used.

Three-dimensional models have been used extensively for simulating endodontic treatment since the beginning of the century (Asmussen et al., 2005; Ausiello et al., 2002; Barjau-Escribano et al., 2006; Boschian Pest et al., 2006; Genovese et al., 2005; Lanza et al., 2005). In recent years some of the most complete three-dimensional models ever developed for studying the biomechanics of endodontic restorations have been reported (Ferrari et al., 2008; Garbin et al., 2010; Gonzalez-Lluch et al., 2009b; Maceri et al., 2009; Mezzomo et al., 2011; Okamoto et al., 2008; Schmitter et al., 2010). In these three-dimensional models, tetrahedral or hexahedral finite elements are used. The mesh is created normally using the mesher of a commercial finite element package software, such as Ansys (Garbin et al., 2010; Hsu et al., 2009; Mezzomo et al., 2011), MSC-Nastran (Gonzalez-Lluch et al., 2009b; Maceri et al., 2009; Rodríguez-Cervantes et al., 2007), MSC-Marc (Okada et al., 2008; Pegoretti et al., 2002) or Cosmos (Ichim et al., 2006). In those cases, a tetrahedral mesh is the typical option because of the complicated geometries of the tooth. As an example, Fig. 4 shows a sagittal section of a mesh using tetrahedral elements for a restored incisor, generated by the authors using the Pro/Engineer FEM mesher. Some works, however, have used hexahedral elements (Ferrari et al., 2008; Okamoto et al., 2008; Schmitter et al., 2010; Zarone et al., 2006), which provide models with good results using fewer degrees of freedom, but at the cost of a more difficult mesh generation. In some models, elements with quadratic interpolation, i.e. 20-node hexahedral or 10-node tetrahedral, are used to improve the results (Maceri et al., 2009; Schmitter et al., 2010). Some attempts have been made in recent years to automate the process of creating high-quality meshes using hexahedral elements from anatomical CT data (Clement et al., 2004).

The use of convergence tests is the most commonly reported method for deciding mesh density in the majority of previous works (Ferrari et al., 2008; Maceri et al., 2009; Schmitter et al., 2010). Some authors report special attention to the convergence of results near the more stressed area, such as the post-cement interface and the cemento-enamel junction (Garbin et al., 2010; Zarone et al., 2006). However, no explicit mention is made of the parameter used to test the convergence in most of the works. Hsu et al. (Hsu et al., 2009) based convergence on the total deformation and established a difference of 1% as the limit to consider convergence. The number of nodes and elements for some three-dimensional models of the endodontically restored tooth are presented in the Table 1. It can be observed that a lower number of elements are used when the mesh is composed of hexahedral elements. The average size of elements in most of these models is close to 0.2 mm or 0.3 mm (Gonzalez-Lluch et al., 2009b; Maceri et al., 2009). The authors have shown that a mesh control of 0.3 mm is a good compromise between accuracy and computation time (Gonzalez-Lluch et al., 2009a).

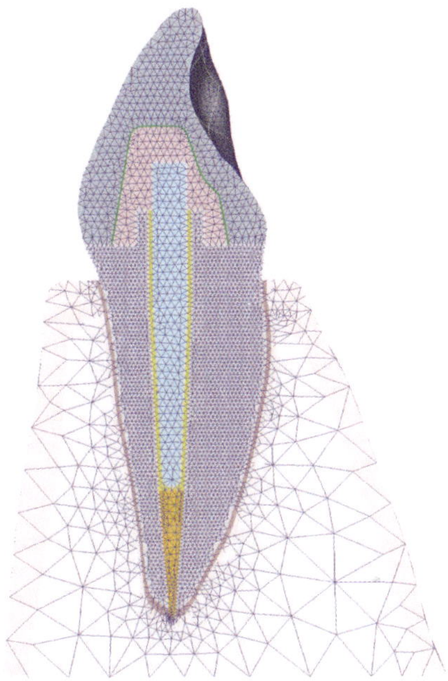

Fig. 4. Sagittal section of a typical mesh with tetrahedral elements for a restored tooth

Reference	# Elements	# Nodes	Type of element
(Zarone et al., 2006)	13272	15152	8-node hexahedral
(Ferrari et al., 2008)	31240	35841	8-node hexahedral
(Gonzalez-Lluch et al., 2009b)	399000	69000	4-node tetrahedral
(Maceri et al., 2009)	130000	185000	10-node tetrahedral
(Schmitter et al., 2010)	95000	100000	20-node hexahedral
(Mezzomo et al., 2011)	23000-33000	30000-42000	4-node tetrahedral

Table 1. Type and number of elements and number of nodes of selected FE models

The assumption of perfect adherence between adjacent components is the rule of thumb for most of the FE models presented in the literature, i.e. nodes located on the contacting surfaces of two components are shared by these components. Post cement is normally supposed to be joined perfectly to the root dentine and to the post. However, some works represent some exceptions to this habitual modelling hypothesis. Ausiello et al. (Ausiello et al., 2002) modelled the adhesive layer in composite restorations of premolars using spring elements, which allow different normal and shear stiffness to be represented, and a good agreement with experimental data was obtained. This representation of cement was also repeated in later works by the same group (Ferrari et al., 2008; Maceri et al., 2009). Schmitter et al. (Schmitter et al., 2010) modelled different debonding states in the adhesive layers, by introducing gaps between components, to investigate possible failure modes and to compare with experimental results and a similar procedure was used by Ichim et al. (Ichim et al., 2006). Asmussen et al. (Asmussen et al., 2005) used contact finite elements to simulate non-bonding states. These contact elements allow a separation between contacting surfaces but not interpenetration between them and can simulate shear friction in the contact area. Finally, in one recent study (Garbin et al., 2010) the cement layer was modelled using shell elements in Ansys.

Different types of finite elements have been used to represent the PDL. Most of the works represent the ligament with solid isotropic elements filling the reduced thickness of the ligament, but other authors use spring elements (Maceri et al., 2009), beam elements (Freitas Junior et al., 2010) or shell elements (Garbin et al., 2010). Finally, in order to represent the viscoelastic behaviour of the ligament better, (Natali et al., 2004) proposed the use of a finite element with customised formulation, using a specific Helmholtz free-energy density. To the authors' knowledge, however, this model has not been used to simulate endodontic restorations.

3.4 Material properties

Material properties are one of the key points in the definition of the model. Accuracy of the results will depend on a good representation of the actual material properties, which are not always well known. Most of the FE models assume the materials of the restored tooth are isotropic, homogeneous, elastic and linear. A material is considered homogenous if its composition can be considered as being the same at all the points, isotropic if the mechanical response is indifferent to the direction of the applied forces, elastic if it returns to the undeformed position after releasing the applied load, and linear if load and deformation are proportional. These four hypotheses are typical in a great part of all FE models in engineering, resulting in linear models for which the response (stress or strain) is proportional to the applied load. Although they allow the definition and interpretation of the model to be simplified to an important extent, these hypotheses can introduce errors in the representation of certain materials. In endodontic restoration, some materials such as bone, dentine, fibre posts or the PDL are known to be anisotropic and even not homogeneous. For example, van-Ruijven et al. (van Ruijven et al., 2006) reported that neglecting the non-homogeneity of the alveolar bone results in important changes in stresses and strains in the model. Moreover, the mechanical response of the PDL has been reported to be non-linear and viscoelastic (Pini et al., 2002). However, not only is the model that is used to represent material important, but also the numerical values of the mechanical properties, such as Young's modulus and Poisson's ratio, are of great importance to obtain an accurate model. Reported values from different sources vary markedly due to the technical problems associated to testing small specimens (Anusavice, 2003). Moreover, some data are not easily available, especially when considering commercial restorative materials. Table 2 shows the range of elastic properties used in different recent biomechanical models in the literature.

Material	Young's modulus (GPa)	Poisson's ratio
Dentine	15-18.6	0.30-0.32
Enamel	41-84.1	0.30-0.33
Cementum	13.7-18.7	0.30
Cancellous bone	0.345-1.37	0.22-0.31
Cortical bone	10.7-13.8	0.22-0.31
Periodontal ligament (PDL)	0.05-0.0689 (*)	0.45-0.49
Resin composite	6-20	0.24-0.35
Cement	4.5-95	0.22-0.35
Glass fibre	20-45	0.25-0.30
Stainless steel	207-210	0.30
Gold alloy	93-120	0.33-0.44
Titanium alloy	107	0.34
Gutta-percha	0.00069(*)-0.1	0.30-0.49
Porcelain	68.8-69	0.28
Amalgam	13.72	0.33
Zirconia	205-210	0.30-0.31
Ceramic	62-380	0.25-0.31

(*) With respect to the value of $6.89 \cdot 10^{-2}$ GPa for the elastic modulus of the PDL and the value of $6.9 \cdot 10^{-4}$ GPa for that of gutta-percha, used in many works, a recent paper (Ruse, 2008) has argued that these data are erroneous and have been disseminated by hundreds of work using FEA in recent years as a consequence of a lack of rigour when it comes to citing and checking original papers. Following Ruse, correct values for the PDL are three orders of magnitude lower and for gutta-percha at least two orders of magnitude greater.

Table 2. Range of values for elastic properties for dental materials used in some FE models (Ferrari et al., 2008; Ferrari et al., 2008; Garbin et al., 2010; Gonzalez-Lluch et al., 2009b; Hsu et al., 2009; Maceri et al., 2009; Mezzomo et al., 2011; Okamoto et al., 2008; Schmitter et al., 2010; Suzuki et al., 2008; Toparli, 2003).

In almost all FE models in the literature, the materials of the natural tooth (dentine and enamel) are considered homogeneous, isotropic and elastic. However, in a critical review of the literature Kinney et al. (Kinney et al., 2003) showed that dentine exhibits an hexagonal anisotropy in the Young's modulus with a greater value (36 GPa) in the direction of the tubules than in the orthogonal direction (29 GPa). Later, Ferrari et al. considered this with an orthotropic model for dentine in the FE model (Ferrari et al., 2008). Kinney et al. (Kinney et al., 2003) also reported that dentine, at small deformations, displays a viscoelastic response, i.e. its deformation depends not only on the load that are applied but also on the time since application. Viscoelastic materials, under a constant stress, continue to deform with time, thereby presenting a time-dependence in the mechanical response. However, little is known about how to characterise this viscoelastic behaviour and in the range of frequencies of physiological interest (0.1-10 Hz) Kinney et al. concluded that dentine can be treated as a perfectly elastic solid.

The PDL is a component that surrounds the root of the tooth and connects it to the bone. It contributes to load distribution and damping from the tooth to the bone. Its mechanical behaviour is anisotropic as a consequence of its composition, with collagen fibres that run in different directions (Zhurov et al., 2007). Between the collagen fibres there are tissue fluids that provide a damping behaviour, which enables the ligament to offer a viscous and time-dependent response (Komatsu, 2010). Some works have shown that the elastic response of the PDL is nonlinear (Pini et al., 2002). The elastic modulus is lower for small strains and increases suddenly for strains greater than near 20%-30% in both tension and compression (Pini et al., 2002). However, some models of the ligament in endodontic simulation simplify this characteristic using an isotropic, linear and perfectly elastic material (Garbin et al., 2010; Mezzomo et al., 2011; Okamoto et al., 2008). This simplification avoids the iterative procedure associated to a non-linear model that entails an important increase in computation time. Rees and Jacobsen (Rees & Jacobsen, 1997) analysed the optimal value of the Young's modulus of the PDL (when using an isotropic and linear constitutive model) which provides a good correlation between experimental results and computations of the FE model. They found an optimal value near 50 MPa. This value is used in several works (Davy et al., 1981; Dejak et al., 2005; Garbin et al., 2010) and a similar value of 68.9 MPa in others (Asmussen et al., 2005; Gonzalez-Lluch et al., 2009b; Holmes et al., 1996; Pegoretti et al., 2002). Some recent works consider the non-linear mechanical response of the ligament using a non-linear stress-strain relationship for the finite elements representing the PDL (Okada et al., 2008; Suzuki et al., 2008; Uddanwadiker et al., 2007). Maceri et al. (Maceri et al., 2009) used a set of different spring elements connecting dentine to the bone to represent the non-linear response of the ligament. In an attempt to represent orthodontic movements better, Qian et al. (Qian et al., 2001) proposed the use of special finite elements including fibres that connect two opposing faces of the element. In a further step, some recent works (Ferrari et al., 2008; Sorrentino et al., 2009) considered a more complicated model that takes into account the non-linearity and the time-dependent response of the ligament, using different stress-strain curves for different values of strain rate. Including viscoelasticity in the model is important to be able to simulate the response under dynamical loads correctly, but the fact that most of the models are used in static simulation explains its absence in the majority of the works. The inclusion of the non-linearity and viscoelasticity of the ligament in the constitutive formulation of customised finite elements has been investigated in recent years (Natali et al., 2004; Zhurov et al., 2007), but to the authors' knowledge it has not yet been implemented in a simulation of endodontic restorations. Maceri et al. (Maceri et al., 2010) proposed recently a method to model the PDL and other materials composed of soft collagen tissues, by means of a nano-scale model and a two-step micro–macro homogenisation technique.

Composite posts, such as glass-fibre or carbon-fibre, exhibit anisotropic behaviour due to the presence of reinforcing fibres oriented in the direction of the post axis. An orthotropic model, with different elastic moduli in the direction of the fibres and in the transverse direction, has been used by several authors to represent this material in FE models of the restored tooth (Barjau-Escribano et al., 2006; Garbin et al., 2010; Maceri et al., 2009; Schmitter et al., 2010; Sorrentino et al., 2007).

3.5 Boundary conditions

Boundary conditions in FEA define the known constraints and forces acting on the system. In endodontic simulation, forces represent the loads acting on the tooth and constraints are limitations to the movement of some parts of the model boundary, which are necessary to obtain a unique solution for the displacement of the different points of the model. A clear definition of the boundary conditions that are employed should be included in the description of any FE model, as any changes in these conditions could introduce important differences in the results. Boundary conditions should represent the actual loads and constraints imposed on the real system as well as possible. In this section, we present a review of how these boundary conditions are defined in the biomechanical models described in the literature.

Most of the models presented in the literature limit the analysis to only one tooth. Some works include a portion of the alveolar bone surrounding that tooth. In these cases, restrictions are imposed on the external surfaces of the solid representing the bone (Gonzalez-Lluch et al., 2009b; Hsu et al., 2009). Other works do not include the bone and consider the outer surface of the PDL to be fixed (Ichim et al., 2006; Maceri et al., 2009). Finally, some models do not include the PDL and constrain the system in the external nodes of the root (Lanza et al., 2005; Sorrentino et al., 2007; Zarone et al., 2006). However, this last solution is not recommended because several works have shown that omission of the PDL implies significant changes in stress distribution (Cattaneo et al., 2005; Davy et al., 1981; Qian et al., 2001). Some studies try to reproduce *in vitro* experiments on endodontically restored teeth using FE models. As the rule of thumb in the experimental setup is to substitute the bone by a resin block, the models used in those studies introduce the constraints in the outline of the block of resin, which is attached to the testing machine in the experiment (Schmitter et al., 2010; Soares et al., 2008b).

To reduce the size of the model or in order to have an easier way to show stresses and strains in the sagittal section of the restored tooth, some works include only half of the tooth in the model by eliminating the mesial or distal half (Ferrari et al., 2008; Schmitter et al., 2010). In those cases, a symmetry boundary condition is imposed on the nodes of the cutting plane, thus preventing its movement out of this plane. Although this simplification could be an interesting way to reduce computational time, the simulation of the total tooth is more realistic, as the tooth is not geometrically symmetric.

A considerable number of works in the literature make no explicit reference to the constraints in the paper (Asmussen et al., 2005; Holmes et al., 1996; Nakamura et al., 2006).

The second type of boundary conditions correspond to forces applied to the system. Oral loads can be variable and several simulations can be performed over the model to simulate different oral situations such as occlusion, grinding, mastication of sticky food, impacts on the tooth, bruxism, and so forth. Most FE models of endodontic restorations simulate a maxillary incisor and introduce a load inclined at 45° to the root axis applied to the palatal surface of the tooth in the vestibular direction to represent the direction of oral loads in type I occlusion (Coelho et al., 2009; Hsu et al., 2009; Mezzomo et al., 2011; Okamoto et al., 2008). Other angles close to this value of 45°, ranging from 30° to 60°, have been used in other works (Barjau-Escribano et al., 2006; Ferrari et al., 2008; Garbin et al., 2010; Ichim et al., 2006; Lanza et al., 2005; Zarone et al., 2006). Apart from masticatory loads, other oral conditions have also been simulated, including impacts, using an angle of 90° to the long axis of the tooth, or bruxism, using an angle of 0° (Genovese et al., 2005; Pegoretti et al., 2002). As far as the position of the applied load is concerned, it is typically applied on the palatal surface, below the incisal edge, near the junction of the incisal third and the medial third (Hsu et al., 2009; Li et al., 2006), distal to the cingulum (Ichim et al., 2006). It is important to note that few details are given in the papers about the size of the area over which the force is applied, although this factor can introduce local changes in stresses and strains near the application zone. Therefore, the authors recommend reporting this information in future works. Two different approaches are used in the selection of the magnitude of the loads applied to the model. Since many of the models are linear, an arbitrary small load of 1 N (Davy et al., 1981) or 10 N (Sorrentino et al., 2007) can be used to analyse the system and to obtain information about the stress distribution, which can be translated to greater force scenarios by a simple scaling operation. This approach is valid to compare stresses among different restorative designs or with respect to the natural tooth. However, other works use a force that represents the expected oral forces in order to obtain stress values that are directly comparable to the stress limits for restorative materials. In these cases, forces of 100 N (Gurbuz et al., 2008; Mezzomo et al., 2011), 200 N (Nakamura et al., 2006; Uddanwadiker et al., 2007) or 300 N (Gonzalez-Lluch et al., 2009b; Hsu et al., 2009) are typical.

For premolars, forces at 0° or 45° were used on the crown (Maceri et al., 2009; Toparli, 2003). Ausiello et al. (Ausiello et al., 2002) distributed an axial load over two different points on the crown using two rigid bars. Okada et al. (Okada et al., 2008) used the data obtained experimentally with a device to measure masticatory forces in vivo to decide the magnitude and direction of the loads in a model of a first premolar. During the experiment a piece of beef jerky was masticated and the resulting load was predominantly directed in the apico-coronal direction (164.3 N) with lower and similar components in the mesial-distal direction and bucco-palatal direction (-28.9 N and -23.9 N respectively). For molars, Imanishi (Imanishi et al., 2003) used three different forces of 225 N to simulate masticatory loads with angles of 0°, 45° and 90° with respect to the radicular axis, and applied it in outer incline of the buccal cusps.

Restored teeth are also subject to thermomechanical loading, because of the transient changes in the temperature of the different components of the restoration when hot or cold foods or liquids are introduced into the mouth. To date very few works included these types of boundary conditions in FE models. Gungor et al. (Gungor et al., 2004) presented a simulation that analysed stresses induced in a first premolar with different all-ceramic crown materials as a consequence of thermal loading.

4. Interpreting FEA results

A correct interpretation of FEA results should be based on the stress and strength of each component in the system. To obtain accurate conclusions from this interpretation, three conditions must be fulfilled: (1) stress values must be reliable, i.e., the FE model should be an adequate representation of the real system, (2) strengths of the different materials present in the model must be known and (3) a suitable failure criterion must be used to compare values of computed stresses, which are bi-axial or tri-axial, with material strengths frequently obtained under conditions of a uniaxial stress state (tension or compression).

The first condition is progressively closer to being fulfilled with the development of more accurate three-dimensional models, with finer meshes and with more components represented in the system. However, as has been commented above, the accuracy of most of the models is still questionable. Many models consider that all materials display linear isotropic behaviour, although this is a simplification for components such as dentine, PDL or fibre posts. A good representation of bonded interfaces is difficult due to their reduced thickness and different ways to model them have been tested, as has been commented in previous sections of this chapter. Moreover, some uncertainty exists about the mechanical properties of different materials. However, the second and third conditions are not met in most of the previous works, due to the lack of consistent and complete data about the strength of some dental materials. More especially, however, the interpretation of results is hampered by the absence of a post-hoc analysis of failure in each component of the model or the use of the Von Mises equivalent strength as the reference value for this analysis.

To meet the second condition, information about compressive and tensile strengths is needed for each material in the restoration. The compressive strength is usually obtained experimentally by a compressive test using cylindrical specimens. The tensile strength is obtained by applying an axial force over specimens with a cylindrical or rectangular cross-section and is a typical test for metals and other ductile materials. This type of test, however, is rarely used for brittle materials. Technical problems related with gripping and aligning the brittle specimens are often cited as an explanation for not measuring the tensile strengths (Ban & Anusavice, 1990; Xie et al., 2000). Alternatively, the diametral tensile test (DTT) is commonly used to obtain the diametral tensile strength (DTS) (Probster et al., 1997; Xie et al., 2000) because of its simplicity and reproducibility (Coelho Santos et al., 2004). The DTT is performed by compressing a cylindrical specimen with its axis perpendicular to the load direction. Tensile strength can also be obtained indirectly as a flexural strength (FS) with three- or four-point flexural tests (FT) (Probster et al., 1997; Xie et al., 2000). However, DTS and FS are obtained in loading states that are not uniaxial and the results of these tests are not equivalent, as numerous previous works have shown for different dental materials (Ban & Anusavice, 1990; Probster et al., 1997; Xie et al., 2000). Despite this, DTS and FS have been used interchangeably in recent works as a reference to compare with computed maximal stresses in finite element models of dental restorations (De Jager et al., 2006; Imanishi et al., 2003). On analysing the stress state in both tests, FS seems preferable as a reference for the tensile strength of a ductile material because the stress state is uniaxial at the failure point, and this can only be said of a DTT if a plain stress state is assumed, which if far from being the actual situation in real tests.

Finally, the third condition for a correct interpretation of the FE results is related to the selection of the proper failure criterion for comparing actual stress with the admissible stress limits of different materials present in the restoration. A stress criterion or failure theory combines principal stresses at a point in a solid with the compressive strength and tensile strength of the material to obtain a safety factor at this point. Safety factor values lower than unity indicate that the material is prone to mechanical failure at this point and values greater than unity indicate a safe condition at this point. Different criteria such as Von Mises (VM), Rankine (R), Coulomb-Mohr (CM) or Modified Mohr (MM), are usually reported in mechanical engineering manuals for isotropic materials (Shigley & Mischke, 2002). Some of these criteria are better suited for ductile materials, whereas others are more accurate for predicting the failure of brittle materials. In a recent study, Christensen (Christensen, 2006) proposed the use of a novel failure criterion that is valid for ductile and brittle materials.

To date, little research has been devoted to the interpretation of FEM results in endodontic restorations. Most previous work analyzed the results of FE simulations from Von Mises maximal stresses (Asmussen et al., 2005; Boschian Pest et al., 2006; Hsu et al., 2009; Pegoretti et al., 2002; Sorrentino et al., 2007), implicitly assuming the validity of the VM criterion for all the materials used in the restoration. However, it is known that the VM criterion is only valid for ductile materials with equal compressive and tensile strength (De Groot et al., 1987), but materials exhibiting brittle behaviour such as ceramics, cements or resin composites are frequently used in endodontic restorations. Even dentine presents reported values of compressive strength that are significantly greater than its tensile strength (Craig & Powers, 2002). Some authors suggest the use of the Rankine or Maximum Normal Stress criterion to evaluate the failure in dentine, using the maximum principal stress to analyse the results (Ichim et al., 2006; Maceri et al., 2009; Nakamura et al., 2006). Others analyse the results of shear stress at the post-dentine interface, and indicate that this value should be compared to the reported shear bond strengths in order to evaluate the risk of loosing retention (Asmussen et al., 2005; Maceri et al., 2009; Pegoretti et al., 2002). Wakabayashi et al. (Wakabayashi et al., 2008) also underline the importance of shear stresses to anticipate the probability of failure in the adhesive joints of the restoration. Okamoto et al. (Okamoto et al., 2008) used an iterative procedure to account for debonding in the cement layer. Their method involved reducing the elastic modulus of the finite elements of the cement with shear or normal stresses beyond their corresponding strength to a value close to zero and then recalculating the model until they reached a final solution with a reduced adhesion surface in the cement layer.

DeGroot et al. (De Groot et al., 1987) compared three criteria to analyse FEM results in composite resin: Von Mises, a modified Von Mises criterion presented by Williams (Williams, 1973), and the Drüker-Prager criterion. From their results, they concluded that the Drüker-Prager criterion is more suitable for describing the failure of this material. Recently, Christensen (Christensen, 2006) proposed a unified failure criterion for ductile and brittle materials, which is equivalent to the modified Von Mises criterion proposed by Williams with an additional modification for brittle materials. The same author also demonstrated some unrealistic behaviour of the Drüker-Prager and Coulomb-Mohr criteria under certain important stress states.

The interpretation of failure probability in anisotropic materials is even more difficult and few researchers address it. Dejak et al. (Dejak et al., 2007) applied the Tsai-Wu criterion for anisotropic materials to dentine, enamel and resin composites in molars with ceramic inlays. From the above discussion, it becomes apparent to the authors that more research is needed to clarify the question of how to interpret the results of FE models correctly. In the authors' opinion, DTS should not be used as a reference for the tensile strength in a failure criterion, and FS is a better option. As regards the failure criterion, a critical review is needed about the extensive use of the Von Mises criterion and the use of the novel Christensen criterion should be taken into consideration as an interesting alternative (Pérez-González et al., 2011).

One of the problems related to the interpretation of FE results is the huge quantity of numerical results obtained by the program, namely the displacements and stresses in all the nodes for every dimension considered (two for planar models and three for three-dimensional models). As there may be several thousands of nodes in current FE models, it is not feasible to present the results in a table or a list, at least not for all the nodes. For a good interpretation of the results, one has to know what to look for and where to look for it. It is clear that maximal stresses are the first option to search for points where the system is prone to failure, although the absolute maximum may not be the initial failure point because stress has to be compared to strength in the different components. For a better understanding of the stress distribution in the tooth, some works present the results by giving a list of stresses for selected points or a plot representing the stress values as a function of point location in some trajectory inside the tooth. For example, Davy et al. (Davy et al., 1981) examined the stresses at selected points located near the cervical with different positions in the coronal-apical direction or in the buccal-labial direction. Posterior works (Hsu et al., 2009; Ichim et al., 2006; Pegoretti et al., 2002) also maintain this method, although complemented with fringe plots. Fringe plots are colour representations of some projection of the model using a coloured scale to represent a particular scalar result. Fringe plots allow the distribution of stress or strain in some part of the model to be seen in one picture. They are the usual way to represent the FE results in most works today (Mezzomo et al., 2011; Okamoto et al., 2008; Silva et al., 2009), although they are better suited for qualitative analysis than for quantitative ones. Maceri et al. (Maceri et al., 2009) employed an averaging function to obtain several mean stress values at each section of the tooth in the coronal-apical direction and considered these functions as indicators of the risk of failure. With this procedure, they can easily compare different restoration methods in a plot with simple curves along the axis of the tooth, although the reliability of this customised parameter as risk indicator is questionable.

Statistical tests have been used in some recent works to compare results from different FE models. Hsu et al. used t-tests over sets of points in the areas of interest to compare different restorative solutions (Hsu et al., 2009). The authors have recently presented a similar approach for using ANOVA tests as a method to assess the significance of different restorative designs (Pérez-González et al., 2010). This option for the interpretation of FE results should be investigated in more detail in the future.

5. Validation of biomechanical models

Validation of biomechanical models employed in numerical simulations should be carried out in order to ensure the validity of the results that are obtained. In other biomechanical ambits, model validation is considered to be of major importance (Dalstra et al., 1995; Gupta et al., 2004). Despite this, very few of the works that make use of FEA for endodontic restoration research include such validations of their models. Moreover, little work has been carried out on validation procedures in this particular field.

Generally speaking, two stages should be accomplished in order to validate the FE models. First, some sort of convergence tests have to be performed, where, according to the FEM theory (Zienkiewicz & Taylor, 1989), subsequent refinements of the mesh should make the results to converge. Second, the numerical results have to be compared with those obtained from experimental tests. This comparison can be achieved in different ways that can be found in the scientific literature. Some works only perform the convergence test for validation (Garbin et al., 2010; Sorrentino et al., 2007) and even in theses cases no detailed information about this stage is offered.

One way to accomplish validation of the model is to compare the relation between the load applied and the displacement obtained from both the numerical and the mechanical tests. In some cases (Ausiello et al., 2001), mechanical tests can be undertaken using a testing machine with a constant rate of displacement, which allows two continuous curves to be compared. In other cases, the comparison is achieved only for some discrete values of load and displacements values (Rappelli et al., 2005). In other works the variables that are compared are the load and the strain values (Magne & Tan, 2008; Tajima et al., 2009) using strain gauges, although the process may be found to be more difficult and tedious. In the work by Tajima et al., the utilisation of the strain gauge technique allows simultaneous comparison of the strain values obtained from FE calculation and from experimental tests at four different points, which can be seen as a more rigorous validation. Furthermore, six occlusal points are concurrently loaded during experiments.

An indirect form of experimental validation may be established when the numerical results of stress distribution obtained by the FE model agree with the results obtained by fracture experiments (Barjau-Escribano et al., 2006; Genovese et al., 2005; Huysmans & Van der Varst, 1993). In this sense, model zones with higher stresses should correspond to a higher probability of reaching the failure at these zones during fracture tests when the same external load is applied. Hence, the fracture modes observed during experiments can be compared with the stress distributions patterns obtained by FEA. In other cases, although both FEA and mechanical tests are implemented (Lang et al., 2001; Schmitter et al., 2010; Soares et al., 2008a), the results are considered complementary and no direct validation of the model is pursued.

When FEA is just a part of a more complex numerical model (Maceri et al., 2007), validation for the whole model has to be performed. In this particular case, validation was carried out by comparison with *in vivo* experimental data found in the literature.

6. Conclusions from previous research with biomechanical models

Conclusions from comprehensive three-dimensional models, that capable of simulating the highly irregular shape of real teeth and the real 3D mastication forces acting on them, are summarized in the following section. These models have mainly contributed to the assessment of the effects of the material and the dimensions of the prefabricated posts on the static biomechanical performance of restored teeth, although other parameters have also been analysed.

6.1 About the effect of post material

A conclusion that can be drawn from different works is that stresses distributed differently in natural teeth than in restored teeth and for the case of restored teeth, the distribution is affected in an important way by the material used for the post (Adanir & Belli, 2007; Coelho et al., 2009). The origin of this different distribution lies in the difference in the elastic modulus of the material (near 18 GPa for dentine, 30 GPa for glass fibre posts, and 210 GPa for stainless steel). Stress concentrates where non-homogeneous material distributions are present, just like interfaces. Interfaces of materials with different moduli of elasticity represent the weak link of restorative systems, as the toughness/stiffness mismatch influences the stress distribution (Barjau-Escribano et al., 2006; Sorrentino et al., 2007; Zarone et al., 2006). FE models that consider teeth under flexural-compressive loads concluded that the high elastic modulus of the metal posts caused the stress to be concentrated at the post-dentine junction (Genovese et al., 2005; Hsu et al., 2009; Okamoto et al., 2008; Pegoretti et al., 2002). Consequently, stresses on the root dentine-cortical bone area were weaker than those of the fibre-post group. The results of the FE model of Barjau-Escribano et al. (Barjau-Escribano et al., 2006) made it possible to identify the difference in the elastic moduli between the post and the dentine and core as the origin of stress concentrations at the post-core-cement interface that weakened the restored tooth when stainless steel posts were used. Other works are consistent with this finding (Boschian Pest et al., 2006; Pegoretti et al., 2002). Most of the studies found the highest stresses in restorations with endodontic posts located near the cervical region (Maceri et al., 2009; Mezzomo et al., 2011; Pierrisnard et al., 2002; Sorrentino et al., 2007), especially for fibre posts, whereas peak stresses tend to move apically when more rigid posts are used (Okamoto et al., 2008).

In the FE models from the literature, a monotonic static load was considered, which does not represent the clinical situation, where a dynamic load is characteristic. In a pioneering work, Sancho-Bru et al. (Sancho-Bru et al., 2009) recently proposed a way to use finite element results for a fatigue analysis of dental restorations. From that work, it was concluded that, although restorations using glass fibre posts are able to bear higher static loads, both stainless steel and glass fibre post systems would have a similar life under dynamic loads, although this conclusion should be confirmed using more detailed models in the future.

6.2 About the effect of post diameter

The effect that post diameter has on the stress distribution over the tooth is not the same for all post materials. Several works (Boschian Pest et al., 2006; Nakamura et al., 2006; Rodríguez-Cervantes et al., 2007) have indicated that the effect of diameter is greater for metallic posts than for fibre posts. This could be explained by the fact that the elastic modulus of fibre posts is more comparable with that of dentine, thus producing a more homogenous restoration that is consequently less affected by a change in the diameter of the tooth. In a work by the authors (Rodríguez-Cervantes et al., 2007), we confirmed with *in vitro* tests and FE models that increases in post diameter for metallic posts tend to reduce the failure loads for the restored tooth without the crown. However, in a later work, it was observed that the inclusion of the crown meant that the post diameter did not influence the biomechanical performance of the post systems no matter what post material was used (Gonzalez-Lluch et al., 2009b). For fibre posts, as has been said, the importance of post diameter is lower and the conclusions of different works vary. Boschian-Pest et al. (Boschian Pest et al., 2006), for example, recommended using small diameters to avoid weakening the root, whereas Okamoto et al. (Okamoto et al., 2008) recommended the use of a large diameter, even assuming that changes in stresses are slight.

6.3 About the effect of post length

Two of the earlier FE works (Davy et al., 1981; Holmes et al., 1996) studied metallic post systems by means of two-dimensional finite element models and reached opposing conclusions. The first predicted minor changes in the stress patterns in dentine for the length variations considered; the only effect of post length was a change in the location of the stress concentrations that occurred at the post apex. In contrast, the second predicted higher shear stresses as the length of the metallic post decreased. This controversy seems to continue in two later works that compared the effect of post length for fibre posts. On the one hand, Boschian Pest et al. (Boschian Pest et al., 2006) suggested using a post inserted as deeply as possible, because shorter posts would increase stresses in the luting materials, although minor effects were recognised in the root. Ferrari et al.(Ferrari et al., 2008), on the other hand, concluded that post length does not influence the biomechanics of restored teeth. The same conclusion about the non-significance of the post length was obtained by the authors in a study with *in vitro* tests and with FEA for both metallic and fibre posts (Rodríguez-Cervantes et al., 2007). More recently Hsu et al. (Hsu et al., 2009) concluded that when a metal post is used, the post should be as long as possible, while the biomechanical performance of a glass-fibre post combined with a composite resin core was less sensitive to post length. Others authors, like Chuang et al. (Chuang et al., 2010), using an FE model supported by an *in vitro* study, concluded that post length is more decisive for root fracture resistance in teeth restored with metal posts than in those restored with fibre posts, since long metal posts give rise to stress concentration in the apical portion of the root. They also concluded that post material has a greater effect on the location of peak stress, and on the resulting fracture pattern, than post length does.

6.4 About the effect of other restoration parameters

FE models have corroborated other experimental results and recommendations, e.g., teeth prepared with a ferrule preparation tend to fail in a more favourable mode and exhibit greater mechanical resistance (Ichim et al., 2006) or crowns with small ferrule heights should be resin-bonded instead of using conventional cements (Schmitter et al., 2010). In a recent work, aimed at trying to find the optimal combination of crown material and luting agent, Suzuki et al. (Suzuki et al., 2008) concluded that polymer-based restorative material for the crown and composite cement were preferable to other restorative alternatives. Sorrentino et al. (Sorrentino et al., 2007) also found that changes in the crown and core materials affected stress distribution and that the stress concentrations in post-dentine interface moved apically when more rigid materials were used. The effect of the crown on stress distribution was also studied by the authors and compared with a restoration without the crown (Gonzalez-Lluch et al., 2009b). We confirmed the conclusion reached by Sorrentino et al., although it was also found that the addition of the crown did not affect the final strength of the restoration to any significant extent for either of the post systems considered (stainless steel and glass fibre). As for the effect of the cement properties, Li et al. (Li et al., 2006) found that the elastic modulus of the cement is an important parameter for stress distribution and concluded that cements with an elastic modulus similar to that of dentine should be used in weakened roots.

7. Conclusions and proposals for future work

In the last decades, biomechanical models of endodontic restorations have been developed increasingly using FEA. FE simulations carried out over this time have made it possible to gain a better understanding of how the restored tooth deforms and what stresses it is subject to under simulated loads. These investigations and others to be expected in the future with more comprehensive models could make a valuable contribution to the development of better restorative solutions in this area. With a view to this objective, future works should concentrate on improving current models in order to eliminate remaining weak points. In the authors' opinion, some of these possible future lines of research are:

- Reliable data about the mechanical properties of the different materials used in clinical endodontic restorations are necessary to be able to have good models and interpret results correctly. The stress-strain curves of all these materials, under both tensile and compressive loads, as well as the failure limits, should be clearly established in the literature. Furthermore, common procedures should also be promoted to obtain these data, and communicate and share them among researchers.
- More comprehensive mechanical models will have to be developed in the future. Of course, they should be three-dimensional and represent all the components present in the restoration, but the model should also consider the possible anisotropy of materials, such as bone, dentine or PDL. Additionally, efforts have to be directed towards developing models that represent the nonlinear response of the restored tooth in a suitable manner, because of the nonlinearity of some components, such as the PDL, or due to the appearance of contacts between components.

- Proper validation methods for FE models should be established and shared among researchers. As validation should be based on well-tested and documented experimental results, it is important to increment the quantity and quality of experimental data. To do so, information such as detailed geometrical data about the restored teeth (with different restorative solutions and subject to different loading situations) and experimental measures of strains or displacements should be available to researchers in order to test their numerical models. A common protocol to promote sharing of these data over the Internet would be an important advance.
- Interpretation of FE results is a key point for the future development and reliability of FE models. Of course, the best options to present the results of the models should be investigated, but more research is also needed to establish correct and validated failure criteria for the different materials and especially for bonded interfaces.

8. References

Adanir, N., Belli, S. (2007). Stress analysis of a maxillary central incisor restored with different posts. *European Journal of Dentistry,* Vol. 1, No.2, pp. 67-71, ISSN 1305-7456.

Anusavice, K. J. (2003). *Phillips' Science of Dental Materials.* Saunders, ISBN: 13: 978-0-7216-9387-3, United States of America.

Asmussen, E., Peutzfeldt, A. & Sahafi, A. (2005). Finite element analysis of stresses in endodontically treated, dowel-restored teeth. *The Journal of Prosthetic Dentistry,* Vol. 94, No.4, pp. 321-329, ISSN 0022-3913.

Assif, D., Gorfil, C. (1994). Biomechanical considerations in restoring endodontically treated teeth. *The Journal of Prosthetic Dentistry,* Vol. 71, No.6, pp. 565-567, ISSN 0022-3913.

Ausiello, P., Apicella, A. & Davidson, C. L. (2002). Effect of adhesive layer properties on stress distribution in composite restorations - A 3D finite element analysis. *Dental Materials,* Vol. 18, No.4, pp. 295-303, ISSN 01095641.

Ausiello, P., Apicella, A., Davidson, C. L. & Rengo, S. (2001). 3D-finite element analyses of cusp movements in a human upper premolar, restored with adhesive resin-based composites. *Journal of Biomechanics,* Vol. 34, No.10, pp. 1269-1277, ISSN 0021-9290.

Aykent, F., Kalkan, M., Yucel, M. T. & Ozyesil, A. G. (2006). Effect of dentin bonding and ferrule preparation on the fracture strength of crowned teeth restored with dowels and amalgam cores. *The Journal of Prosthetic Dentistry,* Vol. 95, No.4, pp. 297-301, ISSN 0022-3913.

Ban, S., Anusavice, K. J. (1990). Influence of test method on failure stress of brittle dental materials. *Journal of Dental Research,* Vol. 69, No.12, pp. 1791-1799, ISSN 0022-0345; 0022-0345.

Barjau-Escribano, A., Sancho-Bru, J. L., Forner-Navarro, L., Rodríguez-Cervantes, P. J., Perez-Gonzalez, A. & Sanchez-Marin, F. T. (2006). Influence of prefabricated post material on restored teeth: fracture strength and stress distribution. *Operative Dentistry,* Vol. 31, No.1, pp. 47-54, ISSN 0361-7734.

Boschian Pest, L., Guidotti, S., Pietrabissa, R. & Gagliani, M. (2006). Stress distribution in a post-restored tooth using the three-dimensional finite element method. *Journal of Oral Rehabilitation,* Vol. 33, No.9, pp. 690-697, ISSN 0305-182X.

Bourauel, C., Vollmer, D. & Jager, A. (2000). Application of bone remodeling theories in the simulation of orthodontic tooth movements. *Journal of Orofacial Orthopedics =*

Fortschritte Der Kieferorthopadie : Organ/official Journal Deutsche Gesellschaft Fur Kieferorthopadie, Vol. 61, No.4, pp. 266-279, ISSN 1434-5293.

Cattaneo, P. M., Dalstra, M. & Melsen, B. (2005). The finite element method: a tool to study orthodontic tooth movement. *Journal of Dental Research,* Vol. 84, No.5, pp. 428-433, ISSN 0022-0345; 0022-0345.

Chan, F. W., Harcourt, J. K. & Brockhurst, P. J. (1993). The effect of post adaptation in the root canal on retention of posts cemented with various cements. *Australian Dental Journal,* Vol. 38, No.1, pp. 39-45, ISSN 0045-0421.

Christensen, G. J. (1998). Posts and cores: state of the art. *Journal of the American Dental Association (1939),* Vol. 129, No.1, pp. 96-97, ISSN 0002-8177.

Christensen, R. M. (2006). A comparative evaluation of three isotropic, two property failure theories. *Journal of Applied Mechanics,* Vol. 73, No.5, pp. 852-859, ISSN 0021-8936.

Chuang, S., Yaman, P., Herrero, A., Dennison, J. & Chang, C. (2010). Influence of post material and length on endodontically treated incisors: an in vitro and finite element study. *The Journal of Prosthetic Dentistry,* Vol. 104, No.6, pp. 379-388, ISSN 0022-3913.

Clement, R., Schneider, J., Brambs, H. -., Wunderlich, A., Geiger, M. & Sander, F. G. (2004). Quasi-automatic 3D finite element model generation for individual single-rooted teeth and periodontal ligament. *Computer Methods and Programs in Biomedicine,* Vol. 73, No.2, pp. 135-144, ISSN 0169-2607.

Coelho Santos, G.,Jr, El-Mowafy, O. & Rubo, J. H. (2004). Diametral tensile strength of a resin composite core with nonmetallic prefabricated posts: an in vitro study. *The Journal of Prosthetic Dentistry,* Vol. 91, No.4, pp. 335-341, ISSN 0022-3913; 0022-3913.

Coelho, C. S., Biffi, J. C., Silva, G. R., Abrahao, A., Campos, R. E. & Soares, C. J. (2009). Finite element analysis of weakened roots restored with composite resin and posts. *Dental Materials Journal,* Vol. 28, No.6, pp. 671-678, ISSN 0287-4547; 0287-4547.

Craig, R. G., Farah, J. W. (1977). Stress analysis and design of single restorations and fixed bridges. *Oral Sciences Reviews,* Vol. 10, pp. 45-74, ISSN 0300-4759.

Craig, R. G., Powers, J. M. (2002). *Restorative dental materials.* Mosby, 0-323-01442-9, United States of America.

Dalstra, M., Huiskes, R. & van Erning, L. (1995). Development and validation of a three-dimensional finite element model of the pelvic bone. *Journal of Biomechanical Engineering,* Vol. 117, No.3, pp. 272-278, ISSN 0148-0731; 0148-0731.

Davy, D. T., Dilley, G. L. & Krejci, R. F. (1981). Determination of stress patterns in root-filled teeth incorporating various dowel designs. *Journal of Dental Research,* Vol. 60, No.7, pp. 1301-1310, ISSN 0022-0345.

De Groot, R., Peters, M. C., De Haan, Y. M., Dop, G. J. & Plasschaert, A. J. (1987). Failure stress criteria for composite resin. *Journal of Dental Research,* Vol. 66, No.12, pp. 1748-1752, ISSN 0022-0345.

De Jager, N., de Kler, M. & van der Zel, J. M. (2006). The influence of different core material on the FEA-determined stress distribution in dental crowns. *Dental Materials : Official Publication of the Academy of Dental Materials,* Vol. 22, No.3, pp. 234-242, ISSN 0109-5641.

Dejak, B., Mlotkowski, A. & Romanowicz, M. (2007). Strength estimation of different designs of ceramic inlays and onlays in molars based on the Tsai-Wu failure criterion. *The Journal of Prosthetic Dentistry,* Vol. 98, No.2, pp. 89-100, ISSN 0022-3913.

Dejak, B., Mlotkowski, A. & Romanowicz, M. (2005). Finite element analysis of mechanism of cervical lesion formation in simulated molars during mastication and parafunction. *The Journal of Prosthetic Dentistry,* Vol. 94, No.6, pp. 520-529, ISSN 0022-3913.

Dejak, B., Mlotkowski, A. & Romanowicz, M. (2003). Finite element analysis of stresses in molars during clenching and mastication. *The Journal of Prosthetic Dentistry,* Vol. 90, No.6, pp. 591-597, ISSN 0022-3913.

Farah, J. W., Craig, R. G. (1974). Finite element stress analysis of a restored axisymmetric first molar. *Journal of Dental Research,* Vol. 53, No.4, pp. 859-866, ISSN 0022-0345.

Farah, J. W., Craig, R. G. & Sikarskie, D. L. (1973). Photoelastic and finite element stress analysis of a restored axisymmetric first molar. *Journal of Biomechanics,* Vol. 6, No.5, pp. 511-514, IN9, 515-520, ISSN 0021-9290.

Fernandes, A. S., Shetty, S. & Coutinho, I. (2003). Factors determining post selection: a literature review. *The Journal of Prosthetic Dentistry,* Vol. 90, No.6, pp. 556-562, ISSN 0022-3913.

Ferrari, M., Sorrentino, R., Zarone, F., Apicella, D., Aversa, R. & Apicella, A. (2008). Non-linear viscoelastic finite element analysis of the effect of the length of glass fiber posts on the biomechanical behaviour of directly restored incisors and surrounding alveolar bone. *Dental Materials,* Vol. 27, No.4, pp. 485-498.

Fokkinga, W. A., Le Bell, A. M., Kreulen, C. M., Lassila, L. V., Vallittu, P. K. & Creugers, N. H. (2005). Ex vivo fracture resistance of direct resin composite complete crowns with and without posts on maxillary premolars. *International Endodontic Journal,* Vol. 38, No.4, pp. 230-237, ISSN 0143-2885.

Fox, K., Wood, D. J. & Youngson, C. C. (2004). A clinical report of 85 fractured metallic post-retained crowns. *International Endodontic Journal,* Vol. 37, No.8, pp. 561-573, ISSN 0143-2885.

Freitas Junior, A. C., Rocha, E. P., Santos, P. H., Ko, C. C., Martin Junior, M. & de Almeida, E. O. (2010). Mechanics of the maxillary central incisor. Influence of the periodontal ligament represented by beam elements. *Computer Methods in Biomechanics and Biomedical Engineering,* Vol. 13, No.5, pp. 515-521, ISSN 1476-8259.

Gallo, J. R.,3rd, Miller, T., Xu, X. & Burgess, J. O. (2002). In vitro evaluation of the retention of composite fiber and stainless steel posts. *Journal of Prosthodontics : Official Journal of the American College of Prosthodontists,* Vol. 11, No.1, pp. 25-29, ISSN 1059-941X.

Garbin, C. A., Spazzin, A. O., Meira-Júnior, A. D., Loretto, S. C., Lyra, A. M. V. C. & Braz, R. (2010). Biomechanical behaviour of a fractured maxillary incisor restored with direct composite resin only or with different post systems. *International Endodontic Journal,* Vol. 43, No.12, pp. 1098-1107, ISSN 01432885.

Genovese, K., Lamberti, L. & Pappalettere, C. (2005). Finite element analysis of a new customized composite post system for endodontically treated teeth. *Journal of Biomechanics,* Vol. 38, No.12, pp. 2375-2389.

Gonzalez-Lluch C, Pérez-González A, Sancho-Bru JL, Rodríguez-Cervantes PJ. Influencia del mallado en la simulación por elementos finitos de un diente incisivo central maxilar restaurado endodónticamente. *CIBIM9*. 2009a.

Gonzalez-Lluch, C., Rodríguez-Cervantes, P. J., Sancho-Bru, J. L., Perez-Gonzalez, A., Barjau-Escribano, A., Vergara-Monedero, M. & Forner-Navarro, L. (2009b). Influence of material and diameter of pre-fabricated posts on maxillary central incisors restored with crown. *Journal of Oral Rehabilitation,* Vol. 36, No.10, pp. 737-747, ISSN 1365-2842.

Gungor, M. A., Kucuk, M., Dundar, M., Karaoglu, C. & Artunc, C. (2004). Effect of temperature and stress distribution on all-ceramic restorations by using a three-dimensional finite element analysis. *Journal of Oral Rehabilitation,* Vol. 31, No.2, pp. 172-178, ISSN 0305-182X.

Gupta, S., van der Helm, F. C., Sterk, J. C., van Keulen, F. & Kaptein, B. L. (2004). Development and experimental validation of a three-dimensional finite element model of the human scapula. *Proceedings of the Institution of Mechanical Engineers.Part H, Journal of Engineering in Medicine,* Vol. 218, No.2, pp. 127-142, ISSN 0954-4119.

Gurbuz, T., Sengul, F. & Altun, C. (2008). Finite element stress analysis of short-post core and over restorations prepared with different restorative materials. *Dental Materials Journal,* Vol. 27, No.4, pp. 499-507, ISSN 0287-4547.

Holmes, D. C., Diaz-Arnold, A. M. & Leary, J. M. (1996). Influence of post dimension on stress distribution in dentin. *The Journal of Prosthetic Dentistry,* Vol. 75, No.2, pp. 140-147, ISSN 0022-3913.

Hsu, M. L., Chen, C. S., Chen, B. J., Huang, H. H. & Chang, C. L. (2009). Effects of post materials and length on the stress distribution of endodontically treated maxillary central incisors: a 3D finite element analysis. *Journal of Oral Rehabilitation,* Vol. 36, No.11, pp. 821-830, ISSN 1365-2842; 0305-182X.

Huysmans, M. C. D. N. J. M., Van der Varst, P. G. T. (1993). Finite element analysis of quasistatic and fatigue failure of post and cores. *Journal of Dentistry,* Vol. 21, No.1, pp. 57-64, ISSN 0300-5712.

Ichim, I., Kuzmanovic, D. V. & Love, R. M. (2006). A finite element analysis of ferrule design on restoration resistance and distribution of stress within a root. *International Endodontic Journal,* Vol. 39, No.6, pp. 443-452, ISSN 0143-2885.

Imanishi, A., Nakamura, T., Ohyama, T. & Nakamura, T. (2003). 3-D Finite element analysis of all-ceramic posterior crowns. *Journal of Oral Rehabilitation,* Vol. 30, pp. 818-822.

Isidor, F., Brondum, K. & Ravnholt, G. (1999). The influence of post length and crown ferrule length on the resistance to cyclic loading of bovine teeth with prefabricated titanium posts. *The International Journal of Prosthodontics,* Vol. 12, No.1, pp. 78-82, ISSN 0893-2174.

Kinney, J. H., Marshall, S. J. & Marshall, G. W. (2003). The mechanical properties of human dentin: a critical review and re-evaluation of the dental literature. *Critical Reviews in Oral Biology and Medicine : An Official Publication of the American Association of Oral Biologists,* Vol. 14, No.1, pp. 13-29, ISSN 1544-1113; 1045-4411.

Komatsu, K. (2010). Mechanical strength and viscoelastic response of the periodontal ligament in relation to structure. *Journal of Dental Biomechanics,* Vol. 2010, pp. 502318. Epub 2009 Dec 15, ISSN 1758-7360.

Lang, L. A., Wang, R. F., Kang, B. & White, S. N. (2001). Validation of finite element analysis in dental ceramics research. *The Journal of Prosthetic Dentistry,* Vol. 86, No.6, pp. 650-654, ISSN 0022-3913.

Lanza, A., Aversa, R., Rengo, S., Apicella, D. & Apicella, A. (2005). 3D FEA of cemented steel, glass and carbon posts in a maxillary incisor. *Dental Materials : Official*

Publication of the Academy of Dental Materials, Vol. 21, No.8, pp. 709-715, ISSN 0109-5641.

Li, L. L., Wang, Z. Y., Bai, Z. C., Mao, Y., Gao, B., Xin, H. T., Zhou, B., Zhang, Y. & Liu, B. (2006). Three-dimensional finite element analysis of weakened roots restored with different cements in combination with titanium alloy posts. *Chinese Medical Journal,* Vol. 119, No.4, pp. 305-311, ISSN 0366-6999.

Maceri, F., Marino, M. & Vairo, G. (2010). A unified multiscale mechanical model for soft collagenous tissues with regular fiber arrangement. *Journal of Biomechanics,* Vol. 43, No.2, pp. 355-363.

Maceri, F., Martignoni, M. & Vairo, G. (2009). Optimal mechanical design of anatomical post-systems for endodontic restoration. *Computer Methods in Biomechanics and Biomedical Engineering,* Vol. 12, No.1, pp. 59-71, ISSN 10255842.

Maceri, F., Martignoni, M. & Vairo, G. (2007). Mechanical behaviour of endodontic restorations with multiple prefabricated posts: A finite-element approach. *Journal of Biomechanics,* Vol. 40, No.11, pp. 2386-2398, ISSN 0021-9290.

Magne, P., Tan, D. T. (2008). Incisor compliance following operative procedures: a rapid 3-D finite element analysis using micro-CT data. *The Journal of Adhesive Dentistry,* Vol. 10, No.1, pp. 49-56, ISSN 1461-5185.

Magne, P. (2007). Efficient 3D finite element analysis of dental restorative procedures using micro-CT data. *Dental Materials,* Vol. 23, No.5, pp. 539-548, ISSN 0109-5641.

Mezzomo, L. A., Corso, L., Marczak, R. J. & Rivaldo, E. G. (2011). Three-dimensional FEA of effects of two dowel-and-core approaches and effects of canal flaring on stress distribution in endodontically treated teeth. *Journal of Prosthodontics,* Vol. 20, No.2, pp. 120-129, ISSN 1059941X.

Middleton, J., Jones, M. & Wilson, A. (1996). The role of the periodontal ligament in bone modeling: the initial development of a time-dependent finite element model. *American Journal of Orthodontics and Dentofacial Orthopedics : Official Publication of the American Association of Orthodontists, its Constituent Societies, and the American Board of Orthodontics,* Vol. 109, No.2, pp. 155-162, ISSN 08895406.

Nakamura, T., Ohyama, T., Waki, T., Kinuta, S., Wakabayashi, K., Mutobe, Y., Takano, N. & Yatani, H. (2006). Stress analysis of endodontically treated anterior teeth restored with different types of post material. *Dental Materials Journal,* Vol. 25, No.1, pp. 145-150, ISSN 0287-4547.

Natali, A., Pavan, P., Carniel, E. & Dorow, C. (2004). Viscoelastic response of the periodontal ligament: an experimental-numerical analysis. *Connective Tissue Research,* Vol. 45, No.4-5, pp. 222-230, ISSN 0300-8207.

Nothdurft, F. P., Pospiech, P. R. (2006). Clinical evaluation of pulpless teeth restored with conventionally cemented zirconia posts: A pilot study. *The Journal of Prosthetic Dentistry,* Vol. 95, No.4, pp. 311-314.

Okada, D., Miura, H., Suzuki, C., Komada, W., Shin, C., Yamamoto, M. & Masuoka, D. (2008). Stress distribution in roots restored with different types of post systems with composite resin. *Dental Materials Journal,* Vol. 27, No.4, pp. 605-611, ISSN 0287-4547.

Okamoto, K., Ino, T., Iwase, N., Shimizu, E., Suzuki, M., Satoh, G., Ohkawa, S. & Fujisawa, M. (2008). Three-dimensional finite element analysis of stress distribution in composite resin cores with fiber posts of varying diameters. *Dental Materials Journal,* Vol. 27, No.1, pp. 49-55, ISSN 0287-4547.

Pegoretti, A., Fambri, L., Zappini, G. & Bianchetti, M. (2002). Finite element analysis of a glass fibre reinforced composite endodontic post. *Biomaterials,* Vol. 23, No.13, pp. 2667-2682, ISSN 0142-9612.

Pereira, J. R., de Ornelas, F., Conti, P. C. & do Valle, A. L. (2006). Effect of a crown ferrule on the fracture resistance of endodontically treated teeth restored with prefabricated posts. *The Journal of Prosthetic Dentistry,* Vol. 95, No.1, pp. 50-54, ISSN 0022-3913.

Pérez-González, A., González-Lluch, C., Sancho-Bru, J. L., Rodríguez-Cervantes, P. J. & Iserte-Vilar, J. L. (2010). FEM and statistical analysis for studying the optimal design of endodontic posts. *Computer Methods in Biomechanics and Biomedical Engineering 2010,* Valencia (Spain).

Pérez-González, A., Iserte-Vilar, J.L., González-Lluch, C. (2011). Interpreting finite element results for brittle materials in endodontic restorations. *Biomedical Engineering Online* 2011, 10:44.

Pierrisnard, L., Bohin, F., Renault, P. & Barquins, M. (2002). Corono-radicular reconstruction of pulpless teeth: A mechanical study using finite element analysis. *The Journal of Prosthetic Dentistry,* Vol. 88, No.4, pp. 442-448, ISSN 0022-3913.

Pini, M., Wiskott, H. W., Scherrer, S. S., Botsis, J. & Belser, U. C. (2002). Mechanical characterization of bovine periodontal ligament. *Journal of Periodontal Research,* Vol. 37, No.4, pp. 237-244, ISSN 0022-3484.

Probster, L., Geis-Gerstorfer, J., Kirchner, E. & Kanjantra, P. (1997). In vitro evaluation of a glass-ceramic restorative material. *Journal of Oral Rehabilitation,* Vol. 24, No.9, pp. 636-645, ISSN 0305-182X.

Qian, H., Chen, J. & Katona, T. R. (2001). The influence of PDL principal fibers in a 3-dimensional analysis of orthodontic tooth movement. *American Journal of Orthodontics and Dentofacial Orthopedics,* Vol. 120, No.3, pp. 272-279, ISSN 0889-5406.

Rappelli, G., Scalise, L., Procaccini, M. & Tomasini, E. P. (2005). Stress distribution in fiber-reinforced composite inlay fixed partial dentures. *The Journal of Prosthetic Dentistry,* Vol. 93, No.5, pp. 425-432, ISSN 0022-3913.

Rees, J. S., Jacobsen, P. H. (1997). Elastic modulus of the periodontal ligament. *Biomaterials,* Vol. 18, No.14, pp. 995-999, ISSN 0142-9612.

Ren, L. M., Wang, W. X., Takao, Y. & Chen, Z. X. (2010). Effects of cementum–dentine junction and cementum on the mechanical response of tooth supporting structure. *Journal of Dentistry,* Vol. 38, No.11, pp. 882-891, ISSN 0300-5712.

Rodríguez-Cervantes, P. J., Sancho-Bru, J. L., Barjau-Escribano, A., Forner-Navarro, L., Pérez-González, A. & Sánchez-Marín, F. T. (2007). Influence of prefabricated post dimensions on restored maxillary central incisors. *Journal of Oral Rehabilitation,* Vol. 34, No.2, pp. 141-152, ISSN 0305-182X.

Ruse, N. D. (2008). Propagation of erroneous data for the modulus of elasticity of periodontal ligament and gutta percha in FEM/FEA papers: A story of broken links. *Dental Materials,* Vol. 24, No.12, pp. 1717-1719, ISSN 0109-5641.

Sahafi, A., Peutzfeldt, A., Ravnholt, G., Asmussen, E. & Gotfredsen, K. (2005). Resistance to cyclic loading of teeth restored with posts. *Clinical Oral Investigations,* Vol. 9, No.2, pp. 84-90, ISSN 1432-6981.

Sancho-Bru, J. L., Rodríguez-Cervantes, P. J., Pérez-González, A. & González-Lluch, C. (2009). Using fatigue analyses from FEA to study the biomechanics of restored teeth with intraradicular posts. *18th IASTED International Conference on Applied Simulation and Modelling, ASM 2009,* ISBN 9780889868083, Palma de Mallorca.

Schmitter, M., Rammelsberg, P., Lenz, J., Scheuber, S., Schweizerhof, K. & Rues, S. (2010). Teeth restored using fiber-reinforced posts: In vitro fracture tests and finite element analysis. *Acta Biomaterialia,* Vol. 6, pp. 3747-3754, ISSN 1742-7061.

Scotti R, Ferrari M. (2004) *Pernos de fibra.* Barcelona: Masson, ISBN 84-458-1358-7

Selna, L. G., Shillingburg, H. T.,Jr & Kerr, P. A. (1975). Finite element analysis of dental structures--axisymmetric and plane stress idealizations. *Journal of Biomedical Materials Research,* Vol. 9, No.2, pp. 237-252, ISSN 0021-9304.

Shigley.J.E. & Mischke, CR. (2002) *Mechanical Engineering Design.* 5th ed. McGraw-Hill, ISBN 0072832096.

Silva, N. R., Castro, C. G., Santos-Filho, P. C., Silva, G. R., Campos, R. E., Soares, P. V. & Soares, C. J. (2009). Influence of different post design and composition on stress distribution in maxillary central incisor: Finite element analysis. *Indian Journal of Dental Research : Official Publication of Indian Society for Dental Research,* Vol. 20, No.2, pp. 153-158, ISSN 1998-3603.

Soares, C. J., Raposo, L. H. A., Soares, P. V., Santos-Filho, P. C. F., Menezes, M. S., Soares, P. B. F. & Magalhães, D. (2010). Effect of different cements on the biomechanical behavior of teeth restored with cast dowel-and-cores - in vitro and FEA analysis. *Journal of Prosthodontics,* Vol. 19, No.2, pp. 130-137, ISSN 1059941X.

Soares, P. V., Santos-Filho, P. C., Gomide, H. A., Araujo, C. A., Martins, L. R. & Soares, C. J. (2008a). Influence of restorative technique on the biomechanical behavior of endodontically treated maxillary premolars. Part II: strain measurement and stress distribution. *The Journal of Prosthetic Dentistry,* Vol. 99, No.2, pp. 114-122, ISSN 0022-3913.

Soares, P. V., Santos-Filho, P. C. F., Queiroz, E. C., Araújo, T. C., Campos, R. E., Araújo, C. A. & Soares, C. J. (2008b). Fracture resistance and stress distribution in endodontically treated maxillary premolars restored with composite resin. *Journal of Prosthodontics,* Vol. 17, No.2, pp. 114-119, ISSN 1059941X.

Sorrentino, R., Apicella, D., Riccio, C., Gherlone, E., Zarone, F., Aversa, R., Garcia-Godoy, F., Ferrari, M. & Apicella, A. (2009). Nonlinear visco-elastic finite element analysis of different porcelain veneers configuration. *Journal of Biomedical Materials Research.Part B, Applied Biomaterials,* Vol. 91, No.2, pp. 727-736, ISSN 1552-4981.

Sorrentino, R., Aversa, R., Ferro, V., Auriemma, T., Zarone, F., Ferrari, M. & Apicella, A. (2007). Three-dimensional finite element analysis of strain and stress distributions in endodontically treated maxillary central incisors restored with different post, core and crown materials. *Dental Materials : Official Publication of the Academy of Dental Materials,* Vol. 23, No.8, pp. 983-993, ISSN 0109-5641.

Suzuki, C., Miura, H., Okada, D. & Komada, W. (2008). Investigation of stress distribution in roots restored with different crown materials and luting agents. *Dental Materials Journal,* Vol. 27, No.2, pp. 229-236, ISSN 0287-4547.

Tajima, K., Chen, K. K., Takahashi, N., Noda, N., Nagamatsu, Y. & Kakigawa, H. (2009). Three-dimensional finite element modeling from CT images of tooth and its validation. *Dental Materials Journal,* Vol. 28, No.2, pp. 219-226, ISSN 0287-4547.

Tan, P. L., Aquilino, S. A., Gratton, D. G., Stanford, C. M., Tan, S. C., Johnson, W. T. & Dawson, D. (2005). In vitro fracture resistance of endodontically treated central incisors with varying ferrule heights and configurations. *The Journal of Prosthetic Dentistry,* Vol. 93, No.4, pp. 331-336, ISSN 0022-3913.

Thresher, R. W., Saito, G. E. (1973). The stress analysis of human teeth. *Journal of Biomechanics,* Vol. 6, No.5, pp. 443-449, ISSN 0021-9290.
Toksavul, S., Zor, M., Toman, M., Gungor, M. A., Nergiz, I. & Artunc, C. (2006). Analysis of dentinal stress distribution of maxillary central incisors subjected to various post-and-core applications. *Operative Dentistry,* Vol. 31, No.1, pp. 89-96, ISSN 0361-7734.
Toms, S. R., Eberhardt, A. W. (2003). A nonlinear finite element analysis of the periodontal ligament under orthodontic tooth loading. *American Journal of Orthodontics and Dentofacial Orthopedics,* Vol. 123, No.6, pp. 657-665, ISSN 0889-5406.
Toparli, M. (2003). Stress analysis in a post-restored tooth utilizing the finite element method. *Journal of Oral Rehabilitation,* Vol. 30, No.5, pp. 470-476, ISSN 0305-182X.
Torbjorner, A., Karlsson, S. & Odman, P. A. (1995). Survival rate and failure characteristics for two post designs. *The Journal of Prosthetic Dentistry,* Vol. 73, No.5, pp. 439-444, ISSN 0022-3913.
Uddanwadiker, R. V., Padole, P. M. & Arya, H. (2007). Effect of variation of root post in different layers of tooth: linear vs nonlinear finite element stress analysis. *Journal of Bioscience and Bioengineering,* Vol. 104, No.5, pp. 363-370, ISSN 1389-1723; 1347-4421.
van Ruijven, L. J., Mulder, L. & van Eijden, T. M. (2006). Variations in mineralization affect the stress and strain distributions in cortical and trabecular bone. *Journal of Biomechanics,* ISSN 0021-9290.
Wakabayashi, N., Ona, M., Suzuki, T. & Igarashi, Y. (2008). Nonlinear finite element analyses: advances and challenges in dental applications. *Journal of Dentistry,* Vol. 36, No.7, pp. 463-471, ISSN 0300-5712.
Walton, R. E., Torabinejad, M. (2002). *Principles and practice of endodontics.* WB Saunders and Company, Philadelphia.
Williams, J. G. (1973). *Stress analysis of polymers.* Logman, London.
Xie, D., Brantley, W. A., Culbertson, B. M. & Wang, G. (2000). Mechanical properties and microstructures of glass-ionomer cements. *Dental Materials : Official Publication of the Academy of Dental Materials,* Vol. 16, No.2, pp. 129-138, ISSN 0109-5641.
Yaman, S. D., Alacam, T. & Yaman, Y. (1998). Analysis of stress distribution in a maxillary central incisor subjected to various post and core applications. *Journal of Endodontics,* Vol. 24, No.2, pp. 107-111, ISSN 0099-2399.
Yaman, S. D., Karacaer, O. & Sahin, M. (2004). Stress distribution of post-core applications in maxillary central incisors. *Journal of Biomaterials Applications,* Vol. 18, No.3, pp. 163-177, ISSN 0885-3282.
Zarone, F., Sorrentino, R., Apicella, D., Valentino, B., Ferrari, M., Aversa, R. & Apicella, A. (2006). Evaluation of the biomechanical behavior of maxillary central incisors restored by means of endocrowns compared to a natural tooth: a 3D static linear finite elements analysis. *Dental Materials : Official Publication of the Academy of Dental Materials,* Vol. 22, No.11, pp. 1035-1044, ISSN 0109-5641.
Zhi-Yue, L., Yu-Xing, Z. (2003). Effects of post-core design and ferrule on fracture resistance of endodontically treated maxillary central incisors. *The Journal of Prosthetic Dentistry,* Vol. 89, No.4, pp. 368-373, ISSN 0022-3913.
Zhurov, A. I., Limbert, G., Aeschlimann, D. P. & Middleton, J. (2007). A constitutive model for the periodontal ligament as a compressible transversely isotropic visco-hyperelastic tissue. *Computer Methods in Biomechanics and Biomedical Engineering,* Vol. 10, No.3, pp. 223-235, ISSN 1025-5842.
Zienkiewicz, O. C., Taylor, R. L. (1989). *The finite element method.* McGraw-Hill, ISBN 0070841744, London ; New York.

Development and Validation of a Three-Dimensional Biomechanical Model of the Lower Extremity

Shihab Asfour and Moataz Eltoukhy
Department of Industrial Engineering, University of Miami
USA

1. Introduction

One of the important applications of the computer modelling of human body is the area of joint replacement where a validated model can be used for surgery planning. It is known that the evolution of total knee and total hip replacement has been influenced to a great extent by the knowledge obtained from gait analysis studies (Andriacchi and Hurwitz, 1997). Many of the mechanical problems associated with these devices have been evaluated in terms of the mechanics of walking where the magnitude and pattern of the forces at the hip and knee joints obtained from gait analysis studies have been used as design criteria of both total hip and total knee replacements.

Gait analysis provides a unique opportunity to obtain objective information that cannot be obtained through other clinical means (Andriacchi and Hurwitz, 1997). For instance, several investigators have advocated the use of gait analysis for planning surgery and therapy treatments for children with cerebral palsy (Lofterod, et al., 2007; Kay, et al., 2000; Molenaers, et al., 2006). Improvement in gait after multi-level surgery using kinematic data has been documented, while kinematics provides information on dynamic joint motion kinetics is essential for differentiating between primary deformities and secondary responses.

The potential benefits of gait analysis are improved treatment decision making, so that surgery and other treatments result in improved walking capability. Also, the information generated from the gait analysis of patients with total joint replacements has been utilized as a tool for assessing recovery following these procedures, where the key to the analysis of functionality following joint replacement is the ability to identify the adaptations corresponding to the joint design features.

It is very difficult to determine muscle force/power output from multiple muscles simultaneously without affecting the pattern of normal movements (Naganoa, et al., 2005). Fortunately, computer modeling can provide useful insights for human biomechanics. Most in-vivo experiments only reveal the forces in the joint and not the surrounding muscle forces or their point of application. It is also known that finding the internal forces in the body by in-vivo experiments alone is difficult and sometime impossible. Because of the inherited redundancy in the musculoskeletal system (Crowninshield and Brand, 1981b) a desired motion can be achieved by an infinite number of activation patterns of the muscles. Because of the additional forces induced by muscles, knowledge of how the muscle forces are applied can be very important for understanding the bone strength and degeneration around the replacement so that replacement joints can be designed and tested with the loading environment in which they will operate.

A number of studies have been conducted to investigate the forces in the different joints in the lower extremities. For instance, with regard to hip joint, a number of studies have been conducted to validate musculoskeletal models using both instrumented hip replacements (Bergmann et al., 2001, Brand et al., 1994) and the activity levels of muscles obtained by means of electromyography (Crowninshield et al., 1978). Others have studied the forces produced in the knee joint (Piazza et al., 1996), and the ankle joint as well (Orendurff et al., 2002).

While these studies have shown that the hip contact forces and muscle activity levels can be represented by computational methods, several theories have been developed (Crowninshield et al., 1978, Rasmussen et al., 2001), but the question of how the body recruits the muscles for a given activity needs more understanding. This question can be better answered through the use of 3D musculoskeletal modeling. Using three-dimensional computer modelling makes it possible to evaluate the behaviour of individual muscles during various human movements (Eltoukhy & Asfour, 2009 and Yamaguchi, 2001).

Although the mechanics of muscles and joints easily become statically indeterminate, which means that there are not enough equilibrium equations describing the muscle activation available to resolve the forces in the system. Another complication is caused by the muscles in the system because they can only pull and some muscles contribute to the joint movements. This constrains the space of possible solutions and adds a fair bit of complexity to the problem.

In principle, resolving forces is a question of setting up the equilibrium equations and solving them. But in biomechanics in particular, there are several complications. There have been several optimization methods used to solve this, the basic requirement to the Inverse Dynamic Analysis solver is that it must be able to cope with both statically indeterminate problems and unilateral forces elements.

1.1 Knee replacement

According to the American Academy of Orthopaedic Surgeons, there are about 270,000 knee replacement operations performed each year in the United States. Although about 70% of these operations are performed in people over the age of 65, a growing number of knee replacements are being done in younger patients. Knee replacement is basically a surgery for people with severe knee damage during which the surgeon removes damaged cartilage and bone from the surface of the knee joint and replaces them with a metal and plastic surface (Figure 1).

In other words, it involves the resurfacing of the worn out parts of the knee using a metal component on the end of the femur and the top of the tibia, with a plastic bearing in between. The total knee replacement had been studied in the literature by a large number of researchers. One of the most relevant studies to our research work was the study conducted by Benedetti et al (2000). In their study the authors determined the gait function as it relates to the residual quadriceps' strength and to the specific components of the quadriceps removed in patients treated with total knee replacement.

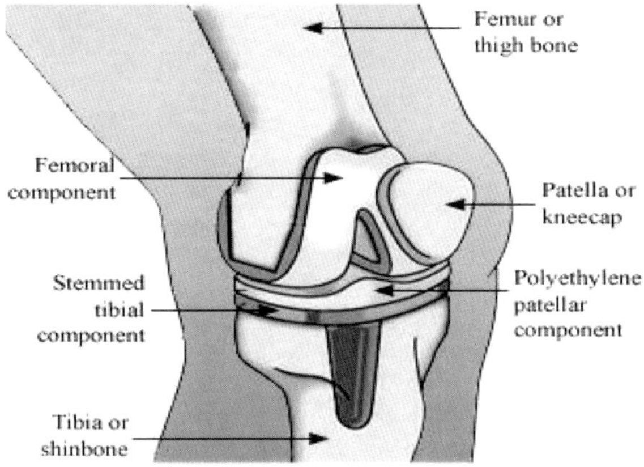

Fig. 1. Total knee replacement surgery (Healthbase)

2. Musculoskeletal modeling

Three-dimensional (3D) computer modeling possesses the advantage of providing useful insights and allowing the 3D-evaluation of the behavior of individual muscles during the different human movements. As it has been shown by a number of researchers such as Alkjaer et al. (2001), 3D vectors better represent the line of action of the different muscles as compared to two-dimensional (2D) vectors specially when investigating the location of both the origin and insertion of muscles.

One of the important applications of the computer modeling of human body is the area of joint replacement where a validated model can be used for instant surgery planning. It is known that the evolution of total knee and total hip replacement has been influenced to a great extent by the knowledge obtained from gait analysis studies.

Many of the mechanical problems associated with these devices have been evaluated in terms of the mechanics of walking where the magnitude and pattern of the forces at the hip and knee joints obtained from gait analysis studies have been used as design criteria of both total hip and total knee replacements. Because of the additional forces induced by muscles, knowledge of how the muscle forces are applied can be very important for understanding the bone strength and degeneration around the replacement so that replacement joints can be designed and tested with the loading environment in which they will operate.

2.1 Model development

One of the main features of the approach used in this study is the possibility to drive a 3D musculoskeletal model entirely from the motion capturing data and to be able to predict the muscle recruitment pattern required to perform a certain task, in this chapter the task studied was a full gait cycle. The gait data collected is used basically for model validation and that is by comparing the data obtained versus the database Hip98 developed by Bergmann et al. (1998).

2.1.1 Subjects and procedures

Five healthy subjects aged 25 ± 2 years participated in this study. The participants were given instructions including an explanation of the test procedures, proper attire, and the expected duration of the testing. The data was collected at the University of Miami Biomechanics Research Laboratory, USA, with an approval from the Institutional Review Board (IRB) at the University of Miami. Forty eight reflective markers were placed at the different land marks (e.g. joints center lines and segments). First, a static trial is conducted where the patient stands at a T- pose; the goal of this static trial is to use it for labelling purposes. Then five dynamics trials were performed. The subject was instructed to walk at his/her normal speed across the laboratory and on top of four force plates (Figure 2).

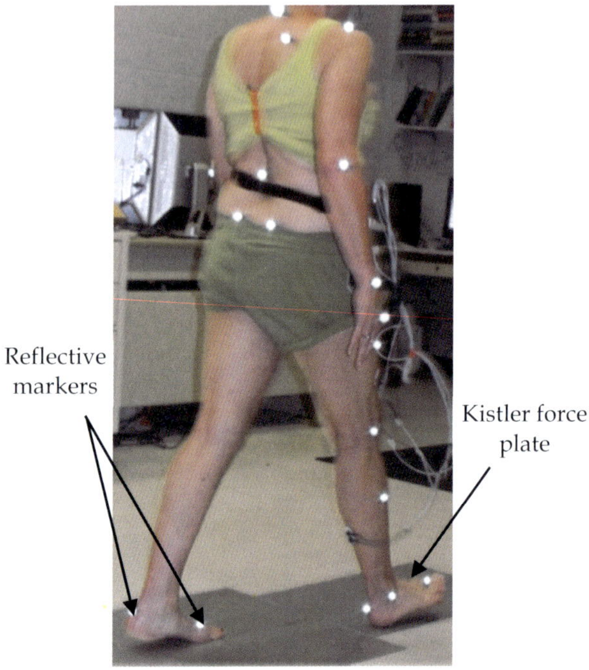

Fig. 2. Actual subject walking across the lab during a gait motion capturing session.

2.1.2 Instrumentation and data collection

The laboratory incorporates a ViconNexus® Motion Capturing System (Oxford Metrics, United Kingdom). The motion capturing system integrates and synchronizes four Kistler force plates (Model: 9253B, sampling rate: 2400 Hz), and eight MX cameras. The MX cameras provide 1024 x 1024 pixel resolution and frame rates up to 250 Hz. The setup including the force plates and the MX cameras is shown in figure 3.

The MX cameras capture the reflected infrared light from the markers placed on the subject's skin and thus the X, Y, and Z coordinates of the body segments and joints at the different time steps are recorded continuously. The reconstructed data output of the motion capturing session is shown in figure 4, which depicts the stick figure of the subject's lower extremity, the reflective markers as recorded by the cameras, the segments' center lines and reference frames, and the ground reaction vectors acting on the subject.

As shown in figure 4, the data collected from the motion capturing (Mocap) system is first reconstructed and each marker is labeled in order to identify the different body segments and joints. Then the segments' center lines are determined accordingly at the same time the synchronized force plates' data is recorded. Body segmental parameter values were derived from Horsman et al. (2007). Hip joints were modelled as universal joints where hip joint flexion/extension, adduction/abduction and internal/external rotation were allowed. Knee joints were modelled as hinge joints, while ankle joints were modelled as biaxial joints, ankle joint dorsi/plantar flexion and inversion/eversion were allowed.

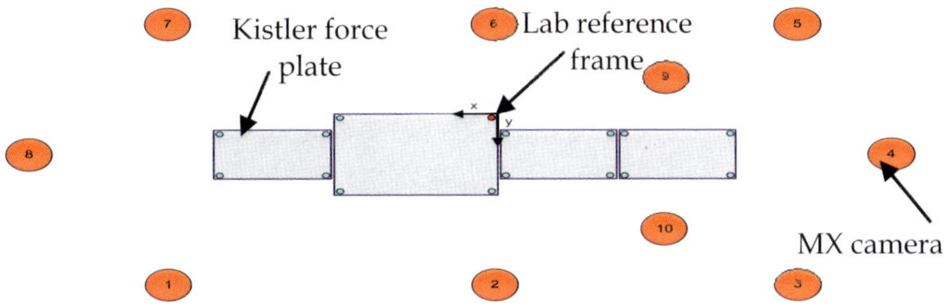

Fig. 3. Force plates and cameras configurations.

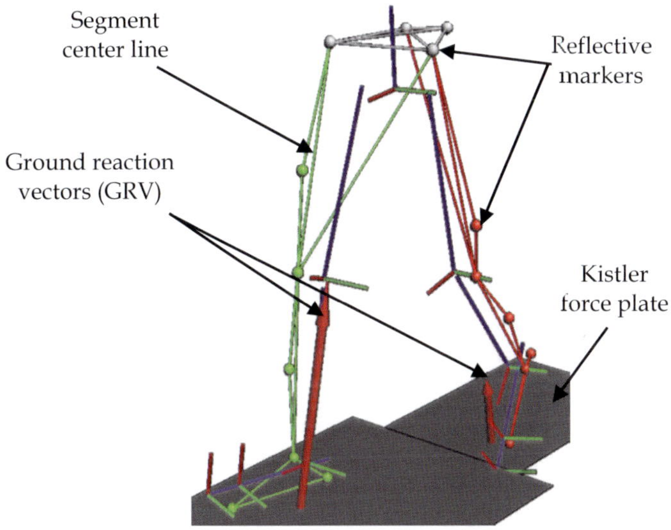

Fig. 4. Lower extremity stick figure and ground reaction vectors with markers and reconstructed segment's center lines.

2.1.3 Model construction

Once the gait session data was reconstructed and all gaps were filled then the C3D file that contains both the X, Y, and Z coordinates of the different markers (those markers was referred to later on as the grey markers) and the force plate data was transferred to the 3D lower extremity modelling phase. The model includes seven segments (Figure 5) that are scalable to the subject's dimensions; with 27 muscles in each leg been included, the exact origin and insertion points as well as the different muscle parameters are all added in the model as well. Some artificial markers (will be referred to as the black markers) are introduced at the same land marks as the ones collected in the Mocap session (Figure 6). Those black markers are driven by the grey markers and the sum of the error squared between the two at each time step was minimized according to the approach by Anderson et.al. (2006).

As shown in figure 5 and 6, by making the black marker as close as possible to the grey marker at all-time steps of the whole gait session it is possible to move the whole system of bones as well as ligaments and muscles attached to those bones in a smooth motion that is as close as possible to the captured motion of the patient. This guarantee that the segments will remain attached together, and the smooth normal motion of the whole system can be achieved which in turn facilitates the accomplishment of the kinematic analysis. After solving for the kinematics problem and the model is deemed to be functioning properly, the muscles' recruitment problem was solved next. This part of the model was trying to mimic the central nervous system (CNS) in recruiting the necessary muscles at the different time stamps during the gait session. Although there are many definitions and indices of muscle fatigue in the literature (Eltoukhy and Asfour, 2009), yet the way selected to approach such a problem was to adopt the idea utilized in human body which is based on minimizing the fatigue (equal to maximizing the endurance), which was done by utilizing the Min/Max criteria, such objective function was introduced in such problem by Rasmussen et al. (2001).

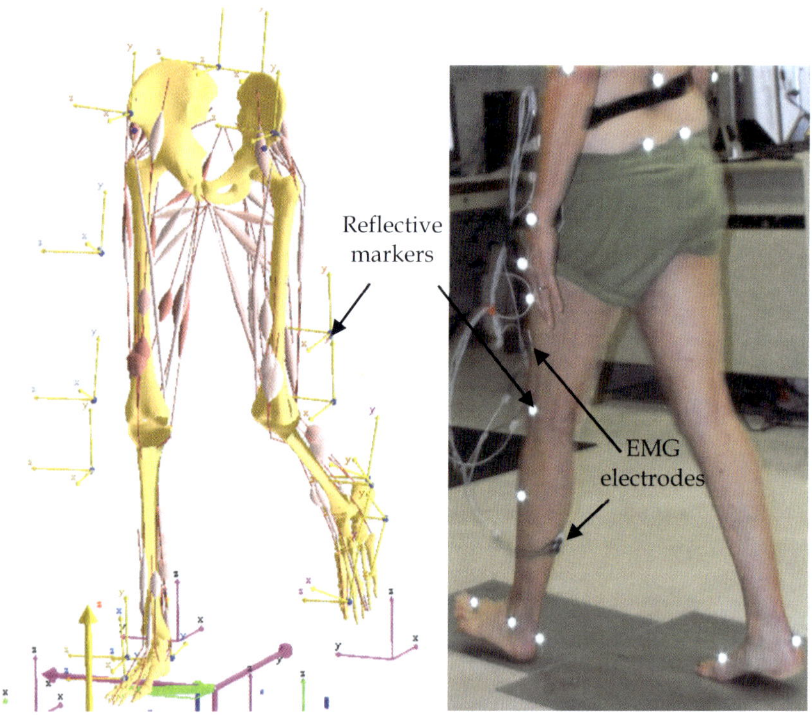

Fig. 5. 3D model of the lower extremity with muscles included and actual subject with EMG electrodes attached.

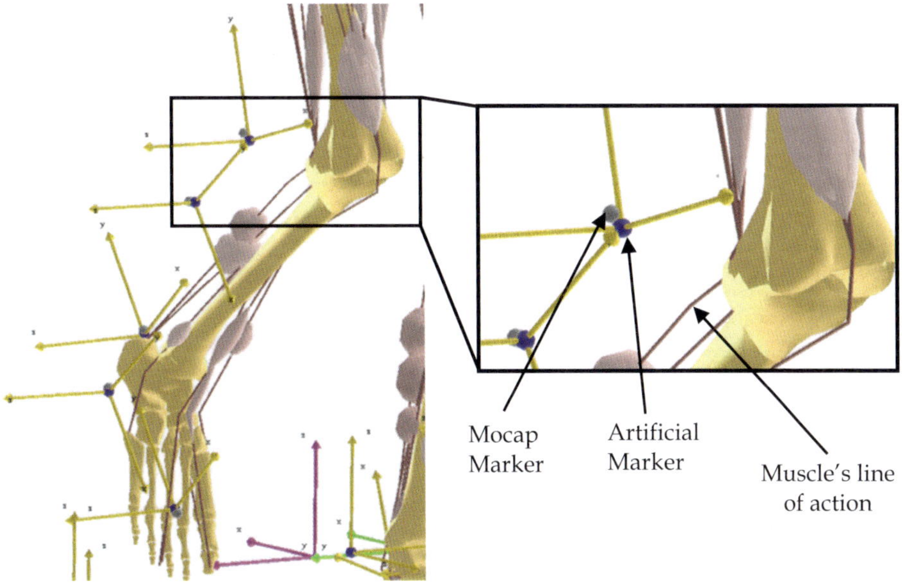

Fig. 6. Lower extremity model with bones and muscles included, each grey marker is followed by a black artificial marker at the same landmark. The sum of error squared between each pair of black and grey markers is minimized at all-time steps.

In their paper, the introduced criteria was applied to a 2D upper limb model composed of only two segments (upper arm and lower arm), three muscles, and one joint (elbow). The motion studied was a simulated motion of lifting a dumbbell and it was not an actual motion capturing experiment data. On the other hand, the developed model adds to that work by utilizing such powerful environment, AnyBody® technology, and provides a 3D model of all right and left legs and a pelvis, the model is driven by actual motion capturing data instead of a simulated (predetermined) motion. Also, the developed model is capable of simultaneously solve the optimization problem of recruiting and disrecruiting of all 54 muscles in both legs during such a complex motion like the gait.

During the muscle recruitment process the solver is trying to reach an optimum solution at each time step where both, the motion needed is achieved and the muscles' fatigue is postponed as much as possible.

A flow chart summarizing the different phases of the developed model is shown in figure 7. The main steps of the developed model can be described as follows:

- Measurement of subject's anthropometric data,
- Motion capturing (Mocap) data collection,
- Noise reduction obtained by a developed in-house LabVIEW signal processing module,
- Data reconstruction and labelling,
- Kinematic analysis utilizing an optimization algorithm by Anderson et al (2006). that minimizes the sum of error squared between any pair of markers (in this study, it's the actual and the artificial markers at the different land marks),

- Muscle recruitment using the capability of AnyBody® modelling environment, where it was possible to simultaneously optimize the recruiting and disrecruiting of 54 muscles in both legs across the whole gait cycle.

The model has a total of 7 bones which resulted in 42 degrees of freedom (d.o.f). On the other hand, only 24 d.o.f. were produced when the joints constraint were put in place, which means that a total of 18 marker coordinates were required to achieve the equilibrium (Table 1). In other words, there are more coordinates in the system than the d.o.f. Therefore, a subset of these coordinates is picked to kinematically drive the model.

Segment	# of Bones	Dofs Per Bone	Total
Foot	2	6	12
Shank	2	6	12
Thigh	2	6	12
Pelvis	1	6	6
			42

Segment	Joint Type	# of Bones	Dofs Per Bone	Total
Ankle	Universal	2	4	8
Knee	Hinge	2	5	10
Hip	Spherical	2	3	6
				24
Number of required marker coordinates				18

Table 1. Model components and degrees of freedom

The human body is composed of more than 200 bones bound and surrounded by soft tissues. To understand such a complex system, certain assumptions, simplifications and approximations must be made.

For instance, the foot is modelled as a single rigid body. The reason for this simplification is due to the complexity of foot anatomy, which is difficult to model mathematically. There are several other assumptions:

- The joint surfaces are frictionless.
- The mass of each segment is concentrated at its centre of mass.
- The estimates of body segment parameters provided by cadaver studies are sufficiently close to the real anthropometry of the person whose gait is being analysed. In practice, the errors from inaccurate segment parameters are thought to be very small, at least in normal gait (Pearsall & Costigan 1999).
- There is no co-contraction of the opposing agonist and antagonist muscles. If this occurs, a net moment will be calculated, which will be the difference between the moments generated by the two muscles.

The following section will describe the details of the kinematic analysis and the muscle recruitment problem. In summary, the model implemented is based on the method of inverse dynamics to determine the muscle forces from the kinematics data, while the muscle recruitment is utilizing the concept of minimizing the maximum muscle activity (Rausmessun et al, 2001), the models' drivers are developed based on the approach by Anderson et al. (2006) of optimizing the captured markers using the ViconNexus® motion capturing system.

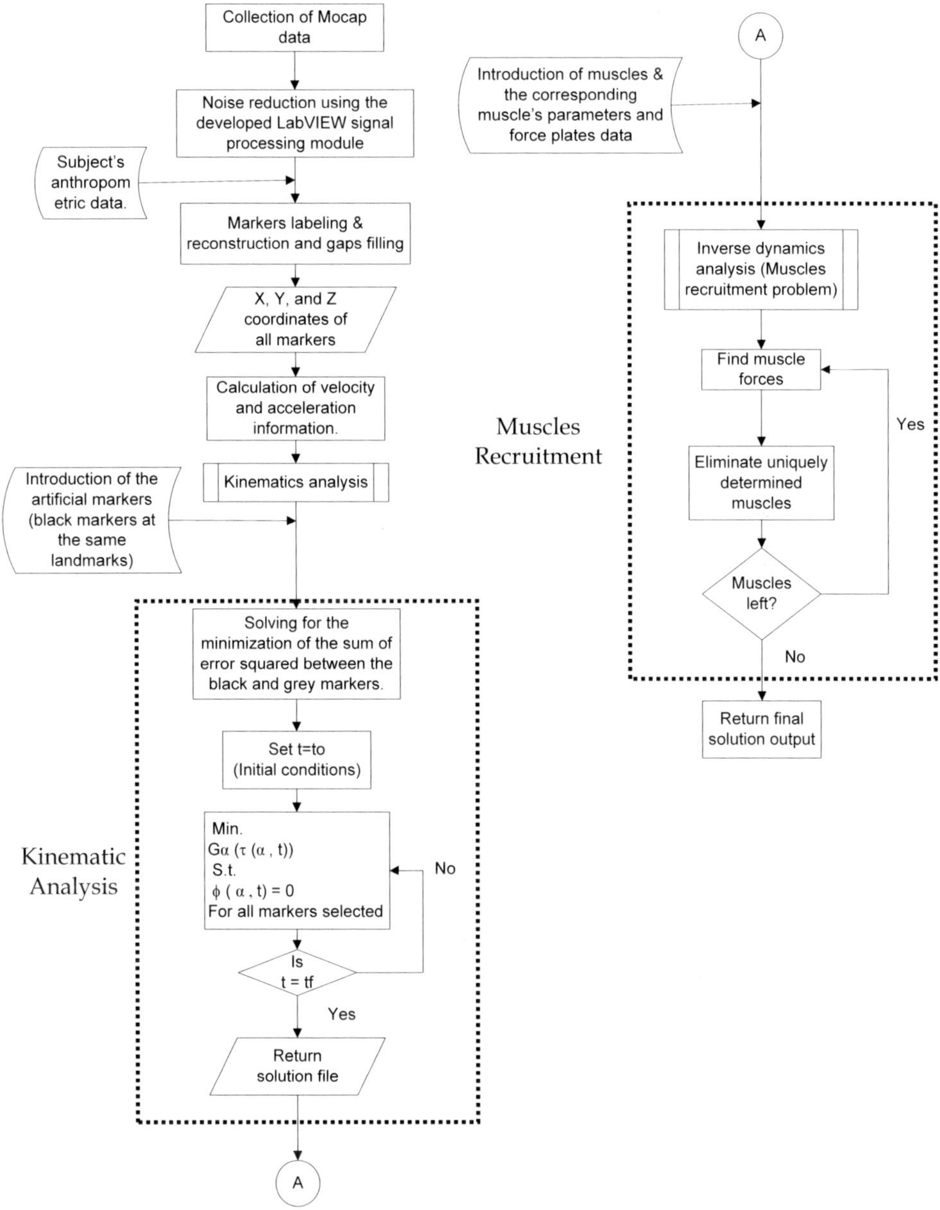

Fig. 7. Flowchart of the modelling steps and phases involved in the analysis of human gait cycle.

2.1.3.1 Kinematic analysis

When developing a musculoskeletal model from motion capture data for inverse dynamics analysis, the resulting set of equations usually will be over-determinate, i.e. the measurement results in more measured degrees-of-freedom than the ones of the model. Several solutions to this problem have been posed in the literature.

They are essentially split into two groups: 1) methods that work on a segment-to-segment basis, and 2) methods that use model information, such as joint constraints, to reduce the effects of skin-artefacts. A general solution to the problem of kinematic over-determinacy when driving a mechanical model from measured data in the form of marker trajectories is implemented in this study.

The solution suggested by Anderson et al. (2006) is based on solving an appropriate constrained weighted least-squares optimization problem for each discrete time step with the system coordinates as unknowns.

The first step in inverse dynamics is always to perform kinematic analysis to find the positions, velocities and acceleration of the time-dependent system coordinates, $\alpha(t) \in \alpha$, i.e. given some system description it is desired to find α (t), $\alpha^{\cdot}(t)$ and $\alpha^{\cdot\cdot}(t)$.

To accommodate this over-determinacy, it is assumed that it is possible to split the position analysis equation into two sets:

$$\chi(\alpha, t) = \begin{bmatrix} \tau & (\alpha, t) \\ \phi & (\alpha, t) \end{bmatrix} \tag{1}$$

Where $\tau \equiv \tau$ (α, t) is a set of equations that only have to be solved "as well as possible" in some sense and the remaining $\phi \equiv \phi$ (α, t) equations have to be fulfilled exactly.

In this study, where the musculoskeletal model was derived from motion capture data, the choice of these sets was that the experimental data belongs to τ and joint constraints and additional driver equations to ϕ.

In other words, it is required to solve the following optimization problem:

$$\text{Min } G\alpha\ (\tau\ (\alpha, t)) \tag{2}$$

$$\text{s.t.} \quad \phi\ (\alpha, t) = 0 \tag{3}$$

This is done by automatically taking all the marker coordinates into account and then taking the minimized deviation between the markers in the model and the markers captured in the motion capturing experiment (Figure 6), i.e., minimizing the square sum of errors. This process is done in an offline mode, where the data is analyzed and then fed back to the model.

Having solved the optimization problem, the system coordinates, α, will be known for the discrete time steps where the optimization problem is solved. However, it still remains to find the velocities and accelerations which are accomplished by differentiating the position data to determine the velocities and a second time to determine the accelerations.

2.1.3.2 Muscle recruitment

The second part of the model is the muscles recruitment problem, where in which the model mimics the CNS in its coordination of muscles during complex activities such as human locomotion.

The basic optimality assumption considered in the model is that the body attempts to use its muscles in such a way that fatigue is postponed as far as possible. Which leads to the idea of minimizing maximum muscle activity (Rasmussen et al., 2001). Thus, the model will recruit muscles according to the following criterion, put in the general form:

Minimize:
Maximum muscle activity
Subject to:

- Equilibrium equations fulfilled.
- Muscles can pull only.

It was also proven by Rasmussen et al. (2001) that the min/max criteria is identical to both soft saturation and polynomial objective functions at high power. And due to the advantages that the min/max possesses, it was decided to apply it as the recruitment criteria.

The effect of implementing the min/max criteria in the muscle recruitment problem is that they tend to form groups; meaning that if there are a number of muscles crossing the same joint and have the same strength; they will form a group in the recruitment. This is because the min/max criteria tries to decrease the activity in all muscles simultaneously, which guarantees that there is no other muscle recruitment pattern that could lead to smaller muscle activity.

2.1.3.3 Noise reduction

The model interpolates the data by a smooth spline interpolation, and it is possible to suppress the noise to some extent by increasing the order of the spline interpolation and/or by down sampling the data. Yet, the best way to minimize the noise is to low pass filter the data before sending them to the model. This will get rid of most of the high frequency noise in the motion capture data, this goal was achieved by developing another module based on LabVIEW programming scheme.

The effect of filtering the data using the developed signal processing module is that it dramatically reduces the time needed by the solver to find the optimum solution of the optimization problem during the kinematic analysis stage (Figure 8). The vertical axis in the

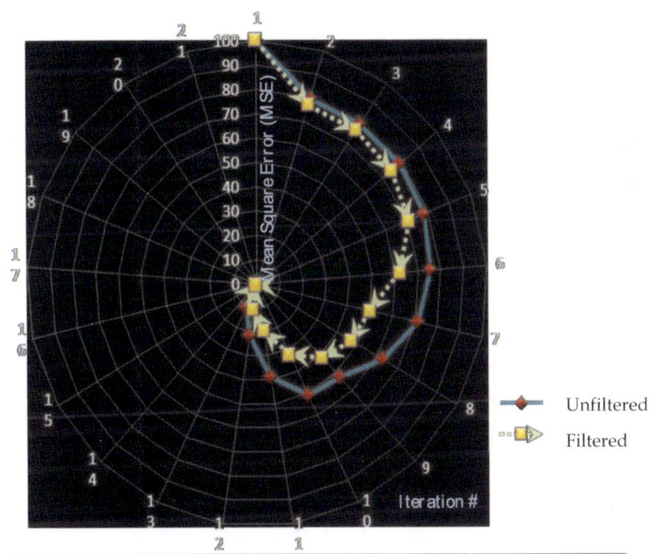

Fig. 8. Mean square error plots of both filtered and unfiltered data

figure depicts the mean squared error (MSE) resulted at each iteration of the solution process of the objective function. The outer circle is the iteration number of the corresponding MSE value.
As shown in figure 8, the dotted curve represents the filtered data indicates that the solver reaches an optimum solution at a fewer number of iterations as compared to the unfiltered data (solid curve), where more iterations were needed to reach an optimum solution for the objective function.
Once the model is validated against measured data it can then be used to analyze the effect of muscles on a hip or knee prosthesis, especially when considering different surgical techniques.

3. Results and discussion

The following section will introduce some of the model outputs obtained in comparison to one of the literature resources available which is the Hip98 data base (Bergmann et al. 2001). All data shown were normalized by the subject's weight. Figure 9 shows a sample of the knee reaction forces obtained from one of the patients studied in the laboratory as compared to the pattern obtained by Harrington (1992).

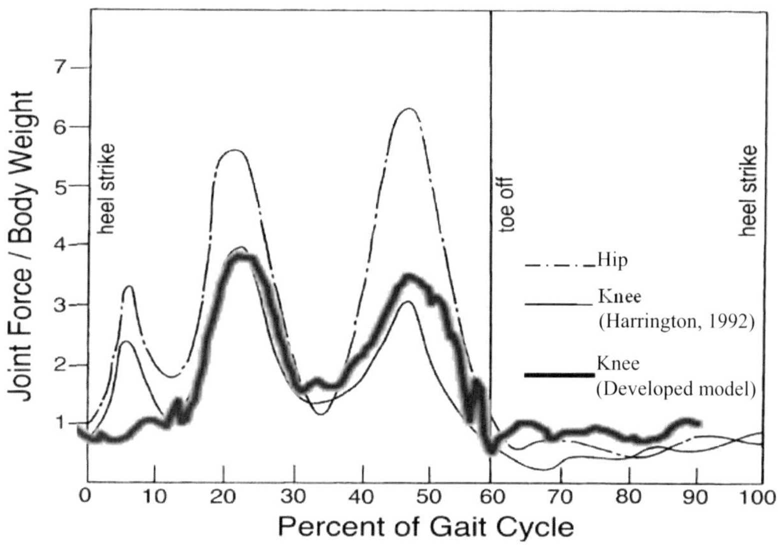

Fig. 9. Knee reaction forces pattern. (Harrington, 1992)

The moments were then calculated. Figure 10 (A, B, and C) shows the hip moments generated in the flexion / extension, internal / external rotation, and abduction / adduction directions respectively.
The force and moment patterns and magnitude predicted were in a great agreement with the measured values in the literature (Hip98). The ground reaction forces utilized in the model were compared to the forces reported in the Hip98 data base as shown in figure 11 (A, B, and C). The figure depicts the ground reaction forces in the inferior, lateral, and anterior directions respectively.

3.1 Case study: Total knee replacement

A total of fifteen subjects participated in this study, five subjects in each group. Based on the statistical analysis conducted it was evident that the allograft group had less significant gait deviations than did those in the metallic group. In particular, the metallic group patients had greater gait deviations both in the loading-response phase, and in the Fore-Aft terminal stance phase. In conclusion, our findings suggest that implantation of hinged total knee prosthesis with removal of one or two of the quadriceps muscles provide good functional results during gait. Additional studies should be performed to evaluate the relationship between the number and extent of the quadriceps heads excised and both the knee mechanics during gait and the long-term survival of the prosthesis.

The comparison between the gait results obtained using the musculoskeletal model and a very relevant experimental research conducted by Benedetti et al. (2000), it was also concluded that the introduced model can provided a high confidence level if used in applications that involves joint replacements which ultimately can be utilized in surgery planning.

3.1.1 Subjects and procedures

Demographics of the Control Group

Five subjects with no history or complaints of known walking problems, knee injuries and postural instability volunteered for this experiment.

Demographics of the Patient Group

Ten patient subjects was the maximum number that was available to participate in this study. All patient subjects had distal femoral knee replacement surgery. Five subjects were allograft patients while the other five were metallic patients. The Following table summarizes the demographics of all three subject groups.

The procedures performed on the study subjects were wide local excision of the tumor and reconstruction using either a Stryker (tm) MRS rotating hinged knee or an osteoarticular allograft. The MRS knee was placed after radical resection of the distal femur. The distal femur was prepared by reaming the intramedullary canal with the appropriate sized reamer to achieve the greatest diameter stem with an appropriate cement mantle (2mm circumferential). The tibia was prepared with standard cutting jigs.

	Control	Metallic	Allograft
No of Subjects	5	5	5
Age (years)	26.6 ± 0.9	42.3 ± 5.9	28.6 ± 5.6
Height (cm)	175.8 ± 1.9	175.8 ± 8.5	163.0 ± 8.0
Weight (kg)	71.8 ± 3.9	89.6 ± 15.5	66.0 ± 8.3

Table 2. Demographics of Subjects

The tibial and femoral canals were filled with cement after pulse irrigation and drying using modern cement techniques. The components were segmental and prepared on the back table to reconstruct the longitudinal dimensions of the defect. The components were assembled using inner bearings an axle and rotating metal hinge. In some cases, a gastrocnemius flap was turned up into the defect to fill the dead space and to help tether the lateral pull of the extensor mechanism. The allografts were prepared differently.

The patient's menisci and portions of the lateral, medial collateral ligaments along with the anterior and posterior cruciate ligaments were retained. The allograft was aseptically

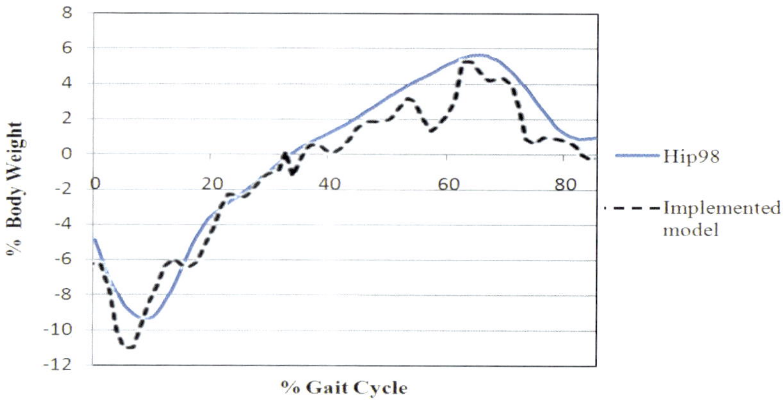

(a)

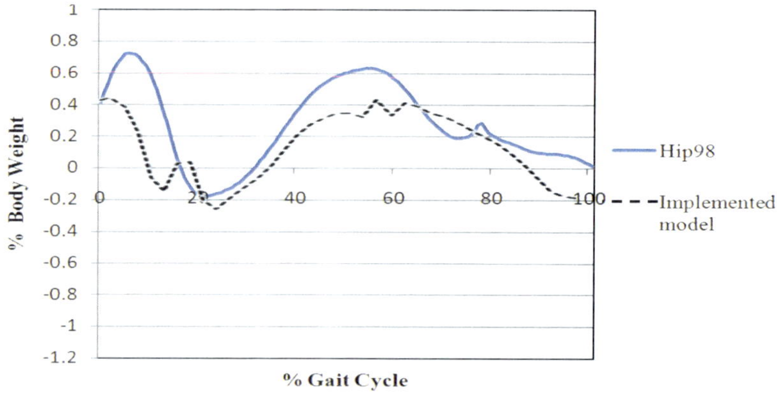

(b)

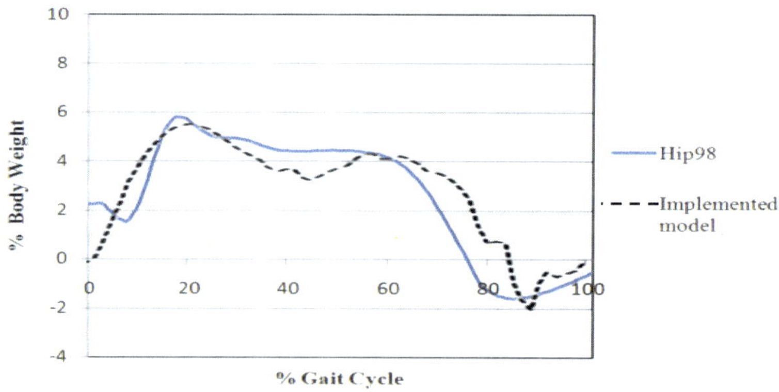

(c)

Fig. 10. Hip moments generated in the following directions: (A) Flexion/Extension, (B) Internal /External rotational, and (C) Abduction/Adduction.

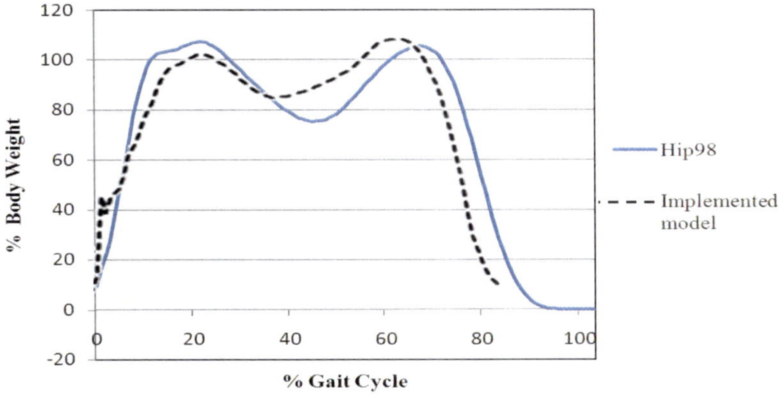

(a)

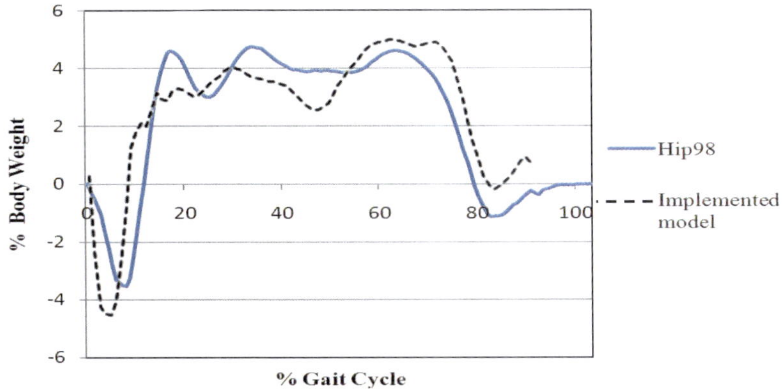

(b)

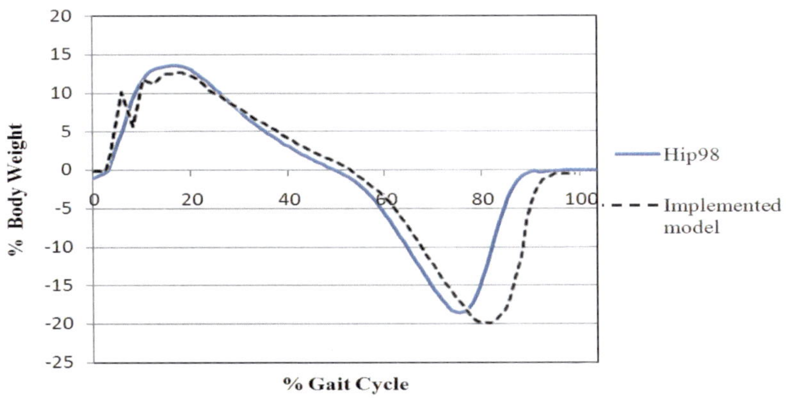

(c)

Fig. 11. Ground reaction forces in the following directions: (A) Inferior, (B) Lateral, and (C) Anterior.

harvested from a suitable donor; the cartilage was preserved with DMSO and frozen in a controlled fashion to -80 degrees for storage. In the operating theatre, this preselected graft was then thawed in lactated ringer solution and cut on the back table to the appropriate length. A plate or plates were then affixed to the graft and the soft tissue structures were then reconstructed. The reconstruction began with the posterior capsule followed by the posterior cruciate, the lateral collateral ligaments and finally the anterior cruciate ligament. The meniscofemoral attachments to the allograft were repaired following this. The graft itself was then anchored to the patient's host bone with plates and screws.

The participants were given instructions including an explanation of the test procedures, proper attire, and the expected duration of the testing. The data was collected at the University of Miami Biomechanics Research Laboratory, USA, with an approval from the Internal Review Board (IRB). 48 reflective markers were placed at the different body land marks (e.g. joints center lines and segments). First, a static trial was conducted where the patient stands at a tee pose which is then used for markers labeling. Then five dynamics trials were performed. Each subject was instructed to walk at his normal speed across the laboratory and on top of the four force plates.

3.1.2 Instrumentation and data collection

The laboratory incorporates a ViconNexus® Motion Capturing System (Oxford Metrics, United Kingdom). The motion capturing system integrates and synchronizes four Kistler force plates (Model: 9253B), ten MX cameras, two high speed reference video cameras, and wireless Noraxon EMG system. The MX cameras provide 1024 x 1024 pixel resolution and frame rates up to 250 Hz.

3.1.3 3D Lower extremity musculoskeletal model

Once the motion capturing data was reconstructed and all gaps were filled then the C3D file, which contains the X, Y, and Z coordinates of the different markers as well as the force plate data, is imported to the 3D lower extremity modeling phase. The three-dimensional musculoskeletal model of the lower extremity introduced by Eltoukhy and Asfour (2009) was utilized in this study.

The model consisted of seven rigid body segments connected with frictionless joints, these segments are the pelvis, right and left thighs, right and left shanks and right and left feet. Hip joints were modeled as universal joints that have three degrees of freedom. Knee joints were modeled as hinge joints, while ankle joints were modeled as biaxial joints. Hip joint flexion/extension, adduction/abduction and internal/external rotation as well as ankle joint dorsi/plantar flexion and inversion/eversion were all allowed (Figure 12). The model is scalable to the subject's dimensions; with 27 muscles in each leg been included, the exact origin and insertion points as well as the different muscle parameters are all added in the model as well.

4. Statistical analysis

Among the different gait variables measured, a specific subset of these variables was carefully selected. These variables were then used in the statistical analysis. Figure 13 shows the ground reaction forces in the X, Y, and Z directions as well as the knee flexion angle measured during the gait session. The figure also depicts the specific force and angle values at the different point of times during the gait cycle that were analyzed in the statistical analysis phase.

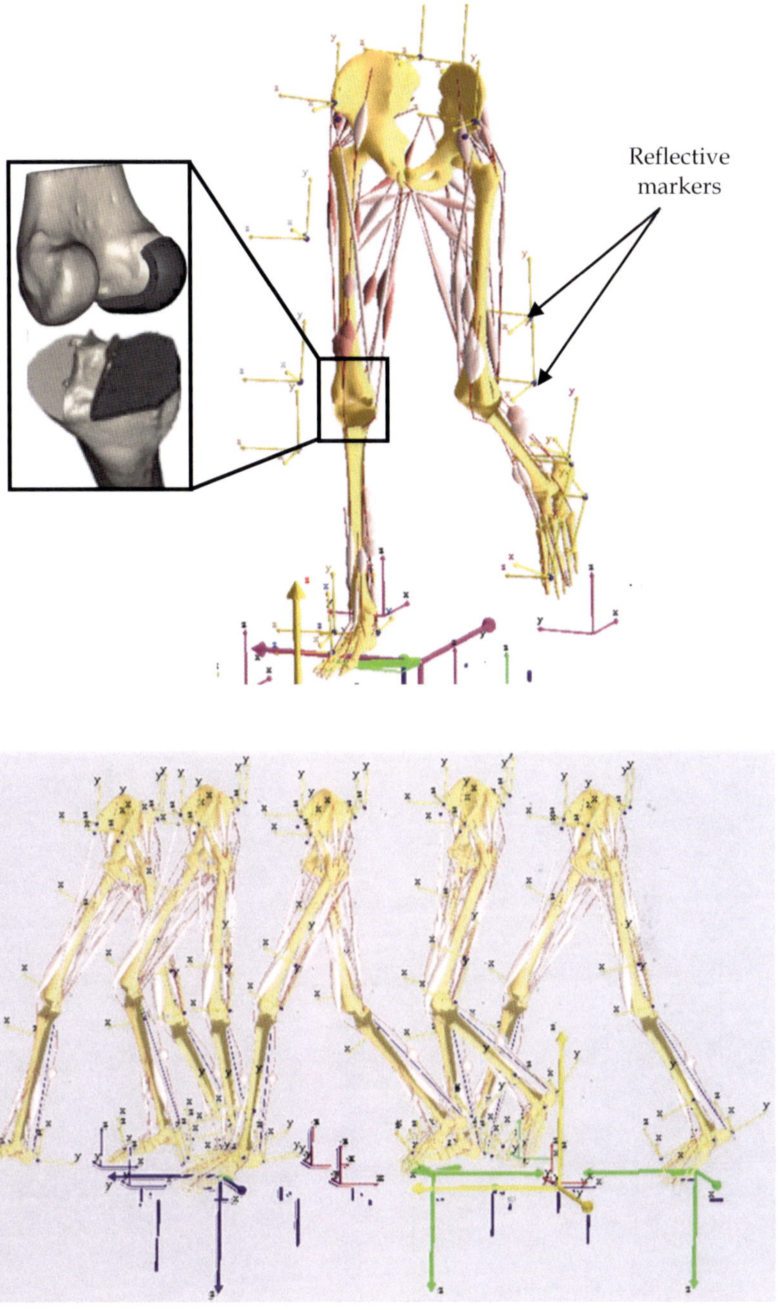

Fig. 12. Modified lower extremity model introduced by Eltoukhy and Asfour, 2009.

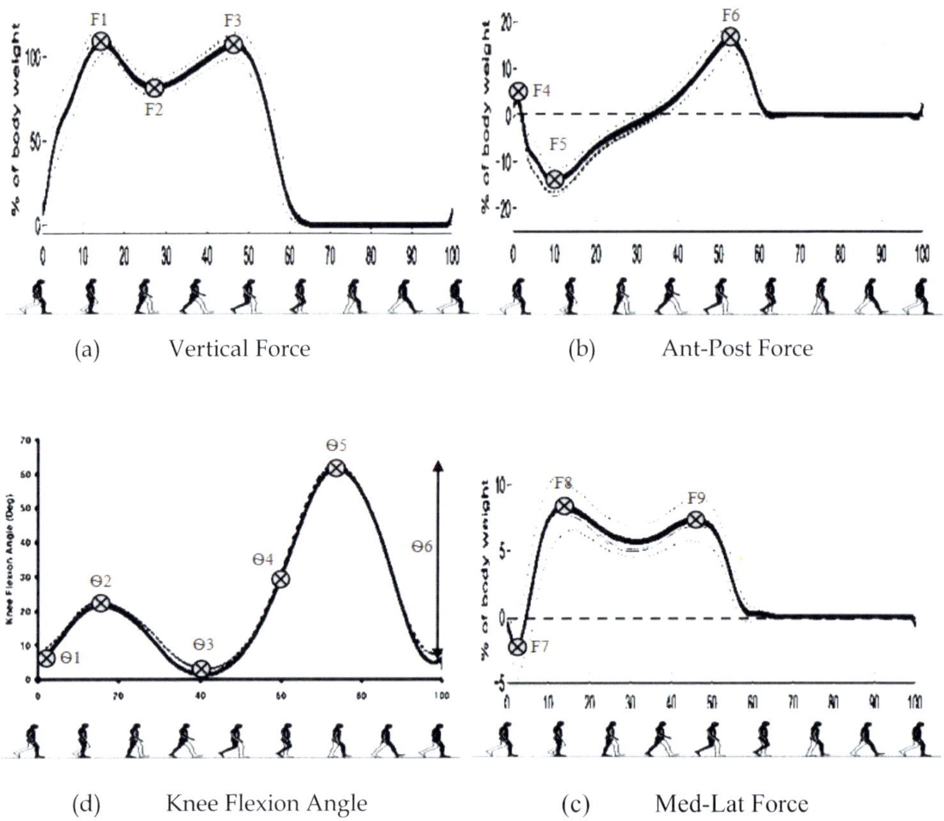

F1:Maximum vertical loading response	F6:Maximum Fore-Aft terminal stance	Θ2:Maximum Flexion loading response
F2:Maximum vertical midstance	F7:Maximum Med-Lat loading response	Θ3:Maximum Extension stance
F3:Maximum vertical terminal stance	F8:Maximum Med-Lat midstance	Θ4:Flexion toe-off
F4:Maximum Fore-Aft loading response	F9 :Maximum Med-Lat terminal stance	Θ5:Maximum Flexion swing
F5:Maximum Fore-Aft midstance	Θ1:Flexion heel-strike	Θ6:Total sagittal plane excursion

Fig. 13. The gait parameters measured.

As shown in the figure, three main points (F1, F2, and F3) in the vertical force component (Figure 6-a); also, F4, F5, and F6 were recorded from the Ant-Post force component (Figure

6-b). The last three force components recorded were the F7, F8, and F9 and that is from the Med-Lat force plot (Figure 6-c). Six angle values were recorded from the knee flexion angle component. These angle components were Θ1 to Θ6 (Figure 6-d).

The data collected from the two patient groups (metallic and allograft knee joints) was plotted along with the control group (normal knee joint). Figure 14 depicts two interval

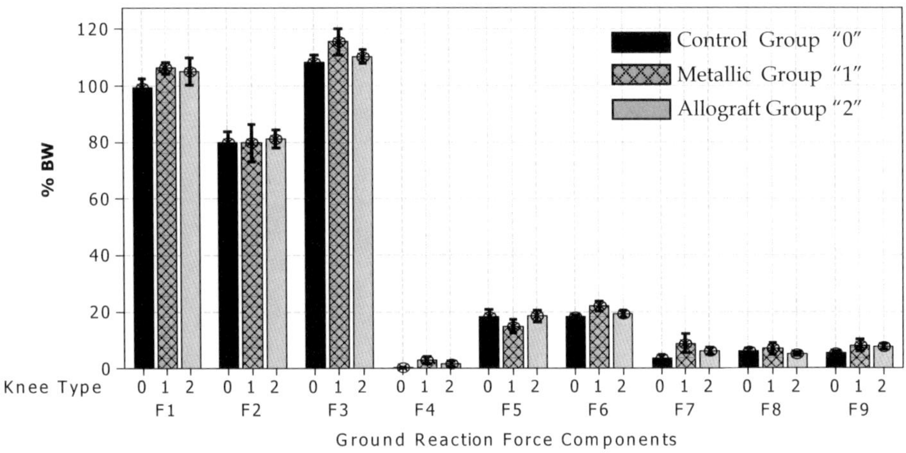

(a)

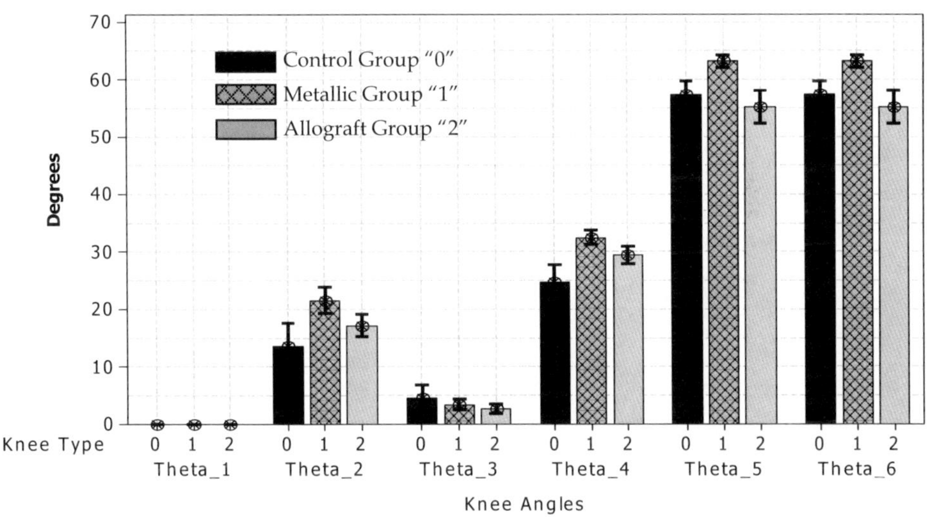

(b)

Fig. 14. Interval plots of (a) the ground reaction forces (F1 to F9) and (b) the knee flexion angle (Θ1 to Θ6) for all three groups, Control "0", Metallic "1", and Allograft "2".

plots for both the ground reaction forces as well as the knee flexion angle measured. As shown in figure 14, each of the force and angle components was plotted in the form of the mean and standard deviation values for all three groups, control, metallic, and allograft.

For the vertical ground reaction force (Z direction) components, both the metallic and allograft groups showed higher average forces when compared to the control group, for the maximum vertical loading response, F1, and the maximum vertical terminal stance, F3 while they showed almost an equal magnitude for the maximum vertical midstance, F2.

The Ant-Post force values (F4-F6) resulted in a similar pattern as the vertical forces where the metallic and allograft groups showed higher values when compared to the control group for both F4 and F6, yet, in case of the maximum Fore-Aft midstance force, F5, the metallic group resulted in lower magnitude while the allograft group resulted in higher forces when compared to the control group. Similar pattern was also obtained in case of the Med-Lat force values, only the F8, maximum Med-Lat midstance, showed higher forces for the metallic group and similar mean value for allograft group when compared to the control group. In regard to the flexion knee angle values, the following conclusions can be drawn. In general, the metallic group showed higher knee flexion angle values (Θ2: Maximum Flexion loading response, Θ3:Maximum Extension stance, Θ4:Flexion toe-off, Θ5:Maximum Flexion swing, and Θ6:Total sagittal plane excursion) as compared to the allograft group, in other words, the allograft group showed stiff-knee gait pattern. Note that only in case of the Θ3 (maximum extension stance), the control group showed higher mean value than the metallic and allograft groups which can be explained because of the range of motion loss resulted from the surgery when compared to the control group.

A statistical analysis of the gait data collected was performed as follows; two Multi-Analysis of Variance (MANOVA) were conducted for both the ground reaction force components as well as the knee joint angle. The factor tested was the knee type (Normal, Metallic, and Allograft), on the other hand the variables tested were the different force components of the three ground reaction forces in the X,Y, and Z directions (F1 to F9) as well as the knee angles (Θ2 to Θ6). The data was first tested for normality. The basic data descriptive statistics as well as the MANOVA results are summarized in table 3, 4, and 5 respectively.

Variable	Count	Mean ± StDev	Variable	Count	Mean ± StDev
F1	30	103.7 ± 5.6	Θ 1	30	0.0
F2	30	80.3 ± 6.6	Θ 2	30	17.5 ± 5.1
F3	30	111.5 ± 5.4	Θ 3	30	3.6 ± 2.1
F4	30	1.6 ± 1.6	Θ 4	30	28.9 ± 4.3
F5	30	17.2 ± 3.5	Θ 5	30	58.5 ± 4.6
F6	30	19.8 ± 2.4	Θ 6	30	58.5 ± 4.6
F7	30	6.1 ± 3.6			
F8	30	6.0 ± 1.9			
F9	30	7.0 ± 2.3			

Table 3. Ground reaction forces and knee angles descriptive statistics

			DF		
Criterion	Test Statistic	F	Num	Denom	P
Wilks'	0.04444	7.903	18	38	0.000
Lawley-Hotelling	7.87640	7.876	18	36	0.000
Pillai's	1.56107	7.904	18	40	0.000
Roy's	5.31098				

s = 2 m = 3.0 n = 8.5

Table 4. MANOVA for Knee Replacement Type (Ground Reaction Forces)

			DF		
Criterion	Test Statistic	F	Num	Denom	P
Wilks'	0.05324	20.003	8	48	0.000
Lawley-Hotelling	9.14198	26.283	8	46	0.000
Pillai's	1.40680	14.822	8	50	0.000
Roy's	8.07144				

s = 2 m = 0.5 n = 11.0

Table 5. MANOVA for Knee Replacement Type (Knee Angles)

As shown in the MANOVA tables and based on the Wilks criteria, the data suggests that the type of knee replacement is associated with changes in gait pattern. As tables 4 and 5 indicate, other similar tests, namely Pillai's Trace, Hotelling's Trace, and Roy's Largest Root test, also lead to the same conclusion. The Wilks' lambda test is used to measure the overall significance of the model. When the overall model is significant, then the significance of the individual variables can be pursued. After statistically significant evidence was obtained from the MANOVA tests, the individual ANOVA analyses for both the ground reaction forces (GRF) and knee flexion angles were performed and the results were summarized in table 6.

Table 6 basically shows the results of the individual ANOVA tests for all GRF components and knee flexion angles. The table also shows the P values, as well as the mean and standard deviations for all variables and that is for each group separately. The table also summarizes the post-hoc analysis results; the post-hoc performed compared the control vs. the metallic, the control vs. the allograft, and the metallic vs. the allograft groups. In general, the allograft showed similar values for both the forces and angles during gait when compared to the control group. In other words, no statistically significant differences were found between the two groups, that is true for all force values (except for F4 and F9) and knee angles (except for Θ4). On the other hand, the metallic group showed statistical differences in most of the force values (except for F8) and knee angles (except for Θ3) when compared to the control group. Finally, to exclude the age factor as a possible reason behind the finding that the allograft group resulted in less gait deviations compared to the metallic group in comparison to the control group, the following statistical analysis was conducted. First a separate MANOVA analysis was conducted with the "Age" set as the factor been modelled and the variable set were the flexion knee angles (Θ2 to Θ5) as shown in table 7.

					P-Value (Post-hoc analysis)		
Variable	P Value*	Control Group	Metallic Group	Allograft Group	Control Group Vs. Metallic Group	Control Group Vs. Allograft Group	Metallic Group Vs. Allograft Group
GRF		Mean±Std	Mean±Std	Mean±Std			
F1	0.010	99.5±4.2	106.3±3.0	105.2±6.8	Sig.	NS	NS
F2	NS	79.8±5.6	79.8±9.2	81.2±4.6	NS	NS	NS
F3	0.006	108.5±3.3	115.6±6.6	110.4±3.2	Sig.	NS	Sig.
F4	0.001	0.2±0.07	2.7±1.8	1.7±1.3	Sig.	Sig.	NS
F5	0.028	18.3±3.3	14.8±3.3	18.4±2.9	Sig.	NS	Sig.
F6	0.001	18.2±1.1	21.9±2.5	19.3±1.8	Sig.	NS	NS
F7	0.004	3.6±1.7	8.7±4.6	6.0±1.9	Sig.	NS	NS
F8	NS	6.2±1.1	6.9±2.7	5.0±0.9	NS	NS	NS
F9	0.007	5.3±1.0	8.0±2.9	7.8±1.3	Sig.	Sig.	Sig.
Knee angles							
Θ 2	0.001	13.6±5.6	21.6±3.2	17.2±2.7	Sig.	NS	NS
Θ 3	NS	4.6±3.1	3.4±1.3	2.7±1.3	NS	NS	NS
Θ 4	0.000	24.7±4.3	32.5±1.8	29.5±2.1	Sig.	Sig.	NS
Θ 5	0.000	57.3±3.2	63.2±1.5	55.1±4.0	Sig.	NS	Sig.
Θ 6	0.000	57.3±3.2	63.2±1.5	55.1±4.0	Sig.	NS	Sig.

* According to analysis of variance unless otherwise indicated. Sig.: significant. NS: not significant.

Table 6. Descriptive Statistics and ANOVA results

			DF		
Criterion	Test Statistic	F	Num	Denom	P
Wilks'	0.00016	1.499	56	9	**0.265**
Lawley-Hotelling	75.73244	0.676	56	2	**0.763**
Pillai's	3.16755	1.359	56	20	**0.227**
Roy's	61.09191				

s = 4 m = 4.5 n = 0.0

Table 7. MANOVA for patients' age (Knee Angles)

As shown in table 7 and based on the three MANOVA indices, there was a clear evidence that no statistically significant effect of the patients' age on the knee kinematics. The second analysis performed was a set of three MANOVA tests of the ground reaction force components (F1 to F9) with the "Age" set as the factor tested. Table 8 summarizes the

MANOVA outputs for these three tests. In was also evident that in case of the kinetics, the patients' age had failed to show any statistically significant effect on the ground reaction force components produced during gait.

Vertical Forces (F1-F3)			DF		
Criterion	Test Statistic	F	Num	Denom	P
Wilks'	0.00209	1.613	42	9	0.227
Lawley-Hotelling	24.80947	0.985	42	5	0.579
Pillai's	2.53192	1.932	42	15	0.084
Roy's	13.96643				
Fore-Aft Forces (F4-F6)			DF		
Criterion	Test Statistic	F	Num	Denom	P
Wilks'	0.00266	1.467	42	9	0.279
Lawley-Hotelling	29.76959	1.181	42	5	0.475
Pillai's	2.39169	1.404	42	15	0.242
Roy's	22.86074				
Med-Lat Forces (F7-F9)			DF		
Criterion	Test Statistic	F	Num	Denom	P
Wilks'	0.00625	20.003	42	9	0.513
Lawley-Hotelling	16.62683	0.660	42	5	0.794
Pillai's	2.33854	1.263	42	15	0.321
Roy's	10.82468				

Table 8. MANOVA for patients' age (Ground Reaction Forces)

5. Conclusions

The goal of this research work shown in the chapter was to introduce the whole process of developing and validating a 3D lower extremity musculoskeletal model and to test the ability of the model to predict the muscles recruitment of the different muscles involved in human locomotion as well as determining the corresponding forces and moments generated around the different joints in the lower extremity. Therefore the model can be applied in one of the important fields of orthopaedics which is joint replacement; the case study used in such application is the total knee replacement. The knee reaction forces were compared to the pattern obtained by Harrington (1992), where the hip moment components (Flexion/extension, internal/external, and abduction/adduction) were all compared to the patterns obtained from the Hip98 data base.

As it was shown in the different forces and moments graphs, the model was able to produce very close results when comparing pattern and magnitude to the literature data. Thus, this 3D biomechanical model is sophisticated enough to be used for surgery evaluation such as in total knee replacement, where the damaged cartilage and bone are removed from the surface of the knee joint and replaced with a man-made surface of metal and plastic.

The three-dimensional (3D) musculoskeletal model of the lower extremity introduced by Eltoukhy and Asfour (2009) has been utilized in the joint replacement applications. The objective of this case study was to test the applicability of the introduced model in situations

that involves joint replacement and to show that the model can be used for such applications such as surgery planning. The case study of the research work presented in this chapter involved the comparison of the gait pattern between two main knee joint types, Metallic and Allograft knee joints against normal subjects (Control group). A total of fifteen subjects participated in this study, five subjects in each group. Based on the results obtained from the MANOVA tests, the allograft group had less significant gait deviations than did those in the metallic group. In particular, the metallic group patients had greater gait deviations both in the loading-response phase, and in the Fore-Aft terminal stance phase.
It was concluded that based on the study conducted and the statistical evidence obtained that the introduced model can be used for applications that involves joint surgeries such as knee replacement that ultimately can be utilized in surgery evaluation.

6. Acknowledgment

The authors would like to thank John Rasmussen, Soren Torholm, Michael Andersen, and Arne Kiis from the AnyBody Co. for their technical support during the implementation of the model. The authors would like to thank Dr. H. T. Temple, M.D. Professor of Orthopaedic and Pathology, Chief of Orthopaedic Oncology Division, and Director of the Tissue Bank at the University of Miami's Leonard M. Miller School of Medicine, for providing all of the subject patients.

7. References

Alkjaer, T., Simonsen, E. and Dyhre-Poulsen, P., 2001. Comparison of inverse dynamics calculated by two- and three-dimensional models during walking, Gait & Posture, pp. 73–77.

American Academy of Orthopaedic Surgeons (AAOS). 6300 North River Road, Rosemont, IL 60018. http://www.aaos.org.

Andersen, M., Damsgaard, M., Tørholm, S., Rasmussen, J., 2006. Kinematic Analysis of Over-determinate Systems. 19th Nordic Seminar on Computational Mechanics, 20-21 October, Lund, Sweden.

Andriacchi,T., Hurwitz, D., 1997. Gait biomechanics and the evolution of total joint replacement, Gait & Posture, 5 (3), pp.256-264.

Benedetti, M., Catani, F., Donati, D., Simoncini, L., and Giannini,S., 2000. Muscle Performance About the Knee Joint in Patients Who Had Distal Femoral Replacement After Resection of a Bone Tumor : An Objective Study with Use of Gait Analysis, J Bone Joint Surg Am., 82(11), pp.1619-1625.

Bergmann, G., Deuretzbacher, G., Heller, M., Graichen, F., Rohlmann, A., Strauss, J. and Duda, G.N., 2001. Hip contact forces and gait patterns from routine activities. Journal of Biomechanics, 34, pp. 859-871.

Brand, R.A., Pederson, D.R., Davy, D.T., Kotzar, G.M., Heiple, K.G. and Goldberg, V.M., 1994. Comparison of hip joint force calculations measured in the same patient. Journal of Arthroplasty, 9, pp. 45-51.

Crowninshield, R.D., Johnston, R.C., Andrews, J.G. and Brand, R.A., 1978. A biomechanical investigation of the human hip. Journal of Biomechanics, 11, pp. 75-85.

Crowninshield, R. and Brand, R., 1981. The prediction of forces in joint structures: distribution of intersegmental resultants, Exercise and Sports Sciences Reviews, 9, pp. 159–181.

Eltoukhy, M. and Asfour, S., 2009. Use of Optimization Theory in the Development of 3D Musculoskeletal Model for Gait Analysis, International Journal of Computational Vision and Biomechanics (IJCV&B), 3 (2), In press.

Eltoukhy, M. and Asfour, S., 2009. Implementation and validation of a detailed three dimensional inverse dynamics lower extremity model for gait analysis applications, Proceedings of the XXIst Annual International Occupational Ergonomics and Safety Conference, 11-12 June, Dallas, Texas, USA, pp.57-62.

Eltoukhy, M. and Asfour, S., 2009. Detection of Muscle Fatigue in Dynamic Tasks using Recurrence Quantification Analysis, International Journal of Computational Vision and Biomechanics (IJCV&B),2 (2), In Press.

Harrington, I.J., 1992. Knee joint forces in normal and pathological gait. In: Niwa S, Perren SW, Hattori T, eds. Biomechanics in orthopaedics, Tokyo, etc. Springer Verlag, pp.121-46.

Healthbase Medical Source: www.healthbase.com/resources/orthopedics/revision-joint-replacement-surgery

HIP98 (2001 Version) Bergmann, G., Graichen F. and Rohlmann A., Biomechanics Lab, Benjamin Franklin School of Medicine, Free University of Berlin, Gemany.

Horsman, M., Koopman, H., van der Helm,F., L. and Veeger,H., 2007. Morphological muscle and joint parameters for musculoskeletal modelling of the lower extremity, Clinical Biomechanics, 22, pp. 239-247.

Kay RM, Dennis S, Rethlefsen S, et al., 2000. The effect of preoperative gait analysis on orthopaedic decision making. Clin Orthop Relat Res., (372), pp.217-222.

Lofterød B, Terjesen T, Skaaret I, et al., 2007. Preoperative gait analysis has a substantial effect on orthopedic decision making in children with cerebral palsy: Comparison between clinical evaluation and gait analysis in 60 patients. Acta Orthop., 78(1), pp.74-80.

Molenaers G, Desloovere K, Fabry G, De Cock P. The effects of quantitative gait assessment and botulinum toxin a on musculoskeletal surgery in children with cerebral palsy. J Bone Joint Surg Am. 2006, 88(1), pp.161-170.

Naganoa, A., Komurab, T., Fukashiroc, S., Himenoa,R., 2005. Force, work and power output of lower limb muscles during human maximal-effort countermovement jumping, 15(4), pp. 367-376.

Orendurff, M., Aiona, M., Dorociak, R. and Pierce, R., 2002. Length and force of the gastrocnemius and soleus during gait following tendo Achilles lengthenings in children with equines, Gait & Posture, 15(2), pp. 130-135.

Pearsall, D. and Costigan, P., 1999. The effect of segment parameter error on gait analysis results. Gait and Posture 9, pp. 173–183.

Piazza, S. and Delp, S., 1996. The influence of muscles on knee flexion during the swing phase of gait. Journal of Biomechanics, 29 (6), pp. 723-733.

Rasmussen, J., Damsgaard, M. and Voigt, M., 2001 Muscle recruitment by the min/max criterion. A comparative numerical study. Journal of Biomechanics, 34(3), pp. 409-415.

Yamaguchi, G., 2001. Dynamic Modeling of Musculoskeletal Motion: A Vectorized Approach for Biomechanical Analysis in Three Dimensions, Kluwer Academic Publishers, Boston.

9

Towards a Realistic and Self-Contained Biomechanical Model of the Hand

Joaquín L. Sancho-Bru et al.*
Universitat Jaume I
Spain

1. Introduction

Most of human mechanical interactions with the surrounding world are performed by the hands. They allow us to perform very different tasks; from exerting high forces (e.g. using a hammer) to executing very precise movements (e.g. cutting with a surgical tool). This versatility is possible because of a very complex constitution: a great number of bones connected through different joints, a complicated musculature and a dense nervous system. This complexity is already evident from the kinematics point of view, with more than 20 degrees of freedom (DOF) controlled by muscles, tendons and ligaments.

Mathematical representations are used in order to perform qualitative or quantitative analyses on this complex reality. These representations are known as biomechanical models of the hand. In biomechanics, their use allows studying problems that cannot be analysed directly on humans or that have an experimental cost that is too high; e.g., the study of new alternatives for restoring hand pathologies. Biomechanical models are a description of the hand as a mechanical device: the different elements of the hand are defined in terms of rigid bodies, joints and actuators, and the mechanical laws are applied. As they are simplified mathematical models of the reality, their use and validity depends on the simplifications considered.

The first biomechanical models of the hand were developed to explain and clarify the functionality of different anatomical elements. In this regard, we can find many works that studied the function of the intrinsic muscles (Leijnse & Kalker, 1995; Spoor, 1983; Spoor & Landsmeer, 1976; Storace & Wolf, 1979, 1982; Thomas et al., 1968) and many others that tried to give an insight into the movement coordination of the interphalangeal joints (Buchner et al., 1988; Lee & Rim, 1990). Models for studying the causes and effects of different pathologies of the hand also appeared early on, such as the swan neck and boutonnière deformities or the rupture of the triangular ligament or the volar displacement of the extensor tendon (Smith et al., 1964; Storace & Wolf, 1979, 1982). All these models were, though, very limited, two-dimensional models allowing only the study of flexion-extension movements, they modelled only one finger, and they included important simplifications. By the year 2000, few three-dimensional models had been developed (Biryukova & Yourovskaya, 1994; Casolo & Lorenzi,

* Antonio Pérez-González, Marta C. Mora, Beatriz E. León, Margarita Vergara, José L. Iserte,Pablo J. Rodríguez-Cervantes and Antonio Morales
Universitat Jaume I, Spain

1994; Chao et al., 1976; Chao & An, 1978; Esteki & Mansour, 1997; Mansour et al., 1994; Valero-Cuevas et al., 1998), and none of them modelled the complete hand.

Since 2000, many three-dimensional biomechanical models can be found in literature, having been developed for very different purposes (Fok & Chou, 2010; Kamper et al., 2006; Kurita et al., 2009; Lee et al., 2008a, 2008b; Qiu et al., 2009; Roloff et al., 2006; Sancho-Bru et al., 2001, 2003a, 2003b, 2008; Valero-Cuevas, 2000; Valero-Cuevas et al., 2000, 2005; Vigouroux et al., 2006, 2008; Wu et al., 2010): to understand the role of the different anatomical elements, to understand the causes and effects of pathologies, to simulate neuromuscular abnormalities, to plan rehabilitation, to simulate tendon transfer and joint replacement surgeries, to analyse the energetics of human movement and athletic performance, to design prosthetics and biomedical implants, to design functional electric stimulation controllers, to name a few. These models, however, do not differ much from the ones developed before 2000, and many limitations are still evident. For example, contact forces and zones need to be measured experimentally and input to the model.

In contrast, much research has been carried out on animation techniques over the past years, mainly for use in developing computer games. Lately, these advances have been cleverly used by some ergonomics researchers to develop improved graphical and kinematics hand models for evaluating the use of products (Endo et al., 2007, 2009; Goussous, 2007; Kawaguchi, 2009), with good results.

On the other hand, robot hand grasps have been extensively studied for years. Although until 2000 little attention was paid to human hand grasping, this too has become a hot topic in robotics. The experience in modelling the robot hand grasps has been used to reach a better understanding of human grasping (Miller & Allen, 2004; Peña-Pitarch, 2007). The hand is considered as the end-effector for humans. These models, however, are not appropriate for studying many of the above-mentioned objectives, as their interest is different. The focus in robotics research is on planning the grasp and finding an optimum grasp, and quality grasp measures that have been developed for robots are used. These models do not include muscles and tendons in the formulation.

The latest developments in ergonomic hand models and human hand grasp models can be used to improve the existing biomechanical models of the hand and extend their functionality. A promising research area lies ahead with scientist, aiming to obtain a more comprehensive model of the hand, integrating knowledge and developments from the fields of biomechanics, ergonomics, robotics, and computer animation.

In this chapter, a review of the literature regarding biomechanical models of the hand, ergonomics hand models and human hand grasp models is presented. The three approaches are used to draw out the rules for developing an improved biomechanical model, able to tackle any of the above-mentioned objectives in a virtual environment, without external experimental data.

2. Literature review

2.1 Biomechanical models of the hand

Over the years, biomechanical models of the hand have been developed for different purposes. Some of them tried to study the functionality of different anatomical elements with the aim of gaining a deeper understanding of the causes and effects of many hand pathologies. These are usually very simplified (mostly two-dimensional) kinematic models (sometimes dynamic) that are used to perform qualitative analyses (Leijnse et al., 1992;

Storace & Wolf, 1979). Others were developed to help in medical planning and surgery for patients; they are usually dynamic models and are used to perform quantitative analyses, such as the study of the tendon excursions in the medical planning of tendon transfers (Giurintano & Hollister, 1991) or to study the nervous stimulation required to restore the grasping ability in muscular dysfunction patients (Esteki & Mansour, 1997). Yet others studied the hand while performing specific tasks with different aims, so as to have approximate values for the articular forces for testing prosthetic designs (Weightman & Amis, 1982). These too are quantitative analyses performed on dynamic models.

Recent models do not differ much from the ones developed before 2000 (Fok & Chou, 2010; Kamper et al., 2006; Kurita et al., 2009; Lee et al., 2008a, 2008b; Qiu et al., 2009; Roloff et al., 2006; Sancho-Bru et al., 2001, 2003a, 2003b, 2008; Valero-Cuevas, 2000; Valero-Cuevas et al., 2000, 2005; Vigouroux et al., 2006, 2008; Wu et al., 2010). All models present a similar configuration. The kinematics are modelled without considering the restraining structure, just the resultant physiological articular movement. The concept of instantaneous centre of rotation has been used to define an axis of rotation in joints with a single predominant DOF. Much effort has also been spent on finding the rotation axes of joints with two DOF (Brand & Hollister, 1992), through the consideration of a virtual link connecting the axes (Giurintano et al., 1995). Thus, all works use fixed axes of rotation; depending on the joint, one or two axes of rotation are considered. This approximation has been found to be good enough for most of the cases, particularly if there is no interest in analysing the role of the articular soft tissue or the articular stresses (Youm et al., 1978).

All works in the literature consider the ideal case of a non-friction belt around a pulley to model the tendons on a joint. Therefore, the tensional force on a tendon is the same along its pathway if no split or connection to other tendon exists. Two different approaches have been used to model tendon action on the joints. The first one considers the tendon freely running when crossing the joint between two points attached one to the proximal segment of the joint and the other to the distal segment. This approach is the basis of the first serious attempt to develop a 3D normative model of the hand (An et al., 1979), in which the position of the tendons with respect the bone segments were obtained from the measurement on 10 fresh cadaveric specimens. The second approach comes from the application of the virtual work principle and considers the moment arm created by the tendon as the first derivative of the tendon excursion with respect to the rotated angle about the rotation axis under study (Storace & Wolf, 1979). This second approach is not strictly correct (Casolo & Lorenzi, 1994), as it does not take into account the work due to the deformation of the sheaths and other structures that constrain the tendon's trajectory along its pathway. Although both approaches present advantages and disadvantages, the second one is difficult to implement in 3D modelling, mainly because of the complexity in the tendon excursion calculation at joints with more than one DOF.

Most of the works in the literature use Hill's model to account for the muscles' mathematical modelling. This simple model allows the consideration of the three main parameters, i.e., muscle activation level and variation of the maximum deliverable muscle force with muscle length and muscle contraction velocity.

Finally, the dynamic equilibrium equations lead to an indeterminate system of equations, with more unknowns (muscle forces) than available equations. Inequality constraints taking into account the maximal forces that may be delivered by each muscle and that tendons cannot support compressive forces have to be considered as well. The problem is usually solved by minimising some cost function. Different functions have been investigated, most of them without any physiological basis. The most often used criterion is the minimisation of the sum of the squared muscle stresses, which has been related to the maximisation of fatigue resistance (Crowninshield & Brand, 1981).

All the effort in biomechanics has been focused on appropriately modelling the different hand components (kinematics, muscles, tendons, etc.). Little effort has been spent on the formulation of the grasping problem when using a biomechanical model. In this sense, many limitations persist. Current models do not allow the estimation of the contact information required to use biomechanical models for simulating the grasping of objects. Forces and zones of contact still need to be measured experimentally and input to the model.

2.2 Hand models in ergonomics

Ergonomics, according to the International Ergonomics Association, is 'the scientific discipline concerned with the understanding of interactions among humans and other elements of a system, and the profession that applies theory, principles, data and methods to design in order to optimise human well-being and overall system performance'. Hand models in Ergonomics are used to simulate postures adopted while grasping objects with different purposes. One of the main goals of physical ergonomics is the study of the size and shape of objects according to the anthropometry of the different people that have to interact with them. Thus, the main feature of a model for Ergonomics is that it has to allow representing different populations and percentiles. People having hands of different sizes and proportions will adopt different postures in grasping the same object for the same functions. For example, pressing a button of a phone with the thumb while holding it with the same hand can be easily achieved for a specific hand size while keeping the grasp. However, other people with different size of hand will need to change the grasping posture to achieve pressing the button. This is a typical problem of reach that needs to be solved in ergonomic assessment.

In recent years, virtual humans have been incorporated into the design process for ergonomic assessment of different types of products, mainly in the aerospace and automotive industry but also in others like product design, tasks simulation, personnel training or simulation of other worker environments (Colombo & Cugini, 2005; Yang et al., 2007). Several commercial software programs such as Jack, RAMSIS, HumanCAD, Safework and SantosHuman are available and other studies have been conducted on digital human models such as SAMMIE (Case et al. 1990) or the Boeing Human Modeling System for the same purposes. A virtual human in these packages is defined as a kinematic chain composed of a number of rigid links connected by joints. These joints have the DOF and allowable motion limits corresponding to the anatomical joint of the human being. Direct and inverse kinematics is incorporated into the models so they can replicate human body movements and also evaluate forces acting in joints. Moreover, different population and percentiles may be selected for the size of the model, usually from known anthropometric databases. With these capabilities the problems of reach and clearance usual in ergonomics may be solved easily. Other useful capabilities of these models are the simulation of the sense of sight with virtual cameras located in the eyes or the possibility to change any particular data of the model, like dimensions of limbs or motion limits of some joints, in order to simulate a particular person or disability. However, the majority of these models focuses on the whole body and does not pay attention to the accuracy of the hand model. Most of them just incorporate a list of hand postures (grasping or others) to be chosen, i.e.

direct kinematics, but do not allow for example inverse kinematics for the joints of the hand, even when it is incorporated for the other joints of the body. In recent developments some attempts to improve the hand model incorporated into some programs have been done (Peña-Pitarch, 2007, Yang et al., 2007).

Early models of the hand (Davidoff & Freivalds, 1993) were actually kinematic models that simulated roughly the external geometry of the hand and its movements. The geometry of the hand has been modelled mainly by jointed cylinders (Fig. 1) and cones (Armstrong, 2009; Sancho-Bru et al., 2003a, 2003b). However, if the geometry of the hand model is not very accurate, the algorithms for inverse kinematics are not precise enough. Recently, some efforts have been made in accurately modelling the surface of real hands to be incorporated into 3D hand models. Rhee et al. (2006) presented an automated method to make a specific human hand model from an image of the palm of the hand. Different algorithms were used in the process: principal creases are extracted, joint locations are estimated from them and the skin geometry of a generic hand model deformed based on hand contours. Rogers et al (2008) made a scalable 3-D geometric model of the hand based on 66 landmarks of the palm surface from 100 subjects in four functional postures. The purpose was to analyse the deformation of the palm surface during the grasp of an object. Recent models incorporate the surface of the hand as a mesh object with more or less realism, obtained from the location of a number of landmarks of the hand or from digital 3D-scanning of the hand (Endo et al., 2007; Peña-Pitarch, 2007, van Nierop et al., 2008). The mesh is linked to a skeleton whose movement controls the deformation of the mesh with different types of algorithms.

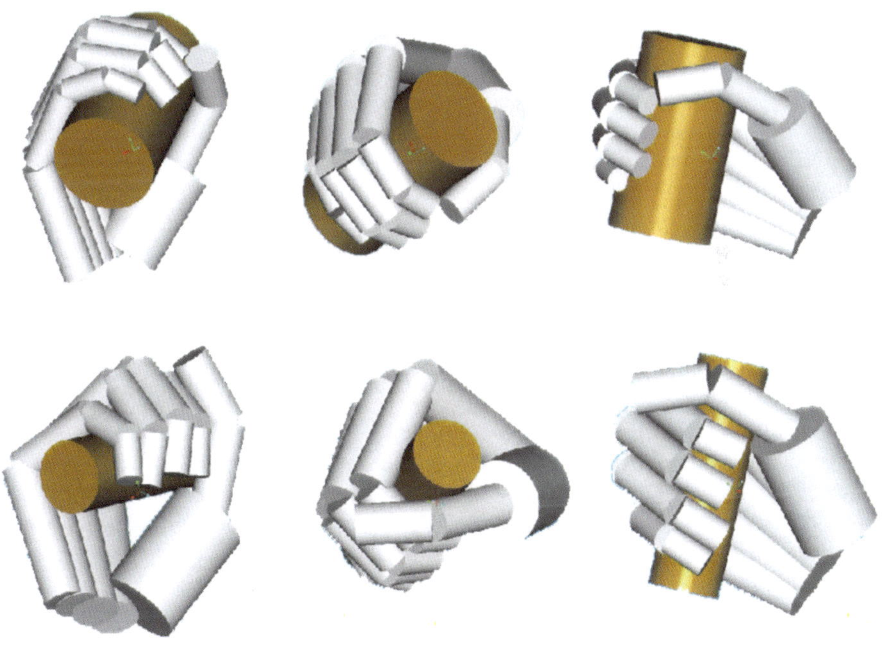

Fig. 1. Different views of the geometric model used in Sancho-Bru et al. (2003a) simulating a hand gripping two cylinders of different diameters.

Other important aspect of hand models for ergonomics is associated with the study of musculoskeletal disorders. Early epidemiological studies (Mital and Kilbom, 1992) showed that the use of hand tools with an improper design for the worker or the task could lead to a high risk of developing cumulative hand trauma disorders (CHTD). The factors influencing the development of CHTD have been reported in different works (Keyserling, 2000; Kong et al., 2006; Muggleton et al., 1999; Schoenmarklin et al., 1994; Spielholz et al., 2001) and different methods have been used in these studies: epidemiological studies, physiological measurements (electromyography activity, pressure in tissues, posture of hand and wrist, tactile sensitivity), biomechanical models of hand and wrist structures and psychophysical assessments. These studies report that CHTD are associated with repetitive tasks, high forces, extreme or awkward postures of hand and wrist, velocity and acceleration of wrist motions and exposure time, among others. Different theories of injury development have been proposed (Kumar, 2001). All of them assume that CHTD and other musculoskeletal disorders are of biomechanical nature.

Therefore, biomechanical hand models able to predict movements, postures and internal forces of hand and wrist structures can be used to assess the risk of developing CHTD. Tendon excursions or maximum gripping strength have been used as index in different works to assess gripping posture for health (Armstrong et al., 2009, Sancho-Bru et al., 2003b).

None of the reported biomechanical models of the hand for ergonomics accounts for all the above-mentioned requirements, although some attempts have been made. Armstrong et al (2009) have developed a scalable kinematic model of the hand with simple geometry (cones and cylinders). The model includes a posture prediction algorithm for fingers that reproduces in a high percentage the observed postures and is able to compute tendon excursions and wrist movements. The model is used to assess how much space is required for hands in an assembly task and to calculate the risk of CHTD from tendon forces and hand strength. Other group of researchers (Endo et al 2007, 2009; Kawaguchi et al., 2009) have developed a scalable digital hand model with an accurate shape of the hand that includes a semiautomatic grasp planning function with robotics indexes of quality (see next section). The model incorporates a 'comfort database' obtained from experimental measurements to assess comfort of postures and is used in the assessment of physical interaction with electronic appliances.

2.3 Grasping in robotics

For many years the robotics community has been studying the autonomous handling of objects by robots. A robot should be able to locate the object and then grasp it, and possibly transport it to a specified destination. The purpose of a grasp is to constrain the potential movements of the object in the event of external disturbances. For a specific robotic hand, different grasp types are planned and analysed in order to decide which one to execute.

A grasp is commonly defined as a set of contacts on the surface of the object. A contact model should be defined to determine the forces or torques that the robot manipulator must exert on the contact areas. Most of the work in robotics assumes point contacts, and larger areas of contact are usually discretised to follow this assumption (Bicchi & Kumar, 2000).

Two main problems can be distinguished in robotic grasping: analysis and synthesis (Mason, 2001). Grasp analysis consists on finding whether the grasp is stable using common closure properties, given an object and a set of contacts. Then, a quality measure can be evaluated in order to enable the robot to select the best grasp to execute. On the other hand, grasp synthesis is the problem of finding a suitable set of contacts given an object and some constrains on the allowable contacts.

In the following sections, a detailed description of the contact models and the most common approaches for grasp analysis and synthesis is presented.

2.3.1 Grasp contact models

A contact can be defined as a joint between the finger and the object. Their shape, stiffness and frictional characteristics define the nature of this joint (Mason, 2001). The force applied by a finger at a contact point generates a *wrench* on the object with force and torque components. The contact model maps the wrench at some reference point of the object, usually the centre of mass. Salisbury (1982) proposed a taxonomy of eight contact models. Among these, the more common contact models used in robotic grasping (Fig. 2) are the point contacts with and without friction and the soft-finger contacts (Roa Garzón, 2009). Point contact models, also named rigid-body contact models, assume rigid-body models for the hand and the grasped object while the soft-finger contact models, also called compliant or regularised models, assume that the hand is a deformable element grasping a rigid body (Kao et al., 2008). The former models assume the collision to be an instantaneous and discontinuous phenomenon (discrete event) and the equations of motion are derived by balancing the system's momenta before and after the impact. In contrast, compliant models describe the normal and tangential compliance relations over time.

A *point contact without friction* can only transmit forces along the normal to the object surface at the contact point. No deformations are allowed at the points of contact between the two bodies and, instead, contact forces arise from the constraint of incompressibility and impenetrability between the rigid bodies. These models do not represent the real contact situations that appear in robotic manufacturing operations (Cutkosky, 1989; Lin et al., 2000) and, when used, the machine accuracy is negatively affected. Moreover, they are not capable of predicting the individual contact forces of a multiple-contact fixture (Bicchi, 1994; Harada et al., 2000).

A *point contact with friction* can also transmit forces in the tangential directions to the surface at the contact point. If Coulomb's friction model is used, all the forces that lie within the friction cone with an angle $atan(\mu)$ can be applied, where μ is the friction coefficient of the contacting materials. Here, contact forces arise from two sources: the rigid-body model assumption for both the hand and the object, and the frictional forces. The use of this contact model in the manipulation planning problem has led to some interesting conclusions. There may be multiple solutions to a particular problem (ambiguity) or there may be no solutions (inconsistency) (Erdmann, 1994).

Finally, the soft contact model is used to model the contact between a soft finger and a rigid object allowing the finger to apply an additional torsional moment with respect to the normal at the contact point (Ciocarlie et al., 2005, 2007; Howe et al., 1988; Howe & Cutkosky, 1996; Kao & Cutkosky, 1992; Kao & Yang, 2004). A typical contact between a soft finger and a contact surface can be modelled by the Hertzian contact model (Hertz, 1882; Johnson, 1985). However, robotic fingertips are made of nonlinear elastic materials. For that reason, the Hertzian contact model does not accurately represent this contact. In Xydas & Kao (1999) and Xydas et al. (2000) a power-law theory is presented for modelling nonlinear elastic contacts present in robotic fingers. It subsumes the Hertzian contact theory. More realistic, and complicated, models have been developed in the last few years that better represent the contact mechanics for soft fingers (Ciocarlie et al., 2005, 2007; Gonthier, 2007). However, it is the hard finger contacts with friction that are used more often in robotics.

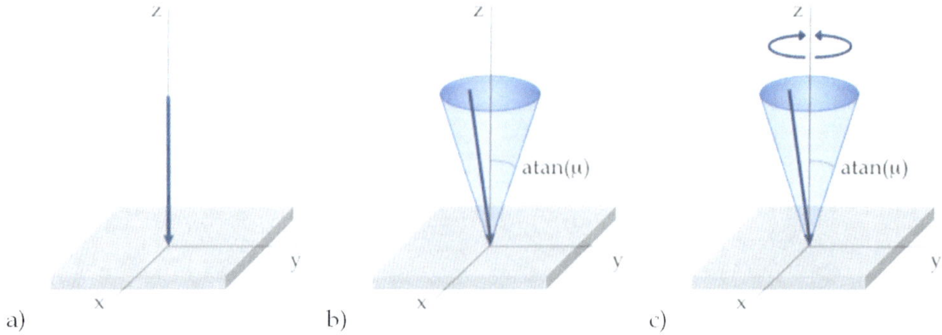

Fig. 2. Contact models commonly used in robotics: a) Point contact without friction; b) Point contact with friction; c) Soft-finger contact

2.3.2 Grasp analysis

After establishing the contact model, the set of contacts defining each grasp can be analysed in order to test its ability to resist disturbances and its dexterity properties. As it is presented afterwards, a grasp can resist disturbances in any direction if it fulfils one of the two closure conditions. However, there is usually more than one grasp that fulfils them. That is why many metrics and approaches have been proposed to evaluate the dexterity of the selected grasps and determine which one is the best to be executed.

Disturbance resistance

The first test for evaluating a grasp consists of determining its ability to constrain the motions of the manipulated object and to apply arbitrary contact forces on the object without violating friction constraints at the contacts (Bicchi, 1995). Two commonly used properties have been proposed to ensure this condition: force and form closure. A grasp is in *force-closure* if the fingers can apply, through the set of contacts, arbitrary wrenches on the object, which means that any motion of the object is resisted by the contact forces (Nguyen, 1988). On the other hand, a grasp is in *form-closure* if the location of the contact points on the object ensures its immobility (Bicchi, 1995).

Form closure is a stronger condition than force closure and it is mostly used when executing power grasps (Siciliano & Khatib, 2008). Force closure is possible with fewer contacts, making it suitable for executing precision grasps, but it requires the ability to control internal forces.

In order to verify the form or force closure property of a grasp, many tests have been proposed (see Liu et al. (2004b) and Roa Garzón (2009) for a review). Most of them define conditions to be satisfied by the grasp wrenches in the wrench space. A *grasp wrench space (GWS)* is the space of wrenches that can be applied to the object at each contact point. The boundary of the wrench space can be calculated as a convex hull. Force-closure then can be determined verifying if the origin of the wrench space lies inside this convex hull (Mishra et al., 1987). Several tests have been proposed to verify this condition, with the one developed by Ferrari & Canny (1992) being the most widely-used. They proposed to calculate the radius of the largest ball inscribed in the convex hull centred in the origin. Force-closure grasps are the ones where the sphere's radius is larger than zero.

Measures of grasp performance

Many approaches have been proposed to measure the quality of a grasp. Some of the measures focus on evaluating the ability to resist external disturbances, others on evaluating the dexterity. These measures can be classified into two groups depending on whether they consider the location of the contact points on the object or the configuration of the end-effector. There are also some that are a combination of these two approaches (see Roa Garzón (2009) for a thorough review).

Measures from the first group take into account the geometric properties of the objects, their materials and closure properties to evaluate the grasp. For example, Li & Sastry (1998) proposed to calculate the smallest singular value of the grasp matrix, which indicates how far the grasp configuration is from losing the capability of withstanding external wrenches. Others have proposed to favour the grasps whose contact points are distributed in a uniform way on the object surface, which improves their stability (Mirtich & Canny, 1994; Park & Starr, 1992). This can be done by measuring either the angles or the area of the polygon whose vertices are the contact points. The centroid of this polygon is also used to calculate its distance to the object centre of mass (Ding et al., 2001; Ponce et al., 1997). The smaller this distance the better the grasp can resist the effect of external forces. In addition, some other measures take into account the uncertainty in the position of the fingers; therefore instead of contact points they calculate contact regions in which force closure grasps are assured (Nguyen, 1988; Roa Garzón, 2009). The quality of the grasp is measured by the size of these regions.

The previous approaches do not consider any limitation on the finger forces, so that in some cases the fingers have to apply very large forces to resist small perturbations. Other measures do consider limitations on the magnitudes of the finger forces. They can limit the force on each finger or the sum of forces applied by all fingers. Ferrari & Canny (1992) used the largest ball not only to evaluate grasp closure but also to measure the grasp quality. This is a geometric representation of the smallest perturbation wrench that breaks the grasp, independently of its direction. It has been widely used by the robotics community (Borst et al., 2003; Miller & Allen, 1999; Roa Garzón, 2009). The volume of the ball is also considered as a quality measure with the advantage that it remains constant independently of the used torque reference system (Miller & Allen, 1999).

When a task is specified to be performed after the object is grasped, the quality of the grasp can be measured with its ability to counteract the expected disturbances during the task execution. The set of all wrenches that are expected to be applied on the object defines the *task wrench space (TWS)* and can be approximated as an ellipsoid (Li & Sastry, 1988) or as a convex polytope (Haschke et al., 2005; Zhu at al., 2001). The problem with these approaches is that modelling the TWS can be quite complicated (Borst et al., 2004). Pollard (2004) introduced the concept of an *object wrench space (OWS),* which is the set of wrenches generated by applying a distribution of disturbance forces on the surface of the object. Borst et al. (2004) proposed the use of the largest factor by which the OWS can fit the GWS as the measure of the grasp quality.

On the other hand, there are measures that consider the configuration of the end-effector, requiring the hand-object Jacobian for their calculation (Roa Garzón, 2009). An example of this group is a measure that favours a grasp that, given certain velocities in the finger joints, produces the largest velocities on the grasped object, calculated with the volume of the manipulability ellipsoid (Yoshikawa, 1985). There is another measure that penalises the joints of the hand being in their maximum limits, calculating the deviation of the joint angles from their centres (Liegeois, 1977). Additionally, there are other measures in this group that also consider the task, giving higher quality indexes to the grasps which ensure the maximum transformation ratio along the direction wrenches more likely to be applied on the object when executing it (Chiu, 1988).

2.3.3 Grasp synthesis

Given an object, grasp synthesis algorithms should provide a suitable set of contacts on the object surface and determine an appropriate hand configuration. Usually they take the geometry of the object as an input to select optimal force-closure contact locations. These contacts are the starting point for grasp analysis and dexterous manipulation methods.

Some approaches give only information about the finger contact locations on the object without considering the hand constraints. They can result in stable grasps that are not reachable in practice by the robot hand. Moreover, even if they are reachable, it is difficult to position the fingers precisely on the contact points because there will be always unavoidable errors locating the end-effector (Morales et al., 2006).

Alternative approaches, called knowledge-based approaches, have considered the configuration of the hand by generating the grasp with a predefined set of hand postures. The idea of hand preshapes started with studies of the human prehension capabilities (Napier, 1956) that introduced the distinction between power and precision grasps. Following this work, Cutkosky (1989) created a taxonomy in which details of the task and the object geometry are taken into account. Since then, several papers have adopted this approach for grasping (Morales et al., 2006; Stansfield, 1991; Wren, 1995). Miller et al. (2003) used a simulator called GraspIt! to test the set of hand preshapes on a 3D model of the object. Using a simulator has many advantages, including the ability to plan grasps in complex environments involving obstacles and also to check the reachability constraints of the robot arm. More recently OpenRAVE, a planning architecture that has a more flexible design, has been proposed to automate this process (Diankov, 2010).

Despite many years of research and all the advances we have reviewed, the robotics community is still not able to build a manipulator with similar capabilities to the human hand. The robot hands constructed until now are only simplifications (Fig. 3), given the complexities not only at the sensor and actuator level, but also at the control level. They vary from the easiest to control, such as 2-jaw grippers, to more anthropomorphic hands like the Salisbury Hand, the Utah-MIT Hand, the Barrett Hand, the ARMAR III Hand or the DLR Hand II (see Biagiotti et al. (2002) and Parada et al. (2008) for a review).

3. Hand biomechanical model proposal

In this section, the current knowledge on biomechanical, ergonomics and robotics hand models is used to draw out the rules for developing a realistic and self-contained biomechanical model of the hand.

Based on the literature review, current hand biomechanical models allow estimating the muscular patterns required to perform a movement while counteracting a system of external forces. But their use for studying object grasping is limited. On the one hand, biomechanical

a) b) c) d)

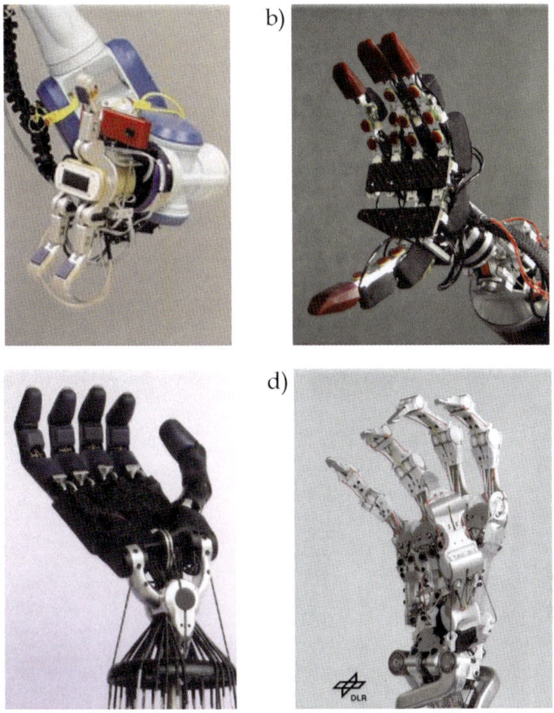

Fig. 3. Anthropomorphic robot hands: a) Barrett Hand (courtesy of the UJI Robotics Intelligent Lab); b) ARMAR III Hand (courtesy of the Institute for Anthropomatics at KIT); c) Shadow Hand C5 (courtesy of Shadow Robot Company); d) Anthropomorphic DLR Hand Arm System (courtesy of DLR Robotics and Mechatronics Center)

models lack realism for assessing the use of handheld products from an ergonomics point of view. Hand models in ergonomics have reached a high level of realism but do not allow for mechanical analyses. On the other hand, biomechanical models are not self-contained, as they need contact information to be input to the model. Current models do not allow predicting grasping postures nor evaluating contact forces and zones, much less predicting the movements while grasp planning. Quality grasp measures in robotics allow comparing different robotic grasping postures and could be adapted to human grasping.

A detailed proposal for modelling the different components of the hand is provided below: joints-kinematics, muscles, ligaments and passive tissues, skin, contact with objects and neuromuscular control. The features that we require in order to create a model are:

- The model has to simulate the complete hand in order to allow the study of any grasp.
- The model has to be scalable to allow the simulation of different population groups.
- The model has to simulate and show the grasping of an object in a realistic way.
- The model has to estimate the muscular patterns required to perform a movement while counteracting the system of external forces that define the object manipulation. Furthermore, the model has to estimate the articular forces at the hand joints.
- The model has to be dynamic in order to allow the study of any grasping task (slow or fast) during the object manipulation.

- The model has to predict feasible grasping postures for a given object and provide the contact information required for evaluating the grasp
- The model has to incorporate quality grasping measures for evaluating the grasp.

The model proposed in this section has been developed in a scalable way, choosing two very well known anthropometric parameters of the hand that are easy to measure and representative of the hand size. The parameters are the hand length (HL) and hand breadth (HB) and are shown in Fig. 4.

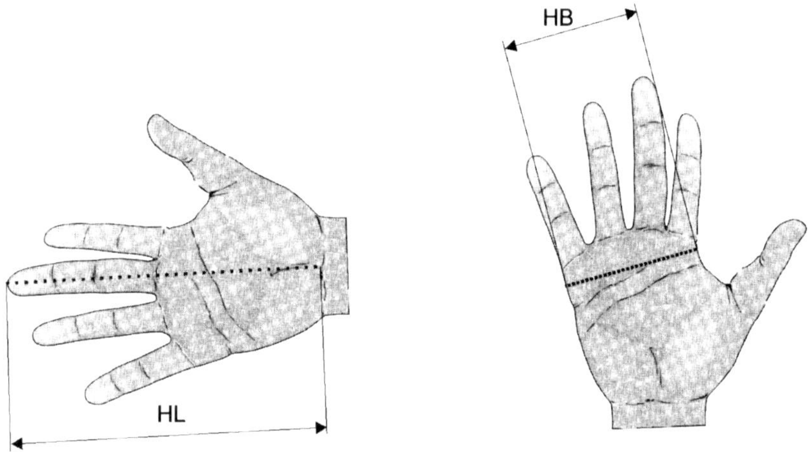

Fig. 4. Parameters used to scale the model: HL (hand length) and HB (hand breadth)

3.1 Kinematics

In order to achieve realistic grasping postures, care has to be taken when selecting the appropriate DOF among the different hand bones. The DOF have to allow the hand model to reach the hand posture for any grasping task. In this sense, it is important that the model considers not only the thumb and finger movements but also the palm arching.

The hand has been considered as five skeletal open chains of rigid bodies connected to the carpus through different joints which characterise the kinematic behaviour of the chains.

Distal and proximal interphalangeal (DIP and PIP) joints of the fingers as well as the interphalangeal (IP) joint of the thumb are trochlear joints, capable only of flexion/extension movements (Brand & Hollister, 1992). These joints are modelled as one DOF joints by means of defining a rotation axis connecting the adjacent phalanxes (hinge joint).

Thumb and fingers metacarpophalangeal (MCP) joints are condylar joints, capable of flexion/extension and abduction/adduction movements (Brand & Hollister, 1992). The thumb carpometacarpal (CMC) joint is a saddle joint, capable also of flexion/extension and abduction/adduction movements (Brand & Hollister, 1992). All these joints are modelled as two DOF joints by defining two axes of rotation connecting the adjacent segments. The axes are neither intersecting nor orthogonal (Brand & Hollister, 1992), so that a virtual link is used to connect both axes (Giurintano et al., 1995).

Finally, the hand model allows the arching of the palm by modelling the CMC joints of the little and ring fingers. These joints are arthrodial joints, with a very limited range of movement (Kapandji, 1998). They have been modelled as one DOF joints by means of

defining a flexion/extension axis of rotation connecting the carpus to each metacarpal. The orientation of the axes is defined oblique in order to appropriately simulate the arching of the palm (Kapandji, 1998). Due to the important role that the shape of the palm plays in grasping, this model is considered more suitable for grasping simulation than others in the literature.
The data for the location and orientation of the rotation axes comes from An et al. (1979), Buchholz et al. (1992) and Hollister et al. (1995). Axes data and link lengths are fully scaled with respect to the hand length and hand breadth (Sancho-Bru, 2000). Limits for the joints have been obtained from Tubiana (1981) and Tubiana et al. (1996).
In order to study the forward and inverse kinematics of the hand, the Denavit- Hartenberg method from the robotics field (Denavit and Hartenberg, 1955) was adapted to define the position of any segment point.

3.2 Musculo-tendon action

Muscles and tendons control the movement of the skeletal chains. Muscles have been considered using a simple Hill three-component model (Hill, 1938) that takes into account the muscle activation level (α) and the force-length and force-velocity relationships, as well as the different index of architecture of muscles. The model considers a contractile element (CE), which is the basic component that generates force, a parallel elastic element (PEE), which is responsible for the passive force generated by the muscle when it is stretched, and a series elastic element (SEE), the muscle tendon unit, which has been considered to be inextensible (Fig. 5).

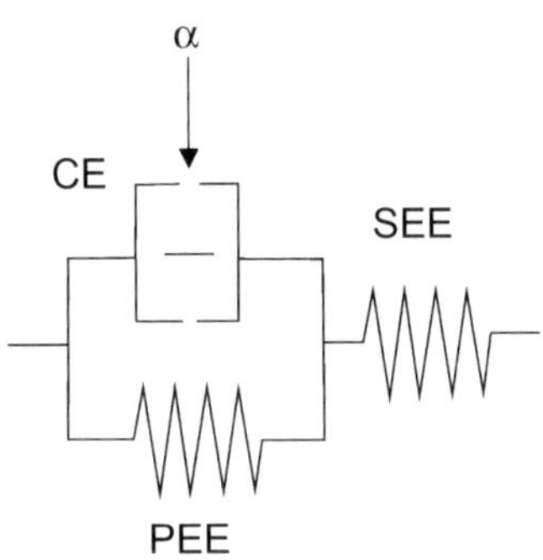

Fig. 5. Hill's three-component model for the muscles

The force a muscle can exert depends on the actual muscle length and contraction velocity. It is widely accepted (An et al., 1991) that the maximum force a muscle can exert in optimal conditions is proportional to its physiological cross-sectional area (PCSA):

$$F_{\max} = PCSA \cdot S_{\max} , \quad (1)$$

where S_{max} is the maximum stress the muscle can bear, which has been considered the same for each muscle (An et al., 1991).
The strain of tendons is insignificant for the magnitude of forces developed by the muscles (Goldstein et al., 1987). Under this consideration, the SEE has been considered to inextensible, so that the force the muscle exerts (F) can be written as:

$$F = F_{max}(F_{CE} + F_{PEE}) \, , \tag{2}$$

where F_{CE} and F_{PEE} are the normalised forces delivered by the CE and PEE, respectively.
The force exerted by the muscle can be decomposed into an active force and a passive force corresponding to the forces delivered by the CE and PEE, respectively. The force delivered by the CE is related to the muscle architecture and is a function of the muscle length l_{CE}, the contraction velocity v_{CE}, and the muscle activation level α (from 0 to 1), which is controlled by the central nervous system (Kaufman et al., 1991):

$$F_{CE} = \alpha \cdot F_l(l_{CE}) \cdot F_v(v_{CE}) \tag{3}$$

where F_l and F_v are the non-dimensional force-length and force-velocity relationships.
A characteristic bell-shaped curve exists between force and length of the muscle. To model this dependence, the expression proposed by Kaufman et al. (1991) has been used:

$$F_l(\varepsilon, i_a) = e^{-\left[\frac{(\varepsilon+1)^{0.96343\left(1-\frac{1}{i_a}\right)}-1.0}{0.35327\cdot(1-i_a)}\right]^2} \quad \text{for } i_a < 1 \tag{4}$$

$$F_l(\varepsilon, i_a) = e^{-[2.727277\cdot\ln(\varepsilon+1)]^2} \quad \text{for } i_a = 1 \tag{5}$$

where i_a is the muscle architecture index, defined as the ratio between the muscle fibre length and the muscle belly length, and ε is the muscle strain due to its lengthening from l_o, the muscle length for the optimal conditions.
The force a muscle can exert decreases when the contraction velocity of the muscle fibres increases. To model this dependence the expression proposed by Hatze (1981) has been used

$$F_v(\dot{\eta}) = \frac{0.1433}{0.1074 + e^{-1.409\cdot\sinh(3.2\cdot\dot{\eta}+1.6)}} \tag{6}$$

where $\dot{\eta}$ is the normalised contractile element velocity, given by the ratio between the lengthening velocity of the muscle ($\dot{\varepsilon}$), and its maximal value ($\dot{\varepsilon}_{max}$).
The force generated by the PEE is a function only of its length. An exponential relationship has been considered in this case (Lee & Rim, 1990; Kaufman et al., 1991), with b_1 and b_2 muscle dependent constants:

$$F_{PEE} = b_1 \cdot e^{b_2\cdot\varepsilon} - b_1 \, , \tag{7}$$

The scalability of the muscular action is achieved by scaling the PCSA of the muscles with respect to the product of hand length and hand breadth parameters (Sancho-Bru et al., 2008) from its value for $\overline{HL}$ = 18.22 cm and $\overline{HB}$ = 8.00 cm.

$$\frac{PCSA(HL,HB)}{PCSA(\overline{HL},\overline{HB})} = 1 + 0.01333\cdot(HB\cdot HL - \overline{HB}\cdot\overline{HL}) \tag{8}$$

The muscles considered on each skeletal chain are listed in Table 1. PCSA data for index finger muscles have been taken from Valero-Cuevas et al. (1998); data for the remaining muscles have been obtained from Brand & Hollister (1992). Muscle stress limit (S_{max}) has been obtained from Zajac (1989). Fibre and muscle lengths and the constants b_1, b_2 for index finger muscles have been taken from Lee & Rim (1990); data for the remaining extrinsic muscles have been obtained from Lemay & Crago (1996) and for the remaining intrinsic muscles from Jacobson et al. (1992). The muscle maximal lengthening velocity ($\dot{\varepsilon}_{max}$) has been taken to be 2.5 s^{-1} (Kaufman et al., 1991).

Index	Medial	Ring	Little	Thumb
1st FP	2nd FP	3rd FP	4th FP	APB
1st FS	2nd FS	3rd FS	4th FS	FPB
1st EDC+EI	2nd EDC	3rd EDC	EDQ	OPP
1st LU	2nd LU	3rd LU	4th LU	ADD
1st DI	2nd DI	4th DI	3rd VI	1st DI
1st VI	3rd DI	2nd VI	FDQ	APL
			ADQ	EPB
				FPL
				EPL

Table 1. Muscles modelled on each skeletal chain (acronyms in the nomenclature section)

Most of the muscles do not act directly on the bones, but transmit the force to the tendons, which finally insert into the bones. To model the tendon action crossing the joints, straight lines connecting 2 points have been considered, one fixed with respect to the proximal bone and the other one with respect to the distal bone (Fig. 6a). This approximation has been found to be close enough to the behaviour of all tendons with the exception of extensors (An et al., 1979), for which Landsmeer's model I has been considered (Fig. 6b). The data for the points defining the tendon actions have been obtained from An et al. (1979).

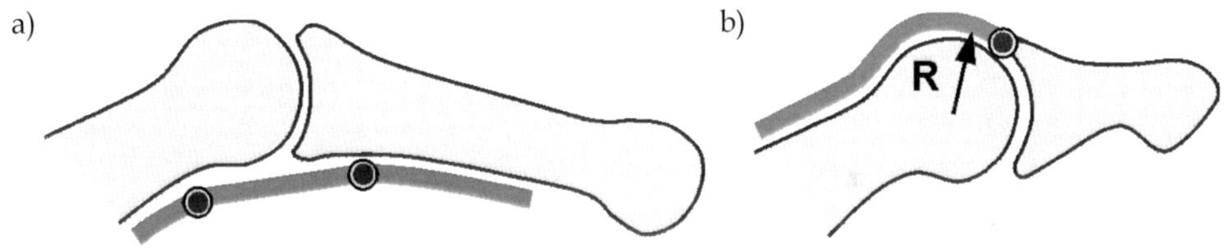

Fig. 6. Models for the tendons crossing the joints: a) Straight lines; b) Landsmeer's model I

The extensor hood mechanisms of the fingers are modelled as a tendon net. The net allows for the connection and division of the tendon paths. The insertions and connection points considered for the tendon nets on each skeletal chain are shown in Fig. 7. Appropriate force balances have been considered in the connecting points of this deformable tendon net. Second DI, fourth DI and ADQ tendons do present a double insertion into the proximal phalanxes and into the extensor aponeuroses. A force distribution proportional to the amount of fibres of each branch (Eyler & Markee, 1954) has been considered.

The muscle force-length and force-velocity relationships presented above require the calculation of the lengthening of the muscles from l_o as a function of time. Having considered the tendons inextensible, the muscle lengthening coincides with the tendon excursion. To calculate the length of the tendon path crossing each joint (l_i), straight lines connecting the points have been considered, except for the extensor tendons, for which a circular path has been considered.

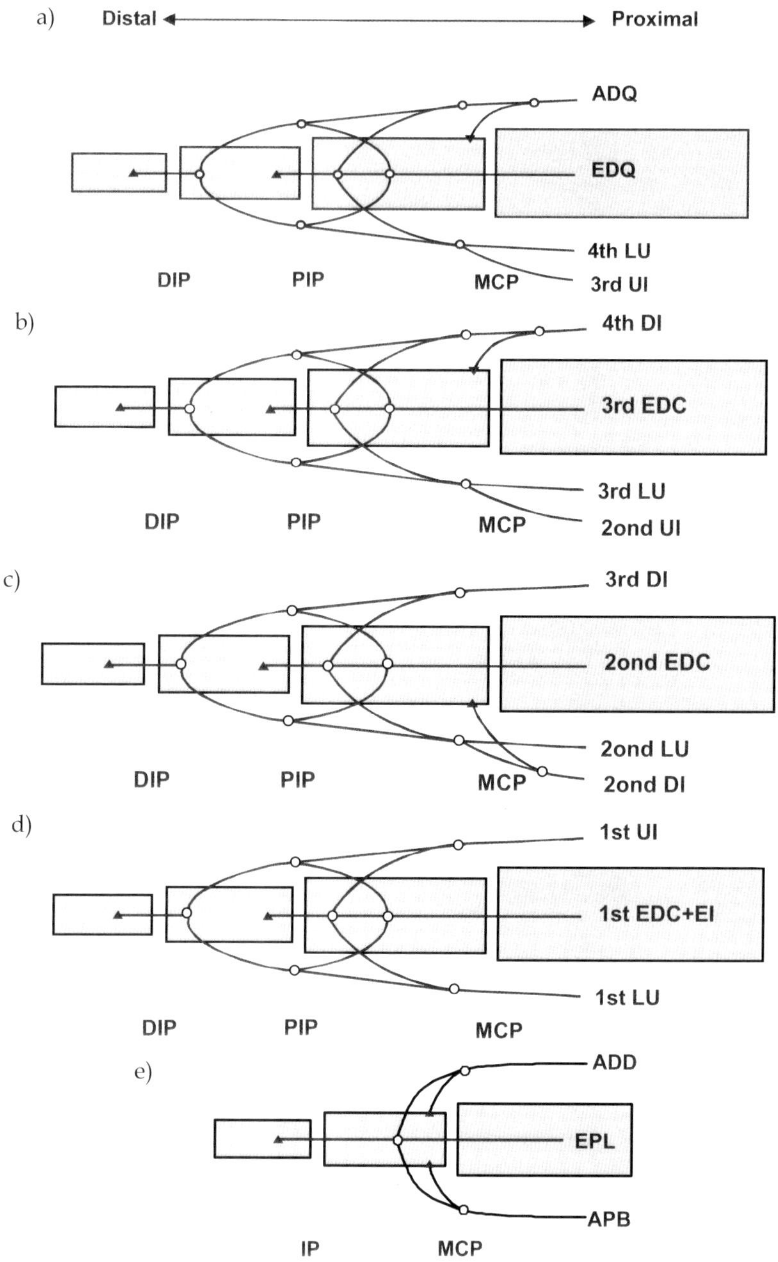

Fig. 7. Sketch of the extensor mechanisms of the fingers and thumb (dorsal view) showing the insertions into the bones (▲) and the connections and splittings considered (○): a) little finger; b) ring finger; c) medial finger; d) index finger; e) thumb.

The data for the location of the points defining the tendon paths comes from An et al. (1979) and Buchholz et al. (1992), and are also scaled with respect to the hand length and hand breadth (Sancho-Bru, 2000).

3.3 Ligaments

In previous work, we showed the importance of modelling the effect of ligaments for studying free finger movements. In the case of grasping, their consideration is not so relevant. Their effect can be neglected for studying power grasps, but they can play an important role in the case of some precision grasps, particularly those involving fast movements.

In the case of DIP and PIP joints of fingers and thumb, the insertion of the collateral ligaments on the proximal segment of the joint corresponds to the flexion-extension axis (Dubousset, 1981). Therefore, they do not develop any flexion-extension moment over the joint and they do not need to be modelled. In the case of MCP joints, the proximal insertion of the lateral ligament on the metacarpal head remains dorsal to the center of the articular curvature (Fig. 8), so that collateral ligaments are lax in extension, but they become taut in flexion, decreasing significantly the range of lateral movement (Craig, 1992; Dubousset, 1981; Kapandji, 1998). Tension on the radial and ulnar ligaments increases with adduction and abduction of the MCP joint, respectively. Furthermore, the line of action of the ligaments remains dorsal to the flexion- extension axis of the joint (Craig, 1992), developing an extension moment over the joint, in addition to the abduction-adduction moment.

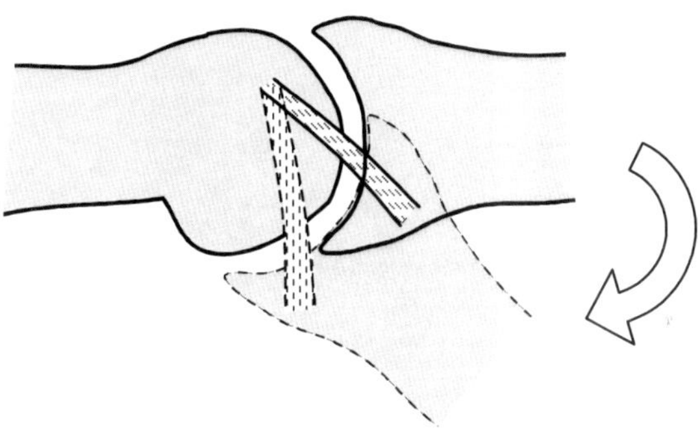

Fig. 8. Collateral ligament over MCP joints becomes taut with flexion.

Both ulnar and radial ligaments over MCP joints have been considered. A unique fibre for each ligament has been considered, joining two points representing the insertions into the bones. One point is fixed with respect to the metacarpal, and the other one with respect to the proximal phalanx. No interaction between bone and ligament has been considered; therefore the ligament path is a straight line between the insertion points. Its non-linear behaviour has been taken into account considering a quadratic relationship between the force developed by the ligament (F_{lig}) and its elongation (Mommersteeg et al., 1996)

$$F_{lig} = K \cdot \left(L_{lig} - L_{lig,o}\right)^2 , \qquad (10)$$

where K is the characteristic constant of the ligament, L_{lig} the length of the fibre representing the ligament, and $L_{lig,o}$ the unstrained length of the ligament.

The data for the ligament insertion points have been obtained from the geometric model presented in Youm et al. (1978), and the stiffness constant has been estimated to be 750 N/cm^2 from Minami et al. (1985).

3.4 Skin and contact with objects

One of the applications of the biomechanical model is its use in assessing the use of handheld products from an ergonomics point of view. To accomplish that goal, the model has to incorporate a realistic model of the skin from the visual point of view. The advances in computer animation have made possible the development of a number of convincing surface skin models.

We propose to use a surface skin model similar to that of Endo et al. (2007) or Goussous (2007). The surface skin model is a 3-dimensional polygonal mesh for the hand surface generated from CT images. The geometry of the skin model is defined at only one opened posture. A surface skin deformation algorithm defines the deformed geometry of the surface skin model when the posture of the kinematic model is changed (Fig. 9). The algorithm assigns each bone a capsule-shaped *envelope*. Vertices of the modified skin within these envelopes move with the bones. Where envelopes overlap, vertex motion is a blend between the envelopes. The influence of each bone for vertices within the intersection of two bones' envelopes is controlled by assigning weight values. The ratio of a vertex's weight values, which always total 1.0, determine the relative extent to which each bone's motion affects the vertex. Furthermore, the model gets scaled when the kinematic model is scaled.

As stated before, the model has to simulate and show the grasping of an object in a realistic way. To satisfy this requirement, it is not enough to have a visually realistic model of the surface skin. The model must also be able to predict feasible grasping postures.

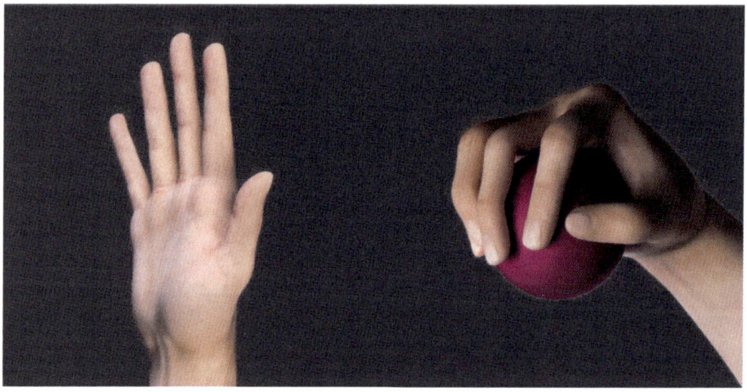

Fig. 9. Surface skin model

In order to generate grasp postures automatically, we propose to use a grasping algorithm based on that of Choi (2008). This algorithm uses a function to automatically generate a natural grasping motion path of the hand model from a fully opened state to a clenched one. The goal is to find contacts between the surface hand skin and the object surface while rotating the joint angles of the fingers. Care has to be taken to properly choose the rotation rate of the finger joints, as it affects the final posture prediction. Based on the results from Choi (2008), we propose to use a variable rotation algorithm, by describing rotations of all joints at observation-based rates. To select the appropriate rotation rate we propose the use of neural networks, similar to those used in Kyota et al. (2005) and Rezzoug & Gorce (2008). This will require intensive experimental work beforehand to record the postures for grasping objects (of different shapes, sizes, weights, etc.) when performing different tasks (power and precision). The experimental data have to be analysed in order to characterise the human grasp and find the parameters affecting the grasping posture. These parameters will be used as input to the neural network to estimate a tentative clenched posture. The rotation rate is defined by the difference between the angles of the fully opened state and the tentative clenched one.

In order to generate the grasp, a contact model is required. We need to check whether the surface skin model makes contact with the surface of the object model. In reality, the surface of a hand is deformed when making contact with the object. Generally, this deformation has a non-linearly elastic property, and it could be simulated using finite element analyses. But this would need a long execution time. This is unacceptable for our model where a large number of different grasp postures have to be generated and tested within a practical time.

Therefore, we propose to consider a simple geometric collision-detection algorithm based on the one used by Endo et al. (2007). The algorithm allows the penetration of the surface skin model and the object model. This penetration is limited by a tolerance that relates to the hand stiffness of each contact region.

The distances between the points on the skin surface and the object are calculated while the joint angles of each joint rotate according to the specific joint rotation algorithm. When the maximum penetration distance between the skin surface points and the object reaches the given tolerance, the contact is achieved and the joint rotation ends. When distal segments of all four fingers make contact with the object, the simulation terminates.

As we have mentioned previously, the model has to provide the contact information required for evaluating the grasp. If a classical robotics quality measure of the grasp is to be performed, the only data needed are the contact points and associated normal vectors at these points, which are easily obtained from the proposed contact model.

When trying to estimate the muscular pattern associated with a grasp, the model needs more contact information. The contact forces between the object and the hand have to be considered in this case. Unlike what happens with robots, real human fingers conform to the grasped object shape. As the contact finger surface is deformable the contact does not occur at just one point but over some finite area that increases as the normal forces increase. Due to this effect, in addition to the normal force and tangential force due to friction, human finger contact may support frictional torsional moments with respect to the normal at the contact point. This clearly shows that the consideration of rigid contact commonly used in robotics is not appropriate for use in studying the human grasp, and a soft contact has to be modelled. Most objects manipulated by human hands are much stiffer than human hands, and it is reasonable to consider the objects to be grasped as rigid bodies, and the hand as a deformable body.

Different soft contact models have been investigated and proposed in order to better account for this deformation effect in the context of soft finger contacts (Ciocarlie et al., 2005, 2007; Gonthier, 2007). In Ciocarlie et al. (2007) friction constraints are derived based on general expressions for non-planar contacts of elastic bodies, taking into account the local geometry and structure of the objects in contact. The following approximation can be used to express the constraint relating the magnitudes of frictional force (f_t) and moment (τ_n):

$$f_t^2 + \frac{\tau_n^2}{e_n^2} \leq \mu^2 \cdot P^2 , \tag{11}$$

where P is the total load applied in the direction of the contact normal, μ is the friction coefficient and e_n is called the eccentricity parameter (height of the ellipsoid described by Eq. 11). Considering a Winkler elastic foundation (Johnson, 1985) of depth h and elastic modulus K, the eccentricity parameter is given by:

$$e_n = \frac{8}{15} \cdot \sqrt{a \cdot b} , \tag{12}$$

where a and b can be calculated from the relative radii of curvature R' and R'' of the objects in contact and the compression δ of the elastic layer:

$$a = \sqrt{2 \cdot \delta \cdot R'} ; b = \sqrt{2 \cdot \delta \cdot R''} ; \delta = \sqrt{\frac{P \cdot h}{K \cdot \pi \cdot (R' \cdot R'')^{1/2}}} , \tag{13}$$

The actual grasping forces for a given posture will be obtained by considering that they have to satisfy the dynamic equilibrium of the grasped object. There is not a unique set of forces that ensures the equilibrium but we have to take into account the biomechanical limitations (maximal muscle forces) and the control performed by the central nervous system. In an effort to minimise the computational cost, we propose to uncouple the computation of the contact forces from the neuromuscular control model. This can be done by considering that the central nervous system is trying to attempt performing the grasp with minimal contact forces, as implemented for robots in the work of Liu et al. (2004a).

3.5 Neuromuscular control

The movement of the skeletal chains, together with the contact forces and the corresponding application points are input to the model. The problem to be solved is the derivation of the muscle activation levels required to produce the given motion under the external loads. It is, therefore, an inverse dynamics problem.

The dynamics equations of the open chain of rigid bodies have been derived using the Lagrange method (García de Jalón & Bayo, 1994). For a system with m generalised co-ordinates q_k, this equation is expressed as:

$$\frac{d}{dt}\frac{\partial L}{\partial \dot{q}_k} - \frac{\partial L}{\partial q_k} = Q_k^{nc} \quad k = 1, \ldots, m , \tag{14}$$

where L is the Lagrangian function and Q_k^{nc} are the generalised non-conservative forces. The generalised coordinates have been considered coincident with the system DOF (m=23).

Eqs. 14 together with the force balances of the tendon nets lead to an indeterminate problem. For example, in the case of the index finger, there are 12 equations (four corresponding to the DOF considered and eight to force balances in the tendon net) and 18 unknowns (six muscle forces and 12 branch forces of the tendon net). There is not a unique combination of muscular efforts that satisfy the dynamic equilibrium constraints. To solve the problem, a criterion chosen by the central nervous system to determine the muscle action control must be introduced. Our proposal is to maximise the endurance. According to Crowninshield and Brand (1981), this is achieved by minimising the non-linear objective function

$$OBJ = \sum \left(\frac{F_i}{PCSA_i} \right)^n , \quad (15)$$

with n between 2.0 and 4.0, and where F_i represents the force exerted by muscle i, and $PCSA_i$ its physiological cross-sectional area. In this case, $n = 2$ will be used. This function is minimised when subjected to Eq. 13 together with the force balances of the tendon nets. Additional constraints are that tendon forces must be non-negative, and the limits of muscle forces obtained from Eqs. 2 and 3 varying the muscle activation level from 0 to 1

$$F_{PEE} \cdot F_{\max} \le F \le (F_l \cdot F_v + F_{PEE}) \cdot F_{\max} . \quad (16)$$

3.6 Grasp evaluation

A global grasp evaluation can be performed through the use of the proposed model, merging the knowledge from ergonomics, robotics and biomechanics. The classical ergonomics evaluation of grasp posture and reachability is possible, for different percentiles of the population represented by the corresponding anthropometric parameters. Furthermore, CHTD evaluation can be performed by using the predicted postures and muscle forces.

It is advisable to use force closure from robotics as a part of the proposed model; once a grasping posture is estimated by the grasping algorithm, force closure should be assured before consuming time in determining the contact forces. Any of the robotics quality measures could be used for evaluating the grasp. Depending on the task to be performed, it would be better to use a grasp quality measure to evaluate the disturbance resistance or a grasp quality measure to evaluate the manipulability.

But the most relevant contribution to grasp evaluation has to come from biomechanics analysis. Grasp measures related to the muscle and articular forces have to be investigated. Just to provide insight into this sense, and to ensure coherence with our model formulation, we propose the use of Eq. 15 as a quality measure related to fatigue that we can call *fatigue index*: the smaller the fatigue index the better will be the grasp. For power grasps, an alternative measure can be the difference between the maximal force the hand can exert on the grasped object for the posture being analysed and the real contact forces estimated by the contact model; this alternative measure can be seen as a safety margin for the muscle forces, that we can call *muscle safety margin index*. Additional measures can be investigated, such as the maximal contact pressure, etc.

4. Conclusion

A realistic and self-contained biomechanical model of the hand has been proposed by merging the current knowledge of biomechanics, ergonomics and robotics. The model simulates the complete hand and can easily be scaled to study different percentiles of populations. It has a realistic representation that allows the ergonomic evaluation of products. The model is dynamic and can be used to study the muscular patterns associated with a specific grasp. It allows predicting feasible grasping postures and provides the contact information required for evaluating the grasp. Finally, the model incorporates original quality grasping measures such as the fatigue index and the muscle safety margin index, in addition to the usual robotics and ergonomics metrics and evaluations. All the abovementioned features are performed in a virtual environment, without external experimental data.

5. Acknowledgment

We are grateful for the financial support of the Fundació Caixa-Castelló and the Universitat Jaume I throughout the project P1-1B2009-40; of the Spanish Research and Innovation Ministry, and the EU (FEDER funds) throughout the project DPI2010-18177; and of European Community's Seventh Framework Programme through the project GRASP, IST-FP7-IP-215821. This research is related to these three projects.

6. Nomenclature

3D	Three-dimensional	FP	Flexor profundus
ADD	Adductor pollicis	FPB	Flexor pollicis brevis
ADQ	Abductor digiti quinti	FPL	Flexor pollicis longus
APB	Abductor pollicis brevis	FS	Flexor superficialis
APL	Abductor pollicis longus	GWS	Grasp wrench space
CE	Contractile element	HB	Hand breadth
CHT	Cumulative hand trauma		
D	disorders	HL	Hand length
CMC	Carpometacarpal	IP	Interphalangeal
DI	Dorsal interosseous	LU	Lumbrical
DIP	Distal interphalangeal	MCP	Metacarpophalangeal
DOF	Degrees of freedom	OPP	Opponens pollicis
EDC	Extensor digitorum communis	OWS	Object wrench space
		PCS	Physiological cross-sectional
EDQ	Extensor digiti quinti	A	area
EFM	Elastic foundation model	PEE	Parallel elastic element
EI	Extensor indicis	PIP	Proximal interphalangeal
EPB	Extensor pollicis brevis	SEE	Series elastic element
EPL	Extensor pollicis longus	TWS	Task wrench space
FDQ	Flexor digiti quinti	VI	Volar interosseous

7. References

An, K.N., Chao, E.Y., Cooney, W.P. & Linscheid, R.L. (1979). Normative model of human hand for biomechanical analysis. *Journal of Biomechanics*, 12, 10, pp. (775-788), ISSN 0021-9290

An, K.N., Chao, E.Y.S. and Kaufman, K.R., 1991. Analysis of muscle and joint loads. In: Mow, V.C and Hayes, W.C. (Eds.), *Basic Orthopaedics Biomechanics*. Raven Press. Ltd., New York, pp. 1-50.

Armstrong, T.J., Best, C., Bae, S., Choi, J., Grieshaber, D.C., Park, D., Woolley, C. & Zhou, W. Development of a Kinematic Hand Model for Study and Design of Hose Installation. *Digital Human Modeling*, HCII 2009, LNCS 5620, pp. 85–94, 2009.

Bernabeu, J. & Tornero, J. (2002). Hough Transform for Distance Computation and Collision Avoidance, *IEEE Transactions on Robotics and Automation*, 18, 3, (June 2002), pp. (393-398), ISSN 1042-296X

Biagiotti, L., Lotti, F., Melchiorri, C. & Vassura, G. (2002). Design Aspects for Advanced Robot Hands, IEEE/RSJ *International Conference on Intelligent Robots and Systems.* Towards Intelligent Robotic Manipulation., pp. (1–16)

Bicchi, A. (1994). On the Problem of Decomposing Grasp and Manipulation Forces in Multiple Whole-limb Manipulation, *Int. Journal of Robotics and Autonomous Systems,* 13, 2, (July 1994), pp. (127-147), ISSN 0921-8890

Bicchi, A. (1995). On the Closure Properties of Robotic Grasping. *International Journal of Robotics Research*, 14, 4, (August 1995), pp. (319–334), ISSN 0278-3649

Bicchi, A. & Kumar, V. (2000). Robotic grasping and contact: a review, *Robotics and Automation, 2000. Proceedings. ICRA '00. IEEE International Conference on*, IEEE, pp. 348–353.

Biryukova, E.V., Yourovskaya, V.Z. (1994). A model of human hand dynamics. *Advances in the Biomechanics of the Hand and Wrist*, Eds. F. Schuind, pp. (107-122), Plenum Press, ISBN: 0-306-44580-8, New York.

Borst, C., Fischer, M. & Hirzinger, G. (2003). Grasping the dice by dicing the grasp, *Proc. IEEE/RSJ IROS, ISBN 0-7803-7860-1, Las Vegas, NV, USA, Octuber 2003*Borst, C., Fischer, M. & Hirzinger, G. (2004). Grasp planning: how to choose a suitable task wrench space, *Proc. IEEE ICRA, ISBN 0-7803-8232-3, New Orleans, LA, USA, April-May 2004*

Brand, P.W. & Hollister, A.M. (1992). *Clinical Mechanics of the Hand*, Elsevier Science Health Science div, third edition, ISBN13 9780815127864, St. Louis

Buchholz, B., T.J. Armstrong, &S.A. Goldstein. Anthropometric data for describing the kinematics of the human hand. *Ergonomics* 35, 3, (March 1992), pp.(261-273), ISSN 0014-0139

Buchner, H.J., Hines, M.J., Hemami, H (1988). A dynamic model for finger interphalangeal coordination. *Journal of Biomechanics*, 21, 6,pp. (459-468), ISSN 0021-9290

Case, K., Porter, J.M. and Bonney, M.C., SAMMIE: a man and workplace modelling system. *Computer Aided Ergonomics*, 1990, 31–56 (Taylor & Francis: London).

Casolo, F., Lorenzi, V. (1994). Finger mathematical modelling and rehabilitation. En Advances in the Biomechanics of the Hand and Wrist, Eds. F. Schuind, pp. 197-223, New York. Plenum Press.

Chao, E.Y., Opgrande, J.D., Axmear, F.E. (1976). Three dimensional force analysis of finger joints in selected isometric hand functions. *Journal of Biomechanics*, 9: 387-395.

Chao, E.Y., An, K.N. (1978). Internal forces in human hand. *Journal of the Engineering Mechanics Division*, ASCE, 104 (EM1): 255-272.

Chiu, S.L. (1988). Task compatibility of manipulator pustures. *Int. J. Robotics Research*, 7, 5) pp. (13-21)

Choi, J. (2008). Doctoral dissertation, University of Michigan.

Ciocarlie, M., Miller, A. & Allen, P. (2005). Grasp Analysis Using Deformable Fingers, 2005 IEEE/RSJ International Conference on Intelligent Robots and Systems (IROS 2005)

Ciocarlie, M., Lackner, C. & Allen, P. (2007). Soft Finger Model with Adaptive Contact Geometry for Grasping and Manipulation Tasks, *Second Joint EuroHaptics Conference and Symposium on Haptic Interfaces for Virtual Environment and Teleoperator Systems (WHC'07)*, ISBN 978-0-7695-2738-3, Tsukuba, Japan, March 2007

Colombo and Cugini, 2005; Virtual humans and prototypes to evaluate ergonomics and safety. *Journal of Engineering Design*, 16, 2, (April 2005), pp. (195–207), ISSN 0954-4828

Craig, S.M., 1992. Anatomy of the joints of the fingers. *Hand Clinics*, 8, 4, (November 1992), pp. (693-700), ISSN 0749-0712

Crowninshield, R.D. & Brand, R.A. (1981). A physiologically based criterion of muscle force prediction in locomotion. *Journal of Biomechanics*. 14: 793-801.

Cutkosky, M. (1989). On grasp choice, grasp models, and the design of hands for manufacturing tasks, IEEE Transactions on Robotics and Automation **5**(3): 269–279.

Davidoff and Freivalds, 1993) Davidoff N.A., Freivalds A. A graphic model of the human hand using CATIA. *International Journal of Industrial Ergonomics*, 1993, 12 (4) 255-264

Denavit, J. and Hartenberg, R.S. (1955) 'A kinematic notation for lower-pair mechanisms based on matrices', *Journal of Applied Mechanics*, Vol. 77, pp.215–221.

Diankov, R. (2010). Automated Construction of Robotic Manipulation Programs, PhD thesis, Carnegie Mellon University, Robotics Institute.

Ding, D., Lee, Y.-H. & Wang, S. (2001). Computation of 3-d form-closure grasps, IEEE Transactions on Robotics and Automation **17**(4): 515 –522.

Dubousset, J.F., 1981. The digital joints. In: Tubiana, R. (Ed.), The Hand. Saunders Company, Philadelphia, pp. 191-201.

Endo, Y., Kanai, S., Kishinami, T., Miyata, N., Kouchi, M., Mochimaru, M. (2007). Virtual grasping assessment using 3D digital hand model. 10th Annual Applied Ergonomics Conference: Celebrating the Past - Shaping the Future.

Endo, Y., Kanai, S., Miyata, N., Kouchi, M., Mochimaru, M., Konno, J., Ogasawara, M., Shimokawa, M. (2009). Optimization-Based Grasp Posture Generation Method of Digital Hand for Virtual Ergonomics Assessment. SAE Int. J. Passeng. Cars - Electron. Electr. Syst. Volume 1, Issue 1, 590-598.

Erdmann, M.A. (1994). On the representation of firction in configuration space. *Int. Journal of Robotics Research*, 13(3),pp. 240-271.

Esteki, A., Mansour, J.M. (1997). A dynamic model of the hand with application in functional neuromuscular stimulation. *Annals of Biomedical Enginnering*, 25: 440-451.

Eyler, D.L. and Markee, J.E., 1954, "The anatomy and function of the intrinsic musculature of the fingers", *The Journal of Bone and Joint Surgery*, Vol. 36-A, pp. 1-18.

Ferrari, C. & Canny, J. (1992). Planning optimal grasps, *Proceedings 1992 IEEE International Conference on Robotics and Automation* pp. 2290–2295.

Fok KS, Chou SM. Development of a finger biomechanical model and its considerations. *Journal of Biomechanics*. 2010 Mar 3;43(4):701-13.

García de Jalón, J. and Bayo, E., 1994. Kinematic and dynamic simulation of multibody systems. Springer-Verlag, New York.

Giurintano, D.J. & Hollister, A.M. (1991). Force analysis of the thumb for a five-link system. ASME Biomechanics Symposium, 120:213-217.

Giurintano, D.J., Hollister, A.M., Buford, W.L., Thompson, D.E. & Myers, L.M. (1995). A virtual 5-link model of the thumb. *Medical Engineering & Physics*, 17, 4, (June 1995), pp. (297-303), ISSN 1350-4533

Goldstein, S.A., Armstrong, T.J., Chaffin, D.B. & Matthews, L.S. (1987). Analysis of cumulative strain in tendons and tendon sheaths. *Journal of Biomechanics*, 20 (1), pp. 1-6.

Gonthier, Y. (2007). Contact Dynamics Modelling for Robotic Task Simulation. Ph. d. thesis. University of Waterloo.

Goussous, F.A. Grasp planning for digital humans. PhD dissertation. Iowa University. 2007

Harada, K., Kaneko, M. & Tsuji, T. (2000). Rolling Based Manipulation for Multiple Objects. *Proc. IEEE Int. Conf. on Robotics and Automation (ICRA)*, pp. 3887-3894.

Haschke, R. Steil, J.J., Steuwer, I. & Ritter, H. (2005). Task-oriented quality measures for dextrous grasping. In: *Proc. 6th IEEE Int. Conf. Computational Intelligence in Robotics and Automation*, pp. 689-694.

Hatze, H., 1981. Myocibernetic control models of skeletal Muscle. University of South Africa, Pretoria.

Hertz, H. (1882). On the Contact of Rigid Elastic Solids and on Hardness, Ch 6: Assorted Papers by H. Hertz . MacMillan, New York, 1882.

Hill, A.V., 1938, "The of shortening and dynamic constants of muscle", Proc R Soc London B, Vol 126, pp. 136-195.

Hollister, A.M., Giurintano, D.J., Buford, W.L., Myers, L.M. & Novich, A. (1995). The axes of rotation of the thumb interphalangeal and metacarpophalangeal joints. *Clinical Orthopaedics*, (320), pp. 188-193.

Howe, R. Kao, I. & Cutkosky, M. (1988). Sliding of robot fingers under combined tornsion and shear loading. Proceedings *IEEE Int. Conf. on Robotics and Automation*, pp. 103-105.

Howe, R. & Cutkosky, M. (1996). Practical force-motion models for sliding manipulation *Int. Journal of Robotics Research* 15(6), pp. 555-572.

Jacobson, M.D., Raab, R., Faxelo. B.M., Abrams, R.A., Botte, M.J. & Lieber, R.L. (1996). Architectutural design of the human intrinsic hand muscles. *The Journal of Hand Surgery*, 17A (5), pp. 804-811.

Johnson, K. L., (1985). Contact Mechanics. Cambridge University Press.

Kamper DG, Fischer HC, Cruz EG. (2006). Impact of finger posture on mapping from muscle activation to joint torque. Clinical Biomechanics. 21(4):361-9.

Kao, I. & Cutkosky, M (1992). Dexterous manipulation with compliance and sliding. *Int. Journal of Robotics Research* 11(1), pp. 20-40.

Kao, I. & Yang, F. (2004). Stiffness and Contact Mechanics for Soft Fingers in Grasping and Manipulation. *IEEE Transactions on Robotics and Automation*, 20(1), pp. 132-135.

Kao, I., Linch, K. & Burdick, J. W. (2008). Contact Modeling and Manipulation. *Handbook of Robotics, chapter 27*, pp. 647-668.

Kapandji, A.I., 1998. *Fisiologie articulaire. Membre Supérieur*. Editions Maloine, Paris.

Kaufman, K.R., An, K.N., Litchy, W.J. and Chao, E.Y.S., 1991. Physiological prediction of muscle forces I. Theoretical formulation. J. Neuroscience 40 (3), 781-792.

Kawaguchi, K., Endo, Y., Kanai, S. (2009). Database-Driven Grasp Synthesis and Ergonomic Assessment for Handheld Product Design. Lecture Notes in Computer Science, Volume 5620/2009, 642-652.

Keyserling, W.M. 2000; Workplace risk factors and occupational musculoskeletal disorders, part 2: A review of biomechanical and Psychophysical research on risk factors associated with upper extremity disorders. AIHA Journal; Mar/Apr 2000; 61 (2) pg. 231-243

Kong, Y., Jang, H. & Freivalds, A. (2006) Wrist and Tendon Dynamics as Contributory Risk Factors in Work-Related Musculoskeletal Disorders. *Human Factors and Ergonomics in Manufacturing*, 16, 1, pp. (83–105), ISSN 1090-8471

Kumar S. 2001. Theories of musculoskeletal injury causation. Ergonomics, 2001, VOL. 44, NO. 1, 17 ± 47

Kurita Y, Onoue T, Ikeda A, Ogasawara T. Biomechanical analysis of subjective pinching effort based on tendon-skeletal model. Conf Proc IEEE Eng Med Biol Soc. 2009;2009:5231-4.

Kyota, F., Watabe, T., Saito, S. & Nakajima, M. (2005). Detection and Evaluation of Grasping Positions for Autonomous Agents. Proceedings of the 2005 International Conference on Cyberworlds (CW'05).

Lee, J.W., Rim, K. (1990). Maximum finger force prediction using a planar simulation of the middle finger. Proc. Instn. Mech. Engnrs. Part H: *Journal of Engineering in Medicine*, 204: 169-178.

Lee SW, Chen H, Towles JD, Kamper DG. (2008a) Effect of finger posture on the tendon force distribution within the finger extensor mechanism. *Journal of Biomechanical Engineering*. 130(5):051014.

Lee SW, Chen H, Towles JD, Kamper DG. (2008b). Estimation of the effective static moment arms of the tendons in the index finger extensor mechanism. *Journal of Biomechanics*. 41(7):1567-73.

Leijnse, J.N.A.L., Bonte, J.E., Landsmeer, J.M.F., Kalker, J.J., Van Der Meulen, J.C., Snijders, C.J. (1992). *Journal of Biomechanics*, 25 (11):1 253-1264.

Leijnse, J.N.A.L., Kalker, J.J. (1995). A two-dimensional kinematic model of the lumbrical in the human finger. *Journal of Biomechanics,* 28 (3): 237-249.

Lemay, M.A. & Crago, P.E. (1996). A dynamic model for simulating movements of the elbow, forearm and wrist. *Journal of Biomechanics*, 29 (19, pp. 1319-1330.

Li, Z & Sastry S. (1988). Task-oriented optimal grasping by multifingered robotic hands. *IEEE Journal of Robotics and Automation*, 4 (1), pp. 32-44.

Li Z., Chang C.-C., Dempsey P. G., Ouyang L., Duan J.. Validation of a three-dimensional hand scanning and dimension extraction method with dimension data. Ergonomics, Vol. 51, No. 11, November 2008, 1672–1692

Liegeois, A. (1977). Automatic supervisory control for the configuration and behavior of multibody mechanisms. *IEEE Trans. System, Man and Cybernetics*, 7 (12), pp. 842-868.

Lin, Q., Burdick, J. M. & Rimon, E. (2000). A stiffness-based quality measure for compliant grasps and fixtures. *IEEE Transactions on Robotics and Automation*, 16(6), pp. 675-688.

Liu, G., Xu, J., & Li, Z. (2004a). On geometric algorithms for real-time grasping force optimization. *IEEE Transactions on Control Systems* Technology, 12 (6): 843–859.

Liu, G., Xu, J., Wang, X. & Li, Z. (2004b). On Quality Functions for Grasp Synthesis, Fixture Planning, and Coordinated Manipulation, *IEEE Transactions on Automation Science and Engineering* **1**(2): 146–162.

Mansour, J.M., Rouvas, C., Sarangapani, J. (1994). Quantitative functional anatomy of finger muscles: Appliction to controlled grasp. *En Advances in the Biomechanics of the Hand and Wrist*, Eds. F. Schuind, pp. 177-188, New York. Plenum Press.

Mason, M. T. (2001). *Mechanics of robotic manipulation*, The MIT Press, Cambridge, MA, USA.

Miller, A. T. & Allen, P. K. (1999). Examples of 3D grasp quality computations, *Robotics and Automation, 1999. Proceedings. 1999 IEEE International Conference on*, Vol. 2, IEEE, pp. 1240–1246.

Miller, A. T., Knoop, S., Christensen, H. & Allen, P. K. (2003). Automatic grasp planning using shape primitives, Robotics and Automation, 2003. Proceedings. ICRA'03. IEEE International Conference on, Vol. 2, IEEE, pp. 1824–1829.

Miller, A., Allen, P.K. (2004). "Graspit!: A Versatile Simulator for Robotic Grasping". *IEEE Robotics and Automation Magazine*, V. 11, No.4, pp. 110-122.

Minami, A., An, K.N., Cooney, W.P. and Linscheid, R.L., 1985. Ligament stability of the MCP joint: A biomechanical study. *J. Hand Surgery* 10A (2), 255-260.

Mirthich, B. & Canny, J. (1994). Easily computable optimum grasps in 2D and 3D. In: *Proc. IEEE ICRA 1994*, pp. 739-747.

Mishra, B., Schwartz, J. T. & Sharir, M. (1987). On the existence and synthesis of multifinger positive grips, *Algorithmica* **2**(1-4): 541–558.

Mital, A. and Kilbom, A., 1992, Design, selection and use of hand tools to alleviate trauma of the upper extremities: Part II- The scientific basis (knowledge base) for the guide, *International Journal of Industrial Ergonomics*, Vol. 10, pp. 7-21

Mommersteeg, T.J.A., Blankevoort, L., Huiskes, R., Kooloos, J.G.M. and Kauer, J.M.G., 1996. Characterization of the mechanical behavior of human knee ligaments: a numerical-experimental approach. J. Biomechanics 29 (2), 151-160.

Morales, A., Sanz, P., Del Poblil, A. & Fagg, A. (2006). Vision-based three-finger grasp synthesis constrained by hand geometry. *Robotics and Autonomous Systems*, 54, 6, (June 2006), pp. (496–512), ISSN 0921-8890

Muggleton, J.M., Allen, R. & Chappell, P.H. Hand and arm injuries associated with repetitive manual work in industry: a review of disorders, risk factors and preventive measures. *Ergonomics*, 1999, VOL. 42, NO. 5, 714 - 739

Napier, J. (1956). The prehensile movements of the human hand, Surger **38**(4): 902–913.

Nguyen, V.-D. (1988). *Constructing force-closure grasps*, Institute of Electrical and Electronics Engineers.

Parada, J. E., Nava, N. E. & Ceccarelli, M. (2008). A Methodology for the Design of Robotic Hands with Multiple Fingers, *International Journal of Advanced Robotic Systems* **5**(2): 177–184.

Park, Y.C. & Starr, G.P. (1992). Grasp synthesis of polygonal objects using a three-fingered robotic hand. *International Journal of Robotics Research*, 11 (3), pp. 163-184.

Peña-Pitarch, E. Virtual human hand. PhD dissertation. Universitat Politècnica de Catalunya. 2007.

Pollard, S.S. (2004). Closure and quality equivalence for efficient synthesis of grasps from examples. *Int. J. Robotics Research*, 23 (6), pp. 595-614.

Ponce, J., Sullivan, S., Sudsang, A., Boissonat, J.D. & Merlet, J.P. (1997). On computing for-finger equilibrium and force-closure grasps of polyhedral objects. *International Journal of Robotics Research*, 16 (1), pp. 11-35.

Qiu D, Fischer HC, Kamper DG. Muscle activation patterns during force generation of the index finger. Conf Proc IEEE Eng Med Biol Soc. 2009;2009:3987-90.

Rezzoug, N. & Gorce, P. (2008). Prediction of fingers posture using artificial neural networks. *Journal of Biomechanics*. 41, pp. 2743-2749.

Rhee T., Neumann U., Lewis J.P. 2006, Human Hand Modeling from Surface Anatomy. I3D '06 Proceedings of the 2006 symposium on Interactive 3D graphics and games, ACM New York

Roa Garzón, M. (2009). *Grasp Planning Methodology for 3D Arbitrary Shaped Objects*, Ph. d. thesis, Universidad Politécnica de Cataluña.

Rogers M. S., Barr A. B., Kasemsontitum B.; Rempel D. M.. A three-dimensional anthropometric solid model of the hand based on landmark measurements. *Ergonomics*, Vol. 51, No. 4, April 2008, 511–526

Roloff I, Schöffl VR, Vigouroux L, Quaine F. Biomechanical model for the determination of the forces acting on the finger pulley system. *Journal of Biomechanics*. 2006;39(5):915-23.

Salisbury, J. (1982). *Kinematics and Force analysis of Articulated Hands*, Ph.d. thesis, Standford University.

Sancho-Bru, J.L., 2000, "Model Biomecànic de la mà orientat al disseny d'eines manuals", Ph.D. thesis, Universitat Jaume I, Castelló.

Sancho-Bru, J.L., Perez-Gonzalez, A., Vergara-Monedero, M., Giurintano,D.J., (2001). A 3-D dynamic model of human finger for studying free movements. *Journal of Biomechanics*, 34, 11, (November 2001), pp. (1491–1500), ISSN 0021-9290

Sancho-Bru, J.L., Perez-Gonzalez, A., Vergara, M., Giurintan, D.J., (2003a). A 3D biomechanical model of the hand for power grip. *Journal of Biomechanical Engineering* 125, 78–83.

Sancho-Bru, J.L., Giurintano, D.J., Pérez-González, A., and Vergara, M., (2003b), "Optimum tool handle diameter for a cylinder grip", *J. Hand. Ther.*, 16(4), pp. 337-342.

Sancho-Bru, J.L, Vergara, M., Rodríguez-Cervantes, P.J., Giurintano, D., Pérez-González, A. (2008). Scalability of the Muscular Action in a Parametric 3D Model of the Index Finger. *Annals of Biomedical Engineering,* 36, 1, (January 2008, pp. (102-107), ISSN 0090-6964

Schoenmarklin R.W., Marras W.S., Leurgans S.E. industrial wrist motions and incidence of hand/wrist cumulative trauma disorders. *Ergonomics*, 1994; 37: 1449-1459

Siciliano, B. & Khatib, O. (eds) (2008). *Springer Handbook of Robotics*, Vol. 15, Springer, Berlin, Heidelberg.

Smith, E.M., Juvinall, R.C., Bender, L.F. Pearson, J.R. (1964). Role of the finger flexors in rheumatoid deformities of the metacarpophalangeal joints. *Arth. Rheum.*, 7: 467-480.

Spielholz et al., 2001; P. Spielholz, B. Silverstein, M. Morgan, H. Checkoway And J. Kaufman. Comparison of self-report, video observation and direct measurement methods for upper extremity musculoskeletal disorder physical risk factors. Ergonomics, 2001, VOL. 44, NO. 6, 588 - 613

Spoor, C.W., Landsmeer, J.M.F. (1976). Analysis of the zigzag movement of the human finger under influence of the extensor digitorum tendon and the deep flexor tendon. *Journal of Biomechanics*, 9: 561-566.

Spoor, C.W. (1983). Balancing a force on the fingertip of a two-dimensional finger model without intrinsic muscles. *Journal of Biomechanics*, 16: 497-504.

Stansfield, S. (1991). Robotic grasping of unknown objects: A knowledge-based approach, *The International Journal of Robotics Research* **10**(4): 314–326.

Storace, A., Wolf, B. (1979). Functional role of the finger tendons. *Journal of Biomechanics,* 12: 575-578.

Storace, A., Wolf, B. (1982). Kinematic analysis of the role of the finger tendons. *Journal of Biomechanics*, 15, 5, pp. (391-393), ISSN 0021-9290

Thomas, D.H., Long, C., Landsmeer, J.M.F. (1968). Biomechanical consideration of lumbricalis behaviour in the human finger. *Journal of Biomechanics*, 1: 107-115.

Tubiana, R (1981), 'The hand', Vol. 1, W.B. Sanders Company, 1981.

Tubiana, R., Thomine, J. and Mackin, E. (1996), 'Examination of the hand and wrist', Second Edition, Martin Dunitz, 1996.

Valero-Cuevas, F.J., Zajac, F.E., Burgar, C.G. (1998). Large index-fingertip forces are produced by subject-independent patterns of muscle excitation. *Journal of Biomechanics*, 31: 693:703.

Valero-Cuevas, F.J. (2000). Predictive modulation of muscle coordinatin pattern magnitude scales fingertip force magnitude over the voluntary range. *Journal of Neurophysiology*, 83 (3): 1469-1479.

Valero-Cuevas, F.J. Towles, JD, Hentz, VR. (2000). Quantification of fingertip force reduction in the forefinger following simulated paralysis of extensor and intrinsic muscles. *Journal of Biomechanics*, 33(12):1601-1609.

Valero-Cuevas, F.J. (2005). An integrative approach to the biomechanical function and neuromuscular control of the fingers. *Journal of Biomechanics*, 38(4): p.673-84.

van Nierop O.A., van der Helm A., Overbeeke K.J., Djajadiningrat T.J.P. A natural human hand model. Visual Comput (2008) 24: 31–44

Vigouroux L, Quaine F, Labarre-Vila A, Moutet F. (2006) Estimation of finger muscle tendon tensions and pulley forces during specific sport-climbing grip techniques. *Journal of Biomechanics*, 39, 14, pp. (2583-2592), ISSN 0021-9290

Vigouroux L, Ferry M, Colloud F, Paclet F, Cahouet V, Quaine F. Is the principle of minimization of secondary moments validated during various fingertip force production conditions? *Hum Mov Sci.* 2008 Jun;27(3):396-407.

Weightman, B. & Amis, A.A. (1982). Finger joint force predictions related to design of joint replacements. *Journal of Biomedical Engineering*. 4:197-205.

Wren, D. & Fisher, R. (1995). Dextrous hand grasping strategies using preshapes and digit trajectories, IEEE International Conference on Systems, Man and Cybernetics, Vol. 1, pp. 910 –915 vol.1.

Wu JZ, An KN, Cutlip RG, Dong RG. A practical biomechanical model of the index finger simulating the kinematics of the muscle/tendon excursions. *Biomed Mater Eng.* 2010;20(2):89-97.

Xydas, N. & Kao, I. (1999). Modeling of contact mechanics and friction limit surface for soft fingers with experimental results, *Int. Journal of Robotics Research*, 18(9), pp. 947-950.

Xydas, N., Bhagavat, M. & Kao, I. (2000). Study of soft-finger contact mechanics using finite elements analysis and experiments, *Proceedings 2000 ICRA. Millennium Conference. IEEE International Conference on Robotics and Automation. Symposia Proceedings (Cat. No.00CH37065)* (April): 2179–2184

Yang, J., Kim, J.H., Abdel-Malek, K., Marler, T., Beck, S. & Kopp, G.R. A new digital human environment and assessment of vehicle interior design. Computer-Aided Design 39 (2007) 548–558

Yoshikawa, T. (1985). Manipulability of robotics mechanisms. *Int. J. Robotics Research*, 4, 2, pp. (735-747)

Youm, Y., Gillespie, T.T., Flatt, A.E. & Sprague, B.L. (1978). Kinematic investigation of normal MCP joint. *Journal of Biomechanics*, 11, 3,pp. (109-118), ISSN 0021-9290

Zajac, F.E., 1989. Muscle and tendon: properties, models, scaling, and application to biomechanics and motor control. *Critical Reviews in Biomedical Engineering* 17 (4), 359-411.

Zhu, X., Ding, H. & Li, H. (2001). A quantitative measure for multifingered grasps. In: *Proc. IEEE/ASME Int. Conf. Advanced Intelligent Mechatronics 2001*, pp. 213-219.

10

Feasible Simulation of Diseases Related to Bone Remodelling and of Their Treatment

Václav Klika[1,2] and František Maršík[1]
[1]*Institute of Thermomechanics, v.v.i., Academy of Sciences of Czech Republic*
[2]*Dept. of Mathematics, FNSPE, Czech Technical Univerzity in Prague*
Czech Republic

1. Introduction

A great advance in understanding mechanosensing and mechanotransduction of bone tissue has occurred in the past years. However, a clear answer is yet to come. There is plentiful evidence that most cells in human body are able to sense their mechanical environment, including osteoblasts and osteocytes. Li et al. found that marrow stromal cells change their proliferation rate and gene expression patterns in response to mechanical stimulation (Li et al, 2004). Ehrlich and Lanyon mention that osteocytes produce significantly higher levels of PGE_2 (prostaglandin E_2) and PGI_2 (prostacylin) than osteoblasts and in vivo inhibition of prostaglandins prevents bone adaptation in response to mechanical strains (Ehrlich and Lanyon, 2002). Further, nitric oxide NO is also a mediator of mechanically induced bone formation. It is released, similarly, as prostanoids, in higher levels after exposure to physiological levels of mechanical loading. Moreover, Rubin discovered that dynamic loading down-regulates osteoclastic formation (Rubin et al, 2000) (more precisely, the strained bone cell downregulates its expression of RANKL (Rubin et al, 2004)), which suggests that mechanical forces play an important role in bone adaptation process.
Candidate mechanoreceptors within a cell are stretch-activated channels, integrins (membrane spanning proteins that couple the cell to its extracellular environment), connexins (membrane spanning proteins that form channels that allow the direct exchange of small molecules with adjacent cells - including intercellular communication via gap junctions), and membrane structure (Rubin, 2006). Nowadays, there is also a completely different possible explanation for transformation mechanical signal into a biochemical function. Valle et al. explain in their review that only a proper mechanical loading may lead to exposure of binding sites and thus enabling further biochemical processes to proceed (Valle, 2007). Most probably multiple mechanosensors are involved in receiving mechanical signals. Moreover, there are other studies showing the importance of many other mechanisms beside those mentioned above (Lemaire et al, 2004).
On tissue level, it is clear that mechanical loading is important in the bone remodelling process. Heřt described an interaction between the mechanical stimulation of local cells and the bone adaptation process in the 1970s (Heřt et al, 1972), Frost observed the same behaviour in his clinical praxis and summed it up in his „Utah paradigm" (Frost, 2004). More recently, the fundamental importance of dynamic loading was accepted. Comparison of the static versus the dynamic loading effects on bone remodelling is given in a nice and

inspectional review by Ehrlich and Lanyon (2002). Further, Robling provides experimental results that confirm the essential importance of the dynamic loading (Robling, 2006). It is worth mentioning that Heřt referred to this fact in his observations more than 35 years ago (Heřt et al, 1972).

From the phenomenological relations for the rate of chemical reaction based on classical irreversible thermodynamics including coupling with mechanical processes, it was shown that, although tissues are exposed to all variety of mechanical factors: straining, shear, pressure, and even dynamic electric fields, the volume variation rate is the most important mechanical stimulus driving the processes in them (Klika, 2010). However, we believe that shear rate might be important for triggering the process. (for details see (Klika, 2010; Klika and Maršík, 2009)). Thus, in the presented manuscript, the mechanical stimulation of bone remodelling was assumed to be proportional to rate of volume change. As it will be seen from the features and results of the model, it seems to capture the response of bone to changes of its mechanical environment on tissue level. Probably, the other ways of mechanosensing are controlling the triggering of bone remodelling process in a given loci. We realize that biochemical reactions are initiated and influenced primarily by genetic effects and then by external biomechanical effects (stress changes). The aim of the presented thermodynamic model is to combine biological and biomechanical factors whereas currently available models of bone remodelling focus only on one of these factors which is actually the reason why this model was developed. It should provide an estimate of the effects of increased physical activity on quality of bone even in several disease states. Such a model may also reflect changes in remodelling behaviour resulting from pathological changes to the bone metabolism or from hip joint replacement and also may help for better assessment of the risk of osteoporosis-related fractures (Lindsay, 2003). Preliminary version of the mentioned approach has been published by our team in the past but not until this considerably improved version was the model applicable to praxis (both qualitative and quantitative results) (Klika and Maršík, 2010; Klika et al., 2010) which is here being extended.

1.1 Available models of bone remodeling

With the development of computer-aided strategies and based on the knowledge of bone geometry, applied forces, and elastic properties of the tissue, it may be possible to calculate the mechanical stress transfer inside the bone (Finite Elements analysis or FE analysis). The change of stresses is followed by a change in internal bone density distribution. This allows to formulate mathematical models that can be used to study functional adaptation quantitatively and furthermore, to create the bone density distribution patterns (Beaupré et al, 1990; Carter, 1987). Such mathematical models have been built in the past. Since they calculate just mechanical transmission inside the bone and not considering cell-biologic factors of bone physiology, they just partially correspond to the reality seen in living organisms. Basically, there are essentially two groups of models for bone remodelling. One assumes that the mechanical loading is the dominant effect, almost to the exclusion of other factors, and treatment of biochemical effects are included in parameter with no physical interpretation (e.g. Beaupré et al, 1990; Carter, 1987; Huiskes et al, 1987; Ruimerman et al, 2005; Turner et al, 1997). The results or predictions of these models yield the correct density distribution patterns in physiological cases. However, they have a limited ability to simulate disease. The second group, the biochemical models, consider control mechanisms of bone adaptation in great detail, but with limited possibilities for including mechanical effects that are known to be essential (Komarova et al, 2003; Lemaire et al, 2004). We realize that biochemical reactions are initiated and influenced primarily by genetic effects and then by external biomechanical effects (stress changes). Our thermodynamic model enables to combine biological and biomechanical factors (Klika and Maršík, 2010). Such a model may also reflect changes in remodelling behaviour resulting from pathological changes to the bone metabolism or from hip joint replacement. However, it is a model and thus it is a great simplification of the complex process of bone remodelling. In this chapter, a more detailed description of biochemical control mechanisms will be added to the mentioned model (Klika and Maršík, 2010; Klika et al, 2010) which in turn leads to possibility to study several concrete bone related diseases using this model.

1.2 Simulation of diseases and of their treatment

In our previous work, the influence of mechanical stimulation on (chemical) interactions in general was studied and it was shown how to comprise this effect into a model of studied biochemical processes (Klika and Maršík, 2009; Klika, 2010). These findings were used to describe the bone remodelling phenomenon (Klika and Maršík, 2010; Klika et al, 2010; Maršík et al, 2010). In this chapter, an extension of the mentioned bone remodelling model (influences of concrete biochemical factors) will be presented where the essential significance of dynamic loading will still be apparent.

Firstly, fundamental control factors will be mentioned. As was mentioned in the introduction, the RANKL-RANK-OPG pathway is essential in the bone remodelling control. Osteoprotegerin (OPG) inhibits binding of ligand RANKL to receptor RANK and thus prevents osteoclastogenesis. Since osteoclasts are the only resorbing agents in bone, osteoprotegerin "protects bone" (osteo-protege). Further, one of the major problems connected to bone remodelling is a rapid bone loss after menopause that affects a significant portion of women after 50 years of age. Menopause is linked to a rapid decrease in estrogen levels. And because estrogen significantly affects bone density, it would be beneficial to be able to simulate the influence of estrogen levels on the bone remodelling process. Similarly, the parathyriod hormone PTH, tumour growth factor TGF-β1, and nitric oxide NO play a significant role during the bone adaptation process.

PTH causes a release of calcium from the bone matrix and induces MNOC differentiation from precursor cells, estrogen has complex effects with final outcome in decreasing bone resorption by MNOC, calcitonin decreases levels of blood calcium by inhibiting MNOC function, and osteocalcin inhibits mineralisation (Sikavitsas et al, 2001). The discovery of the RANKL-RANK-OPG pathway enabled a more detailed study of the control mechanisms of bone remodelling. Robling et al. states that all PTH, PGE (prostaglandin), IL (interleukin), and vitamin D are "translated" by corresponding cells (osteoblasts) into RANKL levels (Robling et al, 2006). Further, nitric oxide NO is known to be a strong inhibitor of bone resorption and recently it has been known that it works in part by suppressing the expression of RANKL and, moreover, by promoting the expression of OPG (Robling et al, 2006). Both these effects eventually lead to a decrease of numbers of active osteoclasts MNOC, which in turn causes decrease of bone resorption. Kong and Penninger mention that the OPG expression is induced by estrogen (Kong and Penninger, 2000). Boyle et al. add that OPG production by osteoblasts is based on anabolic stimulation from TGF-β or estrogen (Boyle et al, 2003). Martin also deals with the question how hormones and cytokines influence contact-dependent regulation of MNOC by osteoblasts. He summaries results from the carried out experiments (mainly in vitro) that PTH, IL-11, and vitamin D ($1.25(OH)_2D_3$ more precisely) promotes RANKL formation, which in turn increases osteoclastogenesis (Martin, 2004).

RANKL-RANK-OPG pathway mediates many of these above mention biochemical factors. Moreover, RANKL levels also reflect microcrack density. Hence, it is essential to incorporate this pathway into our model. The connection will be enabled through the amount RANKL-RANK bonds that are one of the components of developed model, noted as RR, see (Klika and Maršík, 2010).

2. Methods

Bone remodelling is a very complex mechanism. It is necessary to make reasonable simplification to identify the essential control mechanisms. The used model covers the accepted crucial features (Klika and Maršík, 2010).

In this manuscript, several schemes for treating cellular interactions (as interactions among mixtures of chemical substances) are proposed, which are commonly used in similar problems (Keener and Sneyd, 2009; Lemaire et al, 2004). In our model, individual components of bone are substrates and products of biochemical interactions, whose rates are determined by the difference in chemical potentials. The affinity and chemical potential are (in simpler cases) proportional to the logarithm of the molar concentration of the involved substances (deGroot and Mazur, 1962). Here we actually use a modified version of this law of mass action with the additional effect of dynamic loading on the interaction rates (Klika, 2010; Klika and Maršík, 2009). The law of mass action is frequently used in modelling biological processes (Keener and Sneyd, 2009). However, it is only a simplified model that can be justified by agreement between calculated data and clinical observations. From the submitted results, it can be seen that features of the presented model are consistent with clinical and experimental data.

2.1 Incorporation of RANKL-RANK-OPG pathway into the bone remodelling model

A new model for RANKL-RANK-OPG chain kinetics has been formulated and added (Klika et al., 2010) to the mentioned model of bone remodelling (Klika and Maršík, 2010). This section is being RANKL is a ligand molecule and binds to RANK forming a bond, here noted as *RR* and its molar concentration as [RR], between osteoblasts and precursors of osteoclasts. Osteoblasts also secrete a decoy receptor osteoprotegerin OPG that binds with high affinity to RANKL and thus prevents the needed connection between osteoblasts and osteoclastic precursors.

The reaction scheme of interaction of the mentioned molecules can be described as follows:

$$\begin{aligned} RANKL + RANK &\overset{\mathrm{k}_{\pm 1}}{\longleftrightarrow} RR, \\ RANKL + OPG &\overset{\mathrm{k}_{\pm 2}}{\longleftrightarrow} RO_{\text{inactive}}, \end{aligned} \tag{1}$$

where RO_{inactive} represents the bond between the decoy OPG and ligand RANKL. Using the law of mass action (Klika and Maršík, 2009) we may infer kinetics of the above mentioned interactions. Only the simplification, when assuming a relation between forward and backward reaction rates $k_{+i} \gg k_{-i}$, is not applicable here. We get

$$\begin{aligned} \frac{\mathrm{d}n_{RANKL}}{\mathrm{d}\tau} &= -n_{RANKL}(\beta_{\mathrm{RK}}^{\mathrm{RRO}} + n_{RANKL} - n_{OPG}) + \\ &+\delta_{-1}^{\mathrm{RRO}}(\beta_{\mathrm{RR}}^{\mathrm{RRO}} - n_{RANKL} + n_{OPG}) - \\ &\qquad -\delta_{+2}^{\mathrm{RRO}} n_{RANKL} n_{OPG} + \delta_{-2}^{\mathrm{RRO}}(\beta_{\mathrm{RO}}^{\mathrm{RRO}} - n_{OPG}), \\ \frac{\mathrm{d}n_{OPG}}{\mathrm{d}\tau} &= -\delta_{+2}^{\mathrm{RRO}} n_{RANKL} n_{OPG} + \delta_{-2}^{\mathrm{RRO}}(\beta_{\mathrm{RO}}^{\mathrm{RRO}} - n_{OPG}), \end{aligned} \tag{2}$$

where

$$\begin{aligned}
\delta_{-1}^{\mathrm{RRO}} &= \frac{k_{-1}}{k_{+1}[\mathrm{RANKL_{stand}}]},\\
\delta_{-2}^{\mathrm{RRO}} &= \frac{k_{-2}}{k_{+1}[\mathrm{RANKL_{stand}}]},\\
\delta_{+2}^{\mathrm{RRO}} &= \frac{k_{+2}}{k_{+1}},\\
\beta_{\mathrm{RO}}^{\mathrm{RRO}} &= \frac{c_{\mathrm{RO}}}{[\mathrm{RANKL_{stand}}]} = \frac{[\mathrm{RO_0}] + [\mathrm{OPG_0}]}{[\mathrm{RANKL_{stand}}]},\\
\beta_{\mathrm{RR}}^{\mathrm{RRO}} &= \frac{c_{\mathrm{RR}}}{\mathrm{RANKL_{stand}}} = \frac{[\mathrm{RR_0}] + [\mathrm{RANKL_0}] - [\mathrm{OPG_0}]}{[\mathrm{RANKL_{stand}}]}.
\end{aligned} \tag{3}$$

Again $k_{\pm i}$ are reaction rate coefficients, δ_i are interaction rates, and β_j^{RRO} represents the normalised initial molar concentrations of corresponding substances, denoted with index 0 and finally $[\mathrm{RANKL_{stand}}]$ represents standard serum level of RANKL used for normalisation of molar concentrations of substance i, n_i. All the parameters have evidently a physical interpretation and are measurable. However, hardly any such in vivo data for humans is available. Fortunately, the recent progress in the understanding of bone remodelling control enabled in vitro studies of individual factors.

Quinn et al. studied the influence of RANKL and OPG concentration on a number of osteoclasts (more precisely, TRAP positive multinucleated osteoclasts) in a dose-dependent way (Quinn et al, 2001). We would like to use this data to determine the above mentioned parameters of the RANKL-RANK-OPG model. Because the carried out experiments are studying effects of RANKL and OPG separately, the reaction scheme (1) may be splitted into two separate reactions for parameter setting. This is convenient because the kinetics of a single biochemical reaction can be described using a single differential equation (in this case non-linear). Moreover, both normalised differential equations corresponding to these two reactions can be written in the same form:

$$\dot{x} = -Ax^2 - Bx + C, \quad A > 0, C > 0, \tag{4}$$

where $A = 1, B = \beta_{\mathrm{RK}} + \delta_{-1}, C = \delta_{-1}\beta_{\mathrm{RR}}$ for the RANKL reaction and $A = \delta_{+2}, B = \delta_{+2}\beta_{\mathrm{RANKL}} + \delta_{-2}, C = \delta_{-2}\beta_{\mathrm{RO}}$ for OPG reaction. The normalised form is also useful because it decreases the number of unknown parameters. The differential equation (4) has the following solution for positive constants A, C and for initial value x_0:

$$\begin{aligned}
x(\tau) = &\left[\frac{2A}{\sqrt{B^2+4AC}}\left(1 + \frac{1 + \frac{2A}{\sqrt{B^2+4AC}}\left(x_0 + \frac{B}{2A}\right)}{1 - \frac{2A}{\sqrt{B^2+4AC}}\left(x_0 + \frac{B}{2A}\right)} e^{\sqrt{B^2+4AC}\tau}\right)\right]^{-1} \cdot \\
&\cdot \left[\left(1 - \frac{B}{\sqrt{B^2+4AC}}\right) \frac{1 + \frac{2A}{\sqrt{B^2+4AC}}\left(x_0 + \frac{B}{2A}\right)}{1 - \frac{2A}{\sqrt{B^2+4AC}}\left(x_0 + \frac{B}{2A}\right)} e^{\sqrt{B^2+4AC}\tau} - \frac{B}{\sqrt{B^2+4AC}} - 1\right].
\end{aligned} \tag{5}$$

Because we know the analytic form of function describing the kinetics of RANKL (and OPG), we may use the least square method for determination of the unknown parameters according to the carried out experiments. Data from the Quinn et al. in vitro experiment relates RANKL (and OPG) concentration to MNOC concentration (the number of osteoclasts per well). The mentioned reaction scheme (1) of RANKL-RANK-OPG interaction has an output product denoted as RR. Thus, to be able to use the mentioned data from Quinn et al., we need to relate RANKL-RANK bonds ([RR]) to the number of osteoclasts ([MNOC]). To get a precise prediction of this relationship from the presented model we would also need to know the analytical solution of the system of ODEs that describe the bone remodelling process (Klika and Maršík, 2010), which is not possible. On the other hand, the interaction that describes the relation between RANKL-RANK bonds and MNOC concentration is the first one in our bone remodelling scheme (Klika and Maršík, 2010) and it will be assumed that the number of formed and active osteoclasts is proportional to the RR concentration. It means that it was assumed that in vitro, where no remodellation occurs, the formation of osteoclasts may be described by:

$$RR \rightleftarrows MNOC.$$

This assumption will be used just for purposes of parameter setting and from final results it will be possible to see if this simplification was too great or not.

The next issue we have to deal with is finding a possible relation between in vitro and in vivo data. In vivo ones are more or less unavailable, especially in such a detail that is needed for parameter setting. Further, determination of standard serum levels of OPG and RANKL is needed. The problem is that in most cases in vitro concentrations have to be much higher to reach a similar effect as in vivo. Moreover, no such relation may exist. It will be assumed that there is a correspondence among these two approaches and that it is linear, i.e. in vivo data can be gained from in vitro after appropriate scaling of concentrations.

The search for standard serum levels of osteoprotegerin and RANKL was not simple. Studies differ greatly in the presented values. Kawasaki et al states that the standard level of osteoprotegerin is $250\frac{pg}{\mu l}$ (Kawasaki et al, 2006) and Moschen et al. mention $800\frac{pg}{\mu l}$ (Moschen et al, 2005). Further, Eghbali-Fatourechi et al. determined OPG serum levels to be $2.05\frac{pmol}{l}$ (Eghbali-Fatourechi et al, 2003). The probable cause of these discrepancies lies in differently used techniques of gaining osteoprotegerin and measuring its concentration. Kawasaki et al. measured the amount of RANKL in gingival crevicular fluid, Moschen et al. performed collonic explant cultures from biopsies and consequently measured RANKL and OPG levels using an ELISA kit, and Eghbali-Fatourechi used a different cell preparation technique followed by measurement with an ELISA kit. One of the manufacturers of the ELISA kit for assessment OPG levels cites several studies on OPG levels in humans and also submits results from their own research (Elisa OPG kit, 2006). At least all these measurements are carried out by the same measurement technique and are comparable. Therefore, we set standard OPG and RANKL levels according to data that are there referred to - $[\mathrm{RANKL_{stand}}] = 0.84\frac{pmol}{l} = 55 \cdot 0.84\frac{pg}{ml} = 46.2\frac{pg}{ml}$ and $[\mathrm{OPG_{stand}}] = 1.8\frac{pmol}{l} = 20 \cdot 1.8\frac{pg}{ml} = 36\frac{pg}{ml}$ in serum (Kudlacek et al, 2003), where the knowledge of molecular weights $MW_{\mathrm{RANKL}} = 5510^3, MW_{\mathrm{OPG}} = 2010^3$ was used (Elisa OPG kit, 2006; RANKL product data sheet, 2008). Now it is needed to find a reasonable relation with in vitro data from Quinn et al that will be used for the least squares method for parameter estimation. The following consideration will be used: the physiological range of levels of OPG and RANKL will be found and consequently related to studied effective in vitro range by Quinn. OPG serum levels found in human are 12-138$\frac{pg}{ml}$ = 0.6-6.9$\frac{pmol}{l}$ and RANKL serum levels are 0-250$\frac{pg}{ml}$ = 0-4.55$\frac{pmol}{l}$ with standard values of $0.84\frac{pmol}{l}$ for RANKL and $1.8\frac{pmol}{l}$ for OPG, respectively. When we relate these values to the in vitro

ranges of RANKL 0-500$\frac{ng}{ml}$ and of OPG 0-30$\frac{ng}{ml}$, we get the in vitro equivalents for standard values: $[\text{RANKL}_{\text{invitrostand}}] = 92.3\frac{ng}{ml}$, $[\text{OPG}_{\text{invitrostand}}] = 7.83\frac{ng}{ml}$.
A list of parameters that will be determined by least squares from the RANKL experiment are the following:

$$\delta_{-1}^{\text{RRO}}, \tau_{\text{7days}}^{\text{RRO}}, n_{RK_0}, n_{RR_0},$$

where $\tau_{\text{7days}}^{\text{RRO}}$ is the dimensionless time that corresponds to 7 days. Before the parameter setting is by curve fitting (least square method) is carried out, it is reasonable to have at least some estimation of parameter values. Because the normalisation was done by division with term $k_{+1}[\text{RANKL}_{\text{stand}}]^2$ and from (3), we get:

$$\begin{aligned}
\tau_{\text{7days}}^{\text{RRO}} &= tk_{+1}C_{\text{RR}}|_{t=7days} = 6\ 10^5 10^7 10^{-12} \approx 10^0, \\
n_{RR_0} &\approx 10^0, \\
n_{RK_0} &\approx 10^0, \\
\delta_{-1^{\text{RRO}}} &= \frac{k_{-1}}{k_{+1}[\text{RANKL}_{\text{stand}}]} \approx k_{-1}10^5,
\end{aligned}$$

where the value of k_{+1} was estimated from the parameter setting in the bone remodelling model, standard value of RANKL $[\text{RANKL}_{\text{stand}}] \approx 1\frac{pmol}{l}$ was mentioned above, and the k_{-1} value may be anywhere in $(0,10^7)$ but most probably lower than one.
The least square method with the used data from Quinn et al. (Quinn et al, 2001) and the analytic function as described above gives the following estimates:

$$\delta_{-1}^{\text{RRO}} = 4.9210^{-6}, \tau_{\text{7days}}^{\text{RRO}} = 4.64, n_{RK_0} = 1.037, n_{RR_0} = 0.0947. \tag{6}$$

If we compare these values with their order estimation above, we see that the values are acceptable and the curve fit is as well, see Fig. 1a.
Now, we may proceed with OPG parameters. The difference is that if we use only the second reaction of RANKL-RANK-OPG reaction scheme (1), we do not know how initial OPG concentration influences the number of bonds between RANKL and RANK. However, this influence is mediated by a decrease in number of available ligands RANKL by binding with OPG. Because OPG binds with higher affinity to ligand RANKL than this ligand to its receptor RANK (otherwise the decoy effects of OPG would be very limited), it will be assumed that OPG binds to RANKL more rapidly than the competiting reaction. The reason for this is again in the need of analytic solution of differential equations that govern the kinetics of mentioned processes (it was not possible to solve the full system of two differential equations (2) so the mentioned simplification was needed; again, from the results that follow it seems reasonable). Thus, the influence of levels of osteoprotegerin on the *RR* concentration may be mediated by an appropriate modification of initial concentration of RANKL which in turn affects the resulting *RR* concentration. Schematically:

$$2^{\text{nd}} reaction\ in\ (1) \rightarrow [\text{OPG}](t)$$

and consequently $[\text{RANKL}_0] = [\text{OPG}](\tau_{\text{OPG}})$, which is used in

$$1^{\text{st}} reaction\ of\ (1) \rightarrow [\text{RR}][\tau_{\text{7days}}]$$

were τ_{OPG} is a time to be determined.

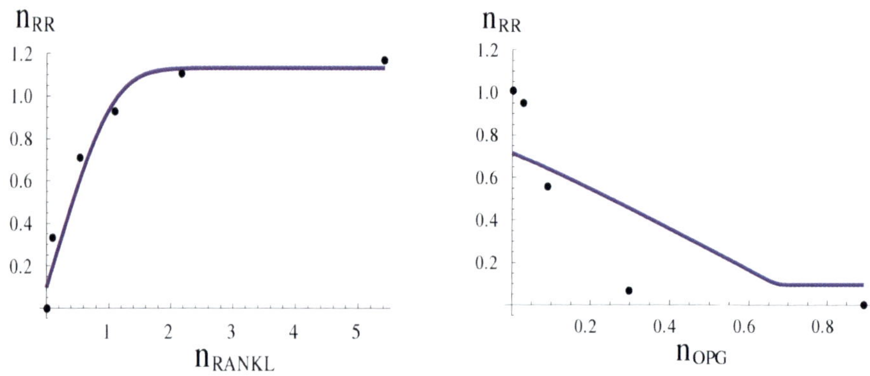

Fig. 1. RANKL and OPG fitted solutions (blue curves) by least squares method to data measured (dots) by Quinn et al. (Quinn et al, 2001). Firstly, n_{RR} as a function of n_{RANKL_0} is determined and consequently n_{RR} as a function of n_{OPG_0}, created by embedding dependency of [RANKL] on [OPG] and of [RR] on [RANKL] concentration, was found.

The already determined parameters from the RANKL setting will be used and only the yet unknown will be determined, i.e.

$$\delta_{-2}^{\mathrm{RRO}}, \delta_{+2}^{\mathrm{RRO}}, \tau_{\mathrm{OPG}}^{\mathrm{RRO}}, n_{RO_0},$$

Again, the least squares in the case of OPG give the following estimates (based on data from Quinn and the fact that molecular weight of RANKL is 55 10^3 and of OPG 20 10^3):

$$\delta_{-2}^{\mathrm{RRO}} = 5.86\ 10^{-19}, \delta_{+2}^{\mathrm{RRO}} = 12.96, \tau_{\mathrm{OPG}}^{\mathrm{RRO}} = 11.36, n_{RO_0} = 6.135. \tag{7}$$

Also, the values are admissible and the curve fit is reasonable (the function here is much more complex because OPG concentration is firstly used to determine an initial RANKL concentration for a consecutive reaction that finally gives [RR] outcome), see Fig 1b.
If the mentioned results of parameter estimation are combined, all the needed values of parameters of RANKL-RANK-OPG model (3) may be inferred:

$$\begin{aligned}
\delta_{-1}^{\mathrm{RRO}} &= \frac{k_{-1}}{k_{+1}[\mathrm{RANKL_{stand}}]} = 4.9210^{-6},\\
\delta_{-2}^{\mathrm{RRO}} &= \frac{k_{-2}}{k_{+1}[\mathrm{RANKL_{stand}}]} = 5.8610^{-19},\\
\delta_{+2}^{\mathrm{RRO}} &= \frac{k_{+2}}{k_{+1}} = 12.96,\\
\beta_{\mathrm{RO}}^{\mathrm{RRO}} &= \frac{C_{\mathrm{RO}}}{[\mathrm{RANKL_{stand}}]} = \frac{[\mathrm{RO_0}] + [\mathrm{OPG_0}]}{[\mathrm{RANKL_{stand}}]} = 6.135 + n_{OPG_0},\\
\beta_{\mathrm{RR}}^{\mathrm{RRO}} &= \frac{C_{\mathrm{RR}}}{[\mathrm{RANKL_{stand}}]} = \frac{[\mathrm{RR_0}] + [\mathrm{RANKL_0}] - [\mathrm{OPG_0}]}{[\mathrm{RANKL_{stand}}]} = 0.0947 + n_{RANKL_0} - [\mathrm{OPG_0}],\\
\beta_{\mathrm{RK}}^{\mathrm{RRO}} &= \frac{C_{\mathrm{RK}}}{[\mathrm{RANKL_{stand}}]} = \frac{[\mathrm{RK_0}] - [\mathrm{RANKL_0}] + [\mathrm{OPG_0}]}{[\mathrm{RANKL_{stand}}]} = 1.037 - n_{RANKL_0} + n_{OPG_0},\\
\tau_{\mathrm{7days}}^{\mathrm{RRO}} &= 4.64.
\end{aligned} \tag{8}$$

The predicted effects of RANKL and OPG serum levels on bone density			
[RANKL] $\left[\frac{\text{pmol}}{\text{l}}\right]$	[OPG] $\left[\frac{pmol}{l}\right]$	n_{RR} [1]	normalised bone density [1]
0.84 (standard)	1.8 (standard)	0.790	100% (0.811)
4.55	1.8	1.132	76.9%(0.624)
0.1	1.8	0.13	**172.6% (1.40)
0.84	6.9	0.276	**152.9% (0.1.24)
0.84	0.6	0.892	92.5% (0.75)

Table 1. The predicted effects of the RANKL-RANK-OPG pathway on bone density. n_{RR} is a result from the RANKL-RANK-OPG pathway model, and consequently, bone density (the number in parentheses in the last column) is predicted from the presented thermodynamic bone remodelling model based on the calculated n_{RR}. The asterisk in the front of values notices that it may be necessary to intermit the treatment after a certain time: * - after a longer time, ** - after a shorter period. Simulated or predicted data by model that are bold are in accordance with data found in literature – (Kudlacek et al, 2003).

Interconnection between this RRO model and bone remodelling model is mediated by [RR]. The concentration of RR influences the value of parameter β_1 in the developed thermodynamic bone remodelling model, see (Klika and Maršík, 2010). There are different normalisations used in these two mentioned models and we assume that in the case of standard values of RANKL and OPG, the parameter β_1 should have its standard value (corresponding to ``healthy'' state). Further, the typical normalised concentration of RR in bone remodelling model is $n_{RR} \in (1.35,1.41)$ in standard state (see (Klika and Maršík, 2010)). Thus:

$$\beta_1 = 1.41/0.79 n_{RR} - 0.81, \tag{9}$$

which gives the value $\beta_1 = 0.6$ for standard values of RANKL and OPG because n_{RR} under these condition equals 0.79 and n_{RR} is a result of the interaction in RANKL-RANK-OPG pathway at time $\tau^{\text{RRO}}_{\text{7days}}$. As can be seen, the value of n_{RR} influences only β_1, i.e. it acts only as a modification of initial conditions of the bone remodelling model. However, it will be seen in the results below that it sufficiently captures the influence of the whole pathway.
The increase in ligand concentration RANKL should lead to an increase in osteoclast formation, and consequently, the decrease of bone tissue density, and conversely, osteoprotegerin OPG prevents osteoclastogenesis. Modelling of this pathway is carried out through solving kinetic equations (2) with the above mentioned parameter values (8). Consequently, the output value of n_{RR} is used as an input variable in the bone adaptation model – (9). Tab. 1 gives an idea of how the added RANKL-RANK-OPG pathway may influence bone density (percentual changes of n_{RR} are more or less in accordance with data found in Quinn et al. (Quinn et al., 2001).

2.2 Incorporation of PTH effects into the bone remodelling model

The parathyroid hormone plays an important role in bone remodelling (see introduction). Again, the discovery of the essential control RANKL-RANK-OPG pathway enabled to describe in higher detail the influence of PTH on bone adaptation process. Robling mentions that PTH effect is ``translated'' into RANKL (Robling et al, 2006), more precisely PTH promotes RANKL formation (Martin, 2004). Fukushima et al. studied in vitro responses of the RANKL expression to PTH (Fukushima et al, 2005). They clearly showed that RANKL levels are dose-dependent on PTH concentrations in vitro (in the studied range $10^{-9}\,M$-$10^{-6}\,M$). Using this data, the influence of PTH into the presented bone remodelling model will be incorporated.

As was mentioned, PTH promotes RANKL expression. Thus, we may describe this fact using the following interaction:

$$PTH + RANKL_{\text{producers}} + Substratum \overset{k_{\pm 1}}{\leftrightarrow} RANKL + RANKL_{\text{producers}}, \tag{10}$$

where $RANKL_{\text{producers}}$ represents the group of cells that are expressing RANKL and a mixture of substances needed for ligand RANKL production is denoted as $Substratum$. Again, the differential equation describing kinetics of PTH concentration can be derived:

$$\frac{\mathrm{d[PTH]}}{\mathrm{d}\tau} = -[\mathrm{PTH}](\beta_{\mathrm{Substr}}^{\mathrm{PTH}} + [\mathrm{PTH}]) + \delta_{-1}^{\mathrm{PTH}}(\beta_{\mathrm{RANKL}}^{\mathrm{PTH}} - [\mathrm{PTH}]), \tag{11}$$

where

$$\begin{aligned} \delta_{-1}^{\mathrm{PTH}} &= \frac{k_{-1}}{k_{+1}[\mathrm{RANKL_{stand}}]}, \\ \beta_{\mathrm{RANKL}}^{\mathrm{PTH}} &= \frac{C_{\mathrm{RANKL}}}{[\mathrm{RANKL_{stand}}]} = \frac{[\mathrm{RANKL_0}] + [\mathrm{PTH_0}]}{[\mathrm{RANKL_{stand}}]}, \\ \beta_{\mathrm{Substr}}^{\mathrm{PTH}} &= \frac{C_{\mathrm{Substr}}}{[\mathrm{RANKL_{stand}}]} = \frac{[\mathrm{Substr_0}] - [\mathrm{PTH_0}]}{[\mathrm{RANKL_{stand}}]}. \end{aligned} \tag{12}$$

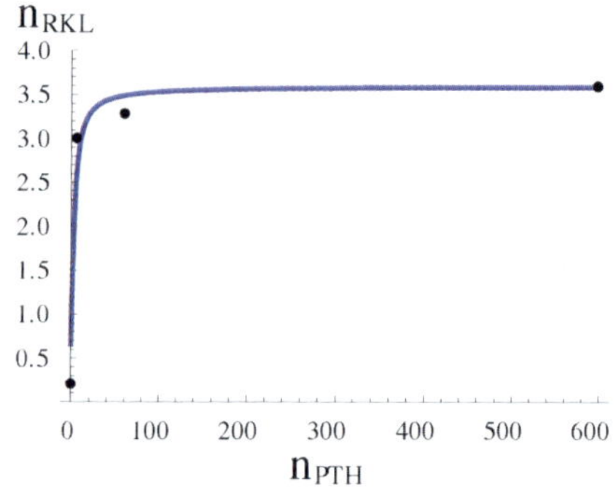

Fig. 2. PTH fitted solution (blue curve) by the least squares method to data measured (dots) by Fukushima et al. (Fukushima et al, 2005).

Again, this differential equation can be rewritten into (4) where $A = 1, B = \beta_{\mathrm{Substr}}^{\mathrm{PTH}} + \delta_{-1}^{\mathrm{PTH}}, C = \delta_{-1}\beta_{\mathrm{RANKL}}$. Thus, the analytical function that describes the evolution of PTH concentration in time from its initial concentration is known. The mentioned in vitro data from Fukushima et al. will be used for estimation of these parameter values using the least square method. Finally, the initial concentration of PTH influences RANKL concentration after 10 days in culture:

$$[\mathrm{RANKL}] = \beta_{\mathrm{RANKL}}^{\mathrm{PTH}} - [\mathrm{PTH}].$$

The least squares method gives the following results (see Fig. 2):

$$\delta_{-1}^{\mathrm{PTH}} = 0.145, \tau_{10\mathrm{days}}^{\mathrm{PTH}} = 26.17, n_{Substr_0}^{\mathrm{PTH}} = 0.018. \quad (13)$$

In vitro behaviour may significantly vary from in vivo observation. Usually, the range of concentration found in humans is much narrower than examined in vitro. A relation between in vitro and in vivo study will be found. Firstly, it is needed to determine standard in vivo serum level of PTH in humans. Khosla et al. state that PTH serum levels in humans are in $0 - 6\frac{pmol}{l}$ (Khosla et al, 1998). Further, Jorde et al. mentions that standard in vivo PTH level in non-smokers is $3.6\frac{pmol}{l} = 33.84\frac{pg}{ml}$ (Jorde et al, 2005), where the fact that $MW_{\mathrm{PTH}} =$ 9400 daltons was used (Potts, 2005). Now, we need to find a study that would capture PTH effects on bone remodelling. Charopoulos et al. studied effects of primary hyperparathyroidism in both calcemic and non-calcemic groups (Charopoulos et al, 2006). They mention normal PTH levels to be $37.13\frac{pg}{ml}$ and in the case of the non-calcemic hyperparathyroidism group, PTH levels were significantly higher $97.09 = \frac{pg}{ml}$. Moreover, these values significantly correlated to BMD (bone mineral density).
The idea is similar as in the previous case, the influence of PTH on bone density is mediated by RANKL-RANK-OPG pathway. The predicted value of RANKL based on PTH level will be used as an input into RRO model that will consequently translate this influence into the appropriate change in number of active osteoclasts.
If one uses in vitro equivalent of in vivo standard level of PTH equal to $5\ 10^{-9}M$ and $n_{RANKL_0} = 1.31$ (again these values are opted to get the described in vivo effect of PTH concentration and that standard PTH values would lead to standard RANKL concentration and consequently also ``healthy'' bone density) we get similar results as observed in Charopoulos et al. study - see Tab. 2.
We see that in normal range of PTH 25-45$\frac{pg}{ml}$ the predicted bone density varies slightly, see Tab. 2. However, disease state such as primary hyper-parathyriodism with PTH levels 3 times higher than normal ($97.09\frac{pg}{ml}$) the BMD dropped by 7-15% in the tibia and by 15% in the lumbar vertebrae (Charopoulos et al, 2006). The presented model estimates a decrease in bone density by 12.8% after such an increase in PTH.

The predicted effects of PTH serum levels on bone density	
[PTH] $\left[\frac{pg}{ml}\right]$	normalised bone density [1]
25	102,8% (0.834)
34 (standard)	**100% (0.811)**
45	97.0%(0.787)
97	**87.3% (0.708)**

Table 2. The predicted effects of PTH serum levels on bone density. PTH influences RANKL expression, which in turn influences osteoclastogenesis. Consequently, bone density is predicted from the presented bone remodelling model based on the calculated [RR]. Simulated or predicted data by model that are bold are in accordance with the data found in literature – (Charopoulos et al, 2006; Jorde et al ,2005).

2.3 Incorporation of NO effects into the bone remodelling model

Nitric oxide is a small molecule that can freely diffuse across cell membrane without any use of channels (and thus without any control from cell). Probably this easy access is reason for its signalling function. Also, because there is no need of passive or even active transportation across membrane it provides very fast communications. From the mentioned nature of signalling molecule NO, it is evident that it plays role in many processes in body, and concretely, it influences bone remodelling.

There has been a quite thorough investigation of NO action on bone remodelling. Before the discovery of the RANKL-RANK-OPG pathway, van't Hof already carried out an in vitro experiment showing that NO plays a significant role in bone resorption by inducing apoptosis of osteoclast progenitors and supressing osteoclast activity (van't Hof and Ralston, 1997). NO also seems to have a significant effect in inflammation-induced osteoporosis (such as rheumatoid arthritis), where NO production is increased, and consequently, bone density decreased (Armour et al, 1997). Wimalawansa et al. studied the effect of NO donor (concretely nitroglycerin) treatment on BMD change in rats. After treatment, they had significantly lower BMD and femur weights and also the influence of NO on the trabecular and cortical bone - loss of trabecular bone volume and decrease in cortical area in cross-section were prevented by the administration of nitroglycerin (Wimalawansa et al, 1997). Van't Hof and Ralston give a very nice overview of the NO role in bone - how nitric oxide is created, in what form, mechanism of NO action on bone remodelling, effects of NO on bone resorption (activation of inducible nitric oxide synthase - iNOS - pathway is essential for IL-1 stimulated bone resorption), and mention several in vivo animal models that exemplify this behaviour (van't Hof and Ralston, 2001). Again, the discovery of RANKL and OPG enabled a more detailed study of NO effects on bone remodelling. Robling mentions that NO suppresses the expression of RANKL and promotes the expression of OPG (Robling et al, 2006). Both these effects lead to the decrease of bone resorption. Fan et al. carried out an in vitro study where a dose-dependent response to NO in both RANKL and OPG production has been shown (Fan et al, 2004). Rahnert et al. studied the influence of 2% exercise ($20000\mu\varepsilon$) with 10 cycles/min (thus approximately $7000\mu\varepsilon s^{-1}$), observed that mechanical loading represses RANKL production (i.e. resorption), and that nitric oxide influences this repression (Rahnert et al, 2008).

Thus the in vitro effects of NO are rather known; however, there is lack of clinical studies with concrete effects of NO on bone quality. Fortunately, there is a group that has recently carried out a control study aimed on NO effects on bones in humans (the NOVEL clinical study - http://clinicaltrials.gov/show/NCT00043719). They performed a pilot study of NO effects on humans (surgically induced menopause women), which had a promising results. Nitroglycerin has similar maintenance effects as estrogen on BMD (Wimalawansa, 2000). Further, there is a nice review by Wimalawansa on the treatment of bone osteoporosis with NO: nitric oxide is a very reactive agent (half life is 1 second) and thus it has a very localised effects; after menopause, the circulating NO is significantly lower than before (can be rectified after hormonal therapy); NO donors have high potential as a novel therapeutic agent in bone diseases (follows from clinical studies of his group); NO seems to have a biphasic effect on bone quality - high levels of NO generation decrease BMD whereas lower levels increase BMD (from here it implies that the possible therapeutic window is $< 35\, mg/day$ - in this range the treatment is beneficial on skeleton); animal studies are confirming that NO has a biphasic effect on BMD. Further, that nitroglycerin is superior to the other 10 studied NO donors, and showing what is the in vivo dose-response to nitroglycerin (Wimalawansa, 2007).

An estimation of NO effects on bone may be carried out (there is yet no clinical study that we may refer to) that will be based on in vitro studies and on studies with NO donor

delivery in humans and animals as mentioned in the previous paragraph (in the animal study with dose response to NO donors, the same levels of nitroglycerin per kilogram of body weight were distributed and the same biphasic effect with the same threshold - $\frac{35mg}{75kg} \approx 0.5\frac{mg}{kg}$ of nitroglycerin per day - were observed as in humans).
For a description of NO influences on bone remodelling, the following reaction scheme will be used. It is based on the previously mentioned observation:

$$\begin{aligned} NO + RANKL &\overset{k_{\pm1}}{\leftrightarrow} Remaining\_product, \\ NO + OPG_{\text{producers}} + Substratum &\overset{k_{\pm2}}{\leftrightarrow} OPG + OPG_{\text{producers}}, \end{aligned} \tag{14}$$

where *Remaining_product* represents inactivated RANKL. Again, we may simply obtain differential equations describing the kinetics of these interactions. Because the influence of NO levels are relatively small (max 6% increase in BMD (Wimalawansa, 2007)), we may separate the influence of NO on RANKL and on OPG, and their collective effect can be obtained by summing the individual ones (confirmed by the numerical solution of both ODEs at once and compared with separated effects). By the same technique (least squares - Fig. 3) as in previous cases, the unknown parameters of the mentioned scheme may be determined (normalisation in the two differential equations is quite different):

$$\begin{aligned} &RANKL\!: \delta_{-1}^{\text{NO,R}} = 2.06\ 10^{-12}, \tau_{\text{24h}}^{\text{NO,R}} = 1.036, n_{Remaining\_product_0} = 0.930, \\ &OPG\!: \delta_{-1}^{\text{NO,O}} = 528.2, \tau_{\text{24h}}^{\text{NO,O}} = 1.6\ 10^{-3}, n_{Substr_0} = 8.50. \end{aligned} \tag{15}$$

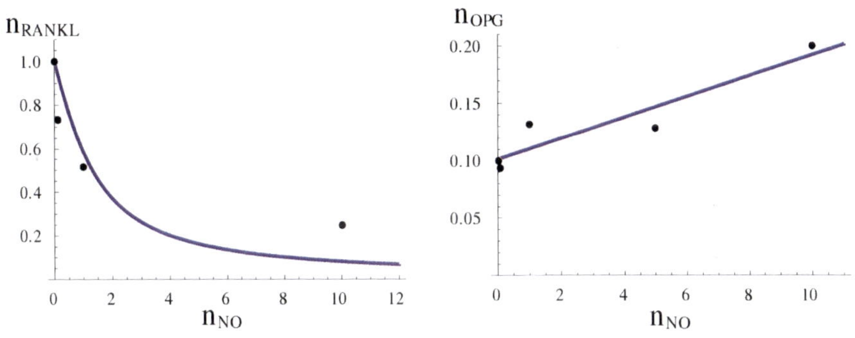

Fig. 3. NO fitted solutions (blue curve) by the least squares method to data measured (dots) by Wimalawansa (Wimalawansa, 2007) - NO influences both RANKL and OPG expression.

The in vivo standard was determined from a graph in (Wimalawansa, 2007): 0.044 $\frac{mg}{kg}$ per day of nitroglycerin - there is no BMD change observed. This dosage of nitroglycerin treatment (and consequently NO levels) in ovariectomized rats is assumed to correspond to standard in vivo levels of NO (or a more stable NO_3). Here, the previously used linear relation between in vitro and in vivo scales does not suitably characterise the observed relationship. Therefore the following logarithmic relation was proposed and served for finding a suitable $[NO_{\text{in\_vitro\_stand}}]$ (so that NO would have the same effects on bone remodelling as observed in vivo):

$$[\mathrm{OPG}_0]^{\mathrm{RRO}} = \frac{n_{OPG_{stand}}}{fitNOOPG([\mathrm{NO}_{\mathrm{in\_vitro\_stand}}])} \cdot$$
$$\cdot fitNOOPG((1 + \ln([\mathrm{NO}_{\mathrm{in\_vivo}}]/[\mathrm{NO}_{\mathrm{in\_vivo\_stand}}])[\mathrm{NO}_{\mathrm{in\_vivo\_stand}}])$$

where $fitNOOPG([\mathrm{NO}_{\mathrm{in\_vitro}}])$ is a function describing in vitro effect of NO concentration on OPG, $n_{OPG_{stand}} = \frac{[\mathrm{OPG}_{\mathrm{stand}}]}{[\mathrm{RANKL}_{\mathrm{stand}}]}$ is a normalised standard OPG molar concentration, $[\mathrm{NO}_{\mathrm{in\_vivo}}]$ represents in vivo NO level corresponding to served dosage of nitroglycerin, $[\mathrm{NO}_{\mathrm{in\_vivo\_stand}}]$ is the standard in vivo NO level, $\frac{n_{OPG_{stand}}}{fitNOOPG([\mathrm{NO}_{\mathrm{in\_vitro\_stand}}])}$ represents a scaling factor guaranteeing linkage between this model of NO influence and RANKl-RANK-OPG model (with different normalisation). Thus, this relation means that a logarithmically different response in vivo to NO levels than in vitro is assumed. Similarly for RANKL:

$$\begin{aligned} RANKL&: [\mathrm{NO}_{\mathrm{in\_vitro\_stand}}]^{\mathrm{NO,R}} = 0.036, \\ OPG&: [\mathrm{NO}_{\mathrm{in\_vitro\_stand}}]^{\mathrm{NO,O}} = 1.01. \end{aligned} \tag{16}$$

From results in Tab. 3, it can be seen that the simulated effects of NO on bone density are very similar to those shown in (Wimalawansa, 2007). As was mentioned, after menopause a decrease in NO levels is observed. As can be seen from Tab. 3, this may also slightly contribute to the increase in bone resorption. Moreover, there seems to be a possibility to

The predicted effects of NG treatment on bone density			
NG (nitroglycerin) $\left[\frac{\mathrm{pg}}{\mathrm{ml}}\right]$ per day	n_{OPG} [1]	n_{RANKL} [1]	normalised bone density [1]
0.001	0.157	1.078	92.4% (0.749)
0.02	0.21	1.016	**98.3% (0.797)**
0.044 (standard)	0.233	1	**100% (0.811)**
0.1	0.250	0.984	**102.0%(0.827)**
0.5	0.281	0.953	**106.0% (0.860)**

Table 3. The predicted effects of nitroglycerin (NO donor) treatment on bone density. NO promotes OPG expression and suppress the RANKL production - the same behaviour can be observed here. Consequently, bone density is predicted from the presented bone remodelling model based on the calculated [RR]. It is worth mentioning that NO has biphasic effect on bone, and in the window here studied, i.e. NO donor nitroglycerin is served up to 0.044 $\frac{\mathrm{mg}}{\mathrm{kg}}$ per day, has anabolic effects. Simulated or predicted data by model that are bold are in accordance with data found in literature – (Wimalawansa, 2007).

decrease these unwanted effects by nitroglycerin treatment, but only to some extent because when the dosage increase approximately over 0.5 $\frac{mg}{kg}$ per day it ceases to be beneficial. On the contrary, it may be deleterious (so-called biphasic effect of NO on skeleton; it may still have a positive impact on cardiovascular system etc.).

2.4 Notes on estradiol $1.25(\mathrm{OH})_2\mathrm{D}_3$(vitamin D) and TGF-$\beta_1$

Estradiol

Analogously to incorporation of PTH effects on bone remodelling through RANKL-RANK-OPG pathway can be carried out so it will be omitted here and can be found in (Klika et al,

2010). However, the simulation results will be shown even with changing levels of estradiol to demonstrate the usage of this model – see section 3.

$1.25(OH)_2D_3$(vitamin D)

Similarly, as in the previous sections, we wanted to incorporate also the influences of vitamin D (more precisely $1.25(OH)_2D_3$) and TGF-β_1 on the bone remodelling phenomenon. However, both these factors had to be omitted (for different reasons).

Vitamin D seems to be quite a significant factor acting on bone remodelling, e.g. seasonal effects due to sun exposure (and consequently increased vitamin D production in body) are observed (Saquib et al, 2006). Tanaka et al. showed that vitamin D promotes active osteoclast formation in vitro (Tanaka et al, 1993). There are in vitro studies that confirm again the mediation of vitamin D effects by the RANKL-RANK-OPG pathway (Martin, 2004). Moreover, it seems that there is a clinical study about to start that documents the mentioned influence on RANKL in humans but not enough of information is available yet.

But the problem is that there are many other studies that do not observe any significant influence of vitamin D levels on bone tissue, e.g. (Lips et al, 2001). One possible reason for these discrepancies in the observed results may lie in problems with its measurement. Carter mentions that there are several different methods for its determination and give significantly different results (Carter et al, 2004). In the year 2007, a thorough recherche was carried out by University of Ottawa, Evidence-based Practice Center for Agency for Healthcare Research and Quality (Cranney et al, 2007). They mention that 11 out of 19 studies are confirming that there is a significant correlation between vitamin D and bone mineral density, but also the remaining 8 are stating that there is no such effect.

Due to this ambiguity in clinical studies, we do not incorporate vitamin D into the presented model. If there is more infomation in future that would clarify these discrepancies, the vitamin D effect may be added by the same procedure as was used in estradiol, PTH, and NO.

TGF-β_1

There is clear evidence that this growth factor plays a significant role in the control of bone remodelling. Murakami et al. showed that the OPG expression is promoted dose-dependently by TGF-β_1 (Murakami et al, 1998) and Quinn et al. further found that RANKL expression is down-regulated by actuation of this growth factor (Quinn et al, 2001). However, clinical data collected by Zhang et al. show a fairly different behaviour of effect (Zhang et al, 2009). This different behaviour may be due to biphasic effect of TGH-β_1 that was observed by Karst et al. in vitro (Karst et al, 2004): TGF-β_1 in lower concentration elevated and in higher decreased the RANKL/OPG ratio. However, still from the mentioned clinical study it follows that actuation of TGF-β on bone remodelling is not mediated only by the RANKL-RANK-OPG pathway because response to TGF-β seems to be more complex. It is known that this factor also induces $MNOC$ apoptosis (Mundy et al, 1995; Murakami et al, 1998), which is described by J_3 in the presented model. Further, TGF-β_1 attracts osteoblastic precursors by chemotaxis to the resorbed site (Mundy et al, 1995). Even though transforming growth factor β is a component of local factors LF in the presented model, the influence of MNOC apoptosis can be described through J_3, and actuation on RANKL-RANK-OPG pathway as well, still the effects on bone tissue are not in accordance with clinically observed behaviour. Thus, the influence of TGF-β on bone remodelling cannot be described by the presented model in enough detail - it is a limitation of the model.

3. Examples of predictions of bone remodelling based on the presented model

We may now simulate the response of bone remodelling to changing environment, both mechanical and biochemical. Similarly, as was described in (Maršík et al, 2010), density distribution patterns may be obtained using Finite Elements Method (FEM). The results from the previous section will be used.

To demonstrate the usage of the presented model, a prediction of density distribution in human femur was carried out (the FE model of femur consists of 25636 3D 10 node tetrahedron elements). As an initial state, a homogeneous distribution of apparent density throughout the whole bone was used (1.8 g/cm^3). Since each iteration is calculated by solving differential equations representing the whole model of bone remodelling, it is actually a time evolution of bone remodelling in bone (Ansys v11.0 program was used to calculate the mechanical stimuli in each element). Real geometry was gained from a CT-scan and external forces were applied in the usual directions and magnitude - including muscle forces acting on the femur (Heller et al., 2005). This technique was used for all computed results included in this chapter. One may observe that cortical bone (the denser part of bone) and cancellous bone are formed (and maintained) as a consequence of mechanical stimuli distribution in human bone.

It was needed to use a relation between predicted bone density and mechanical properties (elastic moduli). There is a great disparity in the proposed elastic-density relationships (Helgason et al, 2008; Rice et al, 1988; Rho et al, 1993; Hodgskinson and Currey, 1992). We used a most common relationship for the human femur because the relation seems to be site-specific (Helgason et al, 2008): $E \propto \rho^2$, which defines through bone density the constitutive relation being considered. If a different power law is used, the pattern of density distribution still remains the same.

As was mentioned in the introduction, the most important mechanical stimulus for maintaining bone tissue is the most common daily activity - walking. Nowadays, many people have sedentary jobs and that is why they spent less hours by walking than would be appropriate. An example of a person whose walking activity is around 55% of a healthy standard (1.5 hours of walking compared to 2.75h) is shown - inappropriate loading leads to decrease in bone density, see Fig. 4. Naturally, a possible treatment would be in spending more time walking (1.25h more) or similar effect can be reached by running, which is a higher osteogenic stimuli - 30 minutes of running every other day will compensate for the disuse - see Fig. 4.

Hyperparathyroidism was chosen as an example of biochemical control of bone remodelling. As was discussed in section 2.2, during this disease, the PTH serum levels are $97\frac{pg}{ml}$, whereas a standard value is $34\frac{pg}{ml}$. This should lead to a significant decrease in bone density. An example of a person who is physically active (correct mechanical stimuli on regular daily basis, i.e. approximately 20 000 steps per day) but suffers from hyperparathyroidism (serum level of PTH is $97\frac{pg}{ml}$) is depicted on Fig. 5. We may observe an expected decrease in bone density. Because mechanical loading has an osteogenic effect even in a disease state, we may try to increase bone density (possibly insufficiently) only with an increase in mechanical stimulation, 30 minute-running per every other day was chosen. The predicted improvement is depicted in Fig.5.

During menopause, a decline in estradiol levels occur. In some women, the decrease is very dramatic (a drop bellow $5\frac{pg}{ml}$ is observed, whereas a standard serum level is 40-60$\frac{pg}{ml}$) while in some not (serum level remains above $20\frac{pg}{ml}$), see (Klika et al, 2010). Further it was observed that, together with estradiol, there is a decline in nitric oxide levels - see section 2.3. An example of a woman who is physically active (correct mechanical stimuli on regular daily basis, i.e. approximately 20 000 steps per day) but in a consequence of menopause has decreased serum levels of estradiol and nitric oxide (as mentioned above - estradiol: $2.5\frac{pg}{ml}$, NO level correspond to $0.02\frac{mg}{kg}$ per day of nitroglycerin) is depicted in Fig. 6. The presented model predicts a decrease of 8% in bone tissue density, which does not seem to be osteoporosis yet. This may be because menopause is accompanied by more effects than these two mentioned and also most probably because they are less physically active (may be caused by pain). If we combine the 8% decrease (Fig. 6) caused by menopause alone with another 9% decline (Fig. 4) caused by improper loading, we get a significant drop by almost 20% in the overall bone density of the femur, which can be considered as osteoporotic state. One possible treatment of bone loss connected with menopause is treated with hormone therapy (HRT). Simulation of such a treatment that increased estradiol serum levels to $20\frac{pg}{ml}$ (or by $0.107\frac{mg}{kg}$ per day of nitroglycerin treatment which is actually less expensive) is given in Fig. 6. Again, the importance of mechanical stimulation shown when increased physical activity (running 30 minutes every other day) increases bone density in similar fashion as HRT treatment (the same figure). And best results are reached when both effects are combined and even the original bone tissue density can be restored - Fig. 6.

4. Conclusion

A natural goal of the modelling of a process in the human body is to help in understanding its mechanisms and ideally to help in the treatment of diseases related to this phenomenon. For this reason, more detailed influences of various biochemical factors were added. Nowadays, the RANKL/RANK/OPG chain is deemed to be one of the most important biochemical controls of the bone remodelling process. The direct cellular contact of osteoclast precursor with stromal cells is needed for osteoclastogenesis. This contact is mediated by the receptor on osteoclasts and their precursor, RANK, and ligand RANKL on osteoblasts. Osteoprotegerin binds with higher affinity to RANK which inhibits the receptor-ligand interaction and as a result, it reduces osteoclastogenesis. Thus, the raise in OPG concentration results in a smaller number of resorbing osteoclasts, which leads to higher bone tissue density. The results discussed in the presented work have exactly the same behaviour. Similarly, the effects of RANKL, RANK, and estradiol were added to the mentioned model. Consequently, simulation capabilities were demonstrated on examples of diseases and their treatment. These results were partially validated by clinical studies found in literature.

However, the impression that the presented model is able to simulate the bone remodelling process in the whole complexity is not correct. It has limitations, as mentioned below, in the spatial precision of the results (i.e. actual structure of bone tissue) and also some control mechanisms cannot be included (e.g. TGF-β effects, as was mentioned at the end of section 2.4). But still, the model can be at least considered as a summary of known important factors, comprising the fundamental aspects of the currently known knowledge of the bone remodelling phenomenon, with some predictive capabilities and encouraging predictive simulations. Since the presented model is a concentration model, it cannot be used arbitrarily. The limitation is, of course, in the spatial precision of results. The minimal volume unit (finite element) should be sufficiently large to contain enough of all the

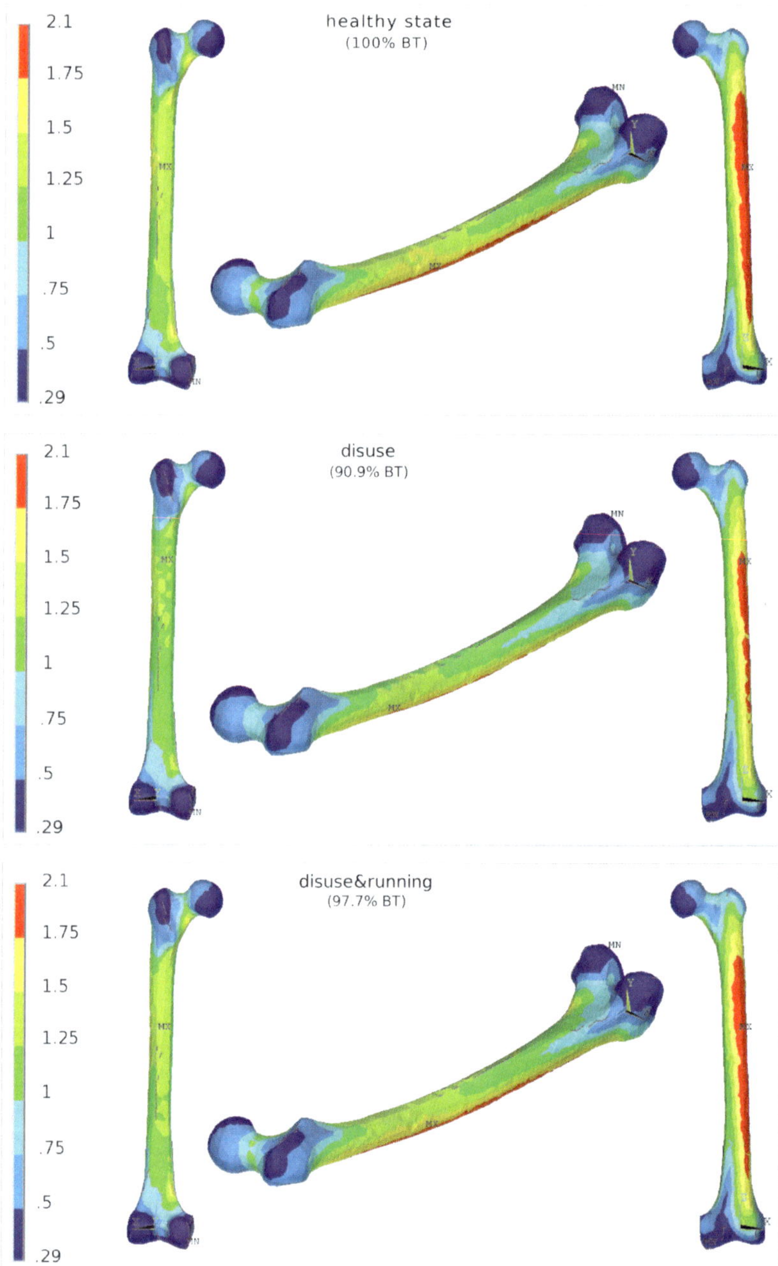

Fig. 4. Prediction of disuse effect on bone quality - simulation of insufficient loading (half of the recommended daily stimulation), treatment proposal - running (30 minutes every other day), and its simulation. Notice the change of bone mass (BM) of the whole femur.

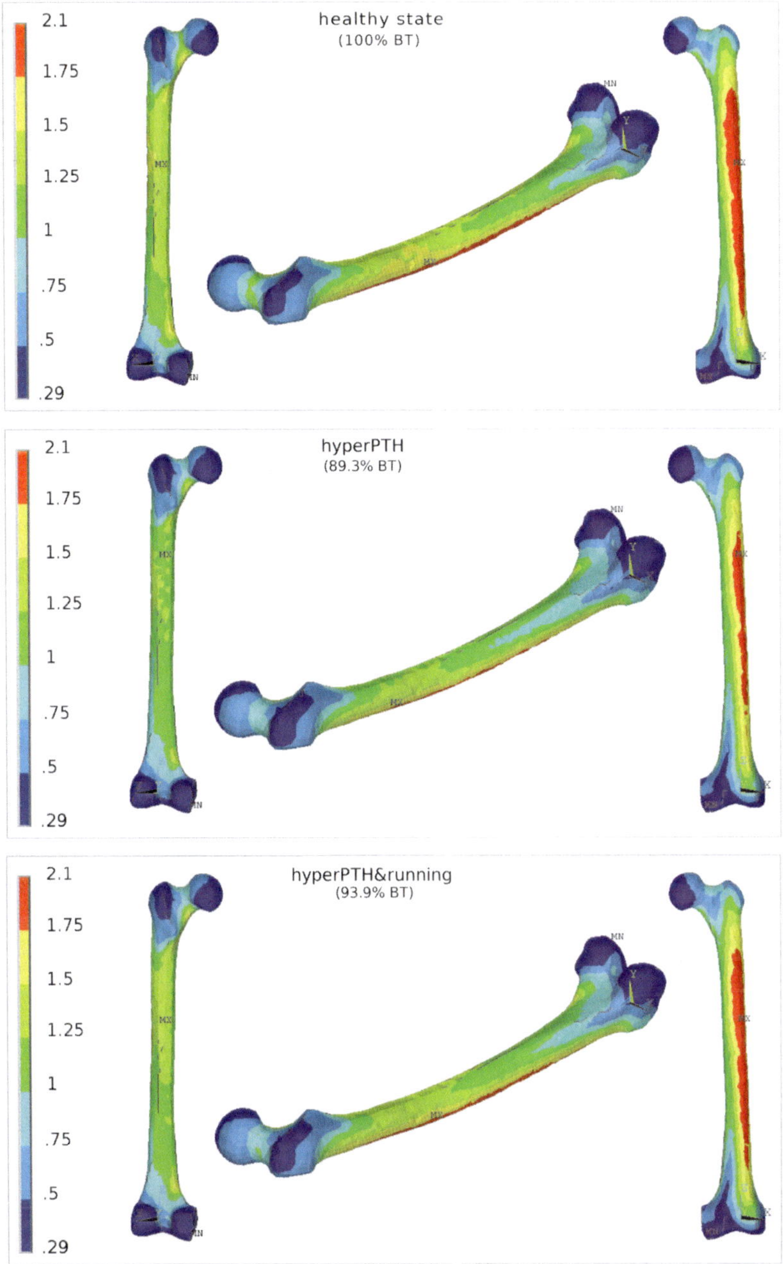

Fig. 5. Prediction of the PTH effect on bone quality - simulation of hyperparathyroidism ($97\,\frac{pg}{ml}$ where normal PTH levels are $34\,\frac{pg}{ml}$), treatment proposal - running (30 minutes every other day), and its simulation. Notice the change of bone mass (BM) of the whole femur.

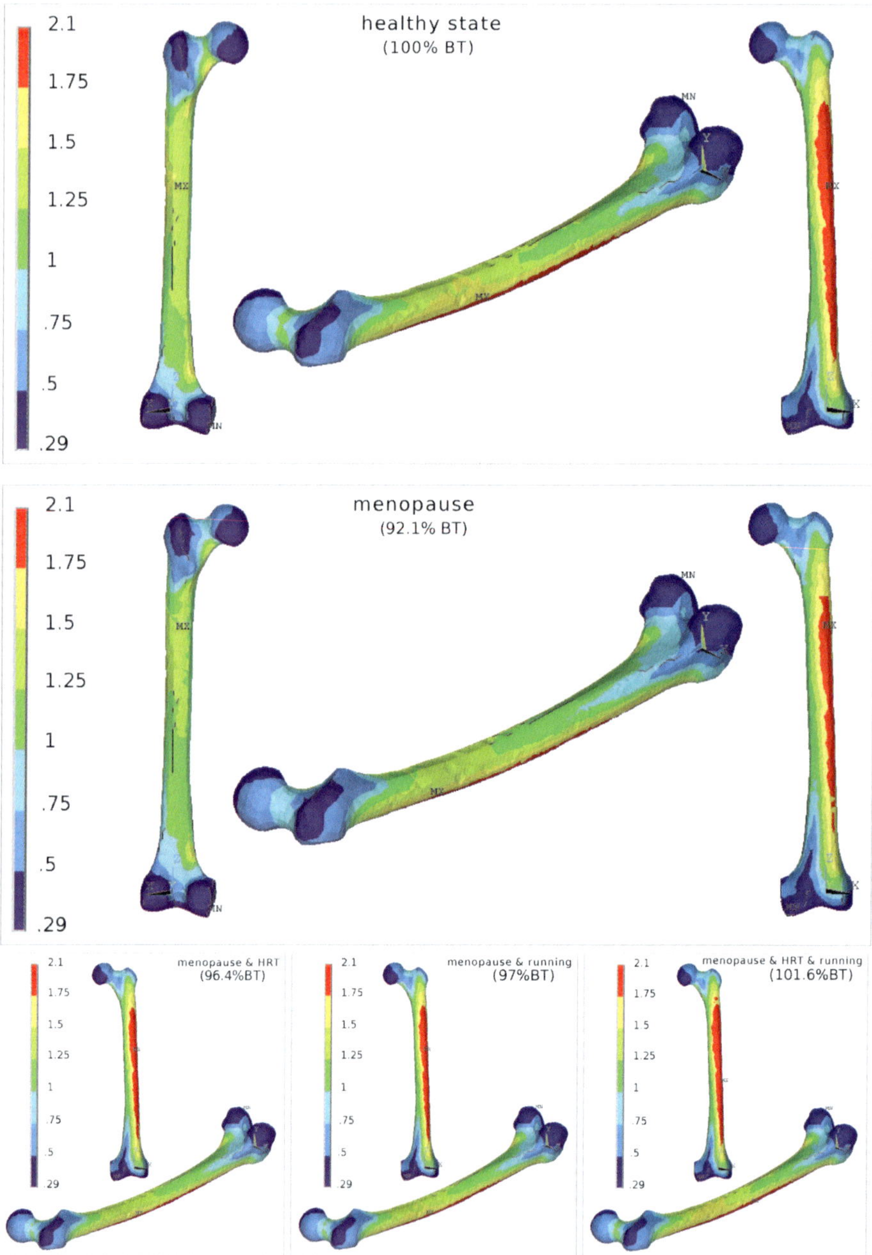

Fig. 6. Prediction of the menopause effect on bone quality (estradiol levels decreased to $2.5\frac{pg}{ml}$ and NO to half of its normal level), treatment proposal, and its simulation - hormonal treatment (HRT), running (30 minutes every other day). Notice the change of bone mass (BM) of the whole femur.

substances entering the reaction schemes, namely osteoclasts and osteoblasts. It surely cannot be used on the length scales of BMU where it is no longer guaranteed that any osteoclast is present. There are approximately 10^7 BMU in a human skeleton present at any moment (Klika and Maršík, 2010) and, because bones have a total volume of 1.75l, there is 1 BMU per 0.175 mm^3 on average at any moment. In other words, the presented model cannot be used for length scales smaller than $\sqrt[3]{0.175}$ mm^3 and we recommend that it is not used on length scales below $\sqrt[3]{0.5}$ $mm^3 \approx 0.8$ mm.

Ongoing applications of the model include simulations of the 3D geometries of the femur and vertebrae (FE models) under various conditions (both biochemical and mechanical). The preliminary results are encouraging and show the correct density distribution. Currently, we are working on bone modelling (change of shape of bone) model that would add the possibility to adapt bone to its mechanical environment as it is observed in vivo. Further, we would like to have a more detailed description of the inner structure of bone as an outcome of the model. Most probably, a homogenisation technique will be used for addressing this goal. Most importantly, a validation of the model's predictions (or finding limits of its application) should start in near future in cooperation with Ambulant Centre for Defects of Locomotor Aparatus in Prague.

5. Acknowledgment

This research has been supported by the Czech Science Foundation project no. 106/08/0557, by Research Plan No. AV0Z20760514 of the Institute of Thermomechanics AS CR, and by Research Plan MSM 6840770010 „Applied Mathematics in Technical and Physical Sciences" of the Ministry of Education, Youth and Sports of the Czech Republic.

6. References

Armour, K. E., van't Hof, R. J., Grabowski, et al. Evidence for a pathogenic role of nitric oxide in inflammation-induced osteoporosis.J Bone Miner Res,14(12): 2137-42, 1997.

Beaupre GS, Orr TE, and Carter DR. An approach for time-dependent bone modeling and remodeling-application: a preliminary remodeling simulation. J Orthopaed Res, 8:662–670, 1990.

Boyle WJ, Simonet WS, and Lacey DL. Osteoclast differentiation and activation. Nature, 423(3):337–342, 2003.

Carter DR. Mechanical loading history and skeletal biology. Journal of Biomechanics, 20:1095–1109, 1987.

Carter GD, Carter R, Jones J et al. How accurate are assays for 25-hydroxyvitamin D data from the international vitamin D external quality assessment scheme, Clin Chem 50 (11), 2195-2197, 2004

Cranney A., Horsley T., O'Donnell S. et al. Effectiveness and Safety of Vitamin D in Relation to Bone Health. Evidence Report/Technology Assessment No. 158 (Prepared by the University of Ottawa Evidence-based Practice Center (UOEPC) under Contract No. 290-02-0021. AHRQ Publication No. 07-E013. Rockville, MD: Agency for Healthcare Research and Quality.

deGroot R. S., Mazur P. Non-equilibrium Thermodynamics. North-Holland, Amsterdam, 1962.

Eghbali-Fatourechi, G. et al. Role of rank ligand in mediating increased bone resorption in early postmenopausal women, J Clin Invest 111: 1221-1230, 2003.

Ehrlich PJ and Lanyon LE. Mechanical strain and bone cell function: A review. Osteoporosis International, (13):688–700, 2002.

ELISA OPG kit, BIOMEDICA OSTEOPROTEGERIN ELISA (BI-20402) FAQ. [online] http://www.bmgrp.com/fileadmin/user_upload/immunoassays/BI-20402_OPG_FAQ_060717.pdf. 2006.

Fan, X., Roy, E., Zhu, L., et al, 2004. Nitric oxide regulates receptor activator of nuclear factor-kappab ligand and osteoprotegerin expression in bone marrow stromal cells. Endocrinology 145 (2), 751-759.

Frost HM. The Utah paradigm of skeletal physiology, volume second. ISMNI, Greece, first edition, 2004.

Frost HM. The utah paradigm of skeletal physiology: an overview of its insights for bone, cartilage and collagenous tissue organs. J Bone Miner Metab, (18):305–316, 2000.

Fukushima H., Jimi E., Kajiya H et al. Parathyroid-hormonerelated protein induces expression of receptor activator of nf-kappab ligand in human periodontal ligament cells via a camp/protein kinase a-independent pathway. J Dent Res 84,329-34, 2005.

Helgason B., Perilli E., Schileo E. et al. Mathematical relationships between bone density and mechanical properties:A literature review. Clin Biomech 23, 135-46, 2008.

Heller M. O., Bergmann G., Kassi J.-P. et al. Determination of muscle loading at the hip joint for use in pre-clinical testing. Journal of Biomechanics 38, 1155-1163. 2005

Heřt J, Přibylová E, and Lišková M. Reaction of bone to mechanical stimuli. part 3: Microstructure of compact bone of rabbit tibia after intermittent loading. Acta Anat, 82:218–230, 1972.

Hodgskinson R., Currey J. D. Young's modulus, density and material properties in cancellous bone over a large density range. J Mater Sci-Mater M 3 (5), 377-381, 1992.

Huiskes R, Weinans H, Grootenboer HJ et al. Adaptive bone-remodeling theory applied to prosthetic-design analysis. Journal of Biomechanics, 20(11):1135–1150, 1987.

Charopoulos I., Tournis S., Trovas G et al.. Effect of primary hyperparathyroidism on volumetric bone mineral density and bone geometry assessed by peripheral quantitative computed tomography in postmenopausal women. J Clin Endocrinol Metab 91 (5), 1748-1753, 2006.

Jorde R., Saleh F., Figenschau Y. et al. Serum parathyroid hormone (PTH) levels in smokers and non-smokers. the fifth Tromso study. Eur J Endocrinol 152, 39-45, 2005

Karst M., Gorny G., Galvin RJS et al. Roles of stromal cell rankl, opg, and m-csf expression in biphasic tgf-b regulation of osteoclast differentiation.J Cell Physiol 200,99-106, 2004.

Kawasaki K., Takahashi T., Yamaguchi M. Et al. Effects of aging on rankl and opg levels in gingival crevicular fluid during orthodontic tooth movement, Orthod Craniofac Res 9: 137-142, 2006.

Keener J and Sneyd J. Mathematical Physiology, I: Cellular Physiology. Springer Science+Business Media, LLC, New York, 2009. ISBN: 978-0-387-75846-6.

Khosla S., Melton LJ., Atkinson EJ et al, Relationship of serum sex steroid levels and bone turnover markers with bone mineral density in men and women: A key role for bioavailable estrogen. J Clin Endocrinol Metab 83 (7), 2266-2274, 1998.

Klika V and Maršík F. Coupling effect between mechanical loading and chemical reactions. Journal of Physical Chemistry B, 113:14689–14697, 2009.

Klika V. Comparison of the Effects of Possible Mechanical Stimuli on the Rate of Biochemical Reactions. Journal of Physical Chemistry B 114(32), 10567-10572, 2010

Klika V, Maršík F, and Mařík I. Dynamic Modelling, chapter Influencing the Effect of Treatment of Disease Related to Bone Remodelling by Dynamic Loading. INTECH, Vienna, February 2010. ISBN 978-953-7619-68-8, [online] http://sciyo.com

Klika V, Maršík F.. A Thermodynamic Model of Bone Remodelling: The Influence of Dynamic Loading Together with Biochemical Control. Journal of Musculoskeletal and Neuronal Interactions 10(3), 210-220, 2010.

Komarova SV, Smith RJ, Dixon SJ et al. Mathematical model predicts a critical role for osteoclast autocrine regulation in the control of bone remodeling. Bone, 33:206–15, 2003.

Kong Y.-Y. and Penninger J. M. Molecular control of bone remodeling and osteoporosis, Experimental Gerontology 35: 947—956, 2000.

Kudlacek S, Schneider B, Woloszczuk W et al. Serum levels of osteoprotegerin increase with age in a healthy adult population, Bone 32: 681-686, 2003.

Lee WCC, Maul TM, Vorp DA et al. Effects of uniaxial cyclic strain on adipose-derived stem cell morphology, proliferation, and differentiation. Biomechan Model Mechanobiol, 6:265–273, 2007.

Lemaire V, Tobin FL, Greller LD et al. Modeling the interactions between osteoblast and osteoclast activities in bone remodeling. J Theor Biol, (229):293–309, 2004.

Li YJ et al. Oscillatory fluid flow affects human marrow stromal cell proliferation and differentiation. Journal of Orthopaedic Research, 22:1283–1289, 2004.

Lindsay R. What have we learned from clinical studies? fractures and the interactions of bone mass and remodeling. Osteoporosis International, 14:S8–S11, 2003.

Lips P., Duong T., Oleksik A et al. A global study of vitamin D status and parathyroid function in postmenopausal women with osteoporosis: Baseline data from the multiple outcomes of raloxifene evaluation clinical trial. J Clin Endocrinol Metab 86 (3), 1212-21, 2001.

Maršík F, Klika V, and Chlup H. Remodelling of living bone induced by dynamic loading and drug delivery - numerical modelling and clinical treatment. Math Comput Simulat., 80:1278–1288, 2010.

Martin TJ. Paracrine regulation of osteoclast formation and activity: Milestones in discovery, Journal of Musculoskeletal and Neuronal Interactions 4(3): 243-253, 2004.

Moschen AR, Kaser A., Enrich B et al. The rankl/opg system is activated in inflammatory bowel disease and relates to the state of bone loss, Gut 54: 479-487, 2005.

Mundy GR, Boyce B, Hughes D et al. The effects of cytokines and growth factors on osteoblastic cells. Bone, 17(2):71S–75S, 1995.

Murakami T, Yamamoto M., Ono K.et al. Transforming growth factor-1 increases mrna levels of osteoclastogenesis inhibitory factor in osteoblastic/stromal cells and inhibits the survival of murine osteoclast-like cells. Biochem Bioph Res Co 252, 747-52, 1998.

Nicolis G and Prigogine I. Selforganization in nonequilibrium systems. Wiley, New York, 1977.

Potts JT. Parathyroid hormone: past and present. J Endocrinol 187, 311-325, 2005.

Quinn JMW, Itoh K., Udagawa N et al. Transforming growth factor beta affects osteoclast differentiation via direct and indirect actions.J Bone Miner Res 16(10): 1787-74,2001.

Rahnert J., Fan X., Case N. et al. The role of nitric oxide in the mechanical repression of rankl in bone stromal cells. Bone 43, 48-54, 2008.

RANKL product data sheet. Product data sheet alx-522-131: Fc (human):rankl, soluble (mouse) (rec.), enzo life sciences. 2008 [online] http://www.enzolifesciences.com/fileadmin/reports/Fc_humanRANKL_Soluble_mouse_rec_rep_Xcq55b.pdf

Rice J. C., Cowin S. C., Bowman J. A. On the dependence of the elasticity and strenght of cancellous bone on apparent density. Journal of Biomechanics 21 (2), 155-168. 1988.

Robling AG, Castillo AB, and Turner CH. Biomechanical and molecular regulation of bone remodeling. Annual Review of Biomedical Engineering, 8:455–498, 2006.

Rubin J, Murphy T, Nanes MS et al. Mechanical strain inhibits expression of osteoclast differentiation factor by murine stromal cells. Am J Physiol-Cell Ph, 278:C1126–32, 2000.

Rubin J, Murphy TC, Zhu L et al. Mechanical strain differentially regulates endothelial nitric-oxide synthase and receptor activator of nuclear kappa b ligand expression via erk1/2 mapk. Journal of Biological Chemistry, 278:34018–34025, 2004.

Rubin J, Rubin C, and Jacobs RC. Molecular pathways mediating mechanical signaling in bone. Gene, 367:1–16, 2006.

Ruimerman R, Hilbers PAJ, van Rietbergen B et al. A theoretical framework for strain-related trabecular bone maintenance and adaptation. J Biomech, (38):931–941, 2005.

Saquib N., von Muhlen D., Garland CF et al. Serum 25-hydroxyvitamin D, parathyroid hormone, and bone mineral density in men: the rancho bernardo study. Osteoporosis International 17, 1734-1741, 2006

Sikavitsas VI., Temenoff JS. and Mikos AG. Biomaterials and bone mechanotransduction, Biomaterials 22: 2581-2593, 2001

Tanaka S., Takahashi N., Udagawa N et al. Macrophage colony-stimulating factor is indispensable for both proliferation and differentiation of osteoclast progenitors. Journal of Clinical Investigation 91, 257-263, 1993

Turner CH, Anne V, and Pidaparti RMV. A uniform strain criterion for trabecular bone adaptation: Do continuum-level strain gradients drive adaptation? J Biomech, 30(6):555–63, 1997.

Valle F, Sandal M, and Samori B. The interplay between chemistry and mechanics in the transduction of a mechanical signal into a biochemical function. Physics of Life Reviews, 4:157–188, 2007.

van't Hof RJ., Ralston SH. Cytokine-induced nitric oxide inhibits bone resorption by inducing apoptosis of osteoclast progenitors and supressing osteoclast activity. Journal of Bone and Mineral Research 12 (11), 1797-1804, 1997.

van't Hof RJ., Ralston SH. Nitric oxide and bone. Immunology 103, 255-261, 2001.

Wimalawansa SJ., Chapa MT., Yallampalli C et al. Prevention of corticosteroid-induced bone loss with nitric oxide donor nitroglycerin in male rats. Bone 21 (3), 275-280, 1997

Wimalawansa SJ. Nitroglycerin therapy is as efficacious as standard estrogen replacement therapy (premarin) in prevention of oophorectomy-induced bone loss: A human pilot clinical study. Journal of Bone and Mineral Research 15 (11), 2240-2244, 2000.

Wimalawansa SJ. Rationale for using nitric oxide donor therapy for prevention of bone loss and treatment of osteoporosis in humans. Ann NY Acad Sci 1117, 283-297, 2007.

Zhang, N. et al. Relationship between age-related serum concentrations of tgf-β1 and tgf- β 2 and those of osteoprotegerin and leptin in native chinese women. Clinical Chimica Acta. Doi:10.1016/j.cca.2009.01.021, 2009.

Part 3

Locomotion and Joint Biomechanics

11

Physical Insights Into Dynamic Similarity in Animal Locomotion. I. Theoretical Principles and Concepts

Valery B. Kokshenev
Departamento de Física, Universidade Federal de Minas Gerais, Belo Horizonte Brazil

1. Introduction

Comparative zoologists, evolutionary biologists, experimental biologists, and mechanical engineers make wonderful generalizations about the movements of different-sized running bipeds and quadrupeds (Heglund et al., 1974; McMahon, 1975; Alexander, 1976; Hoyt & Taylor, 1981; Garland, 1982; McMahon et al., 1987; Rome et al., 1988; Gatesy & Biewener, 1991; Farley et al.,1993; Cynthia & Farley, 1998; Bullimore & Burn, 2006), flying birds and swimming fish (Hill, 1950; Alexander, 2003; Taylor et al., 2003). The dynamic similarity across body mass and taxa of animals maintaining a certain gait in locomotion has been thoroughly investigated (Alexander, 1976, 1985, 1989, 2005; Alexander & Bennet-Clark, 1976; Alexander & Jayes, 1983; Marden & Allen, 2002; Biewener, 2005; Bejan & Marden, 2006a, b; Bullimore & Donelan, 2008). Based on integrative approach to animal locomotion (e.g., review by Dickinson et al., 2000) and using simple physical ideas (e.g., reviews by Lin, 1982 and Alexander, 2003), many cited above researches have demonstrated the importance of scaling biomechanics via reliably established scaling relations for gait characteristics with changes of speed and body mass. Among well known empirical findings of the dynamic similarity in animals observed across body mass are scaling relations established for stride (or stroke) speed and/or frequency (Hill, 1950; Heglund et al., 1974 Greenewalt, 1975; Garland, 1982; Heglund & Taylor, 1988; Gatesy & Biewener, 1991; Farley et al., 1993; Bullen & McKenzie, 2002; Bejan & Marden, 2006a), duty factor and relative stride length (Alexander & Jayes, 1983; Gatesy & Biewener, 1991), body force output (Alexander, 1985; Marden & Allen, 2002; Bejan & Marden, 2006a), limb stress and stiffness (Rubin & Lanyon, 1984; McMahon & Cheng, 1990; Farley & Gonzalez, 1996; Biewener, 2005; Bullimore & Burn, 2006).

Although the concept of *mechanical similarity*, well known in analytical mechanics (e.g., Duncan, 1953; Landau & Lifshitz, 1976), was accurately re-formulated in application to the *dynamic similarity* (Alexander, 1976, 1989, 2003, 2005; Bullimore & Donelan, 2008), its exploration in biomechanics is often controversial. For example, Hill's seminal observation of dynamic similarity through the optimal speeds of birds in flight gaits (Hill, 1950) was found in sharp disagreement (McMahon, 1975) with that revealed through transient (trot-to-gallop) speeds in quadrupeds (Heglund et al., 1974). Then, comparing anatomic consequences of McMahon's elastic similarity (McMahon, 1975) for the stride length, Alexander noted the conceptual inconsistency between the elastic and dynamic similarities (Alexander, 1989, p.1212). Biewener (2005) also claimed confusing biomechanical consequences of McMahon's scaling relations. More recent example is the observation of a new kind of similarity in running humans, simulated on the basis of spring-mass model, no matching the dynamic similarity in running animals (Delattre et al., 2009), reliably established by the same biomechanical model (Farley et al., 1993).

Another example of conceptual controversy concerns the long term standing problem of the origin of empirical scaling laws in biomechanics. The constructal theory by Bejan & Marden (2006a), unifying running, flying, and swimming animals suggested fundamental explanations of intriguing statistically established universal scaling relations for the optimal speed and stride frequency. As a matter of fact, the authors have clearly demonstrated that their principle of minimum useful energy does not provide unifying scaling laws. Instead of searching for new principles, exemplified by recently rediscovered "least-action principle" in human walking (Fan et al., 2009), the design principle of flow systems (Bejan & Marden, 2006a, b), and the basic theorem of dimensional analysis (Bullimore & Donelan, 2008), seemingly resolving the origin of scaling laws in biomechanics, I have addressed the fundamentals of classical analytical mechanics.

In theoretical physics, the mechanical similarity arises from the key principle of minimum mechanical action closely related to Lagrangian's formalism. Examples of successful applications of Lagrangian's method to the dynamics of human walk and the dynamic similarity in animals are explicit descriptions providing, respectively, (i) the conditions of dynamic instability during a walk-to-run crossover obtained regardless of inverted-pendulum modeling (Kokshenev, 2004) and (ii) the whole spectrum of observable scaling laws inferred without recourse to equations of motion (Kokshenev, 2010).

In biomechanics, the dynamic similarity hypothesis (Alexander, 1976; Alexander & Jayes, 1983; Alexander, 1989) stands that similarly in running terrestrial animals should equal their *Froude numbers* (the squared speeds divided by hip heights times the gravitation constant) when tend to change locomotion modes at certain "equivalent speeds" (Heglund et al., 1974) or maintain a certain gait at "preferred speeds" (Heglund & Taylor, 1988). In contrast to *in vivo* established dynamic similarity in the horses trotting at equal Froude numbers (Bullimore & Burn, 2006), the spring-mass model analysis has indicated that the Froude number alone does not yet guarantee the observation of dynamic similarity in the running animals (Donelan & Kram, 1997; Bullimore & Donelan, 2008). Such kind of controversial findings begged a number of questions: whether the sole Froude number (Alexander & Jayes, 1983; Vaughan & O'Malleyb, 2005; Bullimore & Burn, 2006; Delattre et al., 2009), or the sole *Strouhal number* (the limb length, or wing length divided by the speed times stride period, or stroke period) as hypothesized by Whitfield (2003), Taylor et al. (2003) and, likely, Bejan & Marden (2006a), or both the numbers (Delattre et al., 2009), when taken in a certain algebraic combinations (Delattre & Moretto, 2008), e.g., presented by the Groucho number (Alexander, 1989), may warrant the dynamic similarity in animal locomotion? Moreover, when other dimensionless parameters are chosen as the determinants of dynamic similarity, what is the minimal set of independent physical quantities underlying the principle of similarity (Bullimore & Donelan, 2008)?

In this research, a model-independent theoretical framework basically employing Lagrangian's method suggests to establish the validation domains, conditions of observation, criterion, and the minimal set of determinants of dynamic similarity empirically established in different-sized animals.

2. Theory

2.1 Similarity in analytical mechanics

According to the key variational principle of Hamiltonian's classical mechanics, the requirement of minimum mechanical action between two fixed points of the conceivable trajectory of an arbitrary mechanical system determines the Lagrangian function $L(q,v)$ through time-dependent coordinates $q(t)$ and instant velocities $v(t) = dq/dt$. One of the most pronounced properties of the *closed* mechanical systems is preservation of the total energy and momentum, arising respectively from the temporal and spatial homogeneities of the Lagrangian function. The *mechanical similarity* between frictionlessly moving systems also arises from the property of spatiotemporal homogeneity (e.g., Duncan, 1953; Landau & Lifshitz, 1976). Since the property of homogeneity guarantees that the multiplication of Lagrangian on an arbitrary constant does not affect the resulting equations of motion, the *scaling laws* of mechanical similarity can be established without consideration of equations of motion.

More specifically, let us consider the uniform transformation of mechanical trajectories due to linear changing of all coordinates $q' = aq$ and times $t' = bt$ performed via arbitrary in amplitude (positive) linear-transformation factors a and b, resulting in changed velocities $v' = (a/b)v$. The overall-system basic mechanical characteristics, *period* T and *speed* V change as $T' = bT$ and $V' = (a/b)V$, whereas the kinetic energy $\mathcal{K}$, as a quadratic function of velocities, and potential energy $\mathcal{U}$ scale as

$$\mathcal{K}'(v) = \mathcal{K}\left(\frac{a}{b}v\right) = \left(\frac{a}{b}\right)^2 \mathcal{K}(v) \text{ and } \mathcal{U}'(v) = \mathcal{U}(aq) = a^{\lambda}\mathcal{U}(q), \tag{1}$$

where the *dynamic exponent* λ is introduced to distinguish distinct cases of mechanical similarity.

The self-consistency of exploration of the property of homogeneity, determining the property of similarity, requires the proportionality in changes of both the energies of the Lagrangian $\mathcal{L}'(q,v) = \mathcal{K}'(v) - \mathcal{U}'(q)$, *i.e.*, $\mathcal{K}' \backsim \mathcal{U}'$, thus, $(a/b)^2 = a^{\lambda}$, or $b = a^{1-\lambda/2}$, as follows from Eq. (1). Hence, the frictionless propagation of a classical system obeys the *scaling rules* imposed on the overall-system dynamic characteristics (T and V) and mechanical characteristics (*force amplitude* F and $\mathcal{U}$), namely

$$T_{\lambda} \propto L^{1-\lambda/2}, V_{\lambda} \propto L^{\lambda/2}, F_{\lambda} \propto L^{\lambda-1}, \text{and } \mathcal{U}_{\lambda} \propto L^{\lambda}, \tag{2}$$

where L is a characteristic linear size of the *trajectory* , as suggested by Landau & Lifshitz (1976, Eqs. (10.2) and (10.3)).

The well known examples of distinct mechanically similar systems distinguished by dynamic exponent readily follow from Eq. (2): (i) $\lambda = -1$; the case resulting in the third law for planets $T^2 \propto L^3$ that anticipated Newton's theory through interplanetary coupling force $F \propto M^2L^{-2}$; (ii) $\lambda = 2$; the system is driven by the elastic-strain field and has the elastic energy $\mathcal{U}_{elast} = K\Delta L^2$ with $\Delta L \backsim L$, and (iii) $\lambda = 1$; the system moves in the uniform *gravitational field* $g = F_g/M$ and has the potential energy $\mathcal{U}_g = MgH$, with $H \backsim L$. The dimensional factors of proportionality M and K, required by the scaling relations, are analyzed below by dimensional method.[1]

[1] Hereafter I distinguish two symbols of proportionality: $\backsim$ and $\propto$, supporting and not supporting dimensional units that should be read as "is proportional to" and "scales as", respectively.

2.2 Similarity in biomechanics

The exploration of the concept of dynamic similarity generally assumes model-independent relations validated for slow and fast gaits and supporting linear transformations in changing dynamic and mechanical characteristics, namely

$$\Delta L \backsim L \backsim H \backsim L_b \text{ and } \Delta T \backsim T, \Delta F = K\Delta L_b. \quad (3)$$

Here ΔL is a change of the amplitude of *dynamic length* L, e.g., stride length L, or the maximum vertical displacement H of body's center of mass that may be chosen for periodic terrestrial locomotion, or the stroke amplitude of flying and swimming animals (e.g., Alexander, 2003). The dynamic length and its change should be distinguished from the *static length* L_b and its change ΔL_b, that may be also chosen either as of the body length L_b or the corresponding limb, wing, or tail length. Respectively, T^{-1} is the stride, wingbeat, or tailbeat rate attributed to the *frequency* of locomotion. The dynamic length is commonly determined by the measured speed V (*mean* cycle forward velocity) and frequency, i.e., as $L = V/T^{-1}$, whereas the body *propulsion force* ΔF introduces the *body stiffness* $K = \Delta F/\Delta L_b$.[2]

2.2.1 Dimensional analysis

Broadly speaking, the mechanical similarity may be tested by two uniform linear transformations, scaling simultaneously all spatial and temporal characteristics. Extending these two degrees of freedom of *biomechanical mechanical systems* by their *body masses* M, let us introduce the corresponding *ltm class of units* through the independent dimensions $[L] = l$, $[T] = t$, and $[M] = m$, in accord with the standard scaling theory (e.g., Barenblatt, 2002). One can show that the three body-system mechanical quantities

$$\Delta F \backsim LT^{-2}M, V \backsim LT^{-1}, \text{and } K \backsim T^{-2}M \quad (4)$$

are mutually independent. Indeed, following the method of dimensional analysis (e.g., Barenblatt, 2002), let us assume the converse, i.e., that numbers x and y exist such that $F \backsim V^x K^y$. Substituting F, V, and K from Eq. (4) and equating exponents in the ltm class, one finds the solutions $x = 1$ and $y = 1$ not matching with $2x + y = 2$. This proves that the considered set $(\Delta F, V, K)$ consists of three physically independent quantities.

The application of the mathematical concept of geometric similarity (Hill, 1950, Rashevsky, 1948; McMahon, 1975; Lin, 1982) introduced between cylindric-shape bodies through the constraint $\rho_b A L_b = M$ (A is body's *cross-sectional area*), where ρ_b is the invariable *body density* (McMahon, 1975, 1984; Alexander, 2003; Bejan & Marden, 2006a, b), allows one to suggested another equivalent set of candidates to the mutually independent *determinants of mechanical similarity*, namely

$$T^{-1} \backsim \sqrt{\frac{\Delta F}{A}} L_b^{-1}, V \backsim \sqrt{\frac{\Delta F}{A}}, \text{and } \Delta F \backsim KL_b, \quad (5)$$

chosen in the ltf class of unites and also depending neither on locomotor gaits nor biomechanical models.

2.2.2 Unifying contsructal theory revisited

For the case of a running (or flying) animal of mass M with the *constant horizontal speed* $V = L/t$, the constructal law calls for the minimization of the total destruction of work W per stride

[2] These last two and other similar model-independent equations play the role of the definitive basic equations in the scaling theory.

(and stroke) length L, represented as

$$\frac{W}{L} = \frac{W_1}{L} + \frac{W_2}{L} = \frac{MgH}{Vt} + C_D \rho_a V^2 L_b^2. \quad (6)$$

Here W_1 is the vertical loss of energy associated with fall from the height H in the gravitational field and W_2 is the horizontal loss of energy related to the friction with air of density ρ_a (for further details see Eqs. (1)-(4) in Bejan & Marden, 2006a). The minimization procedure of the total loss function results in the optimal speed $V_{opt} \backsim \sqrt[3]{MH/L_b^2 t}$, clearly leaving uncertain a choice of the dynamic variables t and H. Using the linear relation $H \backsim L_b$ discussed in Eq. (3) and postulating for the frictionless vertical motion that

$$t = t_{opt} = \sqrt{\frac{2H}{g}} \backsim \sqrt{\frac{L_b}{g}} \propto M^{1/6}, \quad (7)$$

the constructal theory suggests relations

$$V_{opt} \approx \left(\frac{\rho_b}{\rho_a}\right)^{1/3} g^{1/2} \rho_b^{-1/6} M^{1/6} \text{ and } T_{opt}^{-1} \approx \left(\frac{\rho_b}{\rho_a}\right)^{1/3} g^{1/2} \rho_b^{1/6} M^{-1/6} \quad (8)$$

for the optimal speed and frequency, in the case of fast running and flying animals, as shown, respectively, in Eqs. (5) and (22) and Eq. (23) in Bejan & Marden (2006a). Likewise, the frictionless vertical motion has been postulated in the case of optimal swimming, for which the energy loss $W_1 \backsim MgL_b$ was adopted in Eq. (6). For further details, see Eq. (26) in Bejan & Marden (2006a).

2.2.3 Minimum muscular action

Aiming to apply the principle of mechanical similarity formulated for closed inanimate systems to musculoskeletal systems of different-sized animals, one should consider conditions of the observation of effectively frictionless propagation of almost-closed (weekly open) animate systems. These are all cases of *efficient locomotion* (maximum useful work at minimum power consumption) realized at the *resonant propagation frequency*.

Since the animal locomotion is substantially muscular (e.g., McMahon, 1984; Rome et al., 1988; Dickinson et al., 2000; Alexander, 2003), the body-system relations shown in Eqs. (4) and (5) can be generalized to the muscle subsystem presented by a synergic group of locomotory muscles of the *effective muscle length* L_m and cross-sectional area A_m. In the approximation of fully activated muscle states, the maximum muscle stiffness $K_m = E_m A_m / L_m$ is controlled by the geometry-independent muscle rigidity, i.e., the elastic modulus amplitude E_m, defined by ratio of the peak muscle stress $\sigma_m = \Delta F_m / A_m$ to the peak muscle strain $\varepsilon_m = \Delta L_m / L_m$ (e.g., McMahon, 1975, 1984). Let us treat the mass specific muscular (or relative) force output defined by $\mu_m \equiv \Delta F_m / M_m$ as the *muscular field* generating active force ΔF_m through the *muscle mass* M_m, which being a source of the force field μ_m plays the role of the motor mass (Marden & Allen, 2002).

Dynamic motion parameters of the trajectory of body's center of mass are linked to the characteristic static body's and muscle's lengths via the common in biomechanics *linear* relations, namely

$$\frac{\Delta L}{L} \backsim \frac{\Delta L_b}{L_b} = \varepsilon_b \backsim \frac{\Delta L_m}{L_m} = \varepsilon_m, \frac{\Delta T}{T} = \frac{\Delta T_m}{T_m} = \beta, \text{ and } \Delta F \backsim \Delta F_m. \quad (9)$$

Dynamic regime $\lambda = 0$	Frequency	Length	Speed	Force	Mass
$T_{res}^{-1}, T_m^{-1} = T^{-1} \sim (K/M)^{1/2}$	T^{-1}	$\rho_b^{-\frac{1}{2}} E_0^{\frac{1}{2}} \cdot L_b^{-1}$	$\rho_b^{-\frac{1}{4}} E_0^{\frac{1}{4}} \cdot V^{-\frac{1}{2}}$	F^0	$\rho_b^{-\frac{1}{6}} E_0^{\frac{1}{2}} \cdot M^{-\frac{1}{3}}$
$L_{dyn}^{(\max)} \sim L_b, L = VT$	$\rho_b^{-\frac{1}{2}} E_0^{\frac{1}{2}} \cdot T^1$	L^1	$\rho_b^{-\frac{1}{4}} E_{m0}^{\frac{1}{4}} \cdot V^{\frac{1}{2}}$	F^0	$\rho_b^{-\frac{1}{3}} \cdot M^{\frac{1}{3}}$
$V_{b\text{-}slow}^{(\max)} = \rho_b^{-\frac{1}{2}} E_0^{\frac{1}{2}}, V_{m\text{-}slow}$	T^0	L^0	$\rho_b^{-\frac{1}{2}} E_0^{\frac{1}{2}}$	F^0	M^0
$K_{b\text{-}slow}^{(\max)} \sim K_{m\text{-}slow}^{(\max)}$	$\rho_b^{\frac{1}{2}} E_0^{\frac{1}{2}} A \cdot T^{-1}$	$E_0 A \cdot L_b^{-1}$	$\rho_b^{\frac{1}{4}} E_0^{-\frac{1}{4}} \cdot V^{-\frac{1}{2}}$	$L^{-1} \cdot F$	$\rho_b^{-\frac{1}{3}} E_0 \cdot M^{\frac{1}{3}}$
$\sigma_{m\text{-}slow}^{(\max)} = \varepsilon_m E_{m0}^{(\max)}$	T^0	L_m^0	V_m^0	F_m^0	M_m^0
$F_{b\text{-}slow}^{(\max)} \sim \varepsilon_b A E_{b\text{-}slow}^{(\max)}$	T^0	L^0	V^0	F^0	$\rho_b^{-\frac{2}{3}} \varepsilon_b E_0 \cdot M^{\frac{2}{3}}$
$St_{slow} = T^{-1} L_b / V = L_b L^{-1}$	T^0	$L_b \cdot L^{-1}$	V^0	F^0	M^0
$Fr_{slow} = V^2 / g L_b$	$g^{-1} \rho_b^{-\frac{1}{2}} E_0^{\frac{1}{2}} \cdot T^{-1}$	$g^{-1} \rho_b^{-1} E_0 \cdot L_b^{-1}$	$g^{-1} \rho_b^{-\frac{3}{4}} E_0^{\frac{3}{4}} \cdot V^{-\frac{1}{2}}$	F^0	$g^{-1} \rho_b^{-\frac{2}{3}} E_0 \cdot M^{-1/3}$

Table 1. The scaling rules of dynamic similarity in different-sized animals moving in the *stationary dynamic regime*, associated with the activation of *slow locomotor muscles*. The calculations are made on the basis of Eqs. (11) and (12) for muscular subsystem taken at $\lambda = 0$ and then extended to the body system via Eq. (5). The abbreviations $E_{m0} = E_{m\text{-}slow}^{(\max)}$ and $E_0 = E_{b\text{-}slow}^{(\max)}$ for, respectively, muscle subsystem and body system are adopted.

Here ΔT is the limb ground contact time or the timing ΔT_m of an activated effective locomotory muscle during maximal shortening (or lengthening) resulted in the *duty factor* β. Considering effective muscles and bones (e.g., Kokshenev, 2007) of the musculoskeletal system as whole, one may ignore the relatively small effects in scaling of muscle and bone masses to body mass and thus introduce in Eqs. (3) and (9) the simplified (isometric) approximation by scaling relations

$$L \backsim L_b \backsim L_m \propto M^{1/3} \backsim M_m^{1/3}. \tag{10}$$

When the principle of mechanical similarity is applied to the different-sized *elastic* body musculoskeletal systems, including muscles, tendons, and bones, and moving at resonance in a certain regime λ along geometrically similar body's center of mass trajectories, the following three scaling relations, namely

$$T_{m\lambda}^{-1} = T_\lambda^{-1} \propto \sqrt{E_{m\lambda}} L_m^{-1}, V_{m\lambda} \backsim V_\lambda \propto \sqrt{E_{m\lambda}}, \text{and } \Delta F_{m\lambda} \propto M_m E_{m\lambda} L_m^{-1}, \tag{11}$$

are suggested as the three possible determinants of dynamic similarity discussed in Eq. (5). One can see that the self-consistency between the body system, including locomotor muscle subsystem, activated in the same dynamic regime λ, and the principle of mechanical similarity formulated in Eq. (2), requires the dynamic elastic modulus of locomotory muscles in Eq. (11) to be adjusted with the muscle length L_m and body length L_b through the scaling relations

$$E_{m\lambda} \propto (L_m)^\lambda \propto (L_b)^\lambda \text{ and } \mu_{m\lambda} \propto (L_m)^{\lambda-1} \backsim \mu_\lambda \propto (L_b)^{\lambda-1}. \tag{12}$$

Thereby, the dynamic process of generation of the active force $\Delta F_{m\lambda} = \mu_{m\lambda} M_m$ during muscle contractions at the resonant frequency $T_{m\lambda}^{-1}$ and the optimized contraction velocity $V_{m\lambda}$ is patterned by the single dynamic exponent λ. In Tables 1 and 2, the scaling rules prescribed by the minimum muscular action in efficiently moving animals are provided for two well distinguished patterns of the dynamic similarity regimes $\lambda = 0$ and $\lambda = 1$.

Dynamic regime $\lambda = 1$	Frequency	Length	Speed	Force	Mass
$T_{opt}^{-1}, T_{res}^{-1}, T^{-1} \sim (K/M)^{1/2}$	T^{-1}	$\mu_1^{\frac{1}{2}} \cdot L_b^{-\frac{1}{2}}$	$\mu_1 \cdot V^{-1}$	$(\rho_b \mu_1^2 A)^{\frac{1}{2}} \cdot F^{-\frac{1}{2}}$	$\rho_b^{\frac{1}{6}} \mu_1^{\frac{1}{2}} \cdot M^{-\frac{1}{6}}$
$L_{opt}^{(\max)}, L_{trans}^{(\max)}, L$	$\mu_1 \cdot T^2$	L	$\mu_1^{-1} \cdot V^2$	$(\rho_b \mu_1 A)^{-1} \cdot F$	$\rho_b^{-\frac{1}{3}} \cdot M^{\frac{1}{3}}$
$V_{opt}^{(\max)}, V_{trans}^{(\max)}, V = LT^{-1}$	$\mu_1 \cdot T^1$	$\mu_1^{\frac{1}{2}} \cdot L^{\frac{1}{2}}$	V^1	$(\rho_b A)^{-\frac{1}{2}} \cdot F^{\frac{1}{2}}$	$\rho_b^{-\frac{1}{6}} \mu_1^{\frac{1}{2}} \cdot M^{\frac{1}{6}}$
$K_{b\text{-}fast}^{(\max)} \sim \rho_b \mu_{fast}^{(\max)} A$	T^0	L^0	V^0	F^0	$\rho_b^{-\frac{1}{3}} \mu_1 \cdot M^{\frac{2}{3}}$
$\sigma_{m\text{-}fast}^{(\max)} = \Delta F_m / A_m$	$\rho_m \mu_{m1} \cdot T^2$	$\rho_m \mu_{m1} \cdot L_m$	$\rho_m \cdot V_m^2$	$A_m^{-1} \cdot F_m$	$\rho_m^{\frac{2}{3}} \mu_{m1} \cdot M_m^{\frac{1}{3}}$
$F_{fast}^{(\max)} / gM \sim \mu_1 / g$	T^0	L^0	V^0	F^0	M^0
$St_{fast} = T^{-1} / VL_b^{-1} = L_b L^{-1}$	T^0	$L_b \cdot L^{-1}$	V^0	F^0	M^0
$Fr_{fast} = V^2 / gL_b \sim \mu_1 / g$	T^0	$L_b^{-1} \cdot L$	V^0	F^0	M^0

Table 2. The scaling rules of dynamic similarity between animals moving with gradually changing speeds within the dynamically similar fast gaits. The corresponding dynamic regime $\lambda = 1$ include optimal-speed stationary states and continuous transient dynamic states, all associated with activation of the fast locomotory muscles. The calculations are provided through Eqs. (11), (12), (5), and some other definitive basic equations discussed in the text, all taken at $\lambda = 1$. The abbreviations $\mu_{m1} = \mu_{m\text{-}fast}^{(\max)}$ and $\mu_1 = \mu_{b\text{-}fast}^{(\max)}$ for, respectively, muscle subsystem and body system are adopted.

3. Results and discussion

3.1 Minimum useful energy

Bejan & Marden (2006a, b) employed the principle of generation of the turbulent flow structure to unify gait patterns of running, swimming, and flying. Specifically, the dynamic similarity between animals across taxa is suggested as an optimal balance achieved between the vertical loss of useful energy (lifting the bodyweight, which later drops) and the horizontal loss caused by friction against the surrounding medium. Broadly speaking, the minimization procedure of total energy losses, being consistent with the concept of minimum cost of locomotion (e.g., Alexander, 2005), is underlaid by the minimization of energy consumption, treated here in terms of the efficient locomotion required by resonance conditions. Consequently, it is not surprising that the contsructal theory has demonstrated its general consistency with scaling rules attributed to the special case of dynamic similarity (Table 2). On the other hand, the optimization approach exemplified in Eq. (6), clearly demonstrating that the empirical scaling relations for speed and frequency should be hold in optimal running, flying and swimming, suggests that solely the gravitational field may explain scaling factors in scaling rules shown in Eq. (8). Therefore, a delicate question on the origin of basic scaling rules in the dynamic similarity remains unanswered in contsructal theory.

However, the major disadvantage of the proposed principle is that the proper scaling relations for optimal speed V_{opt} and frequency T_{opt}^{-1} were in fact incorporated into contsructal theory regardless of the minimization procedure. Indeed, the desired relations

$$V_{opt}^{(\max)} \propto T_{opt} \propto \sqrt{L} \backsim \sqrt{L_b} \propto M^{1/6}, \tag{13}$$

underlying the theoretical findings in Eq. (8) could straightforwardly be derived from the postulate adopted in Eq. (7), without recourse to the principle of minimum useful energy.

Strictly, the postulated basic equation $t_{opt} = \sqrt{2H/g}$ discussed in Eq. (7) has been borrowed from frictionless Newtonian's mechanics, arising from the spatiotemporal homogeneity of the gravitational field. Indeed, one can see that Eqs. (7) and (13) is the special case discussed in Eq. (2) at $\lambda = 1$. The proposed theory of dynamic similarity explains that instead of the gravitational field, in fact adopted on *ad hoc* basis in Eq. (7), the muscular field determines spatiotemporal homogeneity through the universal scaling exponents established for dynamic characteristics of animals naturally tuned to the dynamic similarity regime $\lambda = 1$ (Table 2). Without doubts, the gravity is important in terrestrial locomotion and the Froude number related to potential gravitational energy ($Fr = MV_{opt}^{(\max)2}/MgL_b$) plays important role in understanding of dynamic similarity in animate and inanimate systems (e.g.,Vaughan & O'Malleyb, 2005). After Alexander & Jayes (1983), it is widely adopted that instead of scaling relations shown in Eq. (13) the dynamic similarity between fast moving animals may be determined by the requirement for Froude numbers to be constants. Indeed, the universality of Froude numbers, i.e., $Fr \propto M^0$, straightforwardly provides the basic scaling rule for optimal speed, namely

$$V_{opt}^{(\max)} = (Fr \cdot gL_b)^{1/2} \propto L_b^{1/2} \propto M^{1/6}. \tag{14}$$

With regard to the second basic scaling rule shown in Eq. (13), it follows from the definitive basic equation for dynamic length $L = VT$ and Eq. (14) providing

$$T_{opt}^{-1} = V_{opt}^{(\max)} L_{opt}^{-1} \backsim (Fr \cdot gL_b^{-1})^{1/2} \propto M^{-1/6}, \text{ with } L_{opt}/L_b \propto M^0. \tag{15}$$

It is noteworthy that the optimal frequency is obtained under an additional requirement of the relative dynamic length to be invariable with body mass, as shown in Eq. (15).

3.2 Maximum muscular efficiency

3.2.1 Realization of resonant states

During animal locomotion, *chemical energy* released by muscles in the form of muscular force field and *potential energy* of the gravitational field, both being able to be stored in body's system in the corresponding forms of active-force and reactive-force *elastic energy*, are eventually transformed into useful external body work and partially lost as a heat due to internal work and external frictional effects. In a constant-speed walk, run, flight, and swim, attributed to the dynamic similarity regime $\lambda = 0$, the total mechanical energy is almost unchanged and the animate mechanical system is almost closed. In the non-stationary dynamic similarity regime $\lambda = 1$ characteristic of the gradual change in speeds caused by the steady muscular field, the total mechanical energy may be also unchanged because of the permanent consumption of metabolic energy. The efficient propulsion of humans and other animals, in contrast to human-made engines, is accompanied by the tuning of musculoskeletal system to natural (resonant) propagation frequency (McMahon, 1975; Ahlborn & Blake, 2002), resulted in the reduction to minimum the oxygen (Hoyt & Taylor, 1981) and metabolic energy (e.g., Ahlborn & Blake, 2002; Ahlborn et al., 2006) consumption. It has been demonstrated above, that the requirement of minimum action of musculoskeletal system in animals provides the major constraint in realization of dynamically equivalent (similar) states. Nevertheless, the applicability of the key principle in analytical mechanics, driving frictionless systems, to real animate systems characteristic of non-conservative muscle forces required a special physical analysis. In the special case of the stationary ($\lambda = 0$) human walking (Kokshenev, 2004), the speed-dependent frictional effects were shown to be weak and therefore effectively excluded within the scope of a special dynamic perturbation theory. Likewise, the case of efficient locomotion $\lambda = 1$, including *moderate run* and *fast run* modes in the fast gaits of animals, has

required a generalization of Lagrangian's formalism from the closed mechanical systems to the weakly open, moving at resonance biomechanical systems (Kokshenev, 2010).
As the outcome of analytical study, the *slow-walk* and *fast-walk* modes in bipeds emerge as the free-like body's center of mass propagation composed by the forward translation and the elliptic-cyclic backward rotations (Kokshenev, 2004). The optimal-speed stationary regime ($\lambda = 0$) has been found to be consistent with a slow-walk-to-fast-walk *continuous mode transition* between the two walk modes indicated by the highest symmetry (circular) trajectory of body's center of mass (Kokshenev, 2004, Fig. 2). In contrast, the discontinues in humans *fast-walk-to-slow-run* transition is indicated by the absolute instability of the walk-gait trajectory (Kokshenev, 2004, Fig. 2), signaling on the muscular field amplitude exceeding gravitation, i.e., $\mu_{run} > g$. The formal condition $\mu^{(mod)}_{walk\text{-}run} = g$, completed by that for the limb duty factor $\beta^{(mod)}_{walk\text{-}run} = 0.5$, discussed by Ahlborn & Blake (2002) on the basis of the data for humans started run (Alexander & Bennet-Clark, 1976), may be treated as two *indicators* of the model-independent walk-to-run continuous transition, generally uncommon to terrestrial animals. Hence, the provided above estimates for the transient muscle field amplitude suggest the walk-to-run transition as a smoothed crossover between the slow-regime and the fast-regime dynamic resonant states.
The natural ability of muscles to be tuned to various dynamic regimes is incorporated in animate mechanical systems through the elastic active-force muscle modulus $E^{(max)}_{m\lambda}$, as shown in Eqs. (11) and (12). Thereby, the muscle modulus, most likely sensitive to the intrinsic dynamic muscle length (Kokshenev, 2009), establishes an additional dynamic degree of freedom, not existing in skeletal bone subsystem and other inanimate elastic mechanical systems. Conventionally, the stationary slow-speed dynamics ($\lambda = 0$) and optimal and transient fast-speed dynamics ($\lambda = 1$) are attributed to the activation of the slow-twitch-fiber muscles and fast-twitch-fiber muscles respectively recruited by animals during slow and fast locomotion (Rome et al., 1980). As illustrative example in animal swimming, the studies of gait patterns in fish (Videler & Weihs, 1982) revealed that slowly swimming and quickly swimming fish exploit, respectively, red (slow fibre) muscles or white (fast fibre) muscles, showing those contraction velocities at which recruited muscles work most efficiently (Alexander, 1989).

3.2.2 Mechanical similarity against geometric similarity

Broadly speaking, the dynamic similarity observed through the universal scaling exponents in scaling biomechanics is intimately related to the geometric similarity that can directly be observed in animals of the same taxa through the body shape, including body's locomotor appendages, i.e., limbs, wings, and tails or fins. Mathematically, the geometric similarity in animals is due to adopted spatial uniformity, preserving body shapes under arbitrary linear transformations of linear dimensions of animals (Rashevsky, 1948; McMahon, 1975; Lin, 1982). Mechanically, the dynamic similarity between animals across taxa arises from the similarity established between the geometric and kinematic parameters of the body's point-mass trajectories and driving forces.
Following the formalism of analytical mechanics discussed in Eq. (2), the concept of mechanical similarity has been discussed in physics (e.g., Duncan, 1953) and biomechanics (Alexander & Jayes, 1983; Alexander, 1989, 2005) in terms of the three arbitrary linear-transformation factors (a, b, and, say, c) preserving the homogeneity of all spatial (L), temporal (T) and force (F) mechanical characteristics of animals moving in a certain fashion or gait. Although no conceptual gap exists between the similarities in classical mechanics and biomechanics, the fundamental constraints imposed on the initially chosen arbitrary factors

of linear transformation, i.e., $b = a^{1-\lambda/2}$ and $c = a^{\lambda-1}$, underlying Eq. (2) and providing basic scaling rules of the dynamic similarity, namely

$$T_\lambda^{-1} \propto L_b^{\lambda/2-1},\ V_\lambda \propto L_b^{\lambda/2}, \text{ and } \Delta F_\lambda \propto L_b^{\lambda-1}, \text{ with } L/L_b \propto M^0, \qquad (16)$$

are generally ignored in experimental biology and even violated in some theoretical studies mentioned in the Introduction. This analysis shows how the spatial uniformity, achieved via the stabilization of dynamic length in relation to static length, determines the observation of dynamic similarity in any dynamic regime λ.

The provided analysis explains why the model-dependent requirements of strict geometric similarity, e.g., the requirement of the equality of joint angles in running animals (Alexander, 1989) or swinging angles in dynamically similar pendulums (Alexander, 2005), do not reduce the dynamic similarity concept to the so-called *strict dynamic similarity* (Alexander, 1989, 2005). First, one can see that both the angles may be expressed in terms of the *swept angle* $\Theta = \arcsin(\beta/2St)$ introduced in biomechanics of animal locomotion as a relative angle between the leg spring and vertical (see, e.g., Fig. 1 in Farley et al., 1993), which is also known as the maximum *compass angle* (Cynthia & Farley, 1998), modeling in turn the *protraction-retraction angle* in bipeds (Gatesy & Biewener, 1991, Fig. 1). Second, the requirement of observation of the dynamic similarity through scaling laws of the mechanical similarity reproduced in Eq. (16) implies that the Strouhal number St $(= L_b/L)$, as well as some other dimensionless numbers, including the duty factor β $(= \Delta T/T)$, should be invariable across different-sized animals, i.e., $St \backsim \beta \propto M^0$. One may infer that a rigorous requirement of the strict geometric similarity on that the swing or other related angles (as well as relative stride lengths) must be equal constants is the overestimated constraint of the dynamic similarity concept. In other words, the requirement of dynamic angles to be mass independent, i.e., $\Theta \propto M^0$, arising from the the requirement of stabilization of relative dynamic lengths, i.e., $St \propto M^0$, unambiguously determines observation of the *perfect* dynamic similarity (Alexander, 1989).

3.2.3 Criterion, determinants, and indicators of dynamic similarity

Being the major requirement in realization of both universal dynamic regimes unifying animals in a certain gait, the high mechanical efficiency of the musculoskeletal system prescribed by minimum muscular action plays the role of the unique *criterion* of observation of dynamic similarity.

The concept of mechanical similarity in biomechanics, consistent with that in analytical mechanics, allows linear transformations of two dynamic (spatial and temporal) and one mechanical (force or mass) characteristics through the three independent scaling factors. Hence, the set $(T^{-1}, V, \Delta F)$ of mutually independent and model-independent quantities, chosen in Eq. (5) in the ltf class of units, can be treated as tentative candidates for the determinants of dynamic similarity. The optimization of muscle-field interactions by the minimum mechanical action (i) introduces new state-dependent scaling relations for T_λ^{-1}, V_λ, and ΔF_λ , which determine three scaling rules of the dynamic similarity, and (ii) reduces the number of independent determinants from three to one, as discussed in Eq. (16). Since the choice of the optimal speed V_λ by an animal is accomplished by the resonant frequency T_λ^{-1}, the suggested principal set of determinants $(T_\lambda^{-1}, V_\lambda)$ does not generally excludes another set, including the uniform muscular field or the uniform relative dynamic length, both required by the high level mechanical efficiency. However, the observation of just only one of the two basic scaling rules guarantees the observation of other features of dynamic similarity in animals. Indeed, the observation of the scaling rule for stride frequency $T_\lambda^{-1} \propto L_b^{\lambda/2-1}$

indicates stabilization of the relative dynamic length, as shown in Eqs. (15) and (16). Hence, experimental observation of the constant Strouhal number in animals moving efficiently in any similar gaits determines them as dynamically similar. When solely the fast gaits are considered, the universal Strouhal number should be revealed along with the universal Froude number Fr, whose stabilization in animals across body mass is equivalent to the observation of scaling rule for the maximum amplitude of optimal and transient speeds $V_{opt}^{(\max)} \propto L_b^{1/2}$, as follows from Eqs. (14) and (16). If the principal determinants St or Fr, each may play the role of the dynamic similarity criterion, are chosen for the corresponding cases $\lambda = 0$ and $\lambda = 1$, other universal determinants, such as muscle stress, speed, in the first case, and the Strouhal number and relative muscular field, in the second case, play the role of the indicators of stabilization of the universal similar dynamic states. Moreover, in both cases the *indicators of dynamic similarity* can be extended by the universal duty factors $\beta \propto M^0$ and swept angles $\Theta \propto M^0$.

3.2.4 Mechanically efficient slow and fast flyers

The stationary-state mode patterns of flight gaits were likely first noted by Hill (1950). He had established that the wing frequencies of *hovering birds* are in inverse proportionality with the linear size, that corresponds to the predicted frequency $T_{hover}^{(pred)-1} \backsim \sqrt{E_{m0}^{(\max)}/\rho_m} L_m^{-1}$ (Table 1) for wing muscles contracting in the stationary regime $\lambda = 0$. Hill's pioneering observation of the fundamental frequency-length scaling law, determining dynamic similarity in the efficient flyers solely via the universal (speed-, period-, and mass-independent) *slow-muscle* elastic modulus $E_{m0}^{(\max)}$ (Table 1) can be compared with seminal Kepler's law $T_{planet}^{(\exp)-1} \propto L_{planet}^{(\exp)-3/2}$ (see Eq. (2) taken at $\lambda = -1$), determining the mechanical similarity between trajectories of planets driven solely by gravitation. Later, the hovering flight motors were also recognized in birds by observation of the wing frequencies $T_{hover}^{(\exp)-1} \propto M^{-1/3}$ (Ellington, 1991), that is also equivalent to observation of the universal Strouhal numbers $S_{hover} \propto M^0$ (Table 1).

When an animal travels or cruises slowly for long distances, maintaining constant the optimal speed $V_{cruis}^{(\max)} \backsim \sqrt{E_0^{(\max)}/\rho_b}$ invariable with bodyweight and frequency (Table 1), or moves throughout the terrestrial, air, or water environment resisting drag forces, the limbs, wings, and fins are expected to be tuned via elastic muscle modulus to maintain universal muscular pressure (Table 1). In turn, this effect gives rise to the constant limb-muscle *safety factor* (ratio of muscle strength to peak functional stress), foreseeing by Hill (1950). Moreover, the peak body force output $F_{body}^{(\exp)} \propto M^{2/3}$, exerted on the environment during running, flying, and swimming by animals ranged over nine orders of body mass, was documented by Alexander (1985). The theoretical suggestion that the stationary-state mechanics, equilibrating all drag forces, is due to slow locomotory muscles, is corroborated by the statistically regressed data on the force output $F_{m\text{-}slow}^{(\max)} \propto M_m^{2/3}$ remarkably established in both biological and human-made *slow motors* by Marden & Allen (2002).

The optimum-speed regime $\lambda = 1$ has been recognized through the equilibration of the air drag by wings of *flapping birds*, manifesting the basic scaling rule for wing frequencies $T_{flap}^{(\exp)-1} \propto M^{-1/6}$ (Ellington, 1991), also corresponding to the observation of $S_{flap} \propto M^0$ (Table 2). Earlier, the non-stationary flight regime has been foreseen by Hill's notion that larger birds flap their wings more slowly than smaller ones (Hill, 1950).

As explicitly shown in Eq. (16), the stabilization of the uniformity in Strouhal numbers in both dynamic regimes $\lambda = 0$ and $\lambda = 1$ explains empirically puzzled animal flight and swim (Whitfield, 2003). Indeed, Taylor et al. (2003) experimentally established such a kind of the universal similarity through the almost constant Strouhal numbers (laying between 0.2 and 0.4) in cruising with a high power efficiency dolphins, flapping birds, and bats. This observation suggests two patterns of *efficient flyers* distinguished by hovering ($\lambda = 0$) and flapping ($\lambda = 1$) modes of slow and fast flight gaits. The corresponding examples of slow-swimming and fast-swimming motors are the gaits to swim established through different swimming techniques for the same fish, using their pectoral fins to swim slowly, but undulating the whole body to swim fast (Alexander, 1989). Unifying flying and swimming animals in *fast gaits*, the data by Taylor et al. (2003) suggest the dynamic similarity pattern of *efficient flapping flyers* and *undulating swimmers*. These and other introduced patterns of dynamic similarity are studied in Kokshenev (2011).

3.2.5 Mechanically efficient fast animals

In experimental biology, it is well known that forces required for fast gaits in animals are proportional to body weight, but since the force generation is more expensive of metabolic energy in faster muscles, small animals show apparently low efficiencies in running (Alexander, 1989). Efficient fast biological motors in running, flying, and swimming animals were established by Marden & Allen (2002) through the scaling equation $F_{opt}^{(\max)} = \mu_{fast}^{(\max)} M$ (Table 2), where the relative force amplitude $\mu_{fast}^{(\max)} = 2g$ was re-estimated by Bejan & Marden (2006a, Fig. 2C). Given that the muscular field in running, flying, and swimming animals is twice as many as the gravitational field, adopted above for the lower threshold of a slow run in the walk-to-run transition, the statistical data $\mu_{fast}^{(\max)} = 2g$ may be conventionally adopted as a universal threshold of fast modes in fast gaits. This threshold associated with the slow-run-to-fast run transient state $\lambda = 1$ may in turn determine the pattern of efficient fast animals, including fast running mammals, reptiles, insects; flapping birds, bats, and insects; undulating fish and crayfish, according to Marden & Allen (2002) and Bejan & Marden (2006a). The pioneering observations of the transient-state speeds $V_{trans}^{(\exp)}$ and frequencies $T_{trans}^{(\exp)-1}$ at the trot-to-gallop continuous transition in quadrupeds ($V_{trot\text{-}gall}^{(\exp)} \propto M^{0.22\pm0.05}$ and $T_{trot\text{-}gall}^{(\exp)-1} \propto M^{-0.15\pm0.03}$; Heglund et al., 1974; Heglund & Taylor, 1988), make evidence for, within the experimental error, the predicted stabilization of the uniform (body mass independent) muscular field, i.e., $\mu_{run}^{(\exp)} \propto M^{-0.07\pm0.08}$, when tested by the scaling relation $\mu_{trans}^{(pred)} \backsim V_{trans} T_{trans}^{-1}$ prescribed by dynamic regime $\lambda = 1$ (Table 2). Likewise, the same generic dynamic regime explains stabilization of the uniformity in the muscular field activated in 13 running animals (from a mice to horses) observed indirectly by Heglund &Taylor (1988) at experimental conditions of the *preferred* trotting speeds and the preferred galloping speeds, providing respectively the determinants of similarity $\mu_{trot}^{(\exp)} \propto M^{0.09\pm0.07}$ and $\mu_{gall}^{(\exp)} \propto M^{0.02\pm0.07}$. The revealed large experimental error is most likely caused by small quadrupedal species (one laboratory mice, two chipmunks, three squirrels, and three white rats of bodyweight not exceeding one kg), which should be excluded from the dynamic similarity pattern, as potentially having low mechanical efficiency (Alexander, 1989).

Bipeds, showing the resonant frequency $T_{trans}^{(\exp)-1} \propto M^{-0.178}$ near the slow-walk-to-fast-run transition (Gatesy & Biewener, 1991), indicate the dynamic similarity pattern of *efficient fast walkers*. The scaling rule $V_{opt}^{(\exp)} \propto M^{0.17}$ empirically established by Garland (1983) for maximal speeds in running terrestrial mammals ranging in five orders in body mass

(from smallest bipedal rodents to largest quadrupedal elephants) indicates observation of the pattern of *efficient runners in mammals.*
The dynamically similar continuous resonant states were clearly revealed by Farley et al. (1993) in a trotting rat, dog, goat, horse and a hopping tammar wallaby and red kangaroo. The realistic modeling on the basis of leg-spring model of animals of leg length $L_{leg}^{(\exp)}$ ($\backsim L_b^{(\exp)}$) provided the following scaling equations for the stride frequency $T_{run}^{(\exp)-1}$, peak force output $F_{run}^{(\exp)}$, maximum body stiffness $K_{run}^{(\exp)}$, swept angle $\Theta_{run}^{(\exp)}$, and dynamic length change $\Delta L_{run}^{(\exp)}$, namely

$$T_{run}^{-1} \backsim \Delta T_{run}^{-1} \propto M^{-0.19\pm0.06}, F_{run}^{(\exp)} = 30.1 M^{0.97\pm0.14}, K_{run}^{(\exp)} \propto M^{0.67\pm0.15},$$
$$\Theta_{run}^{(\exp)} \propto M^{-0.03\pm0.1}, \text{and } \Delta L_{run}^{(\exp)} \backsim L_b^{(\exp)} \propto M^{0.30\pm0.15}. \quad (17)$$

One can see that all the observed scaling exponents are consistent (within the experimental error) with those predicted by the dynamic similarity regime $\lambda = 1$ described in Table 2. These data introduce the dynamic similarity pattern of *efficient trotters and hoppers.*

4. Concluding remarks

Following the concept of mechanical similarity, underlaid by the key principle of minimum action in analytical mechanics, the theory of dynamic similarity in animal locomotion is proposed. Exploring the intrinsic property of locomotory muscles to be tuned, via the variable muscle elasticity, to the natural cyclic frequency characteristic of high level efficiency of locomotion, the scaling rules driving the dynamic similarity in inanimate mechanical elastic systems are suggested for the special case of active-force animate elastic systems. The linear-displacement dynamic approach to contracting locomotory muscles, whose resonant frequencies are required by the principle of minimum mechanical action, establishes two different universal patterns of the dynamic regimes of similarity in different-sized animals distinguished by the dynamic scaling exponent λ. The determinants of the stationary locomotion of animals moving at optimal constant speeds (the case $\lambda = 0$) and the non-stationary locomotion at gradually changing speeds ($\lambda = 1$), including the transient-mode speed transitions, are self-consistently inferred and described in Tables 1 and 2, respectively. Exemplified by the non-stationary dynamic regime $\lambda = 1$, the two principal sets of determinants of the dynamic similarity are suggested by the universal exponents for the speed and frequency scaled with body mass, which may be equivalently presented by the corresponding Froude and Strouhal numbers or by other universal dimensionless numbers determining the states of dynamic similarity in different-sized animals.
The primary determinant, playing the role of the unique criterion of the linear dynamic similarity, is shown (in Eq. (16)) to be the Strouhal number, whose universality in animals across body mass indicates establishing of the linearity between the stride or stroke length and the body length in each animal, falling into one or other dynamically similar regime. In the special case of non-stationary dynamic similarity controlled by fast locomotory muscles, the Froude number may be equivalently chosen as a unique criterion of similarity, as hypothesized by Alexander (Alexander, 1976; Alexander & Jayes, 1983; Alexander, 1989). Since the scaling theory of similarity deals only with scaling relations, but not with scaling equations, Alexander's strict requirement that dynamic similarly between running animals should equal Froude numbers is not generally required by the theory. Instead, the theory of dynamic similarity stands only that changing with speed Froude numbers should be

invariable with body mass in animals considered in a certain dynamic state or domain of dynamically equivalent states. A generalization of the proposed theory of the discrete-state dynamic similarity to continuous-state similarity in animals, determining, respectively, by discrete equal and different variable magnitudes of the Froude numbers, will be discussed in the next part of this study (Kokshenev, 2011).

The two kinds of dynamic similarity regimes in animals, well distinguished by the scaling rules established for a number of mechanical characteristics, may explain seemingly controversial experimental observations as well as illuminate some theoretical principles conceptually inconsistent with the mechanical similarity principle of analytical mechanics.

Hill's pioneering observation of bodyweight independence of optimal speeds in a hover flight mode of sparrows and humming birds (Hill, 1950), showing a sharp inconsistency (McMahon, 1975; Jones & Lindstedt, 1993) with the scaling rules for speeds in quadrupeds established at the trot-to-gallop transition (Heglund et al., 1974) can readily be understood by the observations of two distinct dynamic similarity regimes $\lambda = 0$ and $\lambda = 1$. Likewise, a more recent claim on that the similarity between humans running at *fixed* speeds, accurately simulated under the requirement of equal Froude numbers, was surprisingly found (Delattre et al., 2009) to be in sharp disagreement with the scaling rules of dynamic similarity in fast running animals reliably established by Farley et al. (1993). A new kind of similarity discovered in running humans arrived the authors to a puzzle conclusion that neither of Froude and Strouhal numbers is appropriate as determinant of dynamic similarity. In this special case, the proposed theory tells us that the dynamic similarity between humans running at the stationary-speed conditions (Table 1) cannot be constrained by constant Froude numbers, as erroneously was adopted in the study by Delattre et al. (2009).

Another Hill's surmise on the constant limb muscle stress, resulted in the universality of the limb safety factor in animals efficiently moving in slow gaits, has been generalized without grounds to all fast gaits by a number of researches. For example, in attempting to introduce "equivalent speed" states $\lambda = 1$ during trot-to-gallop transition McMahon postulated a constant stress in homologous muscles (McMahon, 1975, Table 4), when suggested the uniform muscle stress $\sigma_{m\text{-}slow} \propto M^0$, corresponding to the case of $\lambda = 0$. The postulated stress evidently contrasted with the already existing data on peak isometric stress, linearly varying with sarcomere length (Huxley & Neidergerke, 1954), i.e., $\sigma_{m\text{-}fast} \propto L_m$ (Table 2), and the data on muscle stress later revealed the linearity to fiber length in running and jumping animals (Alexander & Bennet-Clark, 1976). Likewise, when the axial-displacement dynamic similarity (i.e., $\Delta L_{m\text{-}fast} \propto L_m$) discussed for fast locomotory muscles is generalized to non-axial-displacement elastic similarity in long limb mammalian bones ($\Delta L_{bone}^{(bend)} \propto D_{bone}$, where D_{bone} is bone's diameter; Kokshenev, 2007, Eq. (15)) new puzzled consequences of biomechanical scaling may be revealed. One impressive example is the axial compressive stress $\sigma_{bone}^{(axial)} \propto L_{bone}$, estimated as the peak limb bone stress $\sigma_{bone}^{(\exp)} \propto M^{0.28}$ for the avian taxa, matching well the spring-leg data $\sigma_{leg}^{(\exp)} \propto M^{0.30}$ from running quadrupeds following from Eq. (17), has been shown to provide the anecdotal small largest terrestrial giant weight, no much greater than 20 kg (Biewener, 2005). This puzzle was understood by that instead of axial stress, which is in fact non-critical, the bending stress $\sigma_{bone}^{(bend)} \propto D_{bone}/L_{bone}$, having small but non-zero positive exponent, i.e., $\sigma_{bone}^{(bend)} \propto M^{0.08}$, likely establishes the critical mass of terrestrial giants (Kokshenev & Christiansen, 2011).

One more "least-action principle" in biomechanics was recently declared for walk gaits in humans (Fan et al., 2009). The standard variational procedure was worked out to establish a symmetric point $(T/2)$ in the middle of the two-step stride cycle in human gaits, at which all important mechanical characteristics expose the extreme (minimum or maximum) behavior. This misleading principle of the existence of the symmetrical point, even though consistent with the well-known symmetrical nature of a walk and a run, due to which each equivalent leg moves half a stride cycle out of other leg (e.g., Alexander & Jayes, 1983, p.142) was in fact incorporated, likely unconsciously, into the studied model through symmetric mechanics of the supposedly equivalent human legs.

The constructal theory of dynamic similarity by Bejan & Marden (2006a, b) treats the potential energy of the body falling in the gravitational field g as a useful energy of terrestrial locomotion. Considering only the aerial phase in a stride cycle, the theory excludes the ground contact and thereby all muscular forces providing the body propulsion force $\mu_{fast}^{(exp)} M$. It is surprisingly that the same theoretical framework excluding muscle forces has resulted in the muscular field $\mu_{fast}^{(exp)} = 2g$, since the suggested scaling factors in the basic scaling relations, shown in Eq. (8), are weighted solely by the gravitational field. Hence, it has been demonstrated by the authors that consistency between the principle of destruction of minimum useful energy in the gravitational field (the case $\lambda = 1$ in Eq. (2)) may exist under the additional condition postulated in Eq. (7), in fact borrowed from another, more general mechanical principle.

Following the requirement of equality of Froude numbers, experimental biologists mostly study the discrete-state dynamic similarity in animals. For example, Bullimore & Burn (2006) have remarkably established (see their Table 4) the universal criterion of dynamic similarity $St_{trot}^{(exp)}$ (= 0.70, 0.67, and 0.60) from 21 horses trotting at arbitrary chosen fixed Froude numbers $Fr_{trot}^{(exp)}$ (= 0.5, 0.75, and 1). This finding corroborates McMahon's suggestion (acknowledged by Alexander, 1989) on that besides the Froude number the Strouhal number should be simultaneously constant, as followed from the universality of the Groucho number (McMahon et al., 1987). In contrast, the study by Bullimore & Donelan (2008) of the criteria of dynamic similarity in spring-mass modeled animals suggested four independent determinants, at least. Given that the authors have clearly convinced the reader of that the equality of only two dimensionless numbers is not sufficient for establishing of the dynamic similarity between in-plane modeled animals (Bullimore & Donelan, 2008, Fig. 4), a question arises about what kind of dynamic similarity was reported by Bullimore & Burn (2006) established in real trotting horses through the only one determinant Fr?

Bullimore & Donelan (2008, Table 2) have analyzed the well known solutions of the planar spring-mass model through Buckingham's Π-theorem of the dimensional method (e.g., Barenblatt, 2002) and claimed that minimum four independent dimensionless numbers following from the set of mechanical quantities (V, K, V_z, Θ_0) are required for the observation of dynamic similarity in bouncing modes of animals. First, one can see that the landing angle Θ_0 should be excluded from the proposed set of physically independent quantities, since the horizontal landing speed V and the vertical landing speed V_z definitively determine the angle $\Theta_0 = arctg(V/V_z)$, as can be inferred from Fig. 1 by Bullimore & Donelan (2008). Then, the requirement to control vertical speed via the model-independent relation $V_z \backsim \mu\beta T$ allows one to reduce the proposed set to the equivalent set (T^{-1}, V, μ, β), where the body stiffness is substituted by muscular field via the body stiffness $K \backsim \rho_b A \mu$. The resulted set of four quantities (St, Fr, μ, β) is dynamically equivalent to the originally suggested set (V, K, V_z, Θ_0), but among three determinants (St, Fr, μ) the only one is physically independent. Two other dimensionless numbers play the role of auxiliary determinants in the dynamic similarity, whereas the duty factor may indicate transient-mode and crossover-gait universal states of the same dynamic regime $\lambda = 1$. Hence, it has been repeatedly demonstrated that the

application of Buckingham's theorem only provides a way of generating sets of dimensionless parameters, but does not indicate or even substitute most physically meaningful relations. This well known statement is also illustrated by the provided above study of two scaling equations Eq. (2) and (5), suggesting the same set of three possible determinants of dynamic similarity, respectively provided by the physical concept and the dimensional method.
When comparing the frameworks of dynamic similarity and elastic similarity, respectively elaborated to scale the patterns of fast locomotion gaits and the patterns of primary functions (motor, brake, strut, or spring) of locomotory muscles (Kokshenev, 2008, Table 1), belonging to the same body's elastic system, one can see that in both cases the muscle contractions fall into the same dynamic similarity regime $\lambda = 1$ generally governed by the same uniform muscular field. However, the two distinct (gait and function) muscle patters should not provide the same scaling rules for dynamic muscle characteristics, including the dynamic length noted by Alexander (1989, p.1212), since the dynamic conditions of muscle cycling are distinct. Indeed, the dynamic cycling in similar locomotion is synchronized with the collective muscle dynamics, corresponding to the condition of maximum overall-body mechanical efficiency, whereas the elastic similarity between individual muscles specialized to a certain mechanical function is likely governed by the requirement of maximum power, generally not matching the condition of minimal oxygen consumption. The observation by Hill (1950, Fig. 1) that the muscle power and efficiency maxima are rather blunt and close in space makes it possible to work at maximum power with nearly maximum efficiency. Further analysis of non-linear dynamic similarity in muscle functions and animal locomotion, including powering intermittent gaits (Alexander, 1989, p.1200), will be discussed elsewhere.

5. Acknowledgments

The author is grateful to Dr. in Engineering Sciences Illya Kokshenev for discussion and critical comments. Financial support by the national agency FAPEMIG is also acknowledged.

6. References

Ahlborn, B.K. & Blake, R.W. (2002). Walking and running at resonance, *Zoology* 105: 165–174.

Ahlborn, B.K., Blake, R.W. & Megill, W.M. (2006). Frequency tuning in animal locomotion, *Zoology* 109: 43-53.

Alexander, R.McN. (1976). Estimates of speeds of dinosaurs, *Nature* 261: 129-130.

Alexander, R.McN. (1985). The maximum forces exerted by animals, *Journal of Experimental Biology* 115: 231-238.

Alexander, R.McN. (1989). Optimization and gaits in the locomotion of vertebrates, *Physiological Review* 69: 1199- 1227.

Alexander, R.McN. (2003). *Principles of animal locomotion*, Princeton University Press, Princeton and Oxford, pp.53-67.

Alexander, R.McN. (2005). Models and scaling of energy costs for locomotion, *Journal of Experimental Biology* 208: 1645-1652.

Alexander, R.McN. & Bennet-Clark, H.C. (1976). Storage of elastic strain energy in muscle and other tissue, *Nature* 265: 114-117.

Alexander, R.McN. & Jayes, A.S. (1983). A dynamic similarity hypothesis for the gaits of quadrupedal mammals, *Journal of Zoology* 201: 135–152.

Barenblatt, G.I. (2002). Scaling, Self-Similarity, and Intermediate Asymptotics. Cambridge University Press, Cambridge.

Bejan, A. & Marden, J.H. (2006a). Unifying constructal theory for scale effects in running, swimming and flying, *Journal of Experimental Biology* 209: 238-248.

Bejan, A. & Marden, J.H. (2006b). Constructing animal locomotion from new thermodynamics theory, *American Scientist* 94: 342-350.

Biewener, A.A. (2005). Biomechanical consequences of scaling, *Journal of Experimental Biology* 208: 1665-1676.

Bullimore, S.R. & Burn, J.F. (2006). Dynamically similar locomotion in horses, *Journal of Experimental Biology* 209: 455–465.

Bullimore, S.R.& Donelan, J.M. (2008). Criteria for dynamic similarity in bouncing gaits, *Journal of Theoretical Biology* 250: 339–348.

Cartmill, M., Lemelin, P. & Schmitt, D. (2002). Support polygons and symmetrical gaits in mammals, *Zoolological Journal of Linnean Society* 136: 401-420.

Cynthia, R.L. & Farley, C.T. (1998). Determinants of the center of mass trajectory in human walking and running,*Journal of Experimental Biology* 201: 2935-2944.

Delattre, N. & Moretto, P. (2008). A new dimensionless number highlighted from mechanical energy exchange during running, *Journal of Biomechanics* 41: 2895–2898.

Delattre, N., Lafortune, M.A. & Moretto, P. (2009). Dynamic similarity during human running: About Froude and Strouhal dimensionless numbers, *Journal of Biomechanics* 42: 312–318.

Dickinson, M.H., Farley, C.T., Full, J.R., Koehl, M.A.R., Kram R. & Lehman, S. (2000). How animals move: an integrative view, *Science* 288: 100-106.

Donelan, J. M. & Kram, R. (1997). The effect of reduced gravity on the kinematics of human walking: a test of the dynamic similarity hypothesis for locomotion, *Journal of Experimental Biology* 200: 3193–3201.

Duncan, W.J. (1953). *Physical similarity and dimensional analysis*. Edward Arnold and Co., London.

Ellington, C.P. (1991). Limitations on animal flight performance, *Journal of Experimental Biology* 160: 71-91.

Fan, Y. F., Loan, M, Fan, Y. B., Li, Z.Y. & Luo, D.L. (2009). Least-action principle in gait, *Europhysics Letters* 87: 58003-1-4.

Farley, C.T., Glasheen, J. & McMahon, T.A. (1993). Running springs: speed and animal size, *Journal of Experimental Biology* 185:71-86.

Farley, C.T. & Gonzalez, O. (1996). Leg stiffness and stride frequency in humanrunning, *Journal of Biomechanics* 29: 181–186.

Garland, T. (1983). The relation between maximal running speed and body mass in terrestrial mammals, *Journal of Zoology* 199: 157–170.

Gatesy, S. M. & Biewener, A.A. (1991) Bipedal locomotion: effects of speed, size and limb posture in birds and animals, *Journal of Zoology London* 224: 127-147.

Greenewalt, C.H. (1975). The fligt of birds, *Transactions of American Philosophical Society* 65: 1-67.

Heglund, N., McMahon, T.A. & Taylor, C.R. (1974). Scaling stride frequency and gait to animal size: mice to horses, *Science* 186: 1112-1113.

Heglund, N. & Taylor, C. R. (1988). Speed, stride frequency and energy cost per stride: how do thy change with body size and gait? *Journal of Experimental Biology* 138: 301-318.

Hill, A.V. (1950) The dimensions of animals and their muscular dynamics, *Science Progress* 38: 209-230.

Hoyt, D.F. & Taylor, C.R. (1981). Gait and the energetics of locomotion in horses, *Nature* 292: 239-240.

Huxley, A.F. & Niedergerke, R. (1954). Interference microscopy of living muscle fibers, *Nature* 173: 971-973.

Jones, J.H. & Lindstedt, S. (1993). Limits of maximal performance, *Annual Review Physiology* 55: 547-569.
Kokshenev, V.B. (2003). Observation of mammalian similarity through allometric scaling laws, *Physica A* 322: 491-505.
Kokshenev, V.B. (2004). Dynamics of human walking at steady speeds, *Physical Review Letters* 93: 208101-1-4.
Kokshenev, V.B. (2007). New insights into long-bone biomechanics: Are limb safety factors invariable across mammalian species?, *Journal of Biomechanics* 40: 2911–2918.
Kokshenev, V.B. (2008). A force-similarity model of the activated muscle is able to predict primary locomotor functions, *Journal of Biomechanics* 41: 912–915.
Kokshenev, V.B. (2009). Scaling functional patterns of skeletal and cardiac muscles: New non-linear elasticity approach, *arXiv:0909.1444v1*.
Kokshenev, V.B. (2010). Key principle of the efficient running, swimming, and flying, *Europhysics Letters* 90: 48005-1-5.
Kokshenev, V.B. (2011). Physical insights into dynamic similarity in animal locomotion. II. Observation of continuous similarity states, In: *Theoretical Biomechanics*, Vaclav Klika (ed.), pp. 285-302, ISBN 978-953-307-851-9.
Kokshenev, V.B. & Christiansen, P. (2011). Evolution of locomotor trends in extinct terrestrial giants affected by body mass, Biomechanics I: In: *Theoretical Biomechanics*, Vaclav Klika (ed.), pp. 49-74, ISBN 978-953-307-851-9.
Landau, L.D. & Lifshitz, E.M. (1976). *Mechanics,* Vol. 1 (3rd ed.), Butterworth-Heinemann. ISBN 978-0-750-62896-9.
Lin, H. (1982). Fundamentals of zoological scaling, *American Journal of Physics* 50: 72-81.
Marden, J.H. & Allen, L.R. (2002). Molecules, muscles, and machines: universal performance characteristics of motors *Proceedings of National Academy of Science USA* 99: 4161-4166.
McMahon, T.A. (1975). Using body size to understand the structural design of animals: quadrupedal locomotion *Journal of Applied Physiology* 39: 619-627.
McMahon, T.A. (1984). *Muscles, reflexes, and locomotion*, Princeton University Press, Princeton and New Jersey.
McMahon, T.A., Valiant, G. & Frederick, E.C. (1987). Groucho running, *Journal of Applied Physiology* 62: 2326-2337.
McMahon, T.A. & Cheng, G.C.(1990). The mechanics of running: how does stiffness couple with speed? *Journal of Biomechanics* 23: 65–78.
Rashevsky, N. (1948). *Mathematical biophysics*, revised edition, The University of Chicago Press: Chicago, 1948. (New edition. Dover Publications, New York, 1960).
Rome, L.C., Funke, R.P., Alexander, R.McN., Lutz, G., Aldridge, H., Scott F. & Freadman, M. (1988). Why animals have different muscle fibre types?, *Nature* 335: 824-829.
Rubin, C.T. & Lanyon, L.E. (1984). Dynamic strain similarity in vertebrates; an alternative to allometric limb bone scaling, *Journal of Theoretical Biology* 107: 321-327.
Taylor G.K., Nudds, R.L. & Thomas, A. L. (2003). Flying and swimming animals cruise at a Strouhal number tuned for high power efficiency, *Nature* 425: 707-710.
Vaughan, C.L. & O'Malleyb, M. J. (2005). Froude and the contribution of naval architecture to our understanding of bipedal locomotion, *Gait & Posture* 21: 350-362.
Videler, J.J. & Weihs, D. (1982). Energetic advantages of burst-and coast swimming of fish at high speeds, *Journal of Experimental Biology* 97: 169-172.
Whitfield, J. (2003). One number explains animal flight, *Nature* doi:10.1038/news031013-9.

Physical Insights Into Dynamic Similarity in Animal Locomotion. II. Observation of Continuous Similarity States

Valery B. Kokshenev
Departamento de Física, Universidade Federal de Minas Gerais, Belo Horizonte, Brazil

1. Introduction

In previous studies, the physical theory of dynamic similarity in animals was deduced from the concept of mechanical similarity in analytical mechanics (Kokshenev, 2010, 2011). Unlike a mechanistic approach to the problem of dynamic similarity in biomechanics of locomotion treating the animate systems as freely falling in the gravitational field and resisting drag forces (Bejan & Marden, 2006), the model-independent physical theory, unifying running, swimming, and flying animals, can be outlined as follows.

Broadly speaking, animals of different body size L_b are dissimilar in their forward propagation speeds V and stride or stroke frequencies T^{-1}. However, when traveling or cruising for long distances at the proper body's resonant frequency $T_{res}^{-1} \sim \sqrt{\mu_{slow}/L_b}$, the animals are generally exploit the stationary dynamic regime characteristic of the constant uniform body pressure generated by slow locomotory muscles. The relevant muscular field $\mu_{slow} \propto L_b^{-1}$, scaling with body length by the same way as reaction elastic-force field, was observed indirectly (Kokshenev, 2011, Table 1) through the wingbeat frequency in hovering birds T_{res}^{-1}, first by Hill (1950) and then by Ellington (1991). The first direct observation of the body's *slow muscular field* scaling with body mass as $\mu_{slow} \propto M^{-1/3}$ in flying, running, and swimming animals has been established through the body force output by Alexander (1985) and Marden & Allen (2002). When an animal maintains the resonant cyclic conditions (in frequency and phase; Kokshenev, 2010) with increasing speed, the mechanical efficiency of the properly recruited fast locomotory muscles is higher than that of acting slow muscles, at least in adult species (e.g., Alexander, 1989). Moreover, the mechanically universal (i.e., frequency-, speed-, and force-independent) muscle stiffness $K_{fast} \propto M^{2/3}$ results in the body's *fast muscular field* $\mu_{fast} \sim g$, where g is the gravitational field, whose uniformity determines the dynamic similarity between animals across body mass through the basic scaling rules $V_{fast} \propto M^{1/6}$ and $T_{fast}^{-1} \propto M^{-1/6}$.

The *dynamic similarity patterns*, unifying different-sized animals at a certain dynamically similar slow or fast regime, are unambiguously determined by the reliable observation of just one of the basic scaling rules shown respectively in Tables 1 and 2 in Kokshenev (2011). Alternatively, the equivalent *theoretical observation* of just one *uniform* (across body mass) dimensionless determinant, such as the Strouhal number ($St_{slow} \sim St_{fast} \propto M^0$), the Froude number ($Fr_{fast} \propto M^0$), the force-output number ($\mu_{fast}/g \propto M^0$), the limb duty factor ($\beta_{slow} \sim \beta_{fast} \propto M^0$), or the angle ($\Theta_{slow} \sim \Theta_{fast} \propto M^0$) sweeping by legs, wings, or tails during a stride or a stroke, implies the establishing of the discrete (isolated) dynamically similar states in animals moving in certain fast or slow gait.

In the previous chapter, the pattern of *efficient runners in quadrupeds*, unifying trotting and galloping quadrupeds (from a mice to a horse), was theoretically observed by both the basic scaling rules at well experimentally distinguished "equivalent" speeds (Heglund et al., 1974), "preferred" trotting and galloping speeds (Heglund & Taylor, 1988; Perry et al., 1988), as well as trot-to-gallop transient speeds (Heglund et al., 1974, Heglund & Taylor, 1988). When extended by bipeds and described by a whole spectrum of scaling rules, the latter pattern of similarity called by *efficient trotters and hoppers* was been studied in the domain of "physiologically equivalent" speeds (Farley et al., 1993), unifying near the trot-to-gallop transition running quadrupeds (from a rat to a horse) and hopping bipeds (tammar wallaby and red kangaroo).[1] It has been also demonstrated that the direct experimental observation of both two basic scaling rules is equivalent to the theoretical observation of the uniformity of the underlaid muscular field, i.e., $\mu_{fast} \backsim V_{fast}T^{-1}_{fast} \propto M^0$. Other patterns of the established transient (walk-to-run) state and optimum-speed state, called by *efficient walkers in bipeds* and *efficient runners in mammals*, were theoretically observed through the scaling rules for, respectively, frequency and speed measured in bipeds, including humans (Gatesy & Biewener, 1991) and other terrestrial mammals (from the smallest bipedal rodent to the largest quadrupedal elephant, Garland, 1983). Likewise, the dynamic similarity in *efficient flyers and swimmers* associated with the fast dynamic regime of locomotion was established for dolphins, birds, and bats cruising with a high power efficiency (Taylor et al., 2003).

In the previous chapter, Alexander's hypothesis on the dynamic similarity between running different-sized animals, equalling Froude numbers (Alexander, 1976; Alexander & Jayes, 1983; Alexander, 1989), has been studied in the context of *discrete-state* dynamic similarity. These dynamically similar states of animate systems, moving in either the stationary-speed slow-muscle regime or the non-stationary fast-muscle regime, have been specified by optimal-speed, transient-mode, and transient-gait states, resulted in the mentioned above dynamic similarity patterns. Besides the central hypothesis on discrete-state dynamic similarity, the possible existence of gait-dependent characteristic similarity functions (of the *Froude variable* Fr) unifying animals across body mass, speed, and taxa at a certain gait, was also proposed by Alexander & Jayes (1983). From the theoretical point of view, the discrete-state similarity determined by equal Froude constants has been therefore suggested to be generalized to the *continuous-state dynamic similarity*, determined by the *dynamic similarity functions* provided by continuous data on the limb duty factors $\beta(Fr)$ and the Strouhal numbers $St(Fr)$ obtained by Alexander & Jayes (1983).

In this study, the theory of continuous dynamic similarity is developed and tested by the continuous dynamic similarity states revealed in walking and running mammals on the basis of systematic experimental data on the limb duty factor and relative stride length available for quadrupedal (Alexander & Jayes, 1983; Hutchinson et al., 2006) and bipedal (Gatesy & Biewener, 1991) animals. The developed concept of dynamic similarity hopefully provides

[1] Earlier, the continues dynamically similar states were established by Alexander & Jayes (1983) in trotting and galloping cursorial quadrupeds through the Froude numbers lying in the domain $2 \leq Fr \leq 3$. The corresponding local-state trot-gallop transition was estimated at $Fr_{trot-gall} = 2.5$ (Alexander & Jayes, 1983; Alexander, 2003).

further generalizations of the patterns of dynamic similarity revealed in animals across speed and taxa.

2. Materials and methods

2.1 Systematic experimental data

The available experimental data on gait-dependent characteristics of walking and running terrestrial animals based on the study of dimensionless numbers of dynamic similarity, are conventionally separated in two groups, represented by the discrete-state constant and continuous-state variable Froude parameters.

2.1.1 Discrete similarity data

The study by Farley et al. (1993) of the dynamic similarity in trotting quadrupeds (form a rat to a horse through a dog and a goat) extended by hopping bipeds (tammar wallaby and red kangaroo) has been performed near the trot-to-gallop transient states, whose dynamic similarity was revealed by closely spaced Froude numbers $Fr_{trans}^{(exp)}$ $(= V_{trans}^2/gL_b$, where L_b is hip height), limb duty factors $\beta_{trans}^{(exp)}$ $(= \Delta T/T$, with ΔT is the ground contact time of one foot, and T is the stride period), and peak force output $F_{trans}^{(exp)}$, represented here as

$$Fr_{trans}^{(exp)} = 2.25 \pm 0.13,\ St_{trans}^{(pred)} = 0.40,\ \beta_{trans}^{(exp)} = 0.41 \pm 0.2, \text{ with } \mu_{trans}^{(max)}/g = 3.10. \qquad (1)$$

The statistically averaged data for the mean Froude number and the limb duty factor were reported by Farley et al. (1993, p. 74). The relative force output is estimated here on the basis of $F_{trans}^{(exp)}$ discussed in Eq. (17) in Kokshenev (2011) and the failing Strouhal number is predicted below (Fig. 1).

More recently, the discrete-state dynamic similarity was established in 21 trotting horses by Bullimore & Burn (2006) at three constant Froude numbers $Fr_{trot}^{(exp)}$ $(= 0.5, 0.75$, and $1)$. In their Table 4, the authors have shown that besides the stabilization across body mass of two determinants $Fr_{trot}^{(exp)} \propto M^0$ and $St_{trot}^{(exp)} \propto M^0$, the similar dynamic states are also indicated by the invariable duty factor $\beta_{trot}^{(exp)} \propto M^0$. The omitted scaling factors in statistically observed scaling relations are schematically reproduced here as

$$\begin{pmatrix} Fr_{trot}^{(exp)} \\ St_{trot}^{(exp)} \\ \beta_{trot}^{(exp)} \end{pmatrix} = \begin{pmatrix} 0.50\ 0.75\ 1.00 \\ 0.70\ 0.67\ 0.60 \\ 0.47\ 0.44\ 0.39 \end{pmatrix} \cdot M^0. \qquad (2)$$

2.1.2 Continuous similarity data

Treating the estimated Froude numbers as a dynamic variable, changing with speed in walking and running terrestrial animals, the data on the measured gait-dependent mechanical characteristics were obtained by a number of researches. The available systematic data on continuous dynamic similarity in quadrupeds (from a small rodent to a rhinoceros, Alexander & Jayes, 1983), modern elephants (Hutchinson et al., 2006), land-dwelling birds (from a bobwhite to an ostrich) and two humans (Gatesy & Biewener, 1991) are provided in Table 1 in terms of the duty-factor similarity function $\beta_{gait}^{(exp)}$ and the Strouhal similarity function $St_{gait}^{(exp)}$ scaled by Froude variable Fr.

Animals	$a(Fr)^b$	$a_{walk}^{(exp)}$	$b_{walk}^{(exp)}$	$\pm\Delta b_{walk}^{(exp)}$	$a_{run}^{(exp)}$	$b_{run}^{(exp)}$	$\pm\Delta b_{run}^{(exp)}$
Quadrupeds curs.	$\beta_{gait}^{(exp)}$	0.52	−0.16	0.07	0.53	−0.28	0.03
Quadrupeds curs.	$St_{gait}^{(exp)-1}$	2.4	0.34	0.10	1.9	0.40	0.03
Bipeds	$a(Fr)^b$	$a_{walk}^{(exp)}$	$b_{walk}^{(exp)}$	$r_{walk}^{(exp)2}$	$a_{run}^{(exp)}$	$b_{run}^{(exp)}$	$r_{run}^{(exp)2}$
Birds	$\beta_{gait}^{(exp)}$	0.60	−0.09	0.69	0.56	−0.20	0.69
Humans	$\beta_{gait}^{(exp)}$	0.58	−0.08	0.93	0.40	−0.29	0.90
Bipeds	$\beta_{gait}^{(exp)}$	0.59	−0.09	−−	0.47	−0.25	−−
Birds	$St_{gait}^{(exp)-1}$	2.34	0.16	0.72	2.42	0.31	0.72
Humans	$St_{gait}^{(exp)-1}$	2.48	0.28	0.80	2.48	0.38	0.76
Bipeds	$St_{gait}^{(exp)-1}$	2.41	0.22	−−	2.45	0.35	−−
Elephants	$a+b\log(Fr)$	$a_{African}^{(exp)}$	$b_{African}^{(exp)}$	$r_{African}^{(exp)2}$	$a_{Asian}^{(exp)}$	$b_{Asian}^{(exp)}$	$r_{Asian}^{(exp)2}$
Elephants	$\beta_{eleph}^{(exp)}$	0.53	−0.16	0.89	0.51	−0.16	0.84
Elephants	$a(Fr)^b$	$a_{African}^{(exp)}$	$b_{African}^{(exp)}$	$r_{African}^{(exp)2}$	$a_{Asian}^{(exp)}$	$b_{Asian}^{(exp)}$	$r_{Asian}^{(exp)2}$
Elephants	St_{eleph}^{-1}	2.0	0.18	0.84	2.1	0.17	0.86

Table 1. The equations of linear least squares regression for the limb duty factor (β) and relative stride length ($= St^{-1}$, see, e.g., Table 2 below) obtained from walking and running animals. The data on African and Asian elephants are by Hutchinson et al. (2006, Table 3). The data on cursorial quadrupeds (a dog, a sheep, a camel, and a rhinoceros) are by Alexander & Jayes (1983, Table II). For quadrupeds, the limb duty factor data are the arithmetic means of forelimb and hindlimb data. The dynamic similarity functions for birds and humans are obtained here by the standard least squares regression of the continuous-state data reproduced from Figs. 5 and 7 in Gatesy & Biewener (1991). The scaling equations for bipeds are approximated by the geometric mean of those for birds and humans.[2]

2.2 Theory of continuous similarity

2.2.1 Statement of the problem

When Alexander's central hypothesis exemplified in Eq. (2) is applied to the efficiently trotting dogs, a question arises whether the dogs observed at the same three constant Froude numbers will show the same Strouhal numbers and limb duty factors as in the horses? In other words, whether the equivalent dynamic similarity states chosen at certain fixed numbers Fr determine the same dynamic similarity states in horses indicated by the same equalized magnitudes of St and β? Moreover, if a chosen small trotting horse and an estimated big trotting dog show the same Froude number, does it mean that other corresponding determinants and indicators of the dynamic similarity should be equal in magnitudes? All these questions are concern with the concept of continuous-state dynamic similarity justified by the universal gait-dependent dynamic similarity functions hypothesized by Alexander & Jayes (1983).

[2] For example, for the two similarity functions $y_1 = a_1 x^{b_1}$ and $y_2 = a_2 x^{b_2}$ the geometric mean function results in $y = \sqrt{y_1 y_2}$, with the corresponding scaling factor $a = \sqrt{a_1 a_2}$ and exponent $b = (b_1 + b_2)/2$.

Strictly speaking, the theory developed in the previous chapter tells us that the observation across body mass of a certain dynamically universal state through equal determinants is a sufficient, but not necessary condition for realization of the same or dynamically similar state in different-sized animals. Indeed, it has been demonstrated that the continues-state similarity pattern of *efficient runners in quadrupeds* can be equally observed through the close spaced discrete similar states indicated by non-equal Froude numbers in the domain[1] $2 \leq Fr \leq 3$. Since the spectrum of scaling rules of the dynamic similarity theory establishes the universality for solely scaling exponents, leaving aside the problem of scaling factors, the scaling equations empirically established for speed and frequency in dogs and horses may broadly differ in scaling factors, eventually providing different magnitudes in the set of determinants of discrete-state similarity (Fr, St, β) discussed above. Hence, this qualitative analysis suggests the dynamically equivalent states established in different-sized animals can be observed not by solely equal, but also different, generally closely spaced dimensionless numbers unified by the domains of continuous equivalent states distinguished via continues similarity patterns. The developed below theory is discussed in terms of the continuously similar states revealed via the extended set of determinants and indicators of similarity, such as the set (Fr, St, μ, β) exemplified by the transient mode-state *continuous similarity pattern* shown in Eq. (1).

2.2.2 Continuous similarity states

In this study, the discrete states of similarity unified by the generic regime of *fast* locomotion, are going to be generalized to continuous dynamic states described in Table 2.

Fast gait characteristics	Frequency	Length	Speed	Force	Mass
$T_{opt}^{-1}, T_{res}^{-1} \sim \sqrt{K/M}$	T^{-1}	$\mu^{\frac{1}{2}} \cdot L_b^{-\frac{1}{2}}$	$\mu \cdot V^{-1}$	$(\rho_b \mu^2 A)^{\frac{1}{2}} \cdot F^{-\frac{1}{2}}$	$\rho_b^{\frac{1}{6}} \mu^{\frac{1}{2}} \cdot M^{-\frac{1}{6}}$
$L_{gait}^{(\max)} = L$	$\mu \cdot T^2$	L	$\mu^{-1} \cdot V^2$	$(\rho_b \mu A)^{-1} \cdot F$	$\rho_b^{-\frac{1}{3}} \cdot M^{\frac{1}{3}}$
$V_{gait}^{(\max)} = LT^{-1}$	$\mu \cdot T$	$\mu^{\frac{1}{2}} \cdot L^{\frac{1}{2}}$	V	$(\rho_b A)^{-\frac{1}{2}} \cdot F^{\frac{1}{2}}$	$\rho_b^{-\frac{1}{6}} \mu^{\frac{1}{2}} \cdot M^{\frac{1}{6}}$
$K_{gait}^{(\max)} = \Delta F / \Delta L_b$	T^0	L^0	V^0	F^0	$\rho_b^{-\frac{1}{3}} \mu \cdot M^{\frac{2}{3}}$
$\mu_{gait}^{(\max)} / g = \Delta F / gM$	T^0	L^0	V^0	F^0	M^0
$St_{gait} = L_b / L$	T^0	$L_b L^{-1}$	V^0	F^0	M^0
$Fr_{gait} = V^2 / g L_b$	T^0	L^0	V^0	F^0	M^0

Table 2. The determinants suggested for dynamically similar states in animals moving in fast similar gaits. The data are reproduced from Table 2 in Kokshenev (2011). Here L is the dynamic (stride or stroke) length and L_b is the static (leg or wing) length in animals; A is the body's cross-sectional area; ρ_b is the body density; $K_{run}^{(\max)}$ is the maximum amplitude of body stiffness. Other notations are described in the text. The abbreviation for the fast muscular field $\mu = \mu_{run}^{(\max)}$ is adopted.

Before further advancement of the discrete-state similarity theory, it is noteworthy that when a theoretical concept is applied to the real animate systems, several precautions should be taken. The relevant perfect and imperfect qualification in the application of dynamic similarity to real animals was discussed by Alexander (1989). From the theoretical point of view, deviations from the "perfect" uniformity in the dimensionless determinants and the indicators of discrete dynamically similar states may be exemplified by weak body-mass dependence of the swept angle $\Theta_{run}^{(\exp)}$ $(= 0.60M^{-0.03})$ and the *relative body length change* $\varepsilon_{run}^{(\exp)}$ $(= 0.17M^{-0.04})$, revealed by the leg-spring model in quadrupeds and bipeds (Farley et al., 1993). The plausible reasons of deviations from the universality in dimensionless determinants of the similarity are (i) uncompensated external ground reaction forces and internal body reaction forces, resulting in deviation in body's rigidity, (ii) deviations from the condition of maximal locomotor efficiency and (iii) from the isometrically approximated scaling rules for muscle and bone masses with body mass. The latter effects are caused by small but finite mass allometric exponents (Prange et al., 1979) discussed in the problem of the primary locomotor functions of long skeletal bones (Kokshenev et al. 2003; Kokshenev, 2003, 2007) and striated and cardiac muscles (Kokshenev, 2008, 2009).

Following the original version of the dynamic similarity theory (Kokshenev, 2011), the similarity between equivalent discrete states established by the dimensionless determinants is also indicated by the uniform dimensionless scaling parameters, e.g., β, ε, or Θ, generally omitted in the scaling rules (e.g., Table 2). In the version of continuous-state dynamic similarity driven by continuous Froude variable, all other dimensionless parameters are also state-dependent continuous functions, e.g., $St(Fr)$, $\beta(Fr)$, or $\Theta(Fr)$. Following the concept of the unique similarity criterion (Kokshenev, 2011), each of these functions ambiguously determines the dynamic similarity between animals moving in certain gait. Hence, extending scaling relations from the discrete states to continues states, the omitted in Table 2 dimensionless parameters should be restored.

Using the basic definitive equations for resonant frequency and optimum speed (Table 2), one obtains the basic gait-dependent relations of the continuous dynamic similarity, namely

$$T_{res}^{-1} \sim \sqrt{\frac{\mu_{gait}}{\varepsilon_b}} L_b^{-\frac{1}{2}}, \; V_{gait} \sim \sqrt{\frac{\mu_{gait}}{\varepsilon_b}} L_{gait} L_b^{-\frac{1}{2}}, \text{ with } \varepsilon_b = \frac{\Delta L_b}{L_b}, \tag{3}$$

where L_{gait} is the dynamic length. In turn, two corresponding dimensionless numbers

$$Fr_{gait} \sim \varepsilon_b^{-1} \frac{\mu_{gait}}{g} \left(\frac{L_{gait}}{L_b}\right)^2, \; St_{gait} = \left(\frac{L_{gait}}{L_b}\right)^{-1}, \text{ with } \varepsilon_b \sim \frac{L_{gait}}{L_b}, \tag{4}$$

follow from Table 2, along with the relative static length change ε_b approximated here by the basic relation $\Delta L_b \sim L$, common in linear scaling theory.

When the determinant Fr is chosen as an independent dynamic variable of continuous similarity, Eq. (4) yields *muscle-field similarity function*

$$\mu_{gait}(Fr) \sim gFrSt_{gait}(Fr), \tag{5}$$

where the omitted numerical factor is not universal and therefore insignificant in scaling theory. Bearing in mind the experimental data (Table 1), the *Strouhal similarity function* $St_{gait}^{(\exp)}(Fr)$ and the *duty-factor similarity function* $\beta_{gait}^{(\exp)}(Fr)$ can be presented as

$$St_{gait}^{(\exp)}(Fr) \sim (Fr)^{-b_1} \text{ and } \beta_{gait}^{(\exp)}(Fr) \sim (Fr)^{b_2}, \tag{6}$$

where the exponents b_1 and b_2 (observed experimentally in Table 1) are generally constrained by the basic definitive equations. One can therefore infer that the dynamic similarity between animate systems is controlled by the scaling exponents of the gait-dependent similarity functions, determining continuous similarity. Using the experimental data for the exponents, one obtains a scaling prediction for the muscle-field determinant

$$\mu_{gait}^{(pred)}(Fr) \sim gFr^{b_3}, \text{ with } b_3 = 1 - b_1, \quad (7)$$

straightforwardly following from Eqs. (5) and (6).

3. Results and discussion

The continuous dynamic similarity theory is applied below to the data from running quadrupeds and bipeds (Table 1) on the basis of determinants (Table 2) already specified by the optimum-speed, crossover-gait (walk-to-run), and transient-run (trot-to-gallop) discrete states. The analysis is provided in terms of the continuous-state similarity determinants (Fr, St, β, μ) exemplified in Eq. (1) and in part in Eq. (2).

3.1 Quadrupeds including elephants

As mentioned,[1] the continuous dynamic similarity was first observed by Alexander & Jayes (1983) within the domain $2 \leq Fr \leq 3$ of transient trot-to-gallop dynamically similar states in running cursorial quadrupeds (Table 1). Following the authors, quadrupeds move in dynamically similar way, changing their fashion of locomotion at equal Froude numbers. The trot-to-gallop dynamic transitions were determined by the phase difference between the fore feet, indicating a transition between symmetrical (trot or pace) and asymmetrical (gallop or canter) modes of the run gait (Alexander & Jayes, 1983, Fig. 1). Although all transitions between mode patterns of locomotion are indicated by quantities at which one or more change discontinuously (Alexander & Jayes, 1983; Alexander, 1989, 2003), the *symmetry-mode transitions* are considered here as continuous, at least within the scope of relative stride length and limb duty factor functions, for which no abrupt changes were indicated. The continuous *trot-to-gallop transition*, associated in the cursorial quadrupeds (Table 1) with constant[1] $Fr_{trot-gall} = 2.5$, was re-discovered in quadrupeds (form a rat to a horse) by Farley et al. (1993) as shown in Eq. (1) and re-analyzed in Eq. (17) in Kokshenev (2011) by a number of scaling rules equally validating for discrete and continuous similar states (Table 2).

In contrast to run-mode transitions, a walk-to-run crossover in quadrupeds is associated with *discontinues* transient-gait states. In quadrupeds, excluding elephants, a gradual increasing of speed provokes abrupt changes in both the relative stride length and limb duty factors. These changes revealed in the domain $0.61 \leq \beta_{walk-run}^{(\exp)} \leq 0.67$ indicate the universal (mass independent) discontinues transition from a walk to a run determined by the dynamic similarity variable $Fr_{walk}^{(\exp)} = Fr_{run}^{(\exp)} = 0.40$ (Alexander & Jayes, 1983, Figs. 3 and 4). In Fig. 1, the scaling data on continuous dynamic similarity in quadrupeds by Alexander & Jayes (1983) are reproduced and the discontinues walk-to-run transition at $Fr_{walk-run}^{(\exp)} = 0.40$ is shown by *unstable-state* points 1 and 2 (shown by closed stars), whereas the continuous trot-to-gallop transition is shown by the *continuous-state* points 4 and 5 (shown by open stars).

In the case of cursorial quadrupeds, the duty-factor similarity function (Fig. 1) established for trotting and galloping quadrupeds by Alexander & Jayes (1983) is remarkably consistent with the trot-to-gallop continuous transition states statistically described by Farley et al. (1993) and shown in Eq. (1). These transient-mode states, likely first revealed by Heglund et al. (1974), suggest a stabilization of the characteristic Strouhal number (Table 3) unifying quadrupeds and bipeds within the domain $2 \leq Fr \leq 3$ associated with the continuous similarity pattern of

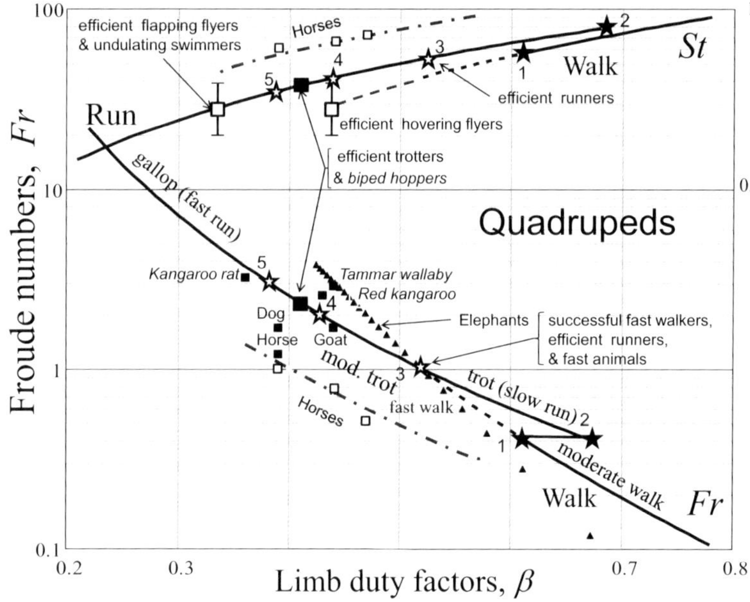

Fig. 1. The comparative analysis of the run-mode and walk-mode dynamic similarity functions in quadrupeds. The *solid lines* are regression data by Alexander & Jayes (1983) described in Table 1. The *dashed lines* are continuously extrapolated data. The *dashed-dotted* lines are the smoothed discrete-state data from trotting horses (shown by *open squares*) by Bullimore & Burn (2006) shown in Eq. (2). The *closed squares* represent those data by Farley et al. (1993, Table 1) for trotting quadrupeds and hopping bipeds (distinguished by *italic style*), which are limited by the experimental error shown in Eq. (1). The *open squares* tentatively represent the data on Strouhal numbers in cruising birds and fish by Taylor et al. (2003). The *closed triangles* are the averaged data from Asian and African elephants (Table 1) by Hutchinson et al. (2006). The open and closed *stars* indicate, respectively, continuous (stable) and discontinues (unstable) dynamic states. For more complete description of these and other characteristic points, see Table 3.

efficient trotters and hoppers (Table 3), evidently including the transient and optimal continuous states established at preferred trotting and preferred galloping speeds (Heglund & Taylor, 1988; Perry et al., 1988).

In the special case of trotting horses, the discrete-state data by Bullimore & Burn (2006), discussed in Eq. (2) and shown Fig. 1 by the open squares, are extended here by the data from a horse by Farley et al. (1993), as shown in Fig. 1 by the closed square. Although the smoothed data on trotting horses (shown by dashed point line in Fig. 1) coincide neither with the duty-factor function $\beta_{run}^{(\exp)}$ nor the Strouhal function $St_{run}^{(\exp)}$, which were suggested to be universal (Alexander & Jayes, 1983), the dynamic continuous similarity between trotting quadrupeds (excluding non-trotting elephants) and trotting horses can theoretically be established. Indeed, the corresponding smoothed lines in Fig. 1 are drawn by the same

Point	Mode states and patterns in animals	Fr	$St_{gait}^{(\exp)}$	$\beta_{gait}^{(\exp)}$	$\mu_{gait}^{(pred)}/g$
1	unstable walk in quadrupeds	0.40	0.57	0.61	0.55
2	unstable run in quadrupeds	0.40	0.76	0.67	1.10
3	efficient runners in quadrupeds	1.00	0.53	0.52	1.91
4	trans. moderate run in quadrupeds	2.00	0.40	0.43	2.90
5	transient fast run in quadrupeds	3.00	0.34	0.38	3.69
4→5	efficient trotters and hoppers$^{(*)}$	2.25	0.40	0.41	3.10
3	successful fast walkers (elephants)	1.00	0.49	0.52	1.00
1	efficient walkers in bipeds (birds)	0.52	0.48	0.64	1.00
1	unstable fast walk in humans	0.40	0.52	0.62	0.85
1	unstable fast walk in bipeds	0.45	0.50	0.63	0.93
2	unstable slow run in humans	0.60	0.49	0.46	1.00
2	unstable slow run in bipeds	0.55	0.50	0.56	1.00
3	efficient runners in bipeds	1.00	0.41	0.47	1.47
4	efficient fast runners in bipeds	1.61	0.35	0.43	2.00
5	successful hoppers in bipeds	4.66	0.24	0.33	4.00

Table 3. The characteristic points, determining continuous and discontinues dynamically similar states in different-sized and different-taxa animals, are analyzed on the basis of the walk similarity and run similarity functions from cursorial quadrupeds (Figs. 1-5). The predictions for relative force output $\mu_{gait}^{(pred)}/g$ are from in Table 4. $^{(*)}$The transient-state pattern introduced via Eq. (1).

$\mu_{gait}^{(pred)}/g = a(Fr)^b$	$a_{walk}^{(pred)}$	$b_{walk}^{(pred)}$	$a_{run}^{(pred)}$	$b_{run}^{(pred)}$	Discussed in
Quadrupeds cursorial	1.00	0.72	1.91	0.60	Fig. 2
Birds	1.73	0.84	1.57	0.69	Fig. 5
Humans	1.57	0.72	1.37	0.62	Fig. 5
Bipeds	1.65	0.78	1.47	0.65	Fig. 5
Elephants modern	1.00	0.82	1.00	0.83	Fig. 2
Elephants extinct	−−	−−	0.29	0.30	Fig. 2

Table 4. The predicted relative force-output similarity function determined in Eq. (7) and described in the text. The equations for bipeds are approximated by geometric mean of the data for birds and humans.[2] The data on the body mobility for extinct elephants are obtained with the help of Eqs. (13) and (14) in Kokshenev & Christiansen (2011).

scaling equations unifying trotting quadrupeds, namely

$$\beta_{trot}^{(\exp)}(Fr) = 0.4\beta_{run}^{(\exp)}(Fr) \text{ and } St_{trot}^{(\exp)}(Fr) = 1.6St_{run}^{(\exp)}(Fr), \qquad (8)$$

which differ in insignificant scaling parameters discussed in Eq. (6).

As mentioned in the Introduction, the revealed continuous dynamic similarity states is expected to provide further generalizations about movements of animals of different size and taxa. The continuous similarity patterns of *efficient flapping flyers* and *efficient hovering flyers* established within the domain $0.2 \leq St \leq 0.4$ for fast and slow flight modes by Taylor et al. (2003, Table 2) in cruising birds are schematically shown in Fig. 1, using, respectively, the run-mode $St_{run}^{(\exp)}$ and walk-mode $St_{walk}^{(\exp)}$ universal Strouhal functions from running and walking quadrupeds by Alexander & Jayes (1983). As the result, the theoretically observed *muscle* duty factor $\beta_{flap}^{(pred)} \approx 1/3$ predicting in turn the muscle timing $\Delta T_{flap}^{(pred)} \approx T_{flap}/3$ (see Eq. (9) in Kokshenev, 2011), indicates that the wing muscle, driving the flap mode in a flight, is activated during one third time of the cycle period T_{flap}. This finding can be explained by the three-step cycling of the flight-motor individual muscles in birds, as clearly revealed by workloop technics (see e.g., Fig. 3B in Dickinson et al., 2000).

Coming back to terrestrial animals, the dynamic similarity predicted by inverted-pendulum model for the *walk-to-run crossover* was expected to be determined by $Fr_{walk\text{-}run}^{(mod)} = 1$ (e.g., Hildebrand, 1980; Cartmill et al., 2002). Also, the universal discrete state indicated by the model-independent duty factor $\beta_{walk\text{-}run}^{(pred)} = 0.5$ (e.g., Alexander & Maloiy, 1989; Alexander, 1992; Usherwood, 2005) could be generally expected, besides the muscular transient field $\mu_{walk\text{-}run}^{(pred)} = g$ (Kokshenev, 2011). However, such a continuous-state transition has been observed neither in bipeds, including humans, nor in quadrupeds, excluding elephants. As indicated by the walk-instability and run-instability points 1 and 2 in Fig. 1, the fast walk mode is avoided by cursorial quadrupeds. But if the fast walk mode would conventionally be activated by the continuous extrapolation of the universal walk-mode similarity function, the desirable continuous *walk-to-run transition* might be theoretically observable, as shown by the dashed line in Fig. 1. Surprisingly, the hypothetical continuous transition was remarkably *in vivo* established by Hutchinson et al. (2006) in modern African and Asiatic elephants, through the dynamic similarity determinant $Fr_{walk\text{-}run}^{(exp)} \approx 1$ and the limb duty factor $\beta_{walk\text{-}run}^{(exp)} \approx 0.5$, indicating dynamic similarity in elephants during the fast-walk-to-moderate-run continuous-state transition. In contrast with other quadrupeds, elephants, having the hindlimb more compliant than the forelimb (Kokshenev & Christiansen, 2010, Fig. 5) are able to avoid abrupt changes in the mean-limb duty factor during the fast-walk-to-run dynamic crossover. Moreover, elephants, being good walkers, most likely can achieve gradually the highest instability point in the fast-walk trajectory of body's center of mass, indicated in the theory of similarity by the transient muscular field $\mu_{walk\text{-}run}^{(pred)} = g$. Hence, the transient similarity state, shown by point 3 in Fig. 1, unifying a gait-crossover transient continuous state in the elephants and a mode-transient continuous state in other quadrupeds, suggests two different patterns of similarity: *successful walkers* and *efficient runners*. The last pattern in quadrupeds is in addition indicated by the universal muscular field evaluated as $\mu_{run}^{(exp)} \approx 2g$ (for details, see Table 3) characteristic of more extent pattern of efficient fast animals, including fast running mammals, reptiles, insects; flapping birds, bats, and insects; swimming fish and crayfish, as reported by Bejan & Marden (2006, Fig. 2C).

When searching for continuous dynamic similarity states through the muscle-force field on the basis of Eq. (7), one obtains the scaling exponent $b_{run}^{(pred)} = 0.60$ using $b_{run}^{(exp)} = 0.40$ from Table 1, in the case of running cursorial quadrupeds. The corresponding scaling factor $a_{run}^{(pred)} = 1.91$ follows from the pattern *efficient trotters and hoppers* (Table 3) reliably established by Taylor et al. (1993) and employed as a reference point in Eq. (7). The resulted universal similarity function $\mu_{run}^{(pred)}(Fr)$ shown in Fig. 2 in turn predicts the data $\mu_{run}^{(pred)} = 1.91g$ failing for *efficient runners in quadrupeds* (Table 3).

In the case of *fast* walking (virtual) quadrupeds, the relative-force continuous similarity function $\mu_{walk}^{(pred)}(Fr)/g$ is obtained by a continuous extrapolation of the moderate-walk mode

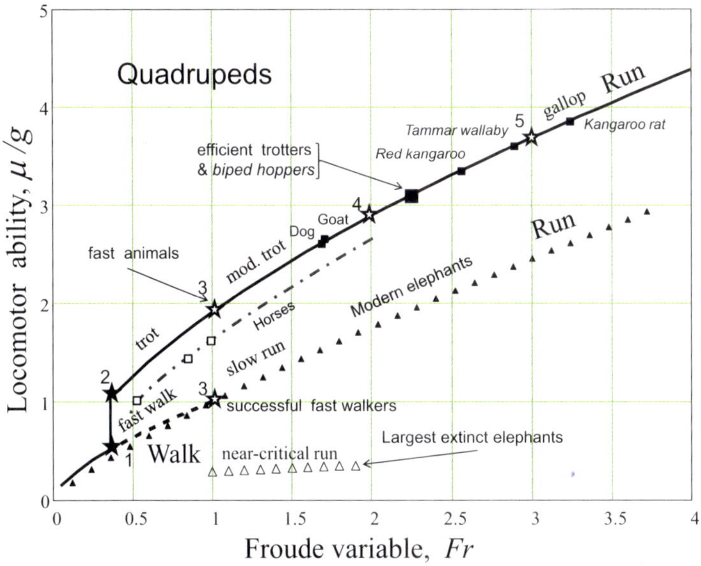

Fig. 2. Locomotor ability similarity function predicted for quadrupeds by the relative force-output. The *solid lines* are estimates for walking and running quadrupeds obtained via Eq. (7) with the help of the corresponding experimental data on the Strouhal similarity function (Tables 1 and 4). The *dashed line* extrapolates the data on slow-walk to fast-walk modes. The *dashed-dotted line* adjusted with *open squares* is a sketched estimate for trotting horses, also discussed in Fig. 1. The characteristic points and the pattern points are those shown in Fig. 1 and described in Table 3. The comparative data for bipeds are indicated by *italic style*. The *closed triangles* and *open triangles* are respectively the predicted data on the body ability in modern elephants and the body mobility in extinct elephants (Table 4).

to the fast-walk mode, where a transient state for the walk-to-run determinant $\mu^{(pred)}_{walk\text{-}run} = g$ predicted in Fig. 1 at $Fr^{(\mathrm{mod})}_{walk\text{-}run} = 1$ is employed as a reference point (Table 4). Likewise, in the case of slow running modern elephants, the relative-force similarity function is obtained on the basis of the data $St^{(\mathrm{exp})}_{eleph}(Fr)$ by Hutchinson et al. (2006) shown in Table 1, with the help of the same transient state in the walk-to-run continuous transition, also employed as the reference point determining the dynamic similarity at $Fr^{(\mathrm{mod})}_{walk\text{-}run} = 1$. One can therefore observe (Fig. 2) the dynamic similarity between poorly running (no trotting) modern elephants (shown by the closed triangles) and other hypothetical quadrupeds using the inverse gradient in the fore-hind limb locomotion function, common to both extant and extinct elephants (Kokshenev & Christiansen, 2010, Fig. 5). The data on low level *mobility* of largest extinct elephants (Kokshenev & Christiansen, 2011, Figs. 4 and 5), shown by open triangles in Fig. 2, are obtained by evaluation of the torsional and bending limb bone elastic forces, acting in running giants (Table 4).

3.2 Bipeds including humans

In humans, a discontinues walk-to-run crossover is generally observed at Froude numbers $Fr^{(\mathrm{exp})}_{walk\text{-}run} \approx 0.5$ (Thorstensson & Roberthson, 1987, Kram et al., 1997; Alexander, 1989;

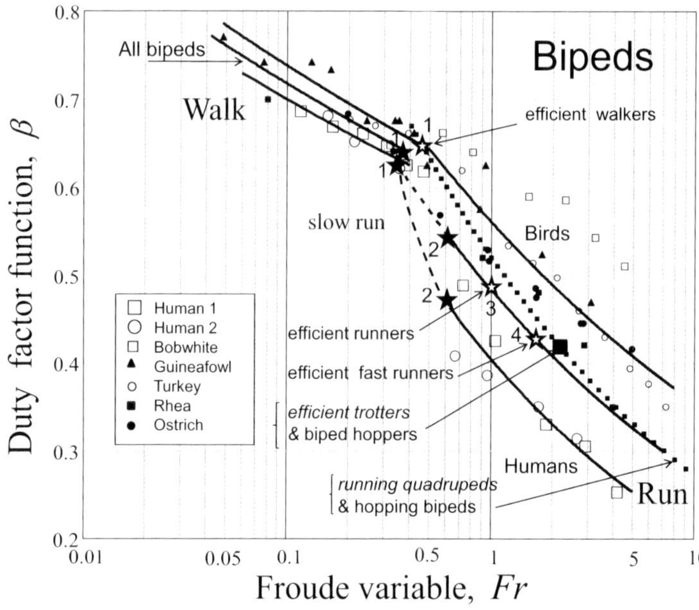

Fig. 3. The limb duty-factor similarity functions in bipeds. The *points* are the data by Gatesy & Biewener (1991) explained in the inset. The *solid lines* are statistical data from walking and running humans, birds, and bipeds as group (Table 1). The *dotted line* represents the continuous-state data from running cursorial quadrupeds (Fig. 1), excluding those for a slow run; other discrete-state data for quadrupeds are shown in *italic style*. The *dashed lines* indicate regions of the unstable slow run. The open and closed *stars* indicate, respectively, stable and unstable transient dynamic states. These and other patterns of similarity are described in the text and Table 3.

Ahlborn & Blake, 2002) and stabilization of the run mode is likely determined by the vertical component of muscular field $\mu_{walk\text{-}run}^{(pred)} = g$ (Ahlborn & Blake, 2002). Unlike elephants and other quadrupeds (Fig. 1), humans and birds expose similar behavior in a number of dynamic characteristics with changes in speed and gait (Gatesy & Biewener, 1991). Although a general consistency between patterns of gaits in humans and birds has been generally established, no clear characterization of the walk-to-run crossover was revealed (Gatesy & Biewener, 1991). The standard least squares analysis of the experimental data on limb duty factor and relative stride length (Gatesy & Biewener, 1991, Figs. 5 and 7) provided here (Table 1) is expected to shed light on the problem of the walk-to-run crossover in bipeds.

In Fig. 3, evident dynamic similarity between the walk modes in humans and birds is observed through the duty-factor similarity functions. Within the domains of continuous states (the solid lines in Fig. 3) treated within context of scaling relations shown in Eq. (6), the dynamic similarity between running humans and running birds can approximately be established on the basis of corresponding experimental data on duty-factor similarity functions (Table 3). As for the walk-to-run discontinues crossover in *bipeds*, the instability of walk modes generally occurs at Froude numbers $Fr_{biped}^{(\exp)} = 0.45 \pm 0.05$ (the closed stars and

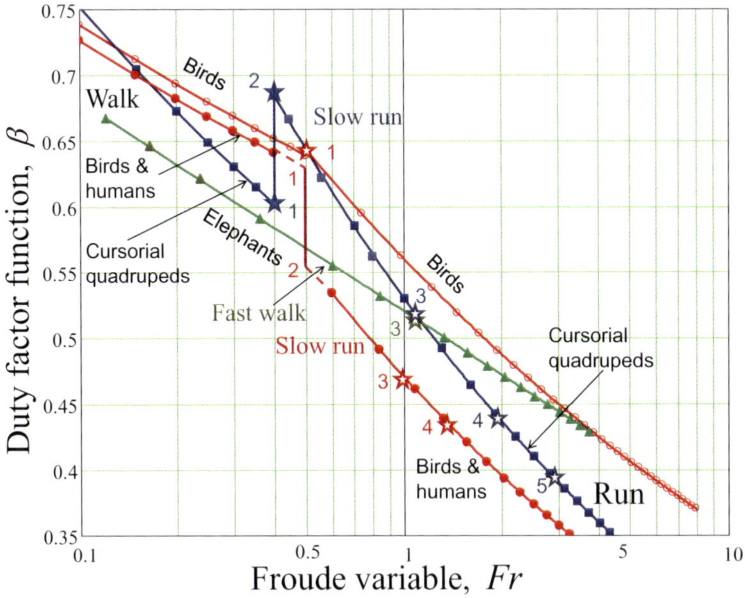

Fig. 4. The comparative analysis of the walk–to-run crossover in bipeds and quadrupeds. The *pointed lines* are the experimental data on duty-factor similarity functions (Table 1). Other notations are the same as in Figs. 1 and 3.

point 1 in Fig. 3), whereas the run modes show features of stabilization at $Fr_{biped}^{(\exp)} = 0.55 \pm 0.05$ (the closed stars and point 2 in Fig. 3). However, when the *birds* are presented by the smoothed experimental data, they exhibit a common point of dynamic-state stabilization determined by a kink in the duty-factor similarity function revealed at $Fr_{bird}^{(\exp)} = 0.52$ (the open star at point 1 in Fig. 3). Although elephants do not show such a kink at the walk-to-run continuous crossover (Fig. 1), the birds as group likely also exhibit a higher leg compliance than humans and most likely also may continuously pass the absolute instability point in the walk-mode trajectory (Kokshenev, 2011), as generally was expected by Ahlborn & Blake (2002) from the elastic-type-pendulum model considered at the conditions $Fr_{walk\text{-}run}^{(\text{mod})} = 0.5$ and $\mu_{walk\text{-}run}^{(pred)} = g$. Since the experimental scaling data on stride frequency in fast walking and slow running birds ($1/T_{trans}^{(\exp)} \propto M^{-0.178}$, Gatesy & Biewener, 1991) obey the scaling criterion of dynamic similarity (Table 2), a new similarity pattern *efficient walkers* may be suggested for birds continuously passing the universal walk-to-run crossover (Table 3).

Specifying the muscle-field similarity functions $\mu_{run}^{(pred)}(Fr)$ through Eq. (7), the continuous similarity transient state determined by $\mu_{run}^{(pred)} = g$ is adopted as a reference point, observed in starting to run humans, birds, and bipeds at $Fr_{run}^{(\exp)} = 0.60, 0.52$, and 0.55, respectively (Table 3). In order to obtain the slow-muscle-field similarity function $\mu_{walk}^{(pred)}(Fr)$ for birds, one uses a kink point equaling both the run and walk similarity functions. In the case of bipeds, the obtained run mode similarity function was interpolated to the corresponding walk mode (the dashed line in Fig. 3), providing scaling parameter in the desirable function $\mu_{walk}^{(pred)}(Fr)$. Then, the relevant data for humans have been obtained as the data adjusting these from birds and bipeds by the geometric mean (Table 4).

The discussed above features of duty-factor similarity functions obtained from walking and running bipeds, including humans, and quadrupeds, including elephants, are reproduced in Fig. 4. One also may infer that bipeds and quadrupeds, showing overall (qualitative) dynamic similarity in a walk and a run gaits, are also generally similar when showing the activation of a slow-run mode within the transient domain, approximated by $0.4 \le Fr \le 1.1$. The exception is not running in a classical sense elephants (Hutchinson et al., 2006), continuously exploiting a fast-walk mode during the walk-to-run crossover.

In Fig. 5, the *efficient fast runners in bipeds* (Table 3) expose transient universal dynamic states close to those in the efficient fast runners in quadrupeds (point 4 in Fig. 5), thereby indicating the universal continuous slow-run-to-fast-run dynamic transition in terrestrial animals. These two patterns are therefore represent the fast running mammals, which belong to the generalized similarity pattern of efficient fast animals (Figs. 1 and 2). Likewise, another dynamic pattern of the continuous fast-walk-to-slow-run dynamic transition is presented by efficient walkers in birds shown by the transient-state point 1 in the inset in Fig. 5.

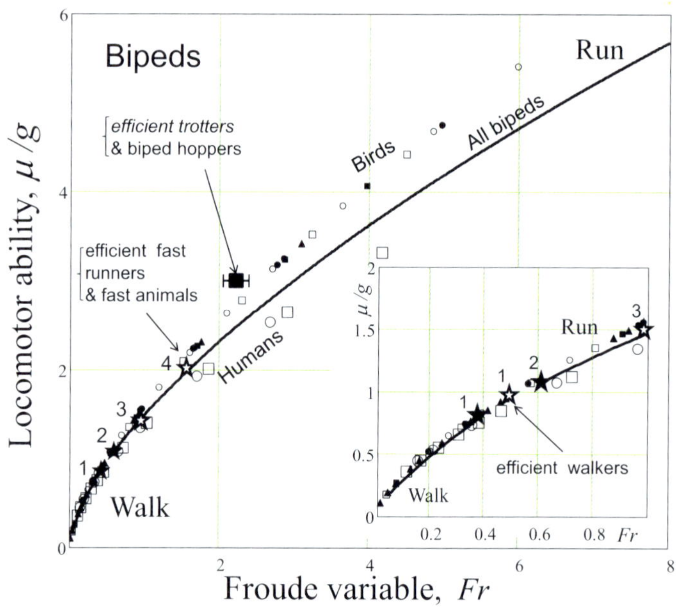

Fig. 5. The observation of the relative force-output similarity function in bipeds. The *solid lines* are the data on continuous dynamic similarity states from walking and running bipeds drawn by the corresponding scaling equations (Table 4). The *experimental points*, corresponding to those in Fig. 3, are drawn through the scaling equations for a run and a walk gaits in birds and humans (Table 4). The *characteristic points* are described in Table 3. The *inset* reproduces the enlarge data near the walk-to-run crossover approximated by continuous similarity states.

One may infer from the provided tentative analysis of continuous similarity states (Table 3) that animals patterned through the one similarity function can be observed slightly different through another one similarity function. Such deviations can be understood by the absence of the reliably established continuous similarity functions, as shown in Fig. 4. Further experimental studies of the domains of equivalent continuous similarity states in animals, moving in dynamically equivalent gaits, statistically searching for the similarity functions controlled by fixed scaling exponents, are needed.

4. Conclusion

Strictly speaking, different-sized animals are not geometrically similar. Moreover, different-taxa animals moving in a certain (slow or fast) gait cannot be patterned by the concept of dynamic similarity until the dynamic conditions unifying running, flying, and swimming are clearly established. In the case of terrestrial animals, when the experimental data from bipeds and quadrupeds, moving in two well distinguished (walk and run) gaits, are compared as two groups of biomechanical systems, no complete dynamic similarity neither inside of each group nor between the two groups can be established. Indeed, inside the bipeds as group, humans contrast to birds, since they are likely unable to explore the slow-run mode continuously near the walk-to-run crossover (Fig. 3). Likewise, cursorial mammals contrast to elephants, compared inside the group of geometrically similar quadrupeds (Fig. 1). When the dynamic similarity is considered between bipeds and quadrupeds, the crossover from a walk gait to a run gait does not occur at the dynamic conditions common to all terrestrial animals (Fig. 4). Less experimental data are available on locomotor mode patterns from flying animals and much less is known about swimming animals. One of the goals of the provided research is to clarify conditions of observation of the dynamic similarity in animals in light of the basic concepts proposed in theoretical biomechanics.

As demonstrated in the first part of this study (Kokshenev, 2011), the dynamic similarity in animals arises from the mechanical similarity existing between frictionlessly moving closed inanimate systems. When mapped onto efficiently moving weakly open dynamically similar biomechanical systems, the animals are conventionally represented (i) as dimensionless center of mass points, possessing a certain body mass M, (ii) propagating with speeds of amplitudes $V_{gait}^{(max)}$ optimized by the variational principle of minimum muscle-field action and (iii) accomplishing rotations at the resonant rate T_{gait}^{-1}. Within the framework of dynamic similarity concept, the geometric similarity between different-sized animals is introduced through the body static length L_b, related (isometrically) to body mass as $L_b \propto M^{1/3}$, that in turn introduces the geometric similarity between linear dimensions of all body's appendages (leg, wing, or tail). The dynamic similarity between animals is thus not due to nonexisting geometric similarity between body's shapes, but is determined by the dynamic-parameter similarity between the compared body's center of mass trajectories (Kokshenev, 2011). When attributed to the similarity temporal uniformity is already established by the resonant conditions, unifying moving animals across mass and taxa, the unique requirement, determining the observable similarity criterion, emerges as a condition of the linearity between the dynamic and static lengths, i.e., $L \sim L_b$, where L plays the role of the primary "geometric" parameter of dynamic trajectories. The accomplished uniformity in the spatial space of dynamic variables is therefore observed through the universal Strouhal numbers $S_{gait} = L_b/L$. Moreover, the scaling rules controlling the dynamic parameters of similarly moving animals are eventually scaled by the body static length, as explicitly shown in Eq. (16) in Kokshenev (2011).

In this chapter, the discrete-state theoretical approach to the dynamic similarity in animals is generalized to the continuous similarity concept on the basis of continuous Froude variable, playing the role of scaling (similarity) parameter. In the discrete-state similarity theory, treating the body mass as scaling parameter, the scaling rules for fundamental observables and some part of dimensionless universal parameters are the determinants of discrete similarity. Another part of dimensionless universal parameters, playing the role of the indicators of discrete-state similarity, is commonly omitted in basic scaling relations of the theory, besides other insignificant scaling factors. In the continuous-state similarity theory, scaling relations should be substituted by more detail dynamically equivalent scaling equations, because all dimensionless indicators, being functions of continuous states through the Froude variable, now turn into the functions of determinants of continuous similarity. Given that the only one determinant is necessary for the observation of dynamically similar states in animals, each observable function of the only one continuous universal variable can determine the dynamic similarity behavior. It has been therefore shown that the surmise by Alexander & Jayes (1983) on the existence of the gait-similarity functions, determining the dynamic similarity in animals at a certain gait, is generally corroborated by the dynamic similarity theory.

The dynamic similarity patterns established in the previous chapter for running, flying, and swimming animals considered in certain localized dynamic states, are re-analyzed here through the experimental data on continuous dynamic similarity functions established for walking and running bipeds and quadrupeds. The three well distinguished domains of continuous dynamic states in terrestrial animals are now suggested to be explored in animals across taxa. These are the domains of optimum-speed (preferred-run, -flight, or -swim) continuous states, the crossover-gait domain of (walk-to-run, hover-to-flap) transient states, and transient-run domain of (moderate-run-to-fast-run, trot-to-gallop etc.) transient states. The analysis of available experimental data in terms of the four-parameter set of determinants of dynamic similarity (Table 3) resulted in further generalizations in patterns of continuous similarity. One evidently generalized pattern suggests to unify efficient trotters in horses and other trotters in cursorial quadrupeds (Fig. 1). Less evident patterns of dynamic similarity are (i) the efficient trotters unified with bipedal hoppers (Figs. 1, 2, 3, and 5) and (ii) the efficient runners in bipeds unified with those in quadrupeds (Fig. 2) and with all other fast flying and swimming animals (Figs. 1, 2, and 5). Another one tentative pattern is proposed for the efficient flapping flyers in birds and the efficient undulating swimmers unified with efficient gallopers in quadrupeds (Fig. 1).

As a predictive preliminary theoretical result, the dynamic similarity function for locomotor ability in animals (associated with the related body force output) is suggested for quadrupeds, including elephants and bipeds, including humans. The locomotor ability in large quadrupeds is twice as many as that in giant quadrupeds, presented by African and Asian elephants (Fig. 2). In turn, the locomotor ability of the 3-5-*ton* efficient modern adult elephants is expected to be three-five times as many as the corresponding body mobility for 10-20-*ton* low-level efficient extinct elephants, running at critical conditions, when compared at close spaced Froude variables (Fig. 2). Likewise, the birds, humans, cursorial and saltatorial mammals show surprisingly close in magnitude muscle-field similarity (Fig. 5), which is twice as many as poorly running modern elephants (Fig. 2).

The discontinuous changes revealed in continuous similarity functions from quadrupeds and bipeds (Figs. 1, 3, and 4) can also be expected in the corresponding relative force-output similarity functions (Figs. 2 and 5). One may figure out that gait-dependent similarity functions in animals are generally piecewise functions, whose continuous-state domains are separated by discontinues transient dynamically similar states attributed to the gait-crossover transient states (Fig. 4). The suggested universal features revealed by continuous similarity approach challenge further experimental and theoretical studies of dynamic similarity in walking, running, hopping, flying, and swimming animals.

5. Acknowledgments

The author acknowledges financial support by the national agency FAPEMIG.

6. References

Alexander, R.McN. (1976). Estimates of speeds of dinosaurs, *Nature* 261: 129-130.

Alexander, R.M., (1989). Optimization and gaits in the locomotion of vertebrates, *Physiological Review* 69: 1199-1227.

Alexander, R.McN. (2003). *Principles of animal locomotion*, Princeton University Press, Princeton and Oxford, pp.53-67.

Alexander, R.McN. & Bennet-Clark, H.C. (1976). Storage of elastic strain energy in muscle and other tissue, *Nature* 265: 114-117.

Alexander, R.M. & Jayes, A.S. (1983). A dynamic similarity hypothesis for the gaits of quadrupedal mammals, *Journal of Zoology* 201: 135–152.

Alexander, R.McN. & Maloiy, G.M.O. (1989). Locomotion of African mammals, *Symposium of Zoological Society in London* 61: 163-180.

Bejan, A. & Marden, J.H. (2006). Unifying constructal theory for scale effects in running, swimming and flying, *Journal of Experimental Biology* 209: 238-248.

Bullimore, S.R. & Burn, J.F. (2006). Dynamically similar locomotion in horses, *Journal of Experimental Biology* 209: 455-465.

Cartmill, M., Lemelin, P. & Schmitt, D. (2002). Support polygons and symmetrical gaits in mammals, *Zoolological Journal of Linnean Society* 136: 401-420.

Ellington, C.P. (1991). Limitations on animal flight performance, *Journal of Experimental Biology* 160: 71-91

Farley, C.T., Glasheen, J. & McMahon, T.A. (1993). Running springs: speed and animal size, *Journal of Experimental Biology* 185: 71-86.

Garland, T. (1983). The relation between maximal running speed and body mass in terrestrial mammals *Journal of Zoology* 199: 157-170

Gatesy, S. M. & Biewener, A.A. (1991) Bipedal locomotion: effects of speed, size and limb posture in birds and animals, *Journal of Zoology London* 224: 127-147.

Heglund, N., McMahon, T.A. & Taylor, C.R. (1974). Scaling stride frequency and gait to animal size: mice to horses, *Science* 186: 1112-1113.

Heglund, N. & Taylor, C. R. (1988). Speed, stride frequency and energy cost per stride: how do thy change with body size and gait? *Journal of Experimental Biology* 138: 301-318.

Hildebrand, M. (1980). The adaptive significance of tetrapod gait selection, *American Zoologist* 20: 255-267.

Hill, A.V. (1950). The dimensions of animals and their muscular dynamics, *Science Progress* 38: 209-230

Hutchinson, J.R., Schwerda, D., Famini, D.J., Dale, R.H.I., Fischer, M.S. & Kram, R. (2006). The locomotor kinematics of Asian and African elephants: changes with speed and size, *Journal of Experimental Biology* 209: 3812-3827.

Kokshenev, V.B., Silva, J.K.L. & Garcia, G.J.M. (2003). Long-bone allometry of terrestrial mammals and the geometric-shape and elastic-force constraints of bone evolution, *Journal of Theoretical Biology* 224: 551-556.

Kokshenev, V.B. (2007). New insights into long-bone biomechanics: Are limb safety factors invariable across mammalian species?, *Journal of Biomechanics* 40: 2911-2918.

Kokshenev, V.B. (2008). A force-similarity model of the activated muscle is able to predict primary locomotor functions, *Journal of Biomechanics* 41: 912-915.

Kokshenev, V.B. (2009). Scaling functional patterns of skeletal and cardiac muscles: New non-linear elasticity approach,*arXiv:0909.1444v1*.

Kokshenev, V.B. (2010). Key principle of the efficient running, swimming, and flying, *Europhysics Letters* 90: 48005-1-5.

Kokshenev, V.B. (2011). Physical insights into dynamic similarity in animal locomotion. I. Observation of continuous similarity states, In: Theoretical Biomechanics, Vaclav Klika (ed.), pp. 267-284, ISBN 978-953-307-851-9.

Kokshenev, V.B. & Christiansen, P. (2011). Evolution of locomotor trends in extinct terrestrial giants affected by body mass, Biomechanics I: In: *Theoretical Biomechanics*, Vaclav Klika (ed.), pp. 49-74, ISBN 978-953-307-851-9.

Kram, R., Domingo, A. & Ferris, D.P. (1997). Effect of reduced gravity on the preferred walk-run transition speed, *Journal of Experimental Biology* 200: 821-826.

Marden, J.H. & Allen, L.R. (2002). Molecules, muscles, and machines: universal performance characteristics of motors, *Proceedings of National Academy of Science USA* 99: 4161-4166.

Perry, A.K., Blickman, R., Biewener, A.A., Heglund, N.C. & Taylor, C.R. (1988). Preferred speeds in terrestrial vertebrates: are they equivalent? *Journal of Experimental Biology* 137: 207-219.

Prange, H.D., Anderson, J.F. & Rahn, H. (1979). Scaling of skeletal mass to body mass in birds and mammals, *American Naturalist* 113: 103-122.

Taylor G.K., Nudds, R.L. & Thomas, A. L. (2003). Flying and swimming animals cruise at a Strouhal number tuned for high power efficiency, *Nature* 425: 707-710.

Thorstensson, A. & Roberthson, H. (1987). Adaptations to changing speed in human locomotion: speed of transition between walking and running, *Acta Physiology Scandinavia* 131: 211–214.

Usherwood, J.R. (2005). Why not walk faster? *Biology Letters* 1: 338–341.

13

Estimating Lower Limb Skeletal Loading

Timo Rantalainen and Adam Kłodowski
Department of Mechanical Engineering, Lappeenranta University of Technology,
Department of Health Sciences, University of Jyväskylä
Finland

1. Introduction

Osteoporosis, accidents and subsequent bone fractures cause suffering on an individual level, as well as an economical burden to the society (Ortiz-Luna et al., 2009; Stevens & Olson, 2000). It has been estimated that, in Finland alone, between 30,000 to 40,000 osteoporosis-related fractures occur annually and that 400,000 Finnish people have osteoporosis (Duodecim, 2008). There are a few potential ways of preventing bone fracture, i.e. strengthening bones and/or preventing falls (Ortiz-Luna et al., 2009; Stevens & Olson, 2000). In order to withstand prevalent loading without breaking; while remaining relatively light in weight to allow for locomotion, bones have the ability to adapt their structure to functional loading (Frost, 2000; 2003; Sievänen, 2005). It has been demonstrated that physical activity affects the weight bearing skeleton more than the non-weight bearing one (Mikkola et al., 2008), and it may therefore be argued that, the skeleton is loaded mainly by locomotory actions that impart strains on bones. Bones are loaded in daily activities by muscles accelerating and decelerating body segments and resisting the pull of gravity (Burr et al., 1996). Since falling is the single most significant bone fracture risk factor (Järvinen et al., 2008) and up to 90% of fractures are caused by falls (Cummings & Melton, 2002; Stevens & Olson, 2000; Wagner et al., 2009), exercise can be viewed as a potential intervention for fracture prevention. Exercise seemingly has a potential of both reducing the fall rate and also increasing bone strength. In agreement, exercise interventions have been shown to successfully decrease the fall rate (Kemmler et al., 2010; Korpelainen et al., 2006), to strengthen the bones and to decrease the fracture rate (Korpelainen et al., 2006; Sinaki et al., 2002).

It is quite obvious, that in some cases even the strongest bone could not withstand the loading associated with falling. Therefore, it is reasonable to question whether strengthening bones makes a significant contribution in preventing fractures. A prospective study has shown that people with higher calcaneal bone mineral density had lower fracture rate even while the fall rates between the groups were relatively similar (Cheng et al., 1997). The differences between the groups in bone mineral density were relatively large (~10%). In agreement, prospective studies have shown that increasing the amount of bone mineral with drugs by about 10% is effective in decreasing fracture rates (Cummings et al., 2009). On the other hand, the increments in bone mineral amount associated with year long exercise interventions are relatively modest, i.e. in the order of 1 - 2% (Nikander et al., 2010). There are examples of fractures for which this kind of relatively modest bone strength increase does play an important role. One of the most convincing examples is vertebral fractures. It has been shown in a prospective study that vertebral bone mineral density (represents bone strength indirectly) may be increased with back strengthening exercise program and that the higher vertebral bone mineral density is also associated with lower incidence of vertebral fractures (Sinaki et al., 2002). Furthermore, exercise induced bone gains may be more appropriately situated in order to maintain bone strength compared to drug induced bone gains. In case of drug therapy, the bone mineral amount increment is distributed rather evenly through the bone[1], while physical activity associated bone increments are situated mechanically advantageously (Leppänen et al., 2010; Ma et al., 2009; Rubin & Lanyon, 1984). In pure compressive or pure tensile loading, the geometry of the bone makes no difference to bone strength (excluding slender structures such as the ones found in trabeculae, which are susceptible to buckling). The only important cross-section parameter is its area. In bending and torsion, however, the geometry of the bone makes a big difference. As a rule of thumb, the further away from the bending/rotation axis the material is situated, the more significant contribution it makes to the strength of the bone (further details given under section 2.1) (Fig. 1). Coincidentally, the toughest part of bone is the external shield, which is also subjected to the highest loads.

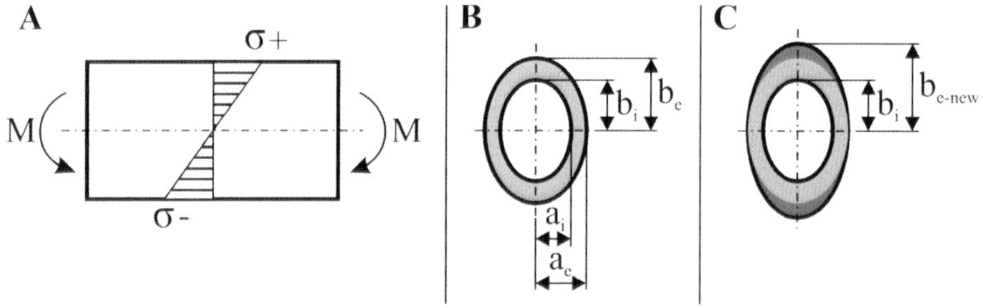

Fig. 1. A) Stress (σ) distribution in a bone subjected to bending moment (M), B) Hollow oval model of tibia mid-shaft cross-section, C) Possible change of tibia mid-shaft cross-section due to exercise.

Since exercise interventions are effective and feasible, how does one optimize the osteogenic loading of the intervention? Strains (Fig. 4) are one of the most important stimulants to bone adaptation Lanyon (1987); Turner (1998), and therefore designing osteogenic interventions could benefit from the knowledge of bone strains at different cross-sections in a wide range of exercises. General rules for bone adaptation are relatively well established, i.e.; bones respond increasingly with increasing 1) strain rate, 2) strain magnitude and 3) number of loading cycles (Lanyon, 1987; Turner, 1998; Whalen et al., 1988). In addition, loading direction affects the response, i.e.; unusual loading direction causes a larger response (Rubin & Lanyon, 1984). In bone adaptation, also the interval between loadings plays an important role. Bone responsiveness to loading decreases relatively rapidly, and dividing the loading bout into smaller bouts separated by several hours is more osteogenic than doing the exercise all in one bout (Umemura et al., 2002). If bone strains are known, the osteogenicity of loading may be

[1] At the moment of writing this chapter, we were unaware of a published article we could cite to confirm this statement. However, the FREEDOM study(Cummings et al., 2009) did include computed tomography measurements, the results of which were presented at least at the ECCEO-IOF11 congress held March 23-26 2011 in Valencia, Spain. Although not mentioned in the presentation, one of the authors of the present chapter was in the audience and queried the presenter (prof. Genant) afterwards whether the bone geometry had changed as a result of the intervention. As one might have expected for an anti-resorptive drug, the geometry had not changed according to the presenter.

estimated by calculating an osteogenic index, OI, (Fig. 2) (adapted from (Turner, 1998; Turner & Robling, 2003)) Eq. 1.

$$OI = \epsilon \frac{\delta \epsilon}{\delta t} ln(i+1)(1-e^{-t/6}) \quad (1)$$

Where ϵ is the magnitude of mechanical strain, $\frac{\delta \epsilon}{\delta t}$ denotes the mechanical strain rate in [Hz], i is the number of loading cycles, and t is the interval between loading expressed in hours.

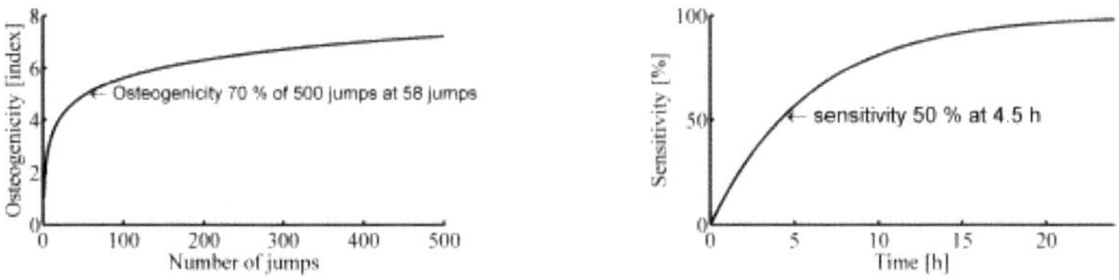

(a) Osteogenicity as a function of repetitions.

(b) Sensitivity as a function of loading interval.

Fig. 2. Osteogenicity of loading is linearly related to strain magnitude and rate, while loading cycle dependency and interval between loadings dependency are non-linear.

However, for human applications, bone strains are generally not known. Furthermore, measuring bone strains in vivo is invasive and limited to superficial bone sites (Hoshaw et al., 1997; Lanyon et al., 1975; Milgrom et al., 2000), thus not feasible in practice. Consequently, indirect estimates have to be used in practical applications. Since, intuitively there is an association between ground reaction force and bone strains, it has been suggested that osteogenic index may be calculated from reaction forces (Turner & Robling, 2003; Whalen et al., 1988). Subsequently, reaction force based osteogenic index has been shown to be able to successfully differentiate two exercise regimes producing differing bone responses from each other in a prospective human study (von Stengel et al., 2007; 2005).

Although, using reaction force as a substitute for bone strains is tempting there are some shortcomings of this approach which will be demonstrated later under heading 3. There are at least a few examples of osteogenic exercise interventions reported, where bone response has been observed on one bone of the lower limb (and spine), while other lower limb bones have not responded (e.g. Vainionpää et al. showed increase in femoral neck bone strength following a high impact exercise intervention in post menopausal women, while tibial mid-shaft bone strength was unaffected by the same intervention (Vainionpää, 2007; Vainionpää et al., 2005). While at first glance it may appear that the aforementioned is unexpected, the phenomenon may be explained by acknowledging that bone response is site specific. High impact exercises are characterized as high impact by the nature of causing high reaction forces. High reaction forces occur in exercises in which the lower limb is mainly compressed (e.g. above 10 times body weight has been measured under one foot in triple jump 2nd jump eccentric phase (Perttunen et al., 2000)), while the leg is straight. This kind of posture enables high reaction forces, since the inertia of the body is efficiently transmitted through hip, knee and ankle joint without the joints giving. If force is not transmitted through the joint centres, the joints give and reaction forces above 6 times body weight are rarely recorded (Ishikawa et al., 2005) even under two feet. In such situation the kinetic energy of the body is damped by muscles and tendons. Bone loading condition (compression or bending) has probably a major effect on bone strains in long bone mid-shaft (Heinonen et al., 1996). Consider a 41 cm long hollow cylinder with an inner radius of 6 mm and an outer radius of 12 mm (corresponds to the dimensions of a rather typical tibia). Should the other end of this cylinder be rigidly fixed and either an axial force (compression) or a perpendicular force (bending moment) with the same magnitude be applied on the other end of the cylinder, the latter would result in 50x greater maximal stress (or strain) at the outer surface of the mid-shaft (furhter details on how stress may be estimated in section 2) (Rantalainen et al., 2010). A force during a high impact exercise, which is compressive for tibia will most likely cause bending in femoral neck and therefore it is plausible that a difference may be observed between femoral neck and tibial mid-shaft bone adaptation (or lack of) following the same high impact exercise intervention.

1.1 Estimating lower limb loading with reaction forces

Several indirect methods have been used in estimating skeletal loading ranging from qualitative analyses to energy expenditure measurements. However, as per the title of the book, only mechanical loading estimates will be considered in the present text[2]. One relatively popular method to estimate loading, and thus strains, caused by locomotory actions on the bones is to examine the ground reaction forces or accelerations of the center of mass registered during these actions Jämsä et al. (2006); Turner & Robling (2003); Vainionpää (2007); Vainionpää et al. (2006). The advantage of measuring reaction forces or accelerations of the center of mass is the relative simplicity of the measurement. However, it is rarely brought into question if estimating skeletal loading from ground reaction forces is reasonable. Joint angles as well as muscle activity have a great influence on the loading of different bones and should be considered. In addition, diverse bone geometry and mineral content also have a significant influence on bone strains. An equal amount of force applied to different bodies will lead to different bone strains if the mineral amount and/or geometry of the loaded bones differ. The next evident step is thus to include the moment arms and joint angles into the calculations in inverse dynamics. This step, however, comes with an increase in the complexity of measurements as kinematics (i.e. movements of body parts in space) need to be recorded in addition to the aforementioned reaction forces. Furthermore the point of force application and direction of force needs to also be determined (detailed description of inverse dynamics is outside of the scope of the present chapter and detailed explanations can be found from other biomechanical textbooks, e.g. (Robertson, 2004)). However, even with inverse dynamics, the whole loading environment is not determined, since only external forces have been considered thus far. Muscles cause the movement of body parts in relation to each other and have relatively short moment arms compared to external forces. Therefore, the muscle (i.e. internal) forces are much higher than the measured reaction forces and neglecting these internal forces affects the loading estimate. This last step of estimating the loading environment is by far the most complex and includes arguably the biggest sources of error. Many muscles cross a given joint causing the same movement of the joint (e.g. soleus and gastrocnemii muscles plantar flex the ankle) making calculating the internal forces an overdetermined (redundant) problem, which means that there are infinite number of possible solutions of muscle forces[3].

[2] And are thought of being the most meaningful estimates by the authors in any case.

[3] We have ignored at least one resourceful way of estimating skeletal loading. A walking simulator using cadaveric specimens has been built (Peterman et al., 2001), which produces reasonable strain results. However, the problem of redundant muscle forces applies also to that application.

2. Stress and strain

It needs to be mentioned that loading, forces, stresses and strains are used somewhat interchangeably in the present text, while generally, forces, stresses and strains should be differentiated. Therefore, the remainder of the paragraph tries to explain what are the differences between forces, stresses and strains and why they should not be mixed. The relationship between the applied load (=force) and relative deformation (Fig. 4) caused by the load can be plotted as a load-deformation curve. The curve may be divided into two parts, the linear elastic region and the non-linear plastic region. The stiffness of the structure is the slope of the elastic region, yield is the load at transition from the linear to elastic region and toughness is the area under curve up to yield or failure (Fig. 3) (Currey, 2001; Martin & Burr, 1989; Turner & Burr, 1993). The load-deformation curve may be converted to stress-strain curve by accounting for the geometry of the structure and the loading situation. The strain by definition is the deformation divided by the original dimension. If the loading force is compressive (or tensile), then the stress is simply force divided by the cross-sectional area of the structure. In bending and torsion, the stress varies throughout a cross-section. The slope of the stress-strain curve in turn is the Young's modulus, i.e. stiffness, of the material. The strength of the structure is defined as the load at which the structure either yields (yield strength) or breaks (breaking strength, which equals ultimate strength in bone). As was the case with stiffness, the strength may be reported as a material property (yield or breaking stress) or structural property (yield or breaking load). Because of the anisotropic structure of bone material, Young's modulus and breaking stress are different in longitudinal and transverse directions. Furthermore, bone ultimate stress is different in tension, compression and shear. While looking at different types of loading: bending, compression and shear, it becomes clear that the geometry of bone is of utmost importance in bending and shear loading (Currey, 2001; Turner & Burr, 1993).

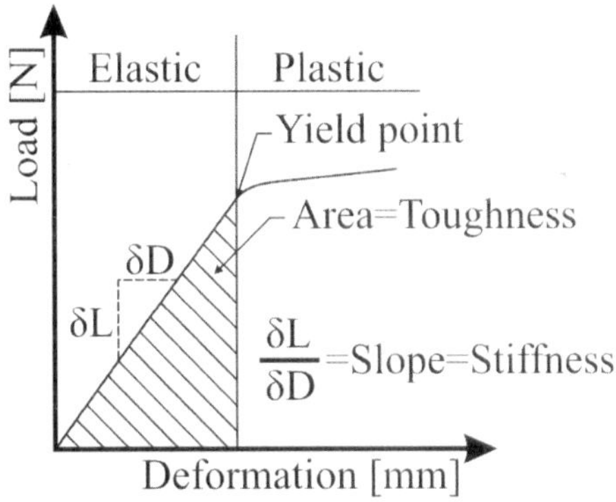

Fig. 3. Schematic illustration of a load-deformation curve.

2.1 Example of how geometry affects bone strength

Bending stress in a bone cross-section in a given loading configuration is determined by the second moment of area (also known as cross-sectional moment of inertia) of the cross-section as shown in (Fig. 1 A). Stress (indicated by the shaded area) is distributed unevenly throughout the cross-section, being by definition zero at the neutral axis and increasing its magnitude linearly while moving away from the neutral axis. The stress (σ) at a given point within the cross-section is determined by multiplying the bending moment (M) with the distance coordinate (y) from the neutral axis (dashed line) and dividing the product with the second moment of area (I) of the cross-section in relation to the neutral axis (i.e. $\sigma = \frac{M}{I}y$). This leads to the conclusion that the bending stress will be positive (tensile) on one side of the neutral axis and negative (compressive) on the other. In case of symmetrical cross-sections the stress magnitudes on both extremes will be equal. In case of a real bone it is rarely the case. Let's simplify the bone mid-shaft cross-section to a hollow oval with external radii a_e, b_e and internal a_i, b_i as depicted in (Fig. 1 B). The area of an oval is equal to πab, where a and b are the radii of the oval and thus the area of an oval ring is given by $\pi(a_e b_e - a_i b_i)$. If the area is increased by 2% in a way observed in association to exercise interventions, only b_e will be increased as shown in figure (Fig. 1 C). Therefore the following relation holds:

$$1.02 \cdot \pi(a_e b_e - a_i b_i) = \pi(a_e b_{e-new} - a_i b_i) \tag{2}$$

and can be transformed to compute the corresponding new external radius, b_{e-new}, with the means of following equation:

$$b_{e-new} = \frac{1.02 \cdot (a_e b_e - a_i b_i) + a_i b_i}{a_e}. \tag{3}$$

The cross-sectional second moment of area of a solid ellipse, I, is equal to:

$$I = \frac{\pi}{4} ab^3 \tag{4}$$

and thus for an elliptic ring, the second moment of area will be:

$$I = \frac{\pi}{4}(a_e b_e^3 - a_i b_i^3). \tag{5}$$

Lets assume $a_i = 0.5$, $b_i = 0.5$ and $a_e = 1.0$, $b_e = 1.5$, which if the units were in cm, corresponds to young adult men tibial mid-shaft. In this particular case the cross-sectional inertia prior to the intervention would have been $2.60 cm^4$ and after $2.74 cm^4$, which is a 5% increase. Accordingly the change would have lead to a 3% decrease in maximal stress. For further details on bone mechanics, please refer to pertinent literature such as prof. Currey's book (Currey, 2002).

3. Reaction forces and inverse dynamics in estimating skeletal loading

Lower limb skeletal loading (bone stresses) may be estimated with a combination of kinetic and kinematic measurements (Anderson et al., 1996). Kinetic measurements are typically the measurement of vertical and horizontal ground reaction forces e.g. during locomotion, whereas the kinematic measurements (displacements, velocities and accelerations of segments and respective angular equivalents of joints) are derived from the motion captured from the subject. The measured kinematics is combined with the measured kinetics in inverse dynamics to calculate joint moments. Judging by the apparent similarity of the patterns of ankle moment and tibial mid-shaft maximal principal strain in walking (Fig. 5), simply looking at joint moments appears to give a reasonable estimate of tibial mid-shaft bone strains. However, it needs to be remembered that tibia is also affected by the knee joint moment and the patterns of the knee joint moments differ quite markedly from the patterns observed at the ankle joint.

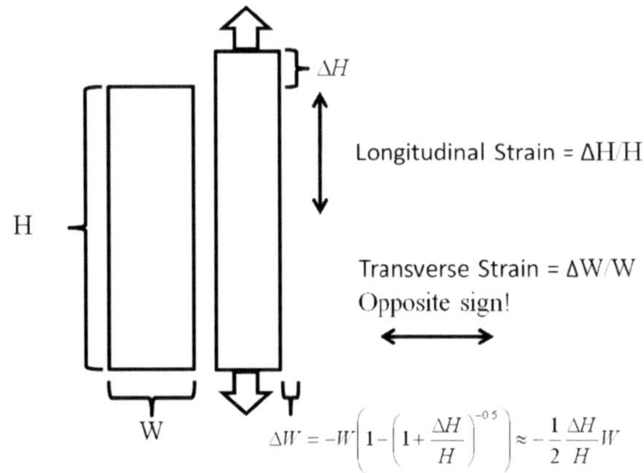

Fig. 4. Strain describes the relative deformation of a structure. If the rectangle (representing a solid structure) on the left is subjected to a tension force as indicated by the arrows on the narrower rectangle (representing the same structure under tension), the rectangle will deform. If the structure is incompressible, the width will change roughly half of the relative change in height but to opposite direction (remember that any given real life structure is three dimensional and volume is maintained if the structure is incompressible, i.e. Poisson's ratio = 0.5), i.e. the rectangle becomes longer but narrower. If the force was compressive, the rectangle would become shorter but thicker. In addition to being subjected to both tensile and compressive strain at the same point, due to being incompressible, the opposite forms of strain also cause shear strain at the same point. Unlike the example given, bone is compressible to some extent (cortical bone Poisson's ratio is somewhere between 0.2 to 0.4). Nevertheless, any given loaded point in bone will nevertheless always develop all forms of strains.

Furthermore, if one were to estimate the magnitude of bone stresses and strains, just calculating based on external forces, (i.e. joint moments), and neglect the internal forces (i.e. muscle forces), the stresses and strains could potentially be greatly miss-characterized (an example is given under section 4). Again, using tibial mid-shaft as an example consider standing on the balls of the feet. If the fact that the moments are caused by muscles were neglected, one would include only ankle joint moment and the weight of the body above tibial mid-shaft in calculating the tibial mid-shaft stresses and strains. However, since the ankle joint moment is in fact produced by the ankle extensors, the compressive and bending forces cause by the muscle activity should be taken into consideration instead of joint moments. Due to the ratio of contact point to ankle joint moment arm and ankle extensor muscles' insertion to ankle joint moment arm, the force required from the ankle extensor musculature is in the order of two to three times body weight (Finni et al., 1998; Ishikawa et al., 2005; Komi et al., 1992). Furthermore, bending moments and compressive forces load the bone in a very different manner and neglecting the muscles as the cause of the joint moment has the potential of greatly influencing the result (Fig. 6). Knowing bone stresses and strains in a single point is useful only to a limited extent and for most practical applications, the stresses and strains need to be estimated across the bone cross-section and at several points through the length of the

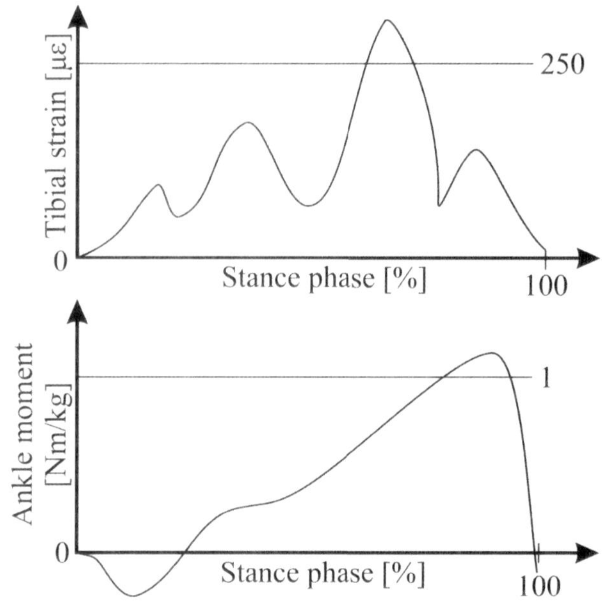

Fig. 5. Schematic illustration of tibial mid-shaft anteromedial aspect maximal principal strain (Lanyon et al., 1975) (upper pane) and ankle sagittal plane joint moment (Silder et al., 2008) during a walking cycle.

bone. Therefore, it quickly becomes evident that building models for individual applications, solving the muscle forces (which are redundant and therefore need to be estimated with some kind of optimization criteria) and calculating the stresses and strains is not feasible and a more general modelling approach needs to be chosen. Flexible multibody dynamics methods can be used as such a generalized modelling method.

3.1 Flexible multibody dynamics

Flexibility can be accounted for in a number of ways in multibody applications. The linear theory of elastodynamics can be considered a traditional approach to account for flexibility. This approach relies on the assumption of small deformations in the flexible bodies. Thus, rigid body simulation is decoupled with the deformation computation. The rigid body simulation is performed to obtain the external, as well as internal, forces acting upon each of the bodies. These forces are later imposed on the finite element model of the body for which deformations, stresses and strains can be obtained (Erdman & Sandor, 1972; Lowen & Chassapis, 1986; Lowen & Jandrasits, 1972; Turcic & Midha, 1984; Turcic et al., 1984; Winfrey, 1971). Standard multibody and finite element solvers can be used for this method, which is a great benefit. Additionally, a considerable increase in computational speed can be achieved if the force application points are known a priori and do not vary over the duration of the simulation. In such cases, the use of linear finite element analysis is reduced to a single computation of the full model. Strains, stresses and deformations can then be computed for each time step as post-processing. Conversely, the flexibility of the bodies does not affect the multibody simulation behaviour, which is the main disadvantage, especially in case of considerable deformations.

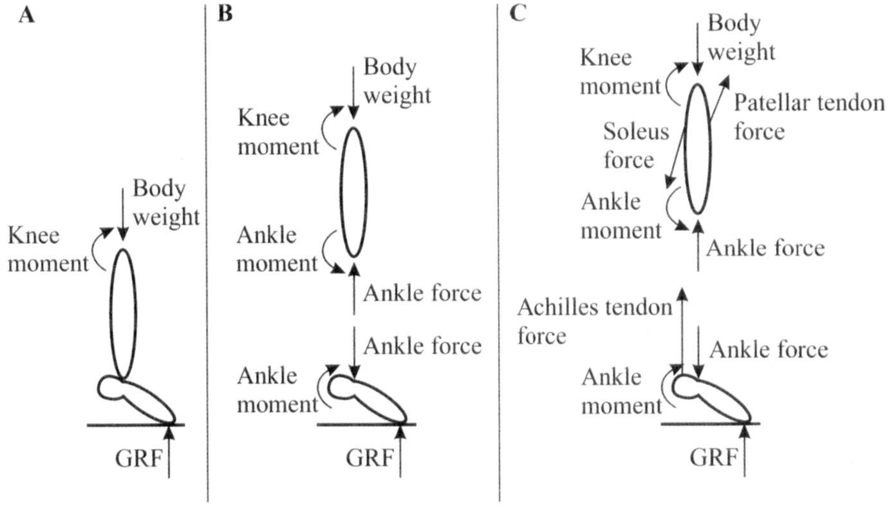

Fig. 6. Freebody diagrams for estimating tibial mid-shaft bone loading while standing on one leg on the ball of the foot. A) Forces accounted for when estimating tibial loading with just the ground reaction force, i.e. ground reaction force (GRF) and its counter force (weight of the subject). B) Estimating tibial loading after inverse dynamics. Compressive loading is accounted for by the GRF and bending is accounted for by the ankle joint moment. It is quite easy to imagine a situation, in which tibial loading is not proportional to ground reaction forces. Consider the situation in pane A and then imagine one standing with the ankle fully plantar flexed. In both cases the GRFs are the same, while ankle joint moment is changed (if one were a ballerina, the ankle joint moment could actually be made to drop to zero). C) Tibial loading is estimated from joint contact forces comprising reaction forces and muscular forces.

Lumped mass formulation is another method that can be used to describe mechanical flexibility (Hughes, 1979; Hughes & Winget, 1980; Huston, 1981; 1991; Kamman & Huston, 2001; Raman-Nair & Baddour, 2003). In this formulation, a flexible body is replaced by a set of point masses connected via springs. Using a sufficient amount of springs and masses allows for reasonably accurate mass distribution, within inhomogeneous bodies as well. Similar to the linear theory of elastodynamics, the lumped mass approach does not require that any changes be made in the standard rigid multibody solver. In contrast to the rigid body representation, the performance decays with the rise of discretization precision. Therefore, this method can only be practically applied to beam structures.

The third major method for introducing flexibility into the multibody formulation is the floating frame of reference (Shabana, 2005). Formulation relies on coordinate partitioning so that one set of coordinates is used to describe the flexible body's reference frame in the global coordinate system and another set of coordinates is used to describe the deformation of the body in the local frame of reference. Originally, the deformation of the body was described in a similar fashion to the finite element method, resulting in a remarkable increase in regards to computational effort. However, Shabana and Wehage (Shabana, 1983) have developed a solution to this problem by replacing the full finite element models of flexible structures with deformation modes description. This allowed for a reduction in the amount of deformation coordinates (in the range of thousands) to a reasonable amount of modal coordinates, making this method an effective compromise between accuracy and computational effort.

3.2 Modelling results obtained with flexible multibody dynamics in human locomotion

There is a relative paucity of dynamic bone loading modelling results in human locomotion in the present literature. One notable exception is the results from Anderson et al. (1996), who modelled femoral neck maximal stresses in several gym exercises. However, Anderson et al. (1996) reported bone stresses from only one location (i.e. the femoral neck). The floating frame of reference method with modal coordinates has been successfully applied in modelling tibial and femoral bone strains during walking (Klodowski et al., 2011; Nazer et al., 2011; Nazer, Klodowski, Rantalainen, Heinonen, Sievänen & Mikkola, 2008; Nazer, Rantalainen, Heinonen, Sievänen & Mikkola, 2008). When looking at femoral neck strain estimates and tibial mid-shaft strain estimates it may be seen that the timing of peak strains differ between these two bone sites. Remembering from the introduction, that literature reports femoral neck adaptation while no adaptation is seen at tibial mid-shaft following an intervention, it certainly appears that modelling based approaches of estimating skeletal loading may prove useful in the future.

4. Numerical example

To illustrate the differences between presented modelling techniques a simple numerical example will be presented. In the example axial stresses and strains at the mid-shaft cross-section of the tibia of a subject standing on the balls of his feet will be estimated. To make the example more realistic, the dimensions of the subject were taken from the LifeMod[4] database and correspond to a male whose height is 180cm, weight 80kg and age 24 years. In the example the subject extends his ankle joints by 20°, and tilts his body forward by 10°. In this condition the center of mass will be slightly ahead of the foot contact, which will add extra torque at joints to make the example more interesting. Only a right half of a lower body will be considered, meaning: pelvis, right upper leg, right lower leg and a right foot. To make simulation models comparable with hand calculations, which are based solely on ground reaction forces, location of the cross-section at which stresses and strains are computed is preserved together with it's geometry described by a polygon. All models share also the material model for the bone which for simplicity is isotropic and homogeneous, with Young's modulus of 17GPa (Dong & Guo, 2004) and Poisson's ratio equal to 0.3 (Reilly & Burstein, 1975).

4.1 Approach based on ground reaction force (model 1)

Let's start the analysis with the simplest 2D (saggital plane) model, which would be the most intuitive first choice (Fig. 7).

In the model the mass is concentrated in a point at the hip joint, represented by body gravity force, F_g. This location is close to the real center of mass for the human. At the same location stabilization force F_s is applied to constrain the model from falling. At the foot-ground contact point, ground reaction force is applied, for simplicity divided into normal, GRF_n, and tangential components, GRF_f which correspond to static friction. Knowing the mass of the subject, $m = 80kg$, we can assume for symmetric case, that the load carried by each leg is equal, thus:

[4] LifeMod plug-in for MSC Adams, version 2008.0.0, LifeModdeler, Inc., San Clemente, California, USA

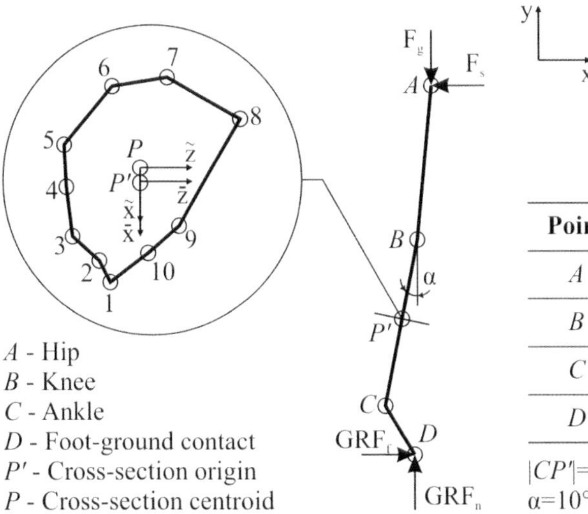

Point	x [mm]	y [mm]
A	-35.33	-24.84
B	-73.27	-416.69
C	-159.55	-840.22
D	-81.47	-964.11

$|CP'|$=225.76mm
α=10°

Fig. 7. Model diagram with tibia cross-section at which the stresses and strains will be computed with the use of ground reaction forces only

$$F_g = \frac{m}{2} \cdot g \tag{6}$$

where g is the gravity constant equal to $9.81066 \frac{N}{kg}$. The unknown stabilization, F_s, and friction forces, GRF_f, as well as vertical component of the ground reaction force, GRF_n can be solved from the equilibrium equations:

$$\Sigma F_{ix} = 0 \Leftrightarrow GRF_f - F_s = 0 \Leftrightarrow GRF_f = F_s \tag{7}$$

$$\Sigma F_{iy} = 0 \Leftrightarrow GRF_n - F_g = 0 \Leftrightarrow GRF_n = F_g \tag{8}$$

$$\begin{aligned} \Sigma M_{iD} = 0 \Leftrightarrow F_g \cdot (A_x - D_x) - F_s \cdot (A_y - D_y) = 0 \\ \Leftrightarrow F_s = \frac{F_g \cdot (A_x - D_x)}{A_y - D_y} \end{aligned} \tag{9}$$

where, A_x, A_y, D_x, D_y are x and y coordinates of hip joint and foot-ground contact point correspondingly. Substituting to equation 6 numerical values F_g can be obtained:

$$F_g = \frac{m}{2} \cdot g = \frac{80kg}{2} \cdot 9.81066 \frac{N}{kg} = 392.43N \tag{10}$$

Knowing the value of F_g from equation 10, value of GRF_n can be obtained from equation 8, yielding $GRF_n = 392.43N$. Substituting numerical values to equation 9, F_s can be solved as:

$$F_s = \frac{F_g \cdot (A_x - D_x)}{A_y - D_y} = \frac{392.43N \cdot (-35.33mm - (-81.47mm))}{-24.84mm - (-964.11mm)} = 19.28N \tag{11}$$

From equation 7 value of GRF_f can be expressed as: $GRF_f = 19.28N$. Knowing all the external forces applied to the model in the equilibrium, internal forces and moments can be computed.

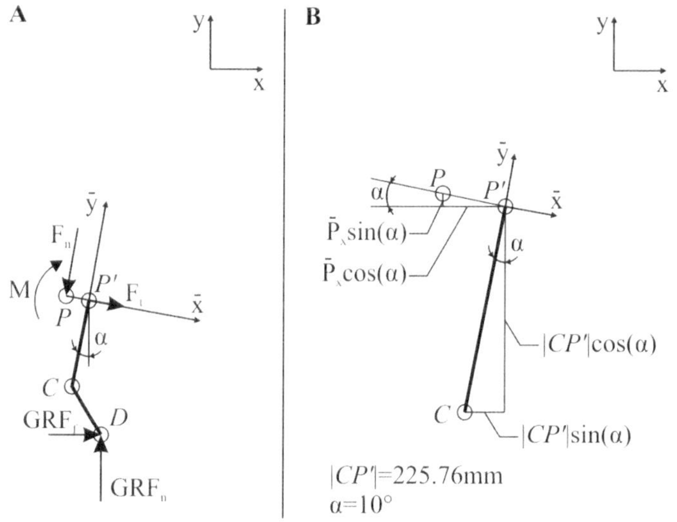

Fig. 8. A) Freebody diagram of the foot and lower part of tibia. B) Lower part of tibia diagram used for calculations of global coordinates of point P

The cross-section at which the stresses and strains will be computed is located at point P, as marked in figure 8. Solving of internal normal force, F_n, transverse force, F_t, and bending moment, M will be based on free body diagram depicted in figure 8.
Equilibrium equations for the bottom part of tibia and a foot can be expressed in the cross-section coordinate system $\bar{x} - \bar{y}$ for simplicity:

$$\begin{aligned} \Sigma F_{i\bar{x}} = 0 &\Leftrightarrow F_t + GRF_f \cdot \cos(\alpha) - GRF_n \cdot \sin(\alpha) = 0 \\ &\Leftrightarrow F_t = GRF_n \cdot \sin(\alpha) - GRF_f \cdot \cos(\alpha) \end{aligned} \tag{12}$$

$$\begin{aligned} \Sigma F_{i\bar{y}} = 0 &\Leftrightarrow -F_n + GRF_f \cdot \sin(\alpha) + GRF_n \cdot \cos(\alpha) = 0 \\ &\Leftrightarrow F_n = GRF_f \cdot \sin(\alpha) + GRF_n \cdot \cos(\alpha) \end{aligned} \tag{13}$$

$$\begin{aligned} \Sigma M_{iP} = 0 &\Leftrightarrow M - GRF_f \cdot (P_y - D_y) - GRF_n \cdot (P_x - D_x) = 0 \\ &\Leftrightarrow M = GRF_f \cdot (P_y - D_y) + GRF_n \cdot (P_x - D_x) \end{aligned} \tag{14}$$

Note that coordinates of points P and D are expressed in the global coordinate system due to the fact, that forces GRF_f and GRF_n act along global coordinate system axes. The resulting moments from those forces around point P are then computed as the force multiplied the moment arm, which is the distance between contact point and point P and is measured along axis perpendicular to the force direction. In this example we assume that moment has a positive sign if it results in clockwise rotation. In order to solve the equilibrium equations location of point P is required. Point P lies at the neutral axis of the bone cross-section. Thus at this point we will compute the cross-sectional parameters: second moment of area along bending axis, centroid location, and area. Bone cross-section is taken from the generic bone model generated by LifeMod. It is described as a polygon (Fig. 7) with vertices coordinates given in table 1.

Point	x̄ [mm]	z̄ [mm]
1	13.11	-4.1
2	10.29	-5.59
3	7.12	-9.23
4	0.67	-10.06
5	-4.84	-10.35
6	-12.45	-3.75
7	-13.61	3.68
8	-8.18	13.6
9	5.76	5.26
10	9.31	1.04

Table 1. Coordinates of the vertices of the polygon defining the cross-section of the bone

Area of a polygon can be obtained using the following equation:

$$A = \frac{1}{2} \sum_{i=1}^{n} (\bar{x}_{i+1} \cdot \bar{z}_i - \bar{x}_i \cdot \bar{z}_{i+1}) \tag{15}$$

where n is the number of points, point $n+1$ refers to point 1 as the polygon must be closed. Note that the equation 15 holds when the points are ordered in clockwise direction, for the anticlockwise order of points the minus sign has to be added. After computations the area of the bone cross-section is $A = 393.07mm^2$. Centroid y coordinate, $\bar{P}_x$, can be obtained from:

$$\bar{P}_x = \frac{1}{6A} \sum_{i=1}^{n} (\bar{x}_i + \bar{x}_{i+1}) \cdot (\bar{x}_{i+1} \cdot \bar{z}_i - \bar{x}_i \cdot \bar{z}_{i+1}) \tag{16}$$

Substituting numerical values to equation 16 yields $\bar{P}_x = -1.84mm$. Global coordinates of point P can be obtained from the geometrical dependencies depicted in figure 8B. Note that $\bar{P}_x$ is a coordinate of the point P with respect to point P′ not a distance (absolute value of a coordinate), thus sign convention in the equations 17 and 18.

$$P_x = C_x + |CP'| \cdot \sin(\alpha) + \bar{P}_x \cdot \cos(\alpha) \tag{17}$$

$$P_y = C_y + |CP'| \cdot \cos(\alpha) - \bar{P}_x \cdot \sin(\alpha) \tag{18}$$

Substituting numerical values to equations 17, 18 yields:

$$P_x = -159.55mm + 225.76mm \cdot \sin(10^\circ) - 1.84mm \cdot \cos(10^\circ) = -122.16mm \tag{19}$$

$$P_y = -840.22mm + 225.76mm \cdot \cos(10^\circ) - (-1.84mm) \cdot \sin(10^\circ) = -617.57mm \tag{20}$$

Second moment of area of the bone cross-section about $\bar{z}$ axis can be defined as:

$$I_{\bar{z}} = \frac{1}{12} \sum_{i=1}^{n} (\tilde{x}_i^2 + \tilde{x}_i \cdot \tilde{x}_{i+1} + \tilde{x}_{i+1}^2) \cdot (\tilde{x}_{i+1} \cdot \bar{z}_i - \tilde{x}_i \cdot \bar{z}_{i+1}); \tag{21}$$

where:

$$\tilde{x} = \bar{x} - \bar{P}_x \tag{22}$$

Substituting numerical values to equations 21 and 22 yields: $I_{\bar{z}} = 15008mm^4$. Finally, having all cross-sectional parameters, and most importantly coordinates of point P in global coordinate system, equilibrium equations 12, 13 and 14, can be solved for: bending moment, M, normal force, F_n and tangential force, F_t as follows:

$$F_t = 392.43N \cdot \sin(10^\circ) - 19.28N \cdot \cos(10^\circ) = 49.16N \tag{23}$$

$$F_n = 19.28N \cdot \sin(10^\circ) + 392.43N \cdot \cos(10^\circ) = 389.82N \tag{24}$$

$$\begin{aligned} M = {} & 19.28N \cdot (-617.57mm - (-840.22mm)) \\ & + 392.43N \cdot (-122.16mm - (-159.55mm)) = 18966Nmm \end{aligned} \tag{25}$$

Each point within the cross-section of the bone is subjected to stresses caused by the normal force, F_n, and bending moment, M. In mechanics tensile stresses are denoted by positive sign, consequently compressive strains are marked by the negative sign. Compressive axial stresses caused by the normal force are uniform within the cross-section and can be calculated using the following relationship:

$$\sigma_{F_n} = -\frac{F_n}{A} \tag{26}$$

Stresses caused by the bending moment vary within the cross-section with respect to the coordinate $\tilde{x}$. The relationship between point location and bending stresses is:

$$\sigma_M = -\frac{M \cdot \tilde{x}}{I_{\tilde{z}}} \tag{27}$$

Total axial strains are sum of stresses caused by the normal force and stresses caused by bending:

$$\sigma = \sigma_{F_n} + \sigma_M = -\frac{F_n}{A} - \frac{M \cdot \tilde{x}}{I_{\tilde{z}}} \tag{28}$$

Substituting numerical values to equation 26 results in:

$$\sigma_{F_n} = -\frac{389.82N}{393.07mm^2} = -0.99MPa \tag{29}$$

Strains are associated with stresses with a linear relationship called the Hook's law:

$$\epsilon = \frac{\sigma}{E} \tag{30}$$

Table 2 contains axial stresses computed at the vertices of bone's cross-section using equations 26, 27, and 28. In the last column of the table total strains are presented computed using the Hooke's law (equation 30). It can be seen that the posterior part of the bone is subjected to tensile strains while the anterior part is in compression. Bending contribution in the loading is dominating, which can be seen from analysis of table 2.

4.2 Inverse dynamics simulation (model 2)

Inverse dynamics simulation is similar to the calculations presented in the previous section. The main difference between the two approaches is the mass distribution within the model and complexity of the mechanical system. Moreover the inverse dynamics model, presented in this section, is three dimensional. This allows to account for bending also in the frontal (coronal) (and transverse) plane(s). In model 2 foot is attached to the ground by a revolute joint. Foot, lower leg and pelvis are interconnected via spherical joints, and pelvis at the center of mass is attached to the ground by planar joint in the sagittal plane. Stabilization force is applied at the center of mass of the body by a constraint restricting translation along the

Point	σ_{Fn} [MPa]	σ_M [MPa]	σ [MPa]	ϵ [μ]
1	-0.99	-18.89	-19.88	-1169
2	-0.99	-15.33	-16.32	-960
3	-0.99	-11.33	-12.32	-725
4	-0.99	-3.17	-4.16	-245
5	-0.99	3.79	2.80	165
6	-0.99	13.41	12.42	731
7	-0.99	14.87	13.88	817
8	-0.99	8.01	7.02	413
9	-0.99	-9.61	-10.6	-623
10	-0.99	-14.09	-15.08	-887

Table 2. Axial stresses resulting from normal force, σ_{Fn}, bending moment, σ_M, total stresses, σ, and total strains, ϵ, at the vertices of the polygon defining the cross-section of the bone

global x axis. In order to maintain the desired body position, ankle, knee and hip joints cannot remain unconstrained, thus at each of this joints torques are applied. In the presented case this corresponds to fixing the body segments together rigidly as only static case is discussed. However in the general case, where motion would be studied, those torques would vary over time in order to reproduce subject's motion. The model used in inverse dynamics simulation is presented in figure 9.

Models used in simulation can be more complex comparing to the simple mechanical calculations. For this reason natural mass distribution along with inertia properties for each body segment can be achieved. Reasonable guess of geometry and mass distribution can be obtained from LifeMod package. According to the subject specification the foot weight 2.14kg, lower leg mass is 4.19kg, upper leg's mass is 7.47kg and the upper body plus pelvis weight 52.4kg. As only half of the model is considered, the upper body and pelvis mass have to be reduced to 26.2kg to maintain symmetry conditions. Stresses and strains calculations could be performed in analogical way like in the model 1 using the multibody model just to obtain the cross-sectional bending moments and normal force. However use of flexible multibody dynamics allows to compute the stresses and strains directly at any nodal location within the flexible bone. To benefit from the flexible multibody approach, the rigid bone at which stresses and strains are to be computed needs to be replaced with it's flexible version. To obtain the most accurate results bone geometry should be reconstructed from medical images to correspond to the subject, however for this example just the simple shell geometry created by LifeMod will be used. After exporting the geometry from Adams[5], it can be imported to any finite element software which is capable of generating modal neutral file. For this example ANSYS 12 will be used.

In the finite element software the initial shell geometry is converted to solid body which can be discretized with solid elements. As in the model 1, it is assumed that bone is homogeneous, thus the whole volume of the bone is meshed with 5mm in size four-node tetrahedral linear solid elements. Each of the elements is assigned Young modulus of 17GPa and Poisson's ratio of 0.3. In order to perform modal analysis rigid beams are added at the distal ends of tibia connecting surface nodes with knee and ankle joint centres respectively. Craig-Bampton (Craig & Bampton, 1968) modal reduction allows to represent large finite element models with the use of several deformation modes, thus remarkable reducing the computational effort in

[5] MSC Adams, version R3, MSC.Software Corporation, Santa Ana, California, USA

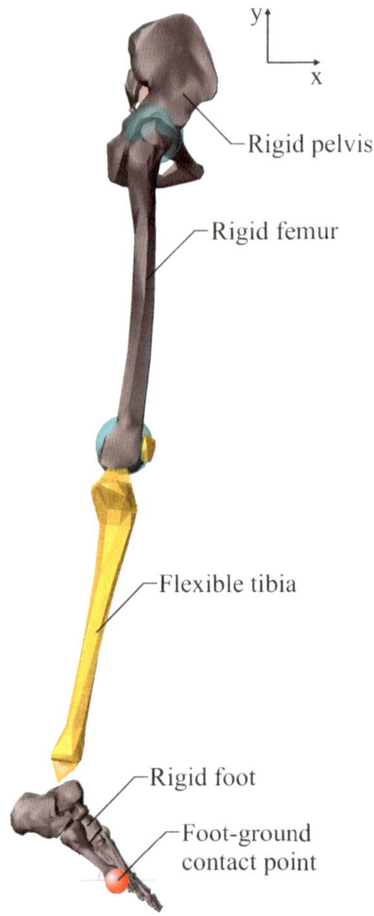

Fig. 9. Illustration of the three-dimensional model used in the inverse dynamics simulation. The model consists of four segments: foot, lower and upper leg, and a pelvis.

the simulation software. Knee and ankle joint center location nodes are used as boundary nodes in the modal analysis. For the current example 42 deformation modes will be computed. In the simulation however only 36 modes are usable, due to the fact that first six deformation modes represent rigid body motion, which is accounted for already in multibody formulation. Ground reaction forces obtained from the model are $GRF_n = 392.27N$ and $GRF_f = 20.50N$. Stress and strain results of inverse dynamics simulation with flexible tibia are grouped in table 3. Comparing table 2 containing results from the simple model with the current results it can be seen that stresses and strains are on average 1.43 times higher in case of a simple model. At the same time, both models predict same deformation mode of the bone, which is bending in the saggital plane causing compressive strains at the anterior site of the bone and tensile strains on the posterior side.

Point	σ [MPa]	ϵ [μ]
1	-13.04	-755
2	-12.14	-713
3	-8.38	-491
4	-4.05	-245
5	2.44	145
6	7.64	447
7	8.65	508
8	4.13	245
9	-7.83	-450
10	-10.56	-617

Table 3. Total axial stresses, σ, and total strains, ϵ, at the vertices of the polygon defining the cross-section of the bone obtained from inverse dynamics model

4.3 Forward dynamics simulation (model 3)

Forward dynamics simulation with the use of flexible multibody dynamics is based on the model presented in inverse dynamics example. However in the model 3, torque actuators at the joints are removed, and in turn muscle actuators are added. Muscle actuators are represented by straight line of action between muscle insertion points. The contraction of each muscle is controlled by the proportional-integral-derivative (PID) controller, which aims at replicating muscle contraction patterns obtained in the inverse dynamics. The model is actuated by 16 muscles: tibialis anterior, soleus, gastrocnemius medialis, gastrocnemius lateralis, rectus femoris, vastus lateralis, vastus medialis, biceps femoris (two actuators), illiacus, semitendinosus, gluteus medialis (two actuators), gluteus maximus (two actuators), adductor magnus. Muscle placement is depicted in figure 10. Adductor magnus is not visible in the picture as it is on the inferior site of the femur.

Forward dynamics simulation requires significant amount of input parameters, among them muscle contraction patterns, that are used as a reference signal for muscle controllers. The easiest way to obtain muscle contraction splines is the inverse dynamics simulation. During the inverse dynamics model is driven by the motion captured from a subject. In the example case, there is no motion, so during the inverse dynamics the model is simply fixed in desired orientation. After gathering muscle contraction splines, which in this case are just initial muscle length values, the forward dynamics simulation can be performed. External constrains are removed, meaning that the joints are free to move if no muscle force is produced. However support hinge at the foot, planar constraint at the pelvis and translation along x axis constrain at the center of mass are preserved.

Simulated ground reaction forces are: $GRF_n = 392.22N$ and $GRF_f = 20.57N$ for the vertical and frictional components respectively. Stresses and strains at the mid-shaft cross-section of the tibia are presented in table 4.

4.4 Summary of the numerical example

It is worth noting that the loading pattern obtained from model 3 is completely different to the ones obtained using models 1 and 2. Model 3 predicts that the posterior part of tibia is subjected to compression while the anterior part is in tension. The magnitude of strains and stresses is around 7.62 times smaller for model 3 compared to model 2. The differences can be explained by analysing differences in mechanics of model 2 and 3. The first one behaves like a rigid structure, where sagittal ankle torque is carried as bending moment by the tibia. Model

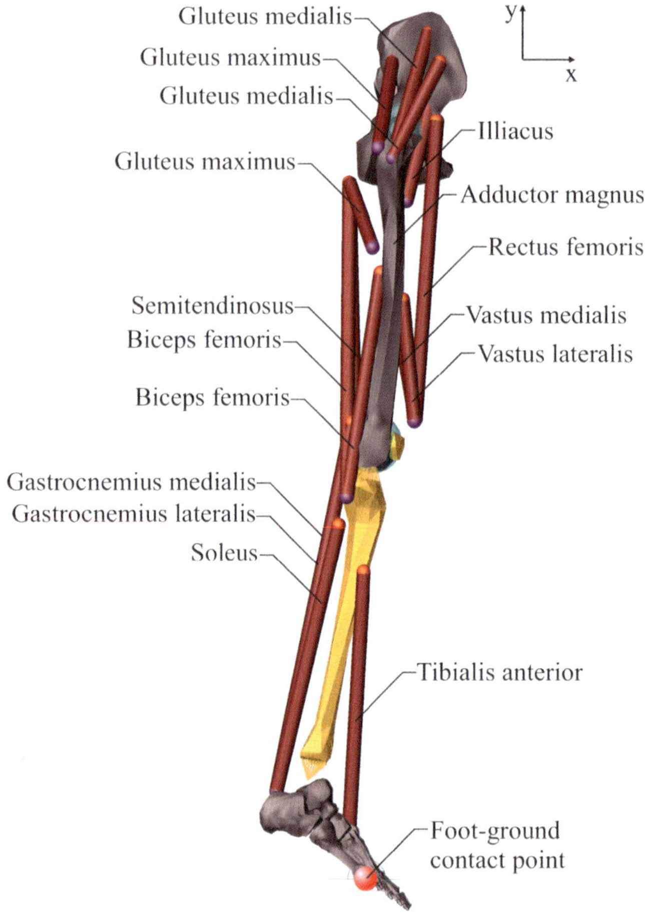

Fig. 10. Illustration of the three-dimensional model used in the forward dynamics simulation. The model consists of four segments: foot, lower and upper leg, and a pelvis; and fifteen muscles.

1 behaves the same way. Comparing the bending stresses at the considered cross-section to normal stresses one can notice that the bending stresses are up to 19 times higher than the normal stresses. In contrast, in model 3 tibia, foot and muscles create a mechanism. Due to the fact that ankle joint is almost frictionless it carries almost no torque at all, and the contact force is transmitted through Achilles tendon, and through ankle joint just as an axial and tangential force. Tibia is then subjected to only transverse and normal forces at the knee and ankle joints, and the bending moment comes mostly from the activity of soleus (545.72N), vastus lateralis (67.6N), vastus medialis (2.39N) and rectus femoris (0.08N) muscles. All of those muscles while contracting create bending moment which creates compressive strains at the posterior site of tibia. Tensile strains from bending moment actually reduce the compressive loading from axial force at the anterior site of tibia. This example demonstrates 1) that internal forces should not be neglected in estimating skeletal loads and 2) that muscle contraction can provide

Point	σ [MPa]	ϵ [μ]
1	1.08	60
2	0.64	37
3	-0.89	-49
4	-2.42	-137
5	-4.73	-275
6	-5.69	-333
7	-5.26	-309
8	-2.75	-164
9	0.19	6
10	0.57	31

Table 4. Total axial stresses, σ, and total strains, ϵ, at the vertices of the polygon defining the cross-section of the bone obtained from forward dynamics model

stress shielding for the bone Sverdlova & Witzel (2010). When it comes to the external forces they were predicted correctly by all three models.

5. Conclusion

Estimating lower limb skeletal loading may be useful e.g. in association to planning osteogenic exercise interventions. Although estimating skeletal loading from ground reaction forces is tempting due to the simplicity of the measurement, more information may be gained from more elaborate approaches. As was demonstrated by the numerical example, accounting for mass distribution in the model (as shown in model 2) can lead to 143% difference in strains. Further difference of up to 19 times can be noted when internal forces are considered in addition to external forces (i.e. joint torque actuators are replaced with muscle models). Even though all of the methods predicted almost identical stabilization force and produced the same ground reaction forces, internal loading was very different. For example in implant design only relatively realistic strain estimates may be expected to be useful. Implant loosening is a well known phenomenon (van Loon et al., 1999) and designing the implant in such a way that appropriate loading levels are attained can be therefore argued to be quite relevant. Furthermore, if a specific (for example clinically relevant) bone site is to be targeted with an exercise intervention, it may be necessary to the estimate the loading in a site specific manner.

6. References

Anderson, D. D., Hillberry, B. M., Teegarden, D., Proulx, W. R., Weaver, C. M. & Yoshikawa, W. (1996). Biomechanical analysis of an exercise program for forces and stresses in the hip joint and femoral neck, *Journal of Applied Biomechanics* 12: 292–312.

Burr, D. B., Milgrom, C., Fyhrie, D., Forwood, M., Nyska, M., Finestone, A., Hoshaw, S., Saiag, E. & Simkin, A. (1996). In vivo measurement of human tibial strains during vigorous activity, *Bone* 18(5): 405–410.

Cheng, S., Suominen, H., Sakari-Rantala, R., Laukkanen, P., Avikainen, V. & Heikkinen, E. (1997). Calcaneal bone mineral density predicts fracture occurrence: a five-year follow-up study in elderly people., *J Bone Miner Res* 12(7): 1075–1082.
URL: *http://dx.doi.org/10.1359/jbmr.1997.12.7.1075*

Craig, R. R. & Bampton, M. C. C. (1968). Coupling of substructures for dynamic analysis, *American Institute of Aeronautics and Astronautics Journal* 6(7): 1313–1319.

Cummings, S. R., Martin, J. S., McClung, M. R., Siris, E. S., Eastell, R., Reid, I. R., Delmas, P., Zoog, H. B., Austin, M., Wang, A., Kutilek, S., Adami, S., Zanchetta, J., Libanati, C., Siddhanti, S., Christiansen, C. & Trial, F. R. E. E. D. O. M. (2009). Denosumab for prevention of fractures in postmenopausal women with osteoporosis., *N Engl J Med* 361(8): 756–765.
URL: *http://dx.doi.org/10.1056/NEJMoa0809493*

Cummings, S. R. & Melton, L. J. (2002). Epidemiology and outcomes of osteoporotic fractures, *Lancet* 359(9319): 1761–1767.

Currey, J. D. (2001). Bone strength: what are we trying to measure?, *Calcified tissue international* 68(4): 205–210.

Currey, J. D. (2002). *Bones: structure and mechanics*, Princeton University Press, Princeton, United Kingdom.

Dong, X. N. & Guo, X. E. (2004). The dependence of transversely isotropic elasticity of human femoral cortical bone on porosity, *Journal of Biomechanics* 37(8): 1281–1287.

Duodecim, S. L. (2008). Osteoporoosi, *Technical report*, Suomalainen Lääkäriseura Duodecim.
URL: *http://www.kaypahoito.fi/*

Erdman, A. G. & Sandor, G. N. (1972). Kineto-elastodynamics – a review of the state of the art and trends, *Mechanism and Machine Theory* 7(1): 19 – 33.
URL: *http://www.sciencedirect.com/science/article/B6V46-482GN85-V/2/ad26341e4743520 3d04178013c171e71*

Finni, T., Komi, P. V. & Lukkariniemi, J. (1998). Achilles tendon loading during walking: application of a novel optic fiber technique, *European journal of applied physiology and occupational physiology* 77(3): 289–291.

Frost, H. M. (2000). Muscle, bone, and the utah paradigm: a 1999 overview, *Medicine and science in sports and exercise* 32(5): 911–917.

Frost, H. M. (2003). Bone's mechanostat: a 2003 update, *The anatomical record.Part A, Discoveries in molecular, cellular, and evolutionary biology* 275(2): 1081–1101.

Heinonen, A., Sievänen, H., Kannus, P., Oja, P. & Vuori, I. (1996). Effects of unilateral strength training and detraining on bone mineral mass and estimated mechanical characteristics of the upper limb bones in young women., *J Bone Miner Res* 11(4): 490–501.
URL: *http://dx.doi.org/10.1002/jbmr.5650110410*

Hoshaw, S. J., Fyhrie, D. P., Takano, Y., Burr, D. B. & Milgrom, C. (1997). A method suitable for in vivo measurement of bone strain in humans, *Journal of Biomechanics* 30(5): 521–524.

Hughes, P. C. (1979). Dynamics of a chain of flexible bodies, *Journal of the Astronautical Sciences* 27: 359–380.

Hughes, T. J. R. & Winget, J. (1980). Finite rotation effects in numerical integration of rate constitutive equations arising in large-deformation analysis, *Int. J. Numer. Meth. Engng.* 15(12): 1862–1867.
URL: *http://dx.doi.org/10.1002/nme.1620151210*

Huston, R. L. (1981). Multi-body dynamics including the effects of flexibility and compliance, *Computers & Structures* 14(5-6): 443 – 451.
URL: *http://www.sciencedirect.com/science/article/B6V28-47X8NJK-11V/2/5a675c9ea3c09 53ea466e0caaabb4861*

Huston, R. L. (1991). Computer methods in flexible multibody dynamics, *Int. J. Numer. Meth. Engng.* 32(8): 1657–1668.
URL: *http://dx.doi.org/10.1002/nme.1620320809*

Ishikawa, M., Komi, P. V., Grey, M. J., Lepola, V. & Bruggemann, G. P. (2005). Muscle-tendon interaction and elastic energy usage in human walking, *Journal of Applied Physiology* 99(2): 603–608.

Jämsä, T., Vainionpää, A., Korpelainen, R., Vihriälä, E. & Leppäluoto, J. (2006). Effect of daily physical activity on proximal femur, *Clin.Biomech.(Bristol, Avon)* 21(1): 1–7.

Järvinen, T. L., Sievänen, H., Khan, K. M., Heinonen, A. & Kannus, P. (2008). Shifting the focus in fracture prevention from osteoporosis to falls, *BMJ (Clinical research ed.)* 336(7636): 124–126.

Kamman, J. W. & Huston, R. L. (2001). Multibody dynamics modeling of variable length cable systems, *Multibody System Dynamics* 5: 211–221.
URL: *http://dx.doi.org/10.1023/A:1011489801339*

Kemmler, W., von Stengel, S., Engelke, K., Häberle, L. & Kalender, W. A. (2010). Exercise effects on bone mineral density, falls, coronary risk factors, and health care costs in older women: the randomized controlled senior fitness and prevention (sefip) study., *Arch Intern Med* 170(2): 179–185.
URL: *http://dx.doi.org/10.1001/archinternmed.2009.499*

Klodowski, A., Rantalainen, T., Mikkola, A., Heinonen, A. & Sievänen, H. (2011). Flexible multibody approach in forward dynamic simulation of locomotive strains in human skeleton with flexible lower body bones, *Multibody System Dynamics* 25: 395–409.
URL: *http://dx.doi.org/10.1007/s11044-010-9240-9*

Komi, P. V., Fukashiro, S. & Järvinen, M. (1992). Biomechanical loading of achilles tendon during normal locomotion, *Clinics in sports medicine* 11(3): 521–531.

Korpelainen, R., Keinanen-Kiukaanniemi, S., Heikkinen, J., Vaananen, K. & Korpelainen, J. (2006). Effect of exercise on extraskeletal risk factors for hip fractures in elderly women with low bmd: a population-based randomized controlled trial, *Journal of Bone and Mineral Research* 21(5): 772–779.

Lanyon, L. E. (1987). Functional strain in bone tissue as an objective, and controlling stimulus for adaptive bone remodelling, *Journal of Biomechanics* 20(11-12): 1083–1093.

Lanyon, L. E., Hampson, W. G., Goodship, A. E. & Shah, J. S. (1975). Bone deformation recorded in vivo from strain gauges attached to the human tibial shaft, *Acta Orthopaedica Scandinavica* 46(2): 256–268.

Leppänen, O. V., Sievänen, H., Jokihaara, J., Pajamäki, I., Kannus, P., Cooper, D. M. & Järvinen, T. L. N. (2010). The effects of loading and estrogen on rat bone growth., *J Appl Physiol* 108(6): 1737–1744.
URL: *http://dx.doi.org/10.1152/japplphysiol.00989.2009*

Lowen, G. & Chassapis, C. (1986). The elastic behavior of linkages: An update, *Mechanism and Machine Theory* 21(1): 33 – 42.
URL: *http://www.sciencedirect.com/science/article/B6V46-482GN2K-NK/2/4ab4249996dbf1be022bcf551d34f9cb*

Lowen, G. G. & Jandrasits, W. G. (1972). Survey of investigations into the dynamic behavior of mechanisms containing links with distributed mass and elasticity, *Mechanism and Machine Theory* 7(1): 3 – 17.
URL: *http://www.sciencedirect.com/science/article/B6V46-482GN85-T/2/037ade3ebbe869634d8d47cb9979d1fa*

Ma, H., Leskinen, T., Alen, M., Cheng, S., Sipila, S., Heinonen, A., Kaprio, J., Suominen, H. & Kujala, U. M. (2009). Long-term leisure time physical activity and properties of bone: A twin study, *Journal of Bone and Mineral Research* .

Martin, R. B. & Burr, D. B. (1989). *Structure, function, and adaptation of compact bone*, Raven Press, New York.

Mikkola, T. M., Sipilä, S., Rantanen, T., Sievänen, H., Suominen, H., Kaprio, J., Koskenvuo, M., Kauppinen, M. & Heinonen, A. (2008). Genetic and environmental influence on structural strength of weight-bearing and non-weight-bearing bone: a twin study, *Journal of Bone and Mineral Research* 23(4): 492–498.

Milgrom, C., Finestone, A., Levi, Y., Simkin, A., Ekenman, I., Mendelson, S., Millgram, M., Nyska, M., Benjuya, N. & Burr, D. (2000). Do high impact exercises produce higher tibial strains than running?, *British journal of sports medicine* 34(3): 195–199.

Nazer, R. A., Klodowski, A., Rantalainen, T., Heinonen, A., Sievanen, H. & Mikkola, A. (2011). A full body musculoskeletal model based on flexible multibody simulation approach utilised in bone strain anaflysis during human locomotion., *Comput Methods Biomech Biomed Engin* p. 1.
URL: *http://dx.doi.org/10.1080/10255842.2010.488223*

Nazer, R. A., Klodowski, A., Rantalainen, T., Heinonen, A., Sievänen, H. & Mikkola, A. (2008). Analysis of dynamic strains in tibia during human locomotion based on flexible multibody approach integrated with magnetic resonance imaging technique, *Multibody System Dynamics* 20: 287–306.
URL: *http://dx.doi.org/10.1007/s11044-008-9120-8*

Nazer, R. A., Rantalainen, T., Heinonen, A., Sievänen, H. & Mikkola, A. (2008). Flexible multibody simulation approach in the analysis of tibial strain during walking, *Journal of Biomechanics* 41(5): 1036–1043.

Nikander, R., Sievänen, H., Heinonen, A., Daly, R. M., Uusi-Rasi, K. & Kannus, P. (2010). Targeted exercise against osteoporosis: A systematic review and meta-analysis for optimising bone strength throughout life., *BMC Med* 8: 47.
URL: *http://dx.doi.org/10.1186/1741-7015-8-47*

Ortiz-Luna, G., Garcia-Hernandez, P. & Tamayo-Orozco, J. A. (2009). Treatment options for osteoporosis and decision making criteria: 2009, *Salud publica de Mexico* 51 Suppl 1: S114–25.

Perttunen, J. O., Kyröläinen, H., Komi, P. V. & Heinonen, A. (2000). Biomechanical loading in the triple jump, *Journal of sports sciences* 18(5): 363–370.

Peterman, M. M., Hamel, A. J., Cavanagh, P. R., Piazza, S. J. & Sharkey, N. A. (2001). In vitro modeling of human tibial strains during exercise in micro-gravity, *Journal of Biomechanics* 34(5): 693–698.

Raman-Nair, W. & Baddour, R. (2003). Three-dimensional dynamics of a flexible marine riser undergoing large elastic deformations, *Multibody System Dynamics* 10: 393–423.
URL: *http://dx.doi.org/10.1023/A:1026213630987*

Rantalainen, T., Nikander, R., Heinonen, A., Suominen, H. & Sievanen, H. (2010). Direction-specific diaphyseal geometry and mineral mass distribution of tibia and fibula: A pqct study of female athletes representing different exercise loading types, *Calcified tissue international* 86(6): 447–454.

Reilly, D. T. & Burstein, A. H. (1975). The elastic and ultimate properties of compact bone tissue, *Journal of Biomechanics* 8(6): 393–405.

Robertson, D. G. E. (2004). *Research methods in biomechanics*, Human Kinetics, Champaign, IL :. URL: *http://www.loc.gov/catdir/toc/ecip0414/2004002355.html*

Rubin, C. T. & Lanyon, L. E. (1984). Regulation of bone formation by applied dynamic loads, *Journal of Bone and Joint Surgery. American volume* 66(3): 397–402.

Shabana, A. A. (2005). *Dynamics of multibody systems*, Cambridge University Press, Cambridge :. URL: *http://libtest.csc.fi:8991/F/?func=direct&doc_number=002760407&local_base=fin01*

Shabana, A. A.; Wehage, R. A. (1983). Coordinate reduction technique for transient analysis of spatial substructures with large angular rotations, *Journal of Structural Mechanics* 11(3): 401–431.

Sievänen, H. (2005). Hormonal influences on the muscle-bone feedback system: a perspective, *Journal of Musculoskeletal & Neuronal Interactions* 5(3): 255–261.

Silder, A., Heiderscheit, B. & Thelen, D. G. (2008). Active and passive contributions to joint kinetics during walking in older adults, *Journal of Biomechanics* 41(7): 1520–1527.

Sinaki, M., Itoi, E., Wahner, H. W., Wollan, P., Gelzcer, R., Mullan, B. P., Collins, D. A. & Hodgson, S. F. (2002). Stronger back muscles reduce the incidence of vertebral fractures: a prospective 10 year follow-up of postmenopausal women., *Bone* 30(6): 836–841.

Stevens, J. A. & Olson, S. (2000). Reducing falls and resulting hip fractures among older women, *MMWR Recomm Rep.* 49(RR-2): 3–12.

Sverdlova, N. S. & Witzel, U. (2010). Principles of determination and verification of muscle forces in the human musculoskeletal system: Muscle forces to minimise bending stress, *Journal of Biomechanics* 43(3): 387–396.

Turcic, D. A. & Midha, A. (1984). Dynamic analysis of elastic mechanism systems. part i: Applications, *Journal of Dynamic Systems, Measurement, and Control* 106(4): 249–254. URL: *http://link.aip.org/link/?JDS/106/249/1*

Turcic, D. A., Midha, A. & Bosnik, J. R. (1984). Dynamic analysis of elastic mechanism systems. part ii: Experimental results, *Journal of Dynamic Systems, Measurement, and Control* 106(4): 255–260. URL: *http://link.aip.org/link/?JDS/106/255/1*

Turner, C. H. (1998). Three rules for bone adaptation to mechanical stimuli, *Bone* 23(5): 399–407.

Turner, C. H. & Burr, D. B. (1993). Basic biomechanical measurements of bone: a tutorial, *Bone* 14(4): 595–608.

Turner, C. H. & Robling, A. G. (2003). Designing exercise regimens to increase bone strength, *Exercise and sport sciences reviews* 31(1): 45–50.

Umemura, Y., Sogo, N. & Honda, A. (2002). Effects of intervals between jumps or bouts on osteogenic response to loading, *Journal of Applied Physiology* 93(4): 1345–1348.

Vainionpää, A. (2007). Bone adaptation to impact loading : significance of loading intensity.

Vainionpää, A., Korpelainen, R., Leppäluoto, J. & Jämsä, T. (2005). Effects of high-impact exercise on bone mineral density: a randomized controlled trial in premenopausal women, *Osteoporosis International* 16(2): 191–197.

Vainionpää, A., Korpelainen, R., Vihriälä, E., Rinta-Paavola, A., Leppäluoto, J. & Jämsä, T. (2006). Intensity of exercise is associated with bone density change in premenopausal women, *Osteoporosis International* 17(3): 455–463.

van Loon, C. J., de Waal Malefijt, M. C., Buma, P., Verdonschot, N. & Veth, R. P. (1999). Femoral bone loss in total knee arthroplasty. a review, *Acta Orthopaedica Belgica* 65(2): 154–163.

von Stengel, S., Kemmler, W., Kalender, W. A., Engelke, K. & Lauber, D. (2007). Differential effects of strength versus power training on bone mineral density in postmenopausal women: a 2-year longitudinal study, *British journal of sports medicine* 41(10): 649–55; discussion 655.

von Stengel, S., Kemmler, W., Pintag, R., Beeskow, C., Weineck, J., Lauber, D., Kalender, W. A. & Engelke, K. (2005). Power training is more effective than strength training for maintaining bone mineral density in postmenopausal women, *Journal of Applied Physiology* 99(1): 181–188.

Wagner, H., Melhus, H., Gedeborg, R., Pedersen, N. L. & Michaelsson, K. (2009). Simply ask them about their balance–future fracture risk in a nationwide cohort study of twins, *American Journal of Epidemiology* 169(2): 143–149.

Whalen, R. T., Carter, D. R. & Steele, C. R. (1988). Influence of physical activity on the regulation of bone density, *Journal of Biomechanics* 21(10): 825–837.

Winfrey, R. C. (1971). Elastic link mechanism dynamics, *Journal of Engineering for Industry* 93(1): 268–272.
URL: *http://link.aip.org/link/?MSE/93/268/1*

14

Induced Acceleration Analysis of Three-Dimensional Multi-Joint Movements and Its Application to Sports Movements

Masaya Hirashima
Graduate School of Education, The University of Tokyo
Japan

1. Introduction

A knowledge of how muscle forces produce joint rotations is fundamental in all fields of human movement science, including rehabilitation and sports biomechanics. Such knowledge is necessary for improving the diagnosis and treatment of persons with movement disabilities and analyzing the techniques used by high-performance athletes (Zajac and Gordon, 1989). However, it is difficult to intuitively understand how muscle forces produce joint rotations in multi-joint movements because of the complexity of inter-joint interactions, especially in three-dimensional (3D) movements. Therefore, although muscle activities, joint torques, and joint rotations themselves have been examined extensively in many sports movements (Barrentine et al., 1998; Elliott et al., 2003; Feltner and Dapena, 1986; Fleisig et al., 1995; Fleisig et al., 1996b; Glousman et al., 1988; Hirashima et al., 2002; Marshall and Elliott, 2000; Matsuo et al., 2001; Nunome et al., 2002; Putnam, 1991; Sakurai et al., 1993; Sakurai and Ohtsuki, 2000; Sprigings et al., 1994), the knowledge about the cause-and-effect relationships between these variables is insufficient.

The purpose of this chapter is to provide the framework to properly understand the cause-and-effect relationship between joint torques and rotations during sports movements. In fast sports movements such as baseball pitching and soccer kicking, joint rotations occur sequentially from proximal joints to distal joints. This kinematic sequence itself or the underlying kinetic mechanism is often called the "proximal-to-distal sequence," "kinetic chain," or "whip-like effect" (Atwater, 1979; Feltner, 1989; Fleisig et al., 1996a; Kibler, 1995; Kindall, 1992; Putnam, 1991). However, the kinetic mechanism has not been properly understood, because previous studies on sports movements have not focused on the fact that a joint rotation is caused by *two different mechanisms*: instantaneous and cumulative effects. The instantaneous effect is an instantaneous angular acceleration induced by a joint torque at that instant, whereas the cumulative effect is an angular acceleration induced by the entire joint torque and gravity torque history until that instant (Hirashima et al., 2008; Zajac et al., 2002). Because the mechanical causes are clearly different between the two effects in terms of time, clear differentiation is necessary to understand the original cause of each joint rotation and develop effective training programs.

In section 2, I will explain the instantaneous effects produced by a joint torque by systematically presenting examples of single-joint movements, multi-joint movements in a two-dimensional (2D) space, and multi-joint movements in a three-dimensional (3D) space. I will not only introduce a mathematical method called "induced acceleration analysis" to derive the joint rotations induced by a joint torque but also provide concrete examples with effective graphics so that the meaning of the mathematical formulations can be easily understood by patients, athletes, and coaches, as well as biomechanics researchers. In section 3, I will explain the difference between instantaneous and cumulative effects. Then, in section 4, by applying the induced acceleration analysis to baseball pitching motions, I will demonstrate that such a distinction is helpful to gain insight into the chain of causation for sports movements and the control strategy adopted by high-performance athletes.

2. Instantaneous effect

2.1 Single-joint movements

I begin the explanation with a single-joint movement in which only one joint is free to rotate around a single axis (e.g., elbow flexion-extension movement in a horizontal plane). Because only one joint angle (θ) is necessary to specify the posture of the system, the number of degrees of freedom (DOF) is one. In such a 1-DOF system, the effect of a torque on the joint rotation is very simple because there is only one equation of motion. The angular acceleration ($\ddot{\theta}$) produced by the joint torque (τ) is determined by the magnitude of that torque and the moment of inertia (I) about the joint axis as follows:

$$\ddot{\theta} = \frac{\tau}{I} \tag{1}$$

2.2 Multi-joint movements in 2D

However, the relation between the torque and acceleration become more complex when multiple joints are involved in the movement. For example, we now consider a 2-DOF (e.g., θ_1, shoulder joint angle; θ_2, elbow joint angle) movement in a vertical plane (Fig. 1). The equations of motion for the upper-arm (Eq. 2) and forearm (Eq. 3) can be written as follows:

$$\begin{aligned}\ddot{\theta}_1[I_1 + I_2 + m_2 l_1^2 + m_1 r_1^2 + m_2 r_2^2 + 2m_2 l_1 r_2 \cos\theta_2] + \ddot{\theta}_2[I_2 + m_2 r_2^2 + m_2 l_1 r_2 \cos\theta_2] \\ = \tau_1 + \dot{\theta}_2^2[m_2 l_1 r_2 \sin\theta_2] + \dot{\theta}_1\dot{\theta}_2[2m_2 l_1 r_2 \sin\theta_2] - g[(m_2 l_1 + m_1 r_1)\cos\theta_1 + m_2 r_2 \cos(\theta_1 + \theta_2)]\end{aligned} \tag{2}$$

$$\begin{aligned}\ddot{\theta}_1[I_2 + m_2 r_2^2 + m_2 l_1 r_2 \cos\theta_2] + \ddot{\theta}_2[I_2 + m_2 r_2^2] \\ = \tau_2 - \dot{\theta}_1^2[m_2 l_1 r_2 \sin\theta_2] - g[m_2 r_2 \cos(\theta_1 + \theta_2)]\end{aligned} \tag{3}$$

where I_i = moment of inertia about the center of gravity, r_i = distance to center of mass from proximal joint of the segment, l_i = length, m_i = mass, τ_i = joint torque (i = 1: upper arm, 2: forearm).

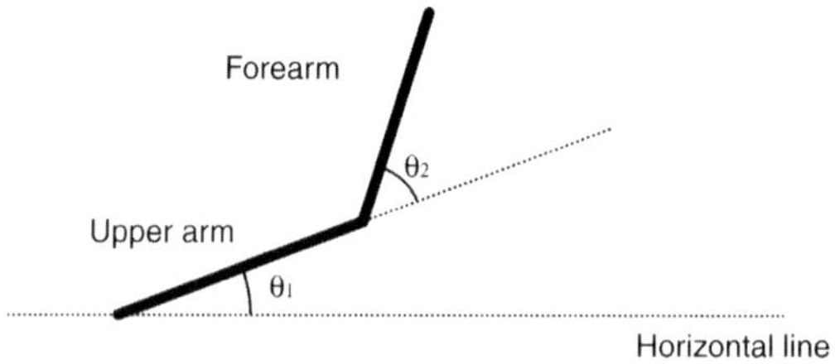

Fig. 1. Two-joint system in a vertical plane.

By using some substitutions, these can be written in the following form:

$$I_{11}\ddot{\theta}_1 + I_{12}\ddot{\theta}_2 = \tau_1 + V_1(\boldsymbol{\theta},\dot{\boldsymbol{\theta}}) + g_1(\boldsymbol{\theta}) \tag{4}$$

$$I_{21}\ddot{\theta}_1 + I_{22}\ddot{\theta}_2 = \tau_2 + V_2(\boldsymbol{\theta},\dot{\boldsymbol{\theta}}) + g_2(\boldsymbol{\theta}) \tag{5}$$

where $\boldsymbol{\theta} = (\theta_1\, \theta_2)^T$ is the joint angle vector, $\dot{\boldsymbol{\theta}} = (\dot{\theta}_1\, \dot{\theta}_2)^T$ is the angular velocity vector, $V_i(\boldsymbol{\theta},\dot{\boldsymbol{\theta}})$ is the angular-velocity-dependent torque, and $g_i(\boldsymbol{\theta})$ is the gravity torque. Now consider the question of how large the angular accelerations ($\ddot{\theta}_1$ and $\ddot{\theta}_2$) are if joint torques (τ_1 and τ_2) are applied at the two joints when the system is in the state of $\boldsymbol{\theta}$ and $\dot{\boldsymbol{\theta}}$. Because unknown variables ($\ddot{\theta}_1$ and $\ddot{\theta}_2$) are present in both equations (Eq. 4 and Eq. 5), we must solve them as simultaneous equations in the following way:

$$\begin{pmatrix} \ddot{\theta}_1 \\ \ddot{\theta}_2 \end{pmatrix} = \begin{pmatrix} I_{11} & I_{12} \\ I_{21} & I_{22} \end{pmatrix}^{-1} \left\{ \begin{pmatrix} \tau_1 \\ \tau_2 \end{pmatrix} + \begin{pmatrix} V_1(\boldsymbol{\theta},\dot{\boldsymbol{\theta}}) \\ V_2(\boldsymbol{\theta},\dot{\boldsymbol{\theta}}) \end{pmatrix} + \begin{pmatrix} g_1(\boldsymbol{\theta}) \\ g_2(\boldsymbol{\theta}) \end{pmatrix} \right\} \tag{6}$$

Accordingly, the angular accelerations of the joints caused by the joint torques can be obtained as follows:

$$\begin{aligned} \ddot{\theta}_1 &= A_{11}(\tau_1 + V_1(\boldsymbol{\theta},\dot{\boldsymbol{\theta}}) + g_1(\boldsymbol{\theta})) + A_{12}(\tau_2 + V_2(\boldsymbol{\theta},\dot{\boldsymbol{\theta}}) + g_2(\boldsymbol{\theta})) \\ \ddot{\theta}_2 &= A_{21}(\tau_1 + V_1(\boldsymbol{\theta},\dot{\boldsymbol{\theta}}) + g_1(\boldsymbol{\theta})) + A_{22}(\tau_2 + V_2(\boldsymbol{\theta},\dot{\boldsymbol{\theta}}) + g_2(\boldsymbol{\theta})) \end{aligned} \tag{7}$$

where A_{11}, A_{12}, A_{21}, and A_{22} are the component of the matrix $\mathbf{I}(\boldsymbol{\theta})^{-1}$:

$$\begin{pmatrix} A_{11} & A_{12} \\ A_{21} & A_{22} \end{pmatrix} = \begin{pmatrix} I_{11} & I_{12} \\ I_{21} & I_{22} \end{pmatrix}^{-1} = \mathbf{I}(\boldsymbol{\theta})^{-1} \tag{8}$$

2.2.1 Joint torque accelerates all joints in multi-joint system

The first important point shown by Eq. 7 is that the angular accelerations of both joints depend on both joint torques. This indicates that, for example, a shoulder joint torque (τ_1) induces angular accelerations not only at the shoulder joint but also at the elbow joint. Figure 2a shows a simulation result where only the shoulder flexor torque is exerted on the 2-DOF (shoulder and elbow) system in a horizontal plane. It is intuitively understandable that the shoulder flexor torque induces the shoulder flexion acceleration, but it should be noted that it also induces the elbow extension acceleration, even though the elbow joint torque is zero. Similarly, an elbow joint torque (τ_2) induces angular accelerations at both joints. Figure 2b shows a simulation result where only the elbow flexor torque is exerted; the elbow flexor torque induces not only elbow flexion acceleration but also shoulder extension acceleration.

Why does a joint torque accelerate not only its own joint but also another remote joint? In fact, interaction forces between body segments occur at the same time as a joint torque is exerted at a certain joint if the body segments are linked by the joints. These interaction forces are the causes of the angular accelerations arising at the remote joints. Because the interaction forces arise instantaneously at the exertion of the joint torque, the angular acceleration at the remote joint also arises at that instant. This phenomenon arising from the mechanical constraint of the joint is called "dynamic coupling" (Zajac and Gordon, 1989).

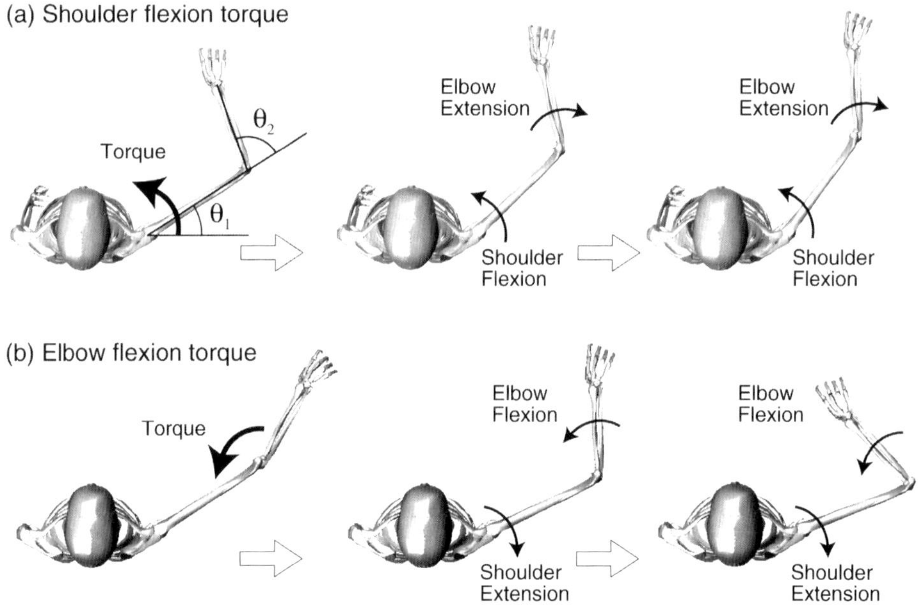

Fig. 2. Simulated motions of two-joint (shoulder and elbow) system in a horizontal plane. Fig. 2a shows angular accelerations induced only by the shoulder flexion torque. Fig. 2b shows angular accelerations induced only by the elbow flexion torque.

2.2.2 Joint torque action depends on system posture

The second important point shown by Eq. 7 is that the angular accelerations produced by a joint torque depend on the system inertia matrix ($\mathbf{I}(\boldsymbol{\theta})$), namely the posture of the system. This indicates that even though the same joint torque is exerted, the angular acceleration induced by the joint torque will vary based on the system's posture when the joint torque is exerted. Figure 3 shows the simulation results when the shoulder flexor torque is exerted on two different postures. The shoulder flexor torque induces the shoulder flexion and elbow *extension* for posture (a), whereas it induces the shoulder flexion and elbow *flexion* for posture (b).

Thus, in order to estimate the angular accelerations induced by joint torques in multi-joint movements, we need to pay attention, not only to the joint torques, but also to the posture of the system. Mathematically speaking, the instantaneous accelerations ($\ddot{\boldsymbol{\theta}}^{\boldsymbol{\tau}} = (\ddot{\theta}_1^{\tau}\ \ddot{\theta}_2^{\tau})^T$) induced by a joint torque can be calculated by multiplying the inverse of the system inertia matrix ($\mathbf{I}(\boldsymbol{\theta})^{-1}$) to the torque vector ($\boldsymbol{\tau} = (\tau_1\ \tau_2)^T$) as follows: $\ddot{\boldsymbol{\theta}}^{\boldsymbol{\tau}} = \mathbf{I}(\boldsymbol{\theta})^{-1}\boldsymbol{\tau}$. This method is often called "induced acceleration analysis." This induced acceleration analysis has been mainly used in gait analysis to determine how individual muscle forces contribute to the forward and vertical acceleration of the body during walking (Anderson and Pandy, 2003; Fox and Delp, 2010; Kepple et al., 1997).

2.3 n-DOF system in 2D

The two properties described above (2.2.1 and 2.2.2) are applicable to a system with more than 2 DOFs. Although the equation of motion with more than 2 DOFs is much more

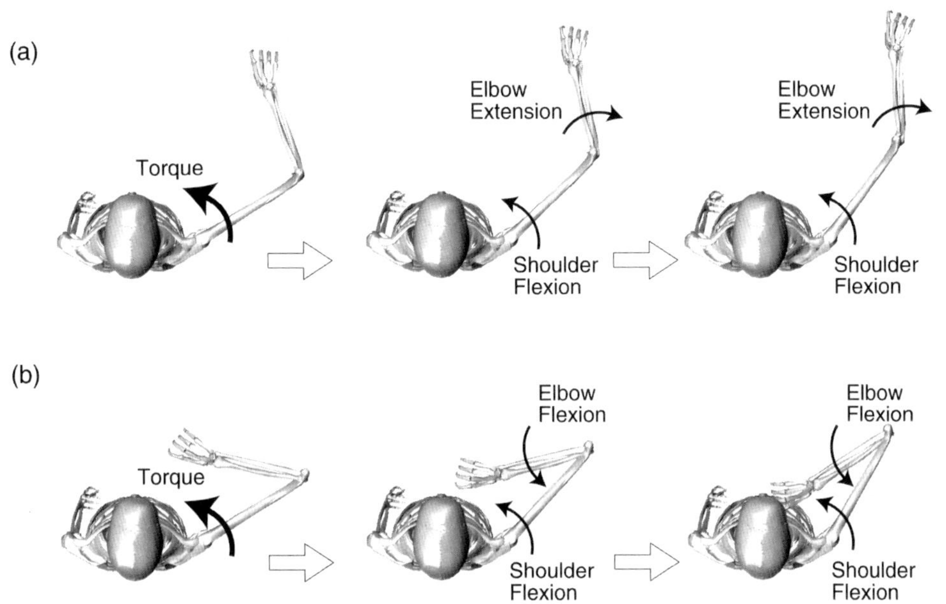

Fig. 3. Simulated motions of two-joint (shoulder and elbow) system in a horizontal plane when the same shoulder flexor torque is exerted on two different postures.

complex than Eq. 2 and Eq. 3, the equation for an n-DOF system (n ≥ 3) can always be written in the following form:

$$\begin{pmatrix} \ddot{\theta}_1 \\ \ddot{\theta}_2 \\ \vdots \\ \ddot{\theta}_n \end{pmatrix} = \begin{pmatrix} I_{11} & I_{12} & \cdots & I_{1n} \\ I_{21} & I_{22} & \cdots & I_{2n} \\ \vdots & \vdots & \ddots & \vdots \\ I_{n1} & I_{n2} & \cdots & I_{nn} \end{pmatrix}^{-1} \left\{ \begin{pmatrix} \tau_1 \\ \tau_2 \\ \vdots \\ \tau_n \end{pmatrix} + \begin{pmatrix} V_1(\boldsymbol{\theta},\dot{\boldsymbol{\theta}}) \\ V_2(\boldsymbol{\theta},\dot{\boldsymbol{\theta}}) \\ \vdots \\ V_n(\boldsymbol{\theta},\dot{\boldsymbol{\theta}}) \end{pmatrix} + \begin{pmatrix} g_1(\boldsymbol{\theta}) \\ g_2(\boldsymbol{\theta}) \\ \vdots \\ g_n(\boldsymbol{\theta}) \end{pmatrix} \right\} \tag{9}$$

It can be written more simply as follows:

$$\ddot{\boldsymbol{\theta}} = \mathbf{I}(\boldsymbol{\theta})^{-1} \left\{ \boldsymbol{\tau} + \mathbf{V}(\boldsymbol{\theta},\dot{\boldsymbol{\theta}}) + \mathbf{g}(\boldsymbol{\theta}) \right\} \tag{10}$$

Because this equation has the same form as Eq. 6 in the 2-DOF system, we can discuss the cause-and-effect relation between joint torques and accelerations in a way similar to the discussion for the 2-DOF system. In general, the mechanism by which joint torques induce angular accelerations can be graphically summarized as shown in Fig. 4. This figure indicates that:

1. A joint torque at each joint induces acceleration not only at its own joint (i.e., direct effect, solid line) but also at the other joints (i.e., remote effect, dotted line).
2. The effects induced by a joint torque depend on the posture of the whole system.

Thus, for example, in the case of a 3-DOF system (shoulder, elbow, and wrist joints), a shoulder joint torque instantaneously accelerates not only the shoulder but also the elbow and wrist joints.

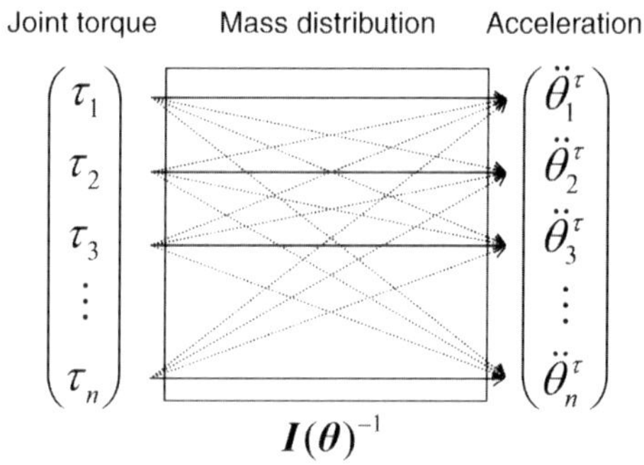

Fig. 4. Schematic figure of how joint torque at each joint induces angular accelerations at all joints in n-DOF system.

2.4 n-DOF system in 3D

The equation of motion for a multi-joint system in 3D is much more complicated than the equation in 2D. Fortunately, however, the equations for 3D movements can also be written in the same form as the equations for 2D movements (Eqs. 9 and 10). The mathematical derivation is described in a reference (Hirashima and Ohtsuki, 2008). It indicates that, similar to 2D multi-joint movements, a joint torque at a certain DOF induces accelerations at all DOFs in 3D multi-DOF movements. Now, let us consider 3D movements, including 3-DOF shoulder joint rotations. In this case, τ_1, τ_2, and τ_3 in Fig. 4 can be regarded as the shoulder joint torques about the internal-external rotation axis, adduction-abduction axis, and horizontal flexion-extension axis, respectively, while $\ddot{\theta}_1$, $\ddot{\theta}_2$, and $\ddot{\theta}_3$ can be regarded as the angular accelerations about the three axes, respectively. Thus, the 3D version of Fig. 4 indicates that, when only the joint torque about the internal-external rotation axis (τ_1) is exerted, it can induce angular accelerations not only about the internal-external rotation axis ($\ddot{\theta}_1$) but also about the other two axes ($\ddot{\theta}_2$ and $\ddot{\theta}_3$). This might seem counterintuitive to some readers, because people tend to intuitively and wrongly believe that the "shoulder internal rotation torque" can only produce a shoulder internal rotation. Actually, however, such a 1-to-1 causal relationship occurs in only a few cases (see below). In almost every case, a joint torque accelerates all of the joint rotations.

2.4.1 Inertial property of 3D objects

To understand this from a mechanical point of view, it is necessary to deepen our understanding of the inertial property of 3D objects. Any object has three orthogonal principal axes of inertia (Zatsiorsky, 2002). If the inertia matrix is expressed in the orthogonal coordinate system (X,Y,Z) whose axes correspond to the principal axes of inertia (Fig. 5a), it can be written as follows:

$$\mathbf{I}_A = \begin{pmatrix} I_{xx} & 0 & 0 \\ 0 & I_{yy} & 0 \\ 0 & 0 & I_{zz} \end{pmatrix} \tag{11}$$

Then, the angular accelerations induced by the torque about the X axis can be expressed as follows:

$$\begin{pmatrix} \ddot{\theta}_x \\ \ddot{\theta}_y \\ \ddot{\theta}_z \end{pmatrix} = \begin{pmatrix} I_{xx} & 0 & 0 \\ 0 & I_{yy} & 0 \\ 0 & 0 & I_{zz} \end{pmatrix}^{-1} \begin{pmatrix} \tau_x \\ 0 \\ 0 \end{pmatrix} = \begin{pmatrix} A_{xx} & 0 & 0 \\ 0 & A_{yy} & 0 \\ 0 & 0 & A_{zz} \end{pmatrix} \begin{pmatrix} \tau_x \\ 0 \\ 0 \end{pmatrix} = \begin{pmatrix} A_{xx}\tau_x \\ 0 \\ 0 \end{pmatrix} \tag{12}$$

Thus, in a case where the axis of the torque vector corresponds to the principal axis of inertia, the torque vector induces angular acceleration about this axis alone. For a human upper limb, this situation occurs only in an ideal simple case where the upper arm, forearm, and hand are linked in line (Fig. 5a) and one of the principal axes of inertia for the entire kinematic chain exactly corresponds to the longitudinal axis of the upper arm. In this case, a torque about the longitudinal axis of the upper arm causes internal-external rotation alone.
On the other hand, when the elbow is at a flexed position (Fig. 5b), the principal axes of inertia for the entire kinematic chain distal to the shoulder deviate from the shoulder joint coordinate system (X,Y,Z). When the inertia matrix is expressed in a coordinate system whose axes do not correspond to the principal axes of inertia, it is written as follows:

$$\mathbf{I}_B = \begin{pmatrix} I_{xx} & I_{xy} & I_{xz} \\ I_{yx} & I_{yy} & I_{yz} \\ I_{zx} & I_{zy} & I_{zz} \end{pmatrix} \tag{13}$$

Then, the angular accelerations induced by the torque about the X axis can be expressed as follows:

$$\begin{pmatrix} \ddot{\theta}_x \\ \ddot{\theta}_y \\ \ddot{\theta}_z \end{pmatrix} = \begin{pmatrix} I_{xx} & I_{xy} & I_{xz} \\ I_{yx} & I_{yy} & I_{yz} \\ I_{zx} & I_{zy} & I_{zz} \end{pmatrix}^{-1} \begin{pmatrix} \tau_x \\ 0 \\ 0 \end{pmatrix} = \begin{pmatrix} A_{xx} & A_{xy} & A_{xz} \\ A_{yx} & A_{yy} & A_{yz} \\ A_{zx} & A_{zy} & A_{zz} \end{pmatrix} \begin{pmatrix} \tau_x \\ 0 \\ 0 \end{pmatrix} = \begin{pmatrix} A_{xx}\tau_x \\ A_{yx}\tau_x \\ A_{zx}\tau_x \end{pmatrix} \tag{14}$$

Thus, when the axis of the joint torque does not correspond to the principal axis of inertia, the torque induces angular accelerations about all three joint axes.

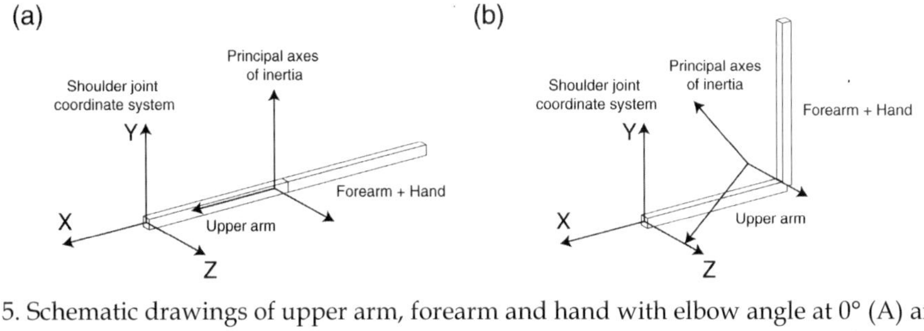

Fig. 5. Schematic drawings of upper arm, forearm and hand with elbow angle at 0° (A) and 90° (B). The shoulder joint coordinate axes (XYZ) and the principal axes of inertia for the entire kinematic chain are drawn [Adapted from (Hirashima et al., 2007a)].

2.4.2 Examples of 3D multi-DOF movements

Computer simulations were used to observe these two situations (Eqs. 12 and 14). Figure 6a shows the simulation results when a shoulder internal rotation torque is exerted on the ideal simple case in which the principal axes of inertia correspond to the shoulder joint coordinate axes. For simplicity, the simulation was conducted in a zero gravity environment. In this case, the shoulder internal rotation torque produces only the shoulder internal rotation. However, when the shoulder internal rotation torque is exerted on a system whose principal axes of inertia do not correspond to the shoulder joint coordinate axes (Fig. 6b), the shoulder internal rotation torque produces not only the internal rotation but also abduction and horizontal extension.

Figure 7 shows another example of exerting the shoulder horizontal flexion torque, which approximately simulates the situation where the anterior deltoid is activated. In a case where the principal axes of inertia correspond to the shoulder joint coordinate axes (Fig. 7a), the shoulder horizontal flexion torque produces only horizontal flexion. However, in the case of the posture shown in Fig. 7b, the shoulder horizontal flexion torque produces not only horizontal flexion but also external rotation. This might be surprising for some readers, because anatomy textbooks never describe the external rotation as a function of the anterior deltoid. Here, I would like to call attention to the fact that anatomy textbooks describe the *torque vector* produced by each muscle, not the *rotation* produced by the muscle: this is a blind spot for novices in the field of biomechanics and motor control. It should be kept in mind that, in order to know how each muscle force produces angular accelerations, we need to consider both the torque vector produced by the muscle (τ) and the inertial property of the system $\mathbf{I}(\boldsymbol{\theta})$ to which the torque is applied.

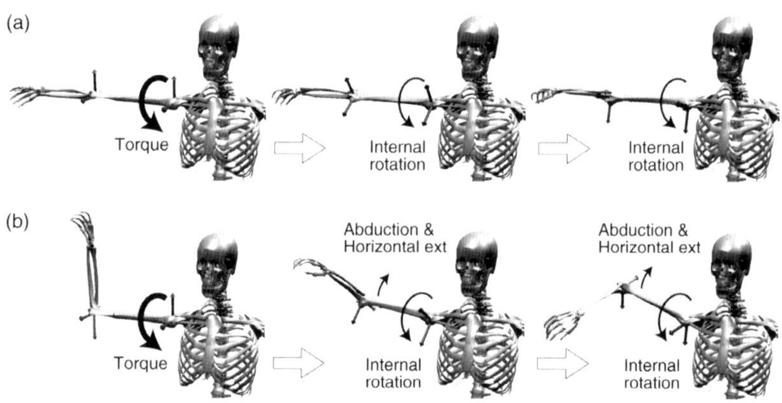

Fig. 6. Simulated motions in zero gravity environment when shoulder internal rotation torque is exerted on two different postures.

3. Cumulative effect

So far, I have explained how a joint torque at a certain instant induces angular accelerations on the system at that instant. However, the effect of the joint torque is not limited to these instantaneous accelerations because the accelerations accumulate and remain in the system as a velocity. The velocity-dependent torques ($\mathbf{V}(\boldsymbol{\theta},\dot{\boldsymbol{\theta}})$) such as Coriolis and centrifugal torques can also induce angular accelerations. The angular acceleration induced by velocity-dependent torques at a certain instant is expressed as follows:

$$\ddot{\boldsymbol{\theta}}^{V} = \mathbf{I}(\boldsymbol{\theta})^{-1}\mathbf{V}(\boldsymbol{\theta},\dot{\boldsymbol{\theta}}) \quad (15)$$

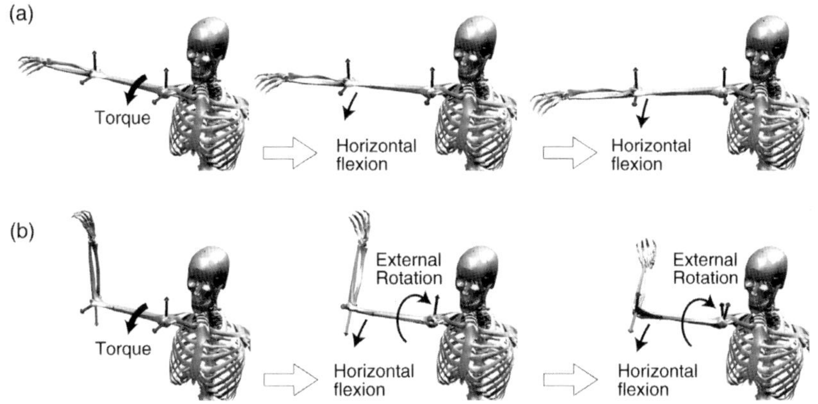

Fig. 7. Simulated motions in zero gravity environment when shoulder horizontal flexion torque is exerted on two different postures.

It should be noted that because the angular velocity is integrated from the angular acceleration, the acceleration induced by the velocity-dependent torque at a certain instant (Eq. 15) reflects the cumulative effects from the history of all the muscles and gravity torques that have been applied to the system until that instant.

In summary, the induced acceleration analysis suggests that the angular acceleration at a certain instant is the sum of 1) the instantaneous effect induced by the joint torques and gravity torque at that instant and 2) the cumulative effect from the history of the joint torques and gravity torque applied to the system until that instant (Fig. 8).

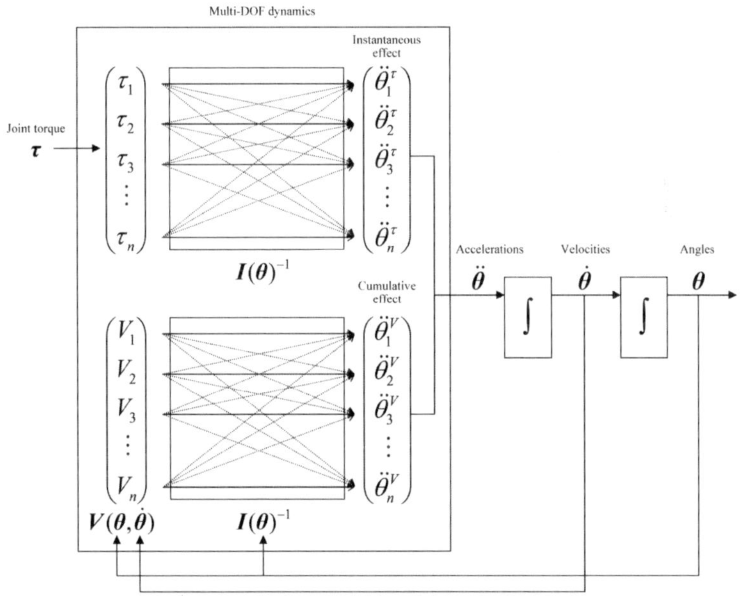

Fig. 8. Block diagram of generation mechanism for multi-DOF human motion [Adapted from (Hirashima et al., 2008)].

4. Application to sports movements

Understanding the cause-and-effect relation between the kinetics (e.g., muscle force, joint torque) and kinematics (e.g., joint rotation) is difficult in multi-joint movements because of the complexity of inter-joint interactions. The induced acceleration analysis provides the framework to show that joint angular acceleration is induced by two different mechanisms (i.e., instantaneous and cumulative effects). Determining whether a joint angular acceleration is caused by the instantaneous or cumulative effect is very important because the original causes of these accelerations are clearly different in terms of time. The cause of the instantaneous effect is the joint torque and gravity torque at that instant, whereas the cause of the cumulative effect is the entire history of the joint torques and gravity torque applied to the system until that instant. However, previous studies on fast sports movements such as baseball pitching and soccer kicking have not clearly differentiated these two effects, and hence the causes of the joint rotations have not been properly understood. In section 4, I apply the induced acceleration analysis to the baseball pitching motion to understand the kinetic mechanism used by skilled baseball players to generate a large ball velocity.

4.1 Kinematic analysis

The first step in understanding how skilled baseball players generate a large ball velocity at ball release is to determine the joint angular velocities that are mostly responsible for the translational velocity of the ball. Here, we consider a serially linked four-segment model of the trunk and upper limb that has 13 degrees of freedom (DOFs) (Fig. 9a). There are three translational DOFs and three rotational DOFs for the trunk, three rotational DOFs for the shoulder, two rotational DOFs for the elbow, and two rotational DOFs for the wrist (for details see the legend of Fig. 9). Suppose the joint rotates only about the i-th DOF axis at an angular velocity of $\dot{\theta}_i$ (Fig. 9b). The translational velocity of the fingertip ($\dot{\mathbf{r}}_i$) produced by this rotation is expressed as

$$\dot{\mathbf{r}}_i = \dot{\boldsymbol{\theta}}_i \times \mathbf{p}_i \tag{16}$$

where $\dot{\boldsymbol{\theta}}_i (= \dot{\theta}_i \mathbf{u}_i)$ is the angular velocity vector ($\mathbf{u}_i$ is the unit vector of the joint axis) and $\mathbf{p}_i$ is the vector from the joint center to the fingertip. Because joints actually rotate about all DOFs, the actual translational velocity of the fingertip ($\dot{\mathbf{r}}$) is expressed as the sum of their effects.

$$\dot{\mathbf{r}} = \sum_{i=1}^{13} \dot{\mathbf{r}}_i \tag{17}$$

We can determine the contribution of each angular velocity to the magnitude of the fingertip translational velocity by projecting each vector ($\dot{\mathbf{r}}_i$) onto the unit vector ($\dot{\mathbf{r}}_u$) of the translational velocity of the fingertip (Feltner and Nelson, 1996; Miyanishi et al., 1996; Sprigings et al., 1994).

$$|\dot{\mathbf{r}}| = \sum_{i=1}^{13} (\dot{\mathbf{r}}_i \cdot \dot{\mathbf{r}}_u) \tag{18}$$

Figure 9c shows the contributions of the 13 DOF velocities to the fingertip velocity at the time of ball release in skilled baseball players (Hirashima et al., 2007b). This analysis reveals that it is mainly produced by the leftward rotation of the trunk, internal rotation of the shoulder, elbow extension, and wrist flexion.

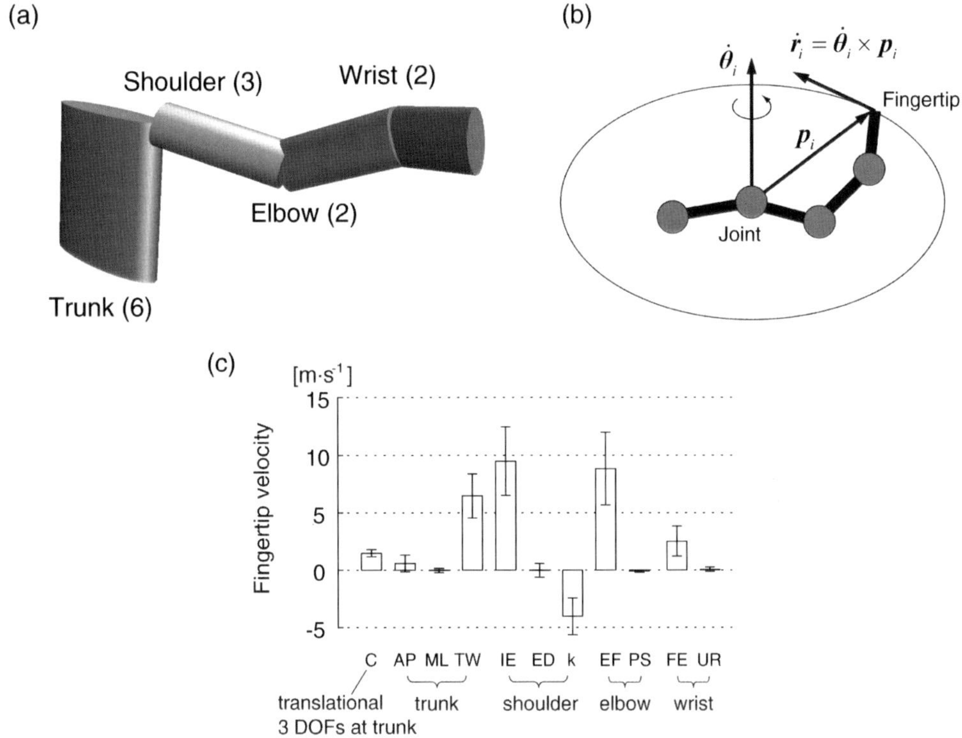

Fig. 9. (a) 13-DOF model. (b) Schematic figure of the relation between joint angular velocity vector $\dot{\boldsymbol{\theta}}_i$ at one joint coordinate axis and the translational velocity vector of the fingertip ($\dot{\mathbf{r}}_i$). (c) Contributions to the translational velocity of the fingertip at the time of ball release. There are 13 contributors to the fingertip velocity: C, translation of the trunk including three degrees of freedom (DOFs) (forward-backward, upward-downward, and right-left); AP, anterior (+)-posterior (-) lean; ML, medial (+)-lateral (-) tilt; TW, left (+)-right (-) twist of the trunk; IE, internal (+)-external (-) rotation; ED, elevation (+)-depression (-); k, third-axis rotation of the shoulder; EF, extension (+)-flexion (-); PS, pronation (+)-supination (-) of the elbow; FE, flexion (+)-extension (-); and UR, ulnar (+)-radial (-) deviation of the wrist [Adapted from (Hirashima et al., 2007b)].

4.2 Induced acceleration analysis

The next step is to understand how baseball players generate a large angular velocity at these joint rotations by coordinating the joint torque and velocity-dependent torque. As described in the above section (2.4), angular accelerations can be calculated by the following equation:

$$\ddot{\boldsymbol{\theta}} = \mathbf{I}(\boldsymbol{\theta})^{-1}\left\{\boldsymbol{\tau} + \mathbf{V}(\boldsymbol{\theta},\dot{\boldsymbol{\theta}}) + \mathbf{g}(\boldsymbol{\theta})\right\} \tag{19}$$

where $\ddot{\boldsymbol{\theta}}$, $\boldsymbol{\tau}$, $\mathbf{V}(\boldsymbol{\theta},\dot{\boldsymbol{\theta}})$, and $\mathbf{g}(\boldsymbol{\theta})$ are the 13-dimensional vectors, and $\mathbf{I}(\boldsymbol{\theta})$ is the 13-by-13 matrix for the 13-DOF model used here. This equation tells us that the j-th angular acceleration ($\ddot{\theta}_j$) is produced by the instantaneous direct effect ($\ddot{\theta}_j^{\tau j}$), instantaneous remote effect ($\ddot{\theta}_j^{\tau k}(k \neq j)$), cumulative effect ($\ddot{\theta}_j^{V}$), and instantaneous effect from gravity torque ($\ddot{\theta}_j^{g}$) as expressed in the following:

$$\begin{aligned}\ddot{\theta}_j &= \sum_{i=1}^{13} A_{ji}\tau_i + \sum_{i=1}^{13} A_{ji}V_i + \sum_{i=1}^{13} A_{ji}g_i \\ &= (\ddot{\theta}_j^{\tau 1} + \ddot{\theta}_j^{\tau 2} + \cdots + \ddot{\theta}_j^{\tau 13}) + \ddot{\theta}_j^{V} + \ddot{\theta}_j^{g}\end{aligned} \tag{20}$$

where A_{ji} is the (j, i) component of the matrix, $\mathbf{I}(\boldsymbol{\theta})^{-1}$.

In baseball pitching, the fastest possible speed at the hand is required, and eventually large angular accelerations are required. Because the instantaneous accelerations induced by the muscle force are limited by the muscle force-producing capacity (i.e., physical capacity), additional utilization of the velocity-dependent torque is a very effective strategy for producing larger angular accelerations than the muscle torque could produce on its own. To what extent do skilled players utilize the velocity-dependent torque? Do they utilize the velocity-dependent torque at all joints?

Figure 10 shows the contributions of the 13 joint torques, velocity-dependent torque, and gravity torque to the trunk forward motion, trunk leftward rotation, shoulder internal rotation, shoulder horizontal flexion, elbow extension, and wrist flexion. This figure indicates that the motions of the trunk (Figs. 10a and b) and shoulder (Figs. 10c and d) are produced by respective joint torques (i.e., instantaneous direct effect): for example, the trunk leftward rotation is accelerated by the trunk leftward rotation torque (Fig. 10b). In contrast, the elbow extension and wrist flexion are mainly produced by the velocity-dependent torque (Figs. 10e and f).

I further examined which segment motion is the source of the velocity-dependent torque acting on the elbow and wrist accelerations by decomposing the velocity-dependent torque into some kinematic sources. The results show that the velocity-dependent torques at the shoulder, elbow, and wrist were produced by the forearm angular velocity that was originally produced by the trunk and shoulder joint torques in an earlier phase (for more details, see Hirashima et al., 2008).

5. Discussion

5.1 Kinetic chain

Taken together, the kinetic chain of baseball pitching can be summarized as follows. First, the trunk forward motion and leftward rotation are accelerated by respective joint torques (instantaneous direct effect) produced by relatively large muscles located at the lower extremity and trunk (Fig. 11a). The shoulder horizontal flexion torque and internal rotation torque during this phase prevent the upper arm from lagging behind relative to the trunk. As a result, the angular velocity of the upper arm also increases with that of the trunk (Fig. 11b). Thus, the motions of the trunk and upper arm in the early phase are produced by the instantaneous direct effect from large proximal muscles. The angular velocities of the trunk and upper arm produced by the above mechanism are the sources of the velocity-dependent torque acting for the elbow extension (Figs. 11c and d). As a result, the elbow joint angular velocity increases, and concurrently, the forearm angular velocity relative to the ground also increases. The forearm angular velocity subsequently accelerates the elbow extension

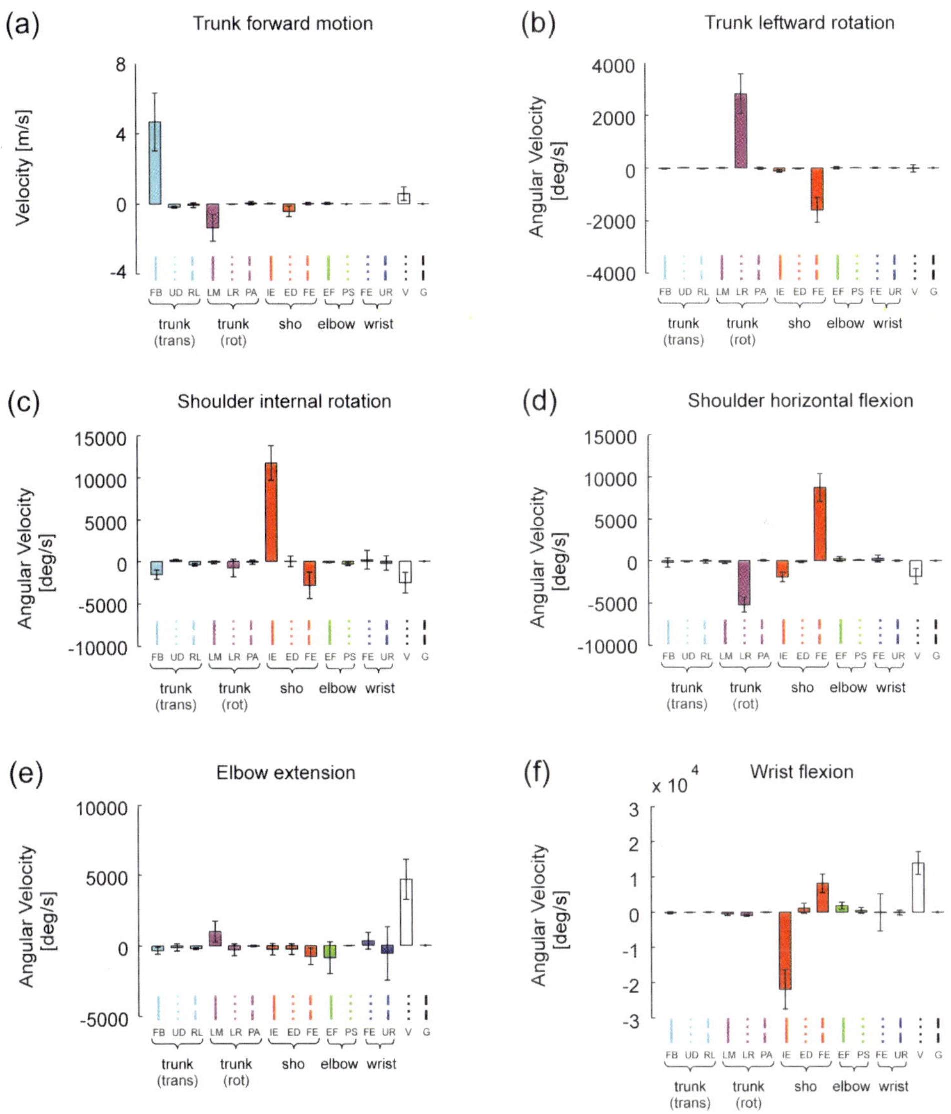

Fig. 10. Contributions of 13 joint torques, velocity-dependent torque, and gravity torque to the trunk forward motion (a), trunk leftward rotation (b), shoulder internal rotation (c), shoulder horizontal flexion (d), elbow extension (e), and wrist flexion (f) during baseball pitching [Adapted from (Hirashima et al., 2008)].

(Fig. 11e) and wrist flexion (Fig. 11f). Thus, the angular velocities of the trunk and upper arm produced by the proximal muscles in the early phase remain in the cumulative effect loop and accelerate the distal joint rotations in the later phase.

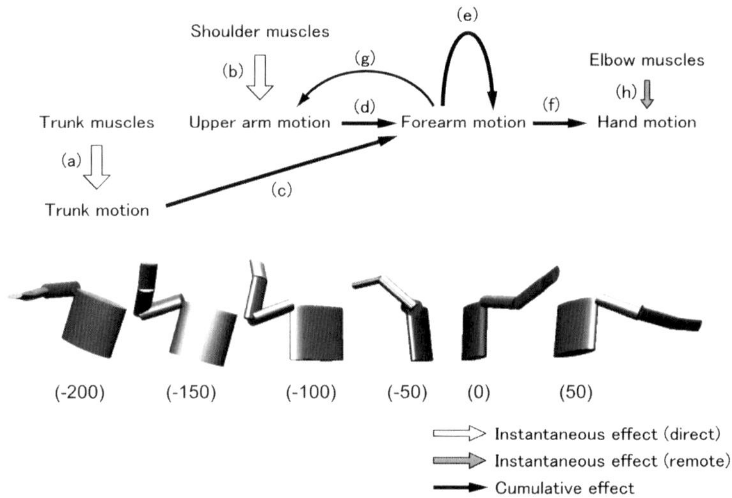

Fig. 11. Kinetic chain of baseball pitching. The number in parentheses indicate the time [msec].

5.2 Instantaneous remote effect vs. cumulative effect

It should be noted that the mechanism for the cumulative effect is different from the mechanism for the "torque reversal" examined by (Chowdhary and Challis, 2001) and (Herring and Chapman, 1992). They demonstrated, using simulations, that the braking of a proximal segment accelerated the distal segment and was effective at generating the fastest throw. In baseball pitching, the elbow joint torque reversed its direction from extension to flexion at about -40 ms (Hirashima et al., 2008). While the elbow flexion torque decelerated the elbow extension, it accelerated the distal wrist flexion (Fig. 11h). Thus, the positive effect of the torque reversal is one of the instantaneous effects from the remote joint torques (dotted line in Fig. 4). Therefore, this effect is not influenced by the proximal joint torques in the early phase, in contrast to the cumulative effect. Until now, however, these two effects have been considered similar because they are caused by torques *other than* the *direct* joint torque. Because the original cause of the instantaneous remote effects is clearly different from that of the cumulative effect in terms of time, in order to develop effective training programs, coaches and athletes should clearly discriminate between these two effects.

5.3 Sequence that does not obey proximal-to-distal sequence

In baseball pitching, almost all of the joint rotations obey the proximal-to-distal sequence. However, one exceptional sequence does not obey the rule. The shoulder internal rotation occurs after the elbow extension. Although this distal-to-proximal sequence has been observed for 20 years, it has been unclear why this sequence is adopted by skilled throwers. One possible reason is that extending the elbow before the shoulder internal rotation can decrease the moment of inertia about the shoulder internal rotation axis. The other reason is that the velocity-dependent torque arising from the elbow extension accelerates the shoulder internal rotation (Fig. 11g): cumulative effects do not always have the proximal-to-distal sequence. Although it has long been believed that the throwing motion is controlled by the role of the proximal-to-distal sequence, here we propose that the throwing motion is controlled by the role of utilizing the cumulative effect. This idea can explain the sequence of joint rotations during the throwing movement without exception.

6. Conclusions

Until now, the kinetic aspect of sports movements has primarily been examined using the *inverse dynamics technique*, which calculates the joint torques that are required to achieve a focused movement. These findings are helpful for specifying the body parts receiving excessive loads and understanding the mechanism underlying sports disorders (Fleisig et al., 1995). However, the cause-and-effect relationship for how these kinetic parameters (joint torque) accelerate joint rotations and how joint rotations affect each other has been unclear. In this chapter, I have shown that the "induced acceleration analysis" method can greatly assist us in understanding the cause-and-effect relationship between joint torques and rotations. In particular, clearly discriminating between the instantaneous direct effect, instantaneous remote effect, and cumulative effect is very important for coaches and athletes, as well as biomechanics researchers, because their causes are clearly different in terms of time and space.

7. References

Anderson, F.C. & Pandy, M.G. (2003). Individual muscle contributions to support in normal walking. *Gait and Posture* 17, 159-169.

Atwater, A.E. (1979). Biomechanics of overarm throwing movements and of throwing injuries. *Exercise and Sport Sciences Reviews* 7, 43-85.

Barrentine, S.W.; Matsuo, T.; Escamilla, R.F.; Fleisig, G.S. & Andrews, J.R. (1998). Kinematic analysis of the wrist and forearm during baseball pitching. *Journal of Applied Biomechanics* 14, 24-39.

Chowdhary, A.G. & Challis, J.H. (2001). The biomechanics of an overarm throwing task: A simulation model examination of optimal timing of muscle activations. *Journal of Theoretical Biology* 211, 39-53.

Elliott, B.; Fleisig, G.; Nicholls, R. & Escamilia, R. (2003). Technique effects on upper limb loading in the tennis serve. *Journal of Science and Medicine in Sport* 6, 76-87.

Feltner, M. & Dapena, J. (1986). Dynamics of the shoulder and elbow joints of the throwing arm during a baseball pitch. *International Journal of Sport Biomechanics* 2, 235-259.

Feltner, M.E. (1989). 3-dimensional interactions in a 2-segment kinetic chain .2. application to the throwing arm in baseball pitching. *International Journal of Sport Biomechanics* 5, 420-450.

Feltner, M.E. & Nelson, S.T. (1996). Three-dimensional kinematics of the throwing arm during the penalty throw in water polo. *Journal of Applied Biomechanics* 12, 359-382.

Fleisig, G.S.; Andrews, J.R.; Dillman, C.J. & Escamilla, R.F. (1995). Kinetics of baseball pitching with implications about injury mechanisms. *American Journal of Sports Medicine* 23, 233-239.

Fleisig, G.S.; Barrentine, S.W.; Escamilla, R.F. & Andrews, J.R. (1996a). Biomechanics of overhand throwing with implications for injuries. *Sports Medicine* 21, 421-437.

Fleisig, G.S.; Escamilla, R.F.; Andrews, J.R.; Matsuo, T.; Satterwhite, Y. & Barrentine, S.W. (1996b). Kinematic and kinetic comparison between baseball pitching and football passing. *Journal of Applied Biomechanics* 12, 207-224.

Fox, M.D. & Delp, S.L. (2010). Contributions of muscles and passive dynamics to swing initiation over a range of walking speeds. *Journal of Biomechanics* 43, 1450-1455.

Glousman, R.; Jobe, F.; Tibone, J.; Moynes, D.; Antonelli, D. & Perry, J. (1988). Dynamic electromyographic analysis of the throwing shoulder with glenohumeral instability. *Journal of Bone and Joint Surgery-American Volume* 70A, 220-226.

Herring, R.M. & Chapman, A.E. (1992). Effects of changes in segmental values and timing of both torque and torque reversal in simulated throws. *Journal of Biomechanics* 25, 1173-1184.

Hirashima, M.; Kadota, H.; Sakurai, S.; Kudo, K. & Ohtsuki, T. (2002). Sequential muscle activity and its functional role in the upper extremity and trunk during overarm throwing. *Journal of Sports Sciences* 20, 301-310.

Hirashima, M.; Kudo, K. & Ohtsuki, T. (2007a). A new non-orthogonal decomposition method to determine effective torques for three-dimensional joint rotation. *Journal of Biomechanics* 40, 871-882.

Hirashima, M.; Kudo, K.; Watarai, K. & Ohtsuki, T. (2007b). Control of 3D limb dynamics in unconstrained overarm throws of different speeds performed by skilled baseball players. *Journal of Neurophysiology* 97, 680-691.

Hirashima, M. & Ohtsuki, T. (2008). Exploring the mechanism of skilled overarm throwing. *Exercise and Sport Sciences Reviews* 36, 205-211.

Hirashima, M.; Yamane, K.; Nakamura, Y. & Ohtsuki, T. (2008). Kinetic chain of overarm throwing in terms of joint rotations revealed by induced acceleration analysis. *Journal of Biomechanics* 41, 2874-2883.

Kepple, T.M.; Siegel, K.L. & Stanhope, S.J. (1997). Relative contributions of the lower extremity joint moments to forward progression and support during gait. *Gait and Posture* 6, 1-8.

Kibler, W.B. (1995). Biomechanical analysis of the shoulder during tennis activities. *Clinics in Sports Medicine* 14, 79-85.

Kindall, J. (1992). Science of coaching baseball. *Human Kinetics Publishers.*

Marshall, R.N. & Elliott, B.C. (2000). Long-axis rotation: The missing link in proximal-to-distal segmental sequencing. *Journal of Sports Sciences* 18, 247-254.

Matsuo, T.; Escamilla, R.F.; Fleisig, G.S.; Barrentine, S.W. & Andrews, J.R. (2001). Comparison of kinematic and temporal parameters between different pitch velocity groups. *Journal of Applied Biomechanics* 17, 1-13.

Miyanishi, T.; Fujii, N.; Ae, M.; Kunugi, Y. & Okada, M. (1996). A three-dimensional study on contribution of torso and throwing arm segments to ball velocity in baseball throwing motion. *Japanese Journal of Physical Education* 41, 23-37.

Nunome, H.; Asai, T.; Ikegami, Y. & Sakurai, S. (2002). Three-dimensional kinetic analysis of side-foot and instep soccer kicks. *Medicine and Science in Sports and Exercise* 34, 2028-2036.

Putnam, C.A. (1991). A segment interaction analysis of proximal-to-distal sequential segment motion patterns. *Medicine and Science in Sports and Exercise* 23, 130-144.

Sakurai, S.; Ikegami, Y.; Okamoto, A.; Yabe, K. & Toyoshima, S. (1993). A 3-dimensional cinematographic analysis of upper limb movement during fastball and curveball baseball pitches. *Journal of Applied Biomechanics* 9, 47-65.

Sakurai, S. & Ohtsuki, T. (2000). Muscle activity and accuracy of performance of the smash stroke in badminton with reference to skill and practice. *Journal of Sports Sciences* 18, 901-914.

Sprigings, E.; Marshall, R.; Elliott, B. & Jennings, L. (1994). A 3-dimensional kinematic method for determining the effectiveness of arm segment rotations in producing racquet-head speed. *Journal of Biomechanics* 27, 245-254.

Zajac, F.E. & Gordon, M.E. (1989). Determining muscles force and action in multi-articular movement. *Exercise and Sport Sciences Reviews* 17, 187-230.

Zajac, F.E.; Neptune, R.R. & Kautz, S.A. (2002). Biomechanics and muscle coordination of human walking - Part I: Introduction to concepts, power transfer, dynamics and simulations. *Gait and Posture* 16, 215-232.

Zatsiorsky, V.M. (2002). *Kinetics of Human Motion, Human Kinetics, Champaign.*

15

Stability During Arboreal Locomotion

Andrew R. Lammers and Ulrich Zurcher
Cleveland State University
USA

1. Introduction

Arboreal locomotion - traveling on the branches, twigs, and trunks of trees and woody shrubs - is very common among mammals. Most primates, many rodents, marsupials, carnivores, and even an occasional artiodactyl travel on arboreal substrates to forage, escape predators, and acquire shelter. Arboreal supports are usually far enough from the ground that a slip or fall could cause serious injury or death, or deprive the animal of a mate, food, or energy. Thus, stability is of great importance for an animal traveling on arboreal supports. The considerable variation among arboreal supports makes stability during locomotion a mechanical challenge. Supports vary in diameter, slope, compliance, texture, direction (that is, bends or curves in a branch), and number and distribution. Furthermore there may be interaction among these variables; for example, compliance varies with diameter - thinner branches are more compliant than thick branches. Also, the thin branches frequently have leaves that act like sails in the wind, causing even more movement in the substrate. Substrate texture often varies with diameter, where narrow twigs have smoother bark than large branches or trunks. Therefore one might expect a considerable number of morphological, behavioral, and biomechanical mechanisms to enhance stability on arboreal supports.

Stability can be divided into two categories: static and dynamic. Static stability is the process by which objects at rest remain stable, i.e., neither move (translation) nor rotate about a point or axis. For example, a table is statically stable because the forces and moments (torques) produced by gravity (weight) are balanced by ground reaction forces and the moments generated by them. One way an animal might remain stable is by not moving and adhering to or gripping the support; this definition is the ultimate example of static stability in an animal. Although this strategy allows no movement, it is nevertheless a valid locomotor strategy for an animal attempting to travel on an arboreal support subjected to a sudden gust of wind or other disturbance (Stevens, 2003). This analysis also applies when the animal walks very slowly, but fails when it walks or runs at considerable speed. Because the distribution of the mass is changing from one instant to the next, the forces and torques necessary to maintain static stability would also change with time. That is, it requires an active control by the nervous system. Because stability is critical, it is very likely that the animal employs both active and passive control (Full et al., 2002). Passive control can be due to dynamic processes of the animal's body, and is referred to as dynamic stability. For example, a hiker might cross a stream or river by running across a fallen log; the rotation of the limbs around the hips and shoulder generates a gyroscopic effect. This gyroscopic effect helps prevent the hiker from toppling off the log. In this chapter we will review the mechanics of static stability during arboreal locomotion. We will then expand on the mechanics of dynamic stability and its importance in arboreal locomotion.

2. Static stability

Slow lorises, as their name implies, usually move very slowly (although see Nekaris and Stevens, 2007). One of the mechanisms these primates use to avoid toppling from narrow arboreal supports is the same method used by the table. At all times the center of mass of the table or slow loris is supported by three or four legs, making toppling less likely (Fig. 1; Hildebrand, 1980).

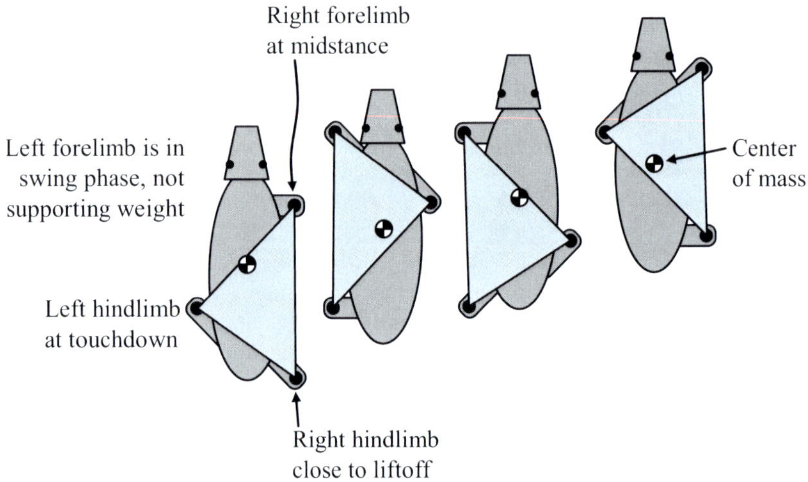

Fig. 1. Base of support (blue triangles) generated by the limbs in contact with the ground or substrate (based on Hildebrand, 1980). The footfall pattern illustrated here is a lateral sequence singlefoot gait (left hind, left fore, right hind, right fore, with footfalls spaced fairly evenly in time). The duty factor is approximately 75%. Note that the center of mass (black and white circle) is supported by three limbs at all times.

Footfall pattern can affect whether the center of gravity passes through the polygon of support. First, at slow speeds, the duty factor usually increases (Fig. 2). Duty factor is the duration of time that a foot or hand contacts a substrate divided by the total stride cycle time. A duty factor of 100% indicates a hand or foot that never leaves the substrate (therefore no movement occurs); a zero duty factor means the animal is flying. Intermediate duty factors indicate how much time within each stride a hand or foot is in contact with the substrate. At slow speeds, when duty factor is high (Fig. 2), the likelihood is higher that three or four limbs are in contact with the substrate at any given moment. Three or four limbs create a support polygon through which the center of gravity may pass, maintaining stability against toppling due to the acceleration of gravity on the animal's mass. However if the branch the animal travels on is very narrow, then the support polygon may be so narrow that the center of mass is frequently outside the polygon. When this occurs, the weight of the animal will create a torque that can make the animal topple.

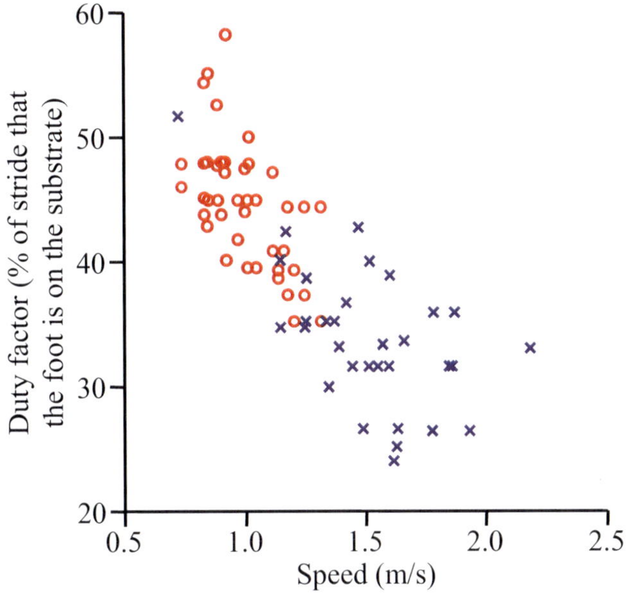

Fig. 2. Duty factor versus speed for gray short-tailed opossums walking and running on branches (red circles) and a flat trackway (blue Xs).

The sequence of footfalls can also affect where the center of gravity falls within a support polygon (Fig. 1). The variation in footfall patterns among taxa, the possible adaptive benefits of different footfall patterns, and the relationship of footfall patterns and walking/running mechanics are elaborated upon by Hildebrand (1976, 1980), Cartmill et al., (2002, 2007), and Reilly and Biknevicius (2003). When animals walk, trot, or pace, the right and left hindlimbs and right and left forelimbs are perfectly out of phase (Fig. 3). For example: assume a stride begins at the time of right lower extremity touchdown, and ends just before the next touchdown of the same limb. At the time the person's right lower extremity touches down while walking, the left lower extremity is halfway through the stride cycle. This also occurs with the right/left hindlimbs and forelimbs of quadrupeds. The phase relationship (limb phase) between the right hindlimb and right forelimb (or left hind and left fore) can be compared as a percentage of synchronization (Fig. 3). For example, if the right hindlimb and forelimb are synchronized (footfall and liftoff occur at the same time), the limb phase is 0%, and the animal is pacing. During a trot, the limb phase is 50% and the right forelimb is 50% ahead or behind whatever the right hindlimb is doing. During a lateral-sequence gait, the limb phase is between 0-50%. (Note: in this chapter, the word *gait* means footfall pattern, which is the definition typically used for non-human locomotor biomechanics. For human locomotor biomechanics, *gait* is any locomotion). After a right hindlimb lands, the right forelimb is the next limb to land. During this gait the center of gravity always passes through the support polygon (as long as three or four limbs are in contact with the ground. The diagonal-sequence gait features a limb phase between 50-100%. After a right hindlimb lands, the *left* forelimb is the next to land. This gait has frequently been observed among arboreal primates, the marsupials Monito del Monte and woolly opossum, and the carnivore kinkajou (Pridmore, 1994; Schmitt and Lemelin, 2002; Lemelin and Cartmill, 2010), although not in the arboreal sugar glider (*Petaurus breviceps*; Shapiro and Young, 2010). The prevalence of diagonal-sequence gaits among arboreal quadrupeds, and the strong lack of prevalence among terrestrial animals, demands an explanation. Cartmill et al. (2002, 2007) suggest that the diagonal sequence gait is an adaptation for increasing stability while walking on narrow arboreal supports. They demonstrate that the diagonal sequence diagonal-couplets gait increases the likelihood that opposing limbs will simultaneously grip the narrow arboreal support (Cartmill et al., 2002, 2007) instead of ipsilateral limbs (limbs on the same side of the body). An animal using this gait will follow a hindlimb contact with a forelimb contact on the opposite side (thus, diagonal sequence). If the hindlimb and diagonal forelimb strike the substrate closely in time, the diagonal sequence gait is also a diagonal couplet gait. Furthermore, Lemelin and Cartmill (2010) point out that the diagonal sequence diagonal couplet gait maximizes the spatial distance between contralateral limbs, which might limit the vertical oscillation of the center of mass. When the opposing limbs of a diagonal sequence diagonal couplet gait (or a trot) apply medially-directed force (Schmitt, 2003; Lammers and Biknevicius, 2004; Schmidt and Fischer, 2010), they squeeze the branch and increase normal force. Friction force is therefore increased, which makes slipping less likely. Furthermore, opposing mediolateral impulses and angular impulses generated by opposing limbs might reduce the mediolateral deviation from the long axis of the branch (Shapiro and Raichlen, 2007). It is also possible, however, that the prevalence of diagonal sequence gaits among many arboreal taxa results from differences in duty factor and stance durations between fore- and hindlimbs (Stevens, 2006).

It is also possible that the stability of an arboreal animal could be affected by the running gait it uses. During *bounding* locomotion, the forelimbs land simultaneously, followed by simultaneous contact of the hindlimbs (or vice-versa). If hindlimbs land simultaneously, but the forelimbs land at separate times, such a gait is referred to as a *half-bound*. A *gallop* is where forelimbs and hindlimbs land at different times; it differs from the gaits described in previous paragraphs (e.g., lateral sequence gait) because although the right and left hindlimbs (or right and left forelimbs) do not land at the same time, the hindlimb footfall contacts both occur before the forelimb contacts occur (or forelimbs can both land before hindlimbs; Bertram and Gutmann, 2008). During any footfall, energy is transmitted from the body of the animal to the substrate. If the animal runs on a narrow branch, the transfer of energy could cause the branch to oscillate, which could destabilize the running animal. Bertram and Gutmann (2008) suggest that a gallop, with its four separate footfalls, can reduce the amount of energy imparted to the ground or branch. We therefore predict that when an arboreal animal's mass relative to branch diameter is substantial enough to cause a branch to oscillate and destabilize the animal, that animal will run with a gallop or half-bound instead of a bounding gait. This prediction is supported by data presented by Young (2009), who showed that running marmosets and squirrel monkeys increase the lead time between right and left limb pairs when running on a narrow cylindrical trackway. For example, if the left forelimb lands first, the time interval (relative to stride duration) between left forelimb and right forelimb touchdowns is greater on the arboreal trackway. It appears that increasing duty factor and crouching during walking gaits has a similar effect of decreasing the vertical oscillation of a narrow arboreal support. Schmitt (1999) found that a wide variety of arboreal primates crouch and walk with a large duty factor, which reduces the peak vertical force and vertical oscillation of the branch; Young (2009) found similar results among running marmosets and squirrel monkeys.

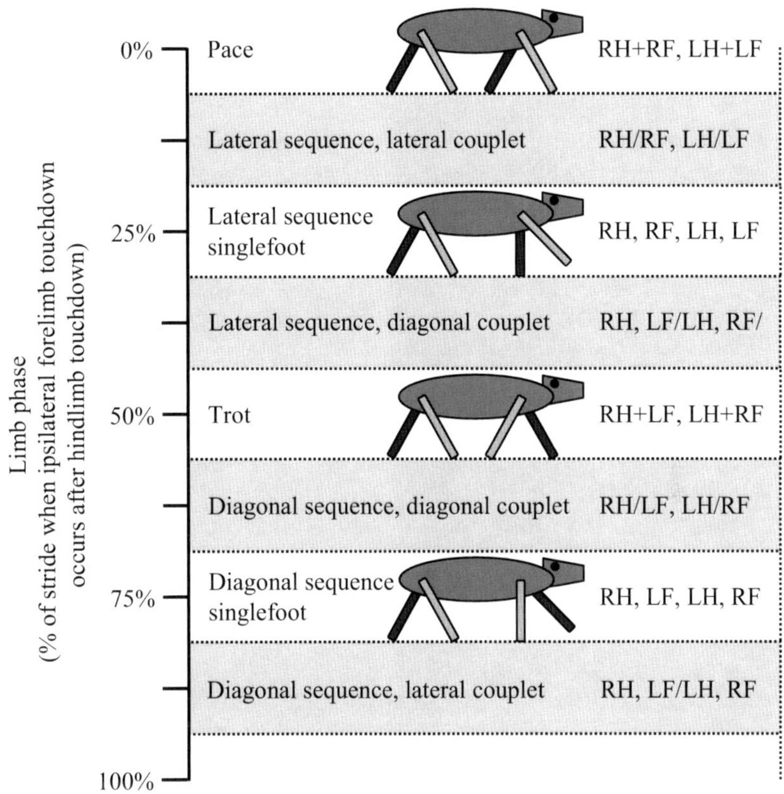

Fig. 3. Limb phase. Note that the configuration of the hindlimbs is the same in each drawing, and that the timing of the forelimb footfalls differs. Right limbs are shown as light gray and left limbs are dark gray. To the right of the quadruped drawings are footfall sequences (R = right, L = left, H = hindlimb, F = forelimb; + indicates footfalls occurring simultaneously, / indicates footfalls occurring close together in time, and a comma designates footfalls occurring relatively far apart in time. In the lateral sequence and diagonal sequence singlefoot gaits, all four footfalls are more or less evenly spaced in time. Each of the eight footfall patterns is defined by a limb phase (e.g., 25%) ± 6.25%. See Hildebrand (1976, 1980) for further detail.

Many arboreal primates, the wooly opossum, and the kinkajou reduce the vertical oscillation of the center of mass while walking on branches (Schmitt, 1999; Schmitt and Lemelin, 2002; Schmitt et al., 2006; Young, 2009; Lemelin and Cartmill, 2010). A gait frequently employed to reduce vertical oscillation is the *amble*, first termed by Schmitt et al. (2006). During ambling locomotion, the duty factor is less than 50% and the footfall pattern is trot-like or diagonal sequence, but there is no aerial phase. In other words, at least one foot is always in contact with the substrate. The lack of an aerial phase means that the center of mass is limited in its dorsal and ventral accelerations, which reduces peak vertical force, which in turn should reduce the vertical oscillation of thin branches (Young, 2009). The effects of branch oscillation or compliance on locomotor kinematics or kinetics are largely unexplored. Stevens (2003) demonstrated that primates change the movements of the limbs very little when a horizontal artificial branch trackway was oscillated in dorsoventral or mediolateral directions. However when the branch underwent twisting (rotating around the long axis), the quadrupedal primates stopped walking and appeared to freeze while branch movement was occurring (Stevens, 2003). Such rotational movement in thin branches could occur during strong winds, with the foliage acting like a sail.

The height of the center of mass over the substrate only matters when the gravitational acceleration vector passing through the center of mass (that is, the center of gravity) falls outside the base of support created by the limbs. The probability of this occurring decreases if the animal crouches. If the center of gravity *does* leave the base of support, then gravitational acceleration acts on the mass, creating a force. The horizontal distance between the center of mass and the outside of the base of support multiplied by the force is a torque that could cause the animal to topple from the support. There are at least three possible solutions (Cartmill, 1985):

1. Generate an opposing torque or other compensation; this requires a strong grip using opposable digits or opposing limbs. The tail may also contribute to reducing the total moment at any given instant (Larson and Stern, 2006).
2. Hang upside-down under the branch; in doing so, the animal will not fall as long as its grip on the branch (via opposable digits, opposable limbs, or both) does not give out. But now the world appears upside down, and the animal must either exert constant force with its musculature, or possess anatomy that allows the grip to be maintained with claws and/or a locking mechanism.
3. Reduce the length of the moment arm by crouching. (Cartmill, 1985, also points out that toppling moment can be reduced over evolutionary time by decreasing overall body size).

Many arboreal taxa grip the supports with long fingers and toes, including an opposable thumb and/or hallux (Cartmill, 1972, 1974, 1985). Strong gripping allows the animal to exert powerful torques on the branch, and the reaction torques stop the animal from toppling off the sides of the branch (Cartmill, 1985). (Strong gripping and exerting torques to keep the center of mass within the base of support formed by the limbs could also be classified as *dynamic stability* because the torque and gripping forces may need to be adjusted as the animal moves). To avoid slipping, arboreal taxa must increase friction force or generated some form of adhesion. Many arboreal taxa have claws to create new contact surfaces that allow normal force to be more efficiently generated (Cartmill, 1985). Some increase friction via pads that possess dermatoglyphic ridges (fingerprints) or other complex micro-structures that interact with the substrate to increase friction force (Cartmill, 1974; Hamrick, 2001) Suction, capillary action, or dry adhesion are other ways that an arboreal animal can make slipping less likely (Cartmill, 1985; Autumn et al., 2006).

The condition of static equilibrium depends on the details of the footfall pattern, details of the anatomy, and the direction and magnitude of the substrate reaction force and torque. This means that the force and torque components necessary for the condition of static stability at one instant during a stride would not provide stability at any other instant.

Therefore the condition of static stability will, in general, be violated except at very slow speeds. Thus another mechanism - dynamic stability - is responsible for the animal's stability when the forces and torques are not fully balanced.

3. Dynamic stability

Dynamic stability can be divided into two categories for analysis: the interaction of the whole, moving body with the substrate, and the internal movements of the various body parts (rotation of the hindlimbs around the hip joints or flexion and extension of the torso, for example). As the whole body moves over an arboreal substrate, the substrate reaction forces act to rotate the body around the center of mass (except during the instances where the substrate reaction force passes directly through the center of mass). Thus the body rotates around the roll, yaw, and pitch axes (Lammers and Zurcher, 2011). Any rotation of the body will increase the likelihood of toppling from a narrow support, especially rotation around the roll axis (around the anteroposterior or craniocaudal axis). Therefore it is necessary that a moment rotating the body in one direction (rolling to the left, for example) is balanced by a moment rolling the body back to the right. This can be quantified by integrating torque or moment during step time (angular momentum or angular impulse). As long as the angular impulse averaged over a stride is zero (or nearly zero), the rotational dynamics prevents the toppling of the animal and it will remain stable. Some data suggest that net zero angular impulses are often not maintained within a single stride, and that two or more strides are necessary to maintain dynamic stability (Belli et al, 1995; Forner-Cordero et al., 2006; Lammers and Zurcher, 2011). Another caveat with maintaining net zero angular impulses is that *at any instant*, it is necessary that moment is non-zero (positive or negative). The condition that the sum of the forces and moments about the center of mass over a stride is tiny or zero is not sufficient to maintain stability because the equilibrium configuration can either be stable, unstable, or indifferent/neutral (Fig. 4; Full et al., 2002). In an unstable equilibrium condition, non-zero moments must be applied to maintain stability. An example of this condition is riding a bicycle.

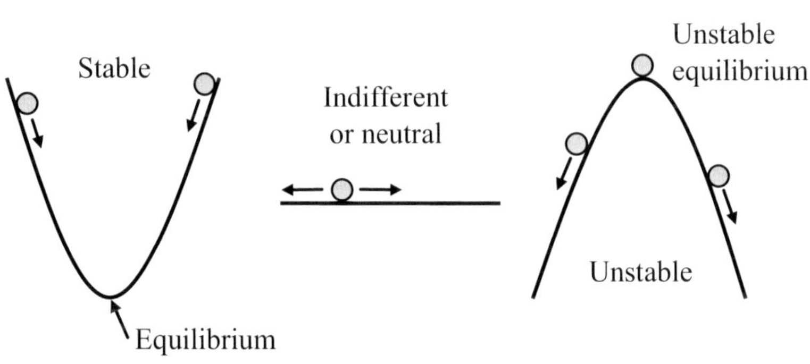

Fig. 4. In the stable configuration, a ball always rolls toward the equilibrium point at the bottom of the valley. In the indifferent or neutral configuration, the ball can roll anywhere and remain equally stable or unstable. In the unstable equilibrium condition, the ball is stable only if it remains perfectly balanced at the top of the hill. (See Full et al., 2002, for further detail).

In the static case, a person sitting on a bicycle will not topple if the person and bicycle are perfectly aligned along the vertical. However the person will fall if he/she and bicycle deviate even slightly from the upright position. On the other hand, a person riding a bicycle does not have any difficulty navigating even a rough terrain. This dynamic stability of the bicycle originates from the angular momentum of the wheels. The wheels rotate about their axis so that their angular momenta are approximately horizontal and perpendicular to the forward motion. If the bicycle is tilted away from the vertical position, the weight exerts a non-zero moment in the horizontal plane and directed in the forward direction. This moment drives the system back towards the equilibrium position. This is sometimes referred to as the "gyroscope effect." The vector of the angular motion of the wheels rotates, or precesses, about the vector of the angular momentum with the angular frequency $\mathbf{\Omega}$ (Fig. 5). The spinning of the wheel provides a *constant angular momentum* for the bicycle. There is, of course, no analogue of a spinning wheel for animal locomotion. For dynamic stability during arboreal locomotion, the non-zero angular momentum stems from small distortions

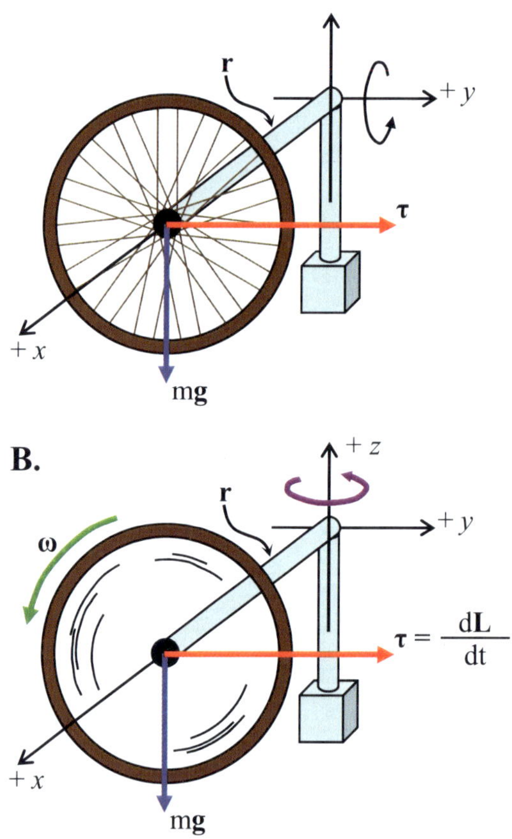

Fig. 5. A., a non-spinning bicycle wheel falls around axis *y* because mg exerts torque τ. B. When the bicycle wheel spins, it precesses around the *z* axis because of angular momentum **L**. (Adapted from Goldenstein, 2001).

of the animal's body. This includes the rotation of the limbs around the hip joint or center of rotation of the scapula; it is possible that the flexion and extension of the animal's trunk during galloping or bounding locomotion can also be included as a source of angular momentum. In human locomotion the angular momentum is due largely to the pendulum motion of legs and arms so the angular momentum must be different in the first and second half of a stride. In this manner, the *average* angular momentum during a stride is (approximately) zero. Indeed, Herr and Popovic (2008) analyzed the role of angular momentum in human walking, and found it to be highly regulated during a stride. The average angular momentum is nearly zero in all three spatial dimensions, but follows a distinct pattern during different phases that contributes to the stability. They found that angular momentum is important for the dynamic stability of human locomotion. Because the mass of the limbs of many quadrupedal arboreal animals (relative to their overall body mass) is small, the pendulum-like motion of the limbs might produce only a small angular momentum. For example, each forelimb of the Siberian chipmunk comprises about 4% of the total body mass, and hindlimbs are each about 6%. However many quadrupedal arboreal primates *do* possess relatively massive fore- and hind limbs, with much of the mass concentrated at the distal ends (Raichlen, 2006). Arboreal primates rely heavily on grasping hands and feet (Cartmill, 1972), and Raichlen (2006) suggests that the distal concentration of muscle mass contributes to the ability of primates' grasping ability. We agree with Raichlen (2006), but we suggest that the distal mass concentration also has the effect of increasing arboreal stability via increased angular momentum of the limbs.

4. Modeling

In the following, we use the convention that vector quantities, e.g., velocity, are printed in bold face. To use our model, we collected kinematic data from Siberian chipmunks (*Tamias sibiricus*) running on a cylindrical trackway 2 cm in diameter. The chipmunks were videotaped using two high-speed video cameras (210 Hz). Each camera captured a different view, and we then used the APAS motion analysis system to digitize 14 points on the head, body, tail, and the right forelimb and hindlimb. Thus we obtained a dataset of 14 three-dimensional points which described the position of the head, body, tail, and limbs every 210th of a second. We chose trials where the chipmunks bounded so that right and left limb pairs were moving more or less synchronously, and their position and movement is symmetrical on either side of the sagittal plane. Using estimates of segment masses obtained from a dead specimen, each segment is assigned a mass (m_i) with coordinate vectors $\mathrm{r}_i(n)$ at the time t_n. Thus the motion of each segment (e.g., body segments, limb segments, etc,) can be described. The digitized coordinates between consecutive video frames determine the coordinate vectors. The velocity vectors are then obtained: $\mathrm{v}_i(n) = [\mathrm{r}_i(n+1) - \mathrm{r}_i(n)] / \Delta t$, where $\Delta t = t_{n+1} - t_n$.
The center of mass [$\mathrm{R}_{CM}(n)$] is then found:

$$\mathrm{R}_{CM}(n) = \frac{\sum_i m_i \mathrm{r}_i(n)}{\sum_i m_i} = \frac{\sum_i m_i \mathrm{r}_i(n)}{M},$$

where M is the total mass. In the following notations, we suppress the discrete time dependence [that is, we eliminate the term n to make the expressions less cumbersome; e.g., R_{CM} rather than $R_{CM}(n)$]. The total linear momentum (P) is:

$$P = MV_{CM} = \sum_i m_i v_i,$$

where V_{CM} is the velocity of the center of mass. The relative coordinates and velocities are defined,

$$r_i = R_{CM} + \delta r_i,$$
$$v_i = V_{CM} + \delta v_i,$$

where δr_i and δv_i are coordinate and velocity vectors with respect to the center of mass. The total angular momentum (L) has a contribution from the center of mass motion and the relative motion of the body segments (Goldstein et al., 2001).

$$L = R_{CM} \times MV_{CM} + \sum_i \delta r_i \times m_i \delta v_i$$

When the center of pressure falls beyond the substrate, the animal is less likely to topple if the angular momentum around the mediolateral axis induces a precession-like rotation of the animal around the vertical axis.

Our preliminary data from Siberian chipmunks running on a narrow (2 cm diameter) cylinder (Fig. 6) suggest that the movement of the head and torso generates very little rolling angular momentum, and that it is largely centered around the zero axis (that is, above the central axis of the cylindrical trackway). Pitch and yaw momentum are relatively large. The pitch momentum results from the flexion and extension of the body, which should contribute to the gyroscopic effect. The yaw momentum is quite unexpected. We noticed that the chipmunks often ran on the left side of the branch trackway, perhaps to avoid the lights or experimenters. The large pitch angular momentum observed here is supported by data from Lammers and Zurcher (2011), which were obtained via a force pole and digitized 240 Hz videography (Fig. 7). Our data show that pitch angular momentum (the area enclosed by the pitch torque versus step time plot) is considerably greater than yaw and rolling angular momenta.

Full et al (2002) argue that neural control best enhances stability when it works with the natural, passive dynamics of the mechanical system. Our preliminary results show that the relative motion of the head, body, and limbs of the chipmunk generate the angular momentum, and thereby replace, partially at least, the role of legs and arms for human locomotion. We believe that the gyroscope effect associated with a non-zero angular momentum is critical for the initial response to a sudden external perturbation (e.g., sway or jerking of a branch) before the hands and feet have a chance to change their grip. Such a passive control is essential for the stability of the animal because it prevents the center of mass from deviating too much outside the base of support. Otherwise the body weight could produce a torque that is too large to be balanced by torques produced by substrate reaction forces and torques generated by the limb musculature.

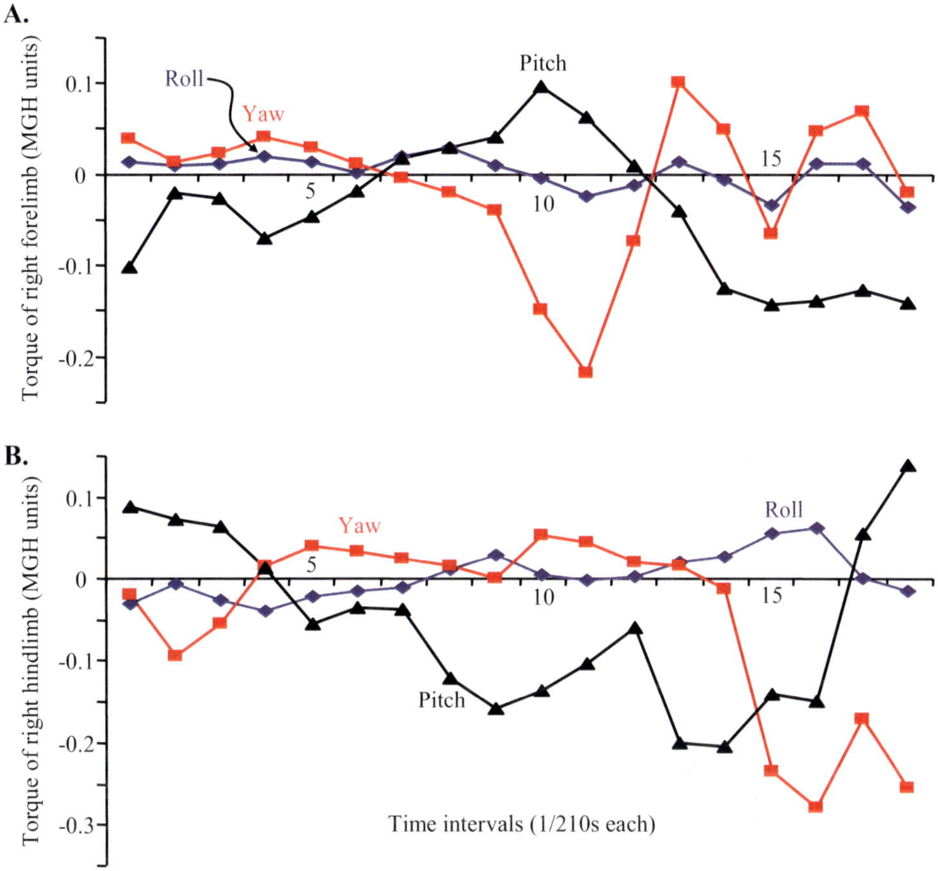

Fig. 6. Torque around three axes during one stride of the Siberian chipmunk. A, right forelimb; B, right hindlimb. Blue triangles represent pitch torque (around a mediolateral axis); red squares represent yaw, and black diamonds are rolling torque. The data points are smoothed by using a moving average; points 1 and 2 are averaged, then 2 and 3, etc. The portions of the stride where yaw torque is large are the swing phases of the limbs, where the limb most likely moves laterally and medially more than during stance phase. Pitch torque reflects the flexion and extension of the limbs and body. Rolling torque remains relatively small.

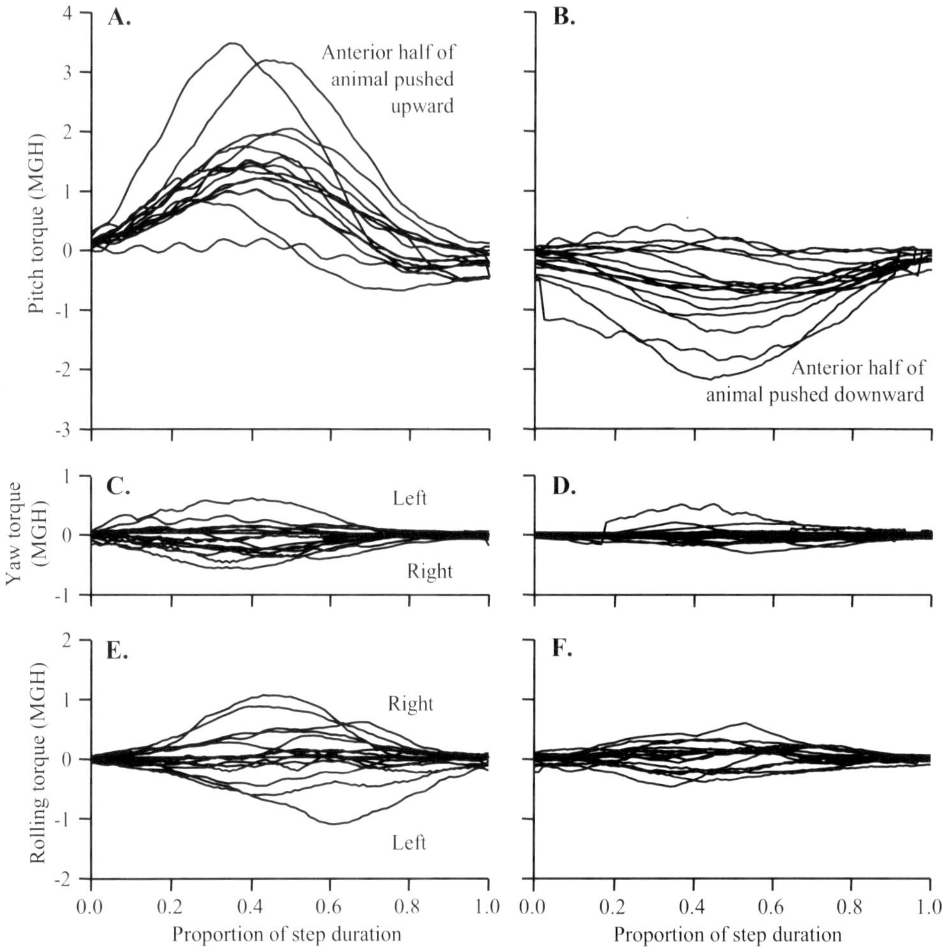

Fig. 7. Torques (MGH = mass · acceleration of gravity · center of mass height) around the center of mass versus percent of step time during forelimb contacts (A, C, and E) and hindlimb contacts (B, D, and F).

5. Dynamic stability analysis

We discuss two different methods of stability analysis. First, we consider only the angular momentum of the center of mass without considering the mass and velocities of the individual parts (**L**'):

$$\mathrm{L}' = \mathrm{R}_{CM} \times M\mathrm{V}_{CM} .$$

Some aspects of the dynamic stability of a bicycle can be used to understand stability during arboreal locomotion. Replacing total angular momentum L with the term L' from the center of mass motion would correspond to a bicycle sliding on a frictionless surface. The wheels do not spin, and the bicycle is mechanically unstable. The body is easily perturbed – if the center of pressure of the hand or foot of the animal or the wheel of the bicycle falls outside the support, a fall or stumble will probably occur. The system (arboreal mammal or bicycle) is dynamically stable if all internal degrees of freedom are included (that is, the mass, positions, and movements of each segment). Here we can add or subtract different modeled parts of the animal to determine their contributions to the angular momentum (and hence, to the dynamic stability):

$$\mathrm{L}'' = \mathrm{R}_{CM} \times M\mathrm{V}_{CM} + \sum_{i \neq k,l,m...} \delta\mathrm{r}_i \times m_i \delta\mathrm{v}_i .$$

In the expression above, the angular momentum of the center of mass *and* the angular momenta of individual parts are taken into account, but we can remove body segments, tail segments, limbs, etc. to determine their contribution. The second term $\delta\mathrm{L} = \sum_{i \neq k,l,m...} \delta\mathrm{r}_i \times m_i \delta\mathrm{v}_i$ provides the necessary angular momentum so that the animal's center of mass precesses around the vertical axis, and thereby prevents the animal from falling from the branch.

The second type of stability analysis uses tools to investigate the stability of dynamic systems for which the underlying equations of motion are not known (Strogatz, 1994). This method is based on the time-dependence of the dynamic variable Q at discrete times $t_n, Q = Q(n)$. For the present study, either the craniocaudal or mediolateral component of the angular momentum are useful choices for the quantity Q. In the phase portrait, the quantity $Q(n+1)$ at time t_{n+1} is plotted versus the same quantity $Q(n)$ at time t_n. If we choose $Q = L_{CC}$ (angular momentum around the craniocaudal axis), the phase portrait will consist of approximate circles, which is the signature of oscillatory motion. Circles in the phase portrait are referred to as "limit cycles" in the mathematical description of dynamic systems. Because the angular momentum (in this example, around the craniocaudal axis of the animal and the branch trackway) maintains a cycle, dynamic stability is maintained. Mathematical tools have been developed to quantify the stability of the system from limit cycles. This method has been used by Blickhan and coworkers (e.g., Seyfarth et al., 2002) to quantify the dynamic stability of human locomotion.

6. The impact of understanding stability during arboreal locomotion

Understanding how arboreal animals utilize static and dynamic stability during arboreal locomotion can provide insights to engineers attempting to build robots with legs.

Biologically-inspired robots might use dynamic stability strategies rather than static stability (Ritzmann et al., 2004). Also, the evolution of an arboreal animal's morphology, behavior, and central nervous system probably assumes dynamic stability mechanisms are used at high speed. This is especially true among animals whose center of mass is relatively far from the ground or substrate. The limb posture of primitive tetrapods was considerably less upright than many modern mammals (including humans); thus we expect that dynamic stability mechanisms were less important to such sprawling animals. A thorough grounding in the importance of dynamic stability during locomotion might help to understand the anatomy and function of motor control systems and brains in general.

7. References

Autumn, K., Dittmore, A., Santos, D., Spenko, M., and Cutkosky, M. 2006. Frictional adhesion: a new angle on gecko attachment. *J Exp Biol* 209, 3569-3579.

Belli, A., Lacour, J.-R., Komi, P.V., Candau, R., and Denis, C. 1995. Mechanical step variability during treadmill running. *Eur J Appl Physiol Occup Physiol* 70, 510–517.

Bertram, J.E.A. and Gutmann, A. 2008. Motions of the running horse and cheetah revisited: fundamental mechanics of the transverse and rotary gallop. *J Roy Soc Interf* 6, 549-559.

Cartmill, M. 1972. Arboreal adaptations and the origin of the order Primates. In *The functional and evolutionary biology of primates*, edited by R. Tuttle. Aldine Atherton Inc., Chicago, pp. 97-122.

Cartmill, M. 1974. Pads and claws in arboreal locomotion. In *Primate locomotion*, edited by F.A. Jenkins, Jr. Academic Press, New York, pp. 45-83.

Cartmill, M. 1985. Climbing. In *Functional vertebrate morphology*, edited by M. Hildebrand, D.M. Bramble, K.F. Liem, and D.B. Wake. Belknap Press of Harvard University Press, Cambridge, pp.73-88.

Cartmill, M., Lemelin, P., and Schmitt, D. 2002. Support polygons and symmetrical gaits in mammals. *Zool J Linn Soc* 136, 401-420.

Cartmill, M., Lemelin, P., and Schmitt, D. 2007. Understanding the adaptive value of diagonal-sequence gaits in primates: a comment on Shapiro and Raichlen, 2005. *Am J Phys Anthrop* 133, 822-825.

Forner-Cordero, A., Koopman, H.J.F.M.,and van der Helm, F.C.T. 2006. Describing gait as a sequence of states. *J Biomech* 39, 948–957.

Full, R.J., Kubow, T., Schmitt, J., Holmes, P., and Koditschek, D. 2002. Quantifying dynamic stability and maneuverability in legged locomotion. *Integ Comp Biol* 42, 149-157.

Goldstein, H., Poole, C.P., and Safko, J.L. 2001. *Classical mechanics*, 3rd edition. Addison Wesley, Reading, MA.

Hamrick, M.W. 2001. Morphological diversity in digital skin microstructure of didelphid marsupials. *J Anat* 198, 683-688.

Herr, H. and Popovic, M. 2008. Angular momentum in human walking. *J Exp Biol* 211, 467-481.

Hildebrand, M. 1976. Analysis of tetrapod gaits: general considerations and symmetrical gaits. In *Neural control of locomotion*, edited by R.M. Herman, S. Grillner, and P.S.G. Stuart. Plenum Press, New York, pp. 203-236.

Hildebrand, M. 1980. The adaptive significance of tetrapod gait selection. *Amer Zool* 20, 255-267.

Jindrich, D.L. and Full, R.J. 2002. Dynamic stabilization of rapid hexapedal locomotion. *J Exp Biol* 205, 2803-2823.

Lammers, A.R. and Biknevicius, A.R. 2004. The biodynamics of arboreal locomotion: the effects of substrate diameter on locomotor kinetics in the gray short-tailed opossum (*Monodelphis domestica*). *J Exp Biol* 207, 4325-4336.

Lammers, A.R. and Zurcher, U. 2011. Torque around the center of mass: dynamic stability during quadrupedal arboreal locomotion in the Siberian chipmunk (*Tamias sibiricus*). *Zool* 114, 95-103.

Larson, S.G. and Stern, J.T. 2006. Maintenance of above-branch balance during primate arboreal quadrupedalism: coordinated use of forearm rotators and tail motion. *Am J Phys Anthrop* 129, 71-81.

Lemelin, P. and Cartmill, M. 2010. The effect of substrate size on the locomotion and gait patterns of the kinkajou (*Potos flavus*). *J Exp Zool* 313A, 157-168.

Nekaris, K.A.I. and Stevens, N.J. 2007. Not all lorises are slow: rapid arboreal locomotion in *Loris tardigradus* of Southwestern Sri Lanka. *Am J Primatol* 69, 112-120.

Pridmore, P.A. 1994. Locomotion in *Dromiciops australis* (Marsupialia: Microbiotheriidae). *Aust J Zool* 42,679-699.

Raichlen, D.A. 2006. Effects of limb mass distribution on mechanical power outputs during quadrupedalism. *J Exp Biol* 209, 633-644.

Ritzmann, R.E., Quinn, R.D., and Fischer, M.S. 2004. Convergent evolution and locomotion through complex terrain by insects, vertebrates and robots. *Arthrop Struct Devel* 33, 361-379.

Schmitt, D., Cartmill, M., Griffin, T.M., Hanna, J.B., and Lemelin, P. 2006. Adaptive value of ambling gaits in primates and other mammals. *J Exp Biol* 209, 2042-2049.

Schmitt, D. and Lemelin, P. 2002. Origins of primate locomotion: gait mechanics of the woolly opossum. *Am J Phys Anthrop* 118, 231-238.

Seyfarth, A., Geyer, H., Günther, M., and Blickhan, R. 2002. A movement criterion for running. *J Biomech* 35, 649-655.

Shapiro, L.J. and Raichlen, D.A. 2007. A response to Cartmill et al.: primate gaits and arboreal stability. *Am J Phys Anthrop* 133, 825-827.

Shapiro, L.J. and Young, J.W. 2010. Is primate-like quadrupedalism necessary for fine-branch locomotion? A test using sugar gliders (*Petaurus breviceps*). *J Hum Evol* 58, 309-319.

Stevens, N.J. 2003. The influence of substrate size, orientation and compliance upon Prosimian arboreal quadrupedalism. Ph.D. dissertation, State University of New York at Stony Brook.

Stevens, N.J. 2006. Stability, limb coordination and substrate type: the ecorelevance of gait sequence pattern in primates. *J Exp Zool* 305A, 953-963.

Strogatz, S.H. 1994. *Nonlinear dynamics and chaos: with applications to physics, biology, chemistry, and engineering.* Westview Press, Boulder, CO.

Young, J.W. 2009. Substrate determines asymmetrical gait dynamics in marmosets (*Callithrix jacchus*) and squirrel monkeys (*Saimiri boliviensis*). *Am J Phys Anthrop* 138, 403-420.

16

The Biomechanics of the Anterior Cruciate Ligament and Its Reconstruction

Christopher D. S. Jones[1] and Paul N. Grimshaw[2]
[1]*School of Medical Sciences*
[2]*School of Mechanical Engineering, University of Adelaide, Adelaide*
Australia

There is a vast amount of literature available discussing the movements of the knee joint and the function of the ligaments controlling these movements.
(Brantigan & Voshell, 1941)

1. Introduction

The anterior cruciate ligament (ACL) continues to be a major topic in orthopaedics and biomechanics. This is due to the high incidence of injury and its disabling consequences. That the disabling consequences have not yet been completely overcome guarantees continued interest.

Injury to the ACL is associated with a range of problems, such as pain, instability, meniscal damage and osteoarthritis (Noyes et al., 1983; Segawa et al., 2001). This can be due to injury to other structures at the time of ACL injury, e.g. meniscus and articular cartilage, as well as developments secondary to the initial injury (Segawa et al., 2001). Although isolated injury to the ACL is considered uncommon, surgical transection of the ACL induces cartilage degeneration so reliably it is used to induce osteoarthritis in experimental animals (Desrochers et al., 2010).

Simple repair is effective for some ligaments, but such repair of the ACL has had poor results, and the orthopaedic world currently awaits the development of a useful scaffold that can be placed between the torn ends of the ligament to promote effective healing (Murray, 2009). In the interim a popular choice of treatment with positive results is surgical reconstruction (replacement), using a graft fashioned typically from the patellar ligament or from hamstring tendons (Woo et al., 2002). But despite positive outcomes from ACL reconstruction problems still persist after 'successful' surgery, especially osteoarthritis (Øiestad et al., 2010). It is only possible to speculate that kinematic differences that remain after, or are caused by, surgical reconstruction lead to osteoarthritis (Scanlan et al., 2010), but post-surgical kinematic differences may lead to cartilage loading differences, which then predispose the knee to osteoarthritis (Andriacchi et al., 2004, 2006). These loading differences may lead to cartilage areas subsequently sustaining higher or lower loads or loads of a different nature (e.g. tension, compression) (Chaudhari et al., 2008).

Development of a suitable ligament substitute is a straightforward matter: (1) determine the nature of the ligament, and (2) design a replacement that replicates this nature tolerably well. But straightforward is not simple, and the following review will highlight what is known, and what yet to be known, about the ACL and its substitutes.

2. Anatomy

The ACL spans the tibiofemoral joint space, and forms a cross with the posterior cruciate ligament. The proximal attachment is located posteriorly on the medial side of the lateral femoral condyle in a semilunar area with the straight border facing forward and slightly down. The ligament attaches distally on the anterior aspect of the tibia, just anterior and lateral to the anterior tibial spine (Fuss, 1989; Girgis et al., 1975).

There is some variation in the description of separate parts of the ligament at the macroscopic level. The pattern with greatest acceptance shows two bundles, anteromedial and posterolateral (Furman et al., 1976; Harner et al., 1999; Inderster et al., 1993; Katouda et al., 2011; Steckel et al., 2007). Harner et al. (1999) and Steckel et al. (2007) described the anteromedial bundle as arising from the proximal part of the femoral attachment, with the posterolateral bundle arising from the distal portion. On the tibia the anteromedial bundle attaches medially and the posterolateral bundle attaches laterally.

But these findings are not unchallenged. Fuss (1989) and Odensten and Gillquist (1985) found no such subdivisions by dissection and histological examination. Clark and Sidles (1990) referred to anteromedial and posterolateral bands but found them "indistinct", and described an anterior furrow that gave the ligament the appearance of being bifid. In the other direction, Amis and Dawkins (1991) and Norwood and Cross (1979) reported three bundles, anteromedial, intermediate and posterolateral.

The acceptance of the two bundle anatomy is so widespread today as to probably make any alternative claim go largely unnoticed. Nevertheless, without rejecting or accepting the preceding descriptions it is biomechanically meaningful to describe anteromedial and posterolateral ligament *fibres*, without assuming a plane of separation, as the cross-sectional shape of the ligament has an anteromedial-posterolateral long axis (Harner et al., 1995).

3. Normal function

The function of a ligament is to resist movement by resisting elongation caused by that movement, which may be rotational, translational or both. To understand the function of a ligament during a rotational movement, some consideration must be given to the relationship of the ligament to the axis of rotation. It is fundamental then to understand normal knee kinematics and ACL behaviour during knee motion.

3.1 Kinematics of the normal knee

The principal motion at the knee joint is flexion-extension in the sagittal plane, with a normal passive range of 130 to 140° and an associated 5 to 10° of hyperextension (Nordin & Frankel, 1989). The knee also has smaller ranges of motion in the horizontal and coronal planes, with passive and active ranges of approximately 70° of combined internal-external rotation in the horizontal plane, and minimal valgus-varus rotation in the coronal plane, although these figures are dependent upon the amount of flexion and extension in the joint (Hollister et al., 1993). The ranges of internal and external rotation are minimal and maximal at zero and 90° of flexion, respectively (Bull & Amis, 1998).

With reference to flexion-extension, there is still debate about the exact location of this axis of rotation (Smith et al., 2003). However, four schools of thought have emerged that present different arguments as to the nature and location of this axis.

The *instantaneous axis* is thought to lie in both the coronal and horizontal planes and moves in a curved or elliptical pathway as the knee undergoes rotation and translation. This approach positions the centre of mass of the joint and the movement of the joint primarily within the sagittal plane. The articular surface of the lateral femoral condyle has a greater variation than that of the medial femoral condyle. In the fully flexed position this axis is closest to the joint surface, which allows the ligaments of the joint (ACL and collateral ligaments) to slacken. In extension the axis is further away from the joint line and the same ligaments become tense (Brantigan & Voshell, 1941). The major criticism of this approach resides in the fact that condyles of the femur are varied in three dimensions rather than two dimensions, the latter of which is the only way to place the axis of rotation purely in the sagittal plane.

More recently a *fixed axis* of rotation offset to both the frontal and horizontal planes has been proposed (Hollister et al., 1993; Martelli & Pinskerova, 2002). The first of two fixed axes, the posterior condylar axis, runs from the medial to the lateral side of the joint and is also inclined posteriorly and distal to the joint centre. This first axis is effective from 15 to 150° of knee flexion and is defined as passing through the origins of both the medial and lateral collateral ligaments and the intersection of the anterior and posterior cruciate ligaments. This axis is considered to also be inclined at an angle of 7° to the sagittal plane, thus closely equating its position to the epicondylar line of the joint (Churchill et al 1998). As the knee moves into extension this axis changes to a second fixed axis of rotation, the distal condylar axis, that is located proximal to the distal aspect of the intercondylar notch (Elias et al., 1990).

The *helical axis* of rotation can perhaps be more easily described and understood as simultaneous rotation around and translation along a specified axis, like the action of a nut rotating and translating along a threaded bolt. This axis defines motion of the joint as a series of displacements rather than relative positions (Bull & Amis, 1998). This approach represents an instantaneous axis that the joint can both translate and rotate about (Blankevoort et al., 1988; Soudan et al., 1979). The *screw-home* mechanism of the joint, where there is an internal rotation and posterior translation of the femur on the tibia during extension is an example of the need for a helical axis of rotation. The main criticism with the helical axis approach to joint motion is one associated with accuracy. For example, for the helical axis to be consistent there would be a requirement that the motion of the joint is firstly described precisely in order to determine the exact location of the helical axis. However, in order to define exact movement of a joint (flexion-extension, internal-external rotation or abduction-adduction rotation) an axis of rotation is required.

The final school of thought incorporates an *infinite axis* of rotation theory where the exact knee motion depends on a number of factors such as ligament and soft tissue restraints, bony architecture, passive motions and external loads and forces during weight bearing. Blankevoort et al. (1988) and La Fortune et al. (1992) found no screw-home mechanism during weight bearing in vivo, and suggested that the knee has a range of motion that is specifically dependent upon passive characteristics. For example, the screw-home mechanism can be found to be overcome by external passive forces during movement (Sanfridsson et al., 2001; Smith et al., 2003).

The choice of axis for the principal motion of knee depends largely on the degree of accuracy that is needed in whatever application it is being used. For the installation of total knee joint prosthesis the complex axis of rotation of the knee is usually replaced by a fixed axis of rotation. However, in this application careful selection of the type of prosthesis is required (Kurosawa et al., 1985; Siu et al., 1996). Alternatively, if the accuracy of determining the axes is not so stringent, as in the case of a clinical test, then the first approach, an instantaneous axis in the frontal and transverse plane, is seen as acceptable.

In the horizontal plane the knee joint rotates about a longitudinal axis that extends through the tibia, however variations in the understanding of the location of this axis still exist within the scientific literature. This axis does not intersect with the flexion-extension axis of the knee and it is firmly located within the tibia. This axis runs close to the medial inter-condylar tubercle (Lehmkuhl & Smith, 1983) and also very close to the ACLs tibial attachment. Furthermore, it is directed posteromedially close to the femoral attachment site of the posterior cruciate ligament (Zatsiorski, 2002). Rotations around this axis are termed internal and external rotations of the tibia and are specified as such unless the coupled motions of the femur are also included (Smith et al., 2003). This axis of rotation is present due to the incongruence of the femoral and tibial articulating surfaces and is affected by ligamentous insufficiency. With the knee in full extension rotation around this axis is minimal as the ligaments are taut and the menisci are firmly held between the articulating surfaces. In addition, the tibial spines are lodged in the intercondylar notch (Levangie & Norkin, 2001). During knee flexion the complex arrangement changes and the condyles of the tibia and femur are free to move. At approximately 90° of knee flexion around 30° internal and 45° external rotation is present at the joint (Nordin & Frankel, 1989).

Several variations exist as to the exact location of this axis. Some research (Brantigan & Voshell, 1941; Hollister et al., 1993; Matsumoto et al., 2001; Shaw & Murray, 1974) has suggested that the axis is either fixed, passing through the medial femoral condyle or the intercondylar eminence, or as an instantaneous centre of rotation. Such wide contrasting opinion has resulted from the fact that the longitudinal axis of rotation in the knee is dependent upon many other factors than bony architecture.

3.2 ACL behaviour

The kinematics of the knee are complex and the ACL crosses the joint obliquely in three planes. There is the potential then that the function of the ACL is also complex, and this is shown by a voluminous literature. To try to impose order on a vast body of knowledge, the main movements relevant to ACL function are presented below first as separate, then combined where appropriate.

3.2.1 Flexion-extension

The ACL is not usually considered a restraint at end of range flexion or extension, but its load or strain behaviour is influenced by the knee's position within these limits and is therefore of interest. The findings presented here do not relate to the entire ligament, as many authors have found the behaviour to differ between the anteromedial and posterolateral bands.

Several studies show reciprocal behaviour of the two bands, in that flexion causes the anteromedial band to lengthen and the posterolateral band to slacken, at least up to 120° (Amis & Dawkins, 1991; Bach et al., 1997; Hollis et al., 1991; Takai et al., 1993; Wang et al.,

1973). But this picture of simple reciprocity may be an over-simplification. Two of the above studies show that the anteromedial band length decreases in the first 10 to 30° of flexion before increasing further into flexion (Amis & Dawkins, 1991; Bach et al., 1997). And Bach and Hull (1998) showed the strains in both bundles dropped in initial flexion (15 to 30°), and then remained at zero; only after 90° did the anteromedial band strain increase. Inderster and coworkers' (1993) results show that the length of the anteromedial band remains roughly constant to 90°, with the posterolateral band slackening from full extension.

3.2.2 Anterior translation

The ACL is the primary restraint to anterior translation, bearing 80 to 90% of the load (Abbott et al., 1944; Butler et al., 1980; Furman et al., 1976; Takai et al., 1993). Ligament strain (Ahmed et al., 1987; Bach & Hull, 1998; Berns et al., 1992; Beynnon et al., 1992; Beynnon et al., 1997; Fleming et al., 2001; Gabriel et al., 2004; Sakane et al., 1997; Takai et al., 1993; Torzilli et al., 1994) or load (Livesay et al., 1995; Markolf et al., 1995) increases with an anterior force on the tibia. When the ACL is cut anterior translation increases (Diermann et al., 2009; Fukubayashi et al., 1982; Hsieh & Walker, 1976; Markolf et al., 1976; Oh et al., 2011; Reuben et al., 1989; Wroble et al., 1993; Yoo et al., 2005; Zantop et al., 2007), or a given translation is resisted by a lesser force (Butler et al., 1980; Li et al., 1999; Lo et al., 2008; Wu et al., 2010).

And while the function of the whole ligament is beyond question here, that of the two bands is another matter. Studies have shown that posterolateral band loading on anterior force is either greater than or equal to that in the anteromedial band in extension, and with slackening of the posterolateral band in flexion a greater proportion of load is borne by the anteromedial band (Amis & Dawkins, 1991; Gabriel et al., 2004; Sakane et al., 1997; Takai et al., 1993). In support of this concept of the posterolateral band being more functional in flexion than extension, Zantop et al. (2007) measured the anterior translation on anterior force in a series of cadaveric knees before and after resection of either the anteromedial or posterolateral band. Deficiency of the posterolateral band led to greater translation increase at 30° flexion, with greater increases seen with anteromedial band deficiency at 60 and 90°.

The findings of two other studies make the relation between the two bundles less clear. Bach and Hull (1998) found no difference in strain between bands on anterior force through flexion. Wu and colleagues (2010) calculated that ligament forces were greater in the anteromedial band than the posterolateral band at all flexion angles, with the peak anteromedial band force at 30° flexion, and the posterolateral band contribution peaking full extension. So although Wu and co-workers' findings on the posterolateral band function reflected those above, their finding that anteromedial band force was greatest at low flexion led them to conclude that the sharing of load bearing is not so much reciprocal, with the anteromedial and posterolateral bands functioning in high and low flexion, respectively, but complementary, meaning here that peaks and troughs are much more similar.

3.2.3 Internal rotation

The ACL may act as a restraint to internal rotation, but there is no widespread agreement. Studies where ACL-intact knees have been subjected to an internal rotation torque have shown increases in ACL strain, both in vitro (Ahmed et al., 1987; Bach & Hull, 1998) and in vivo (Fleming et al., 2001), and ACL force in vitro (Kanamori et al., 2000; Markolf et al., 1990). Results from an in vivo patient study, as well as transection studies in cadaver knees have shown an increase in internal rotation range compared to the ACL-intact state (Hemmerich et al., 2011; Kanamori et al., 2000; Lipke et al., 1981; Markolf et al., 2009; Oh et al., 2011; Wroble et al., 1993). These differences though were typically small though statistically significant; Wroble et al. (1993) concluded their results were "clinically unimportant".

However other transection studies in cadaver knees have not shown an increase in internal rotation range (Lane et al., 1994; Reuben et al., 1989; Wünschel et al., 2010), and Lo et al. (2008) showed no increase in ACL force on internal rotation in vitro. In an in vivo study, Hemmerich and colleagues (2011) found that ACL-deficient patients showed an increase in internal rotation range, but at 0° flexion and not at 30°.

So the effect of the ACL on the range of internal rotation is unclear. Lane et al. (1994) and Oh et al. (2011) concluded that the ACL is unlikely to resist rotation as its central position in the knee is too close to the rotational axis. Interestingly then, Lipke et al. (1981) transected the lateral collateral ligament and posterolateral structures in addition to the ACL. While cutting these other structures in the ACL-intact knee had no effect on internal rotation range, after they were cut in the ACL-deficient knee there was an increase in range. They concluded that cutting the ACL shifted the rotation axis medially. This is supported by other findings that show a medial shift of the rotation axis in the ACL-deficient knee (Mannel et al., 2004; Matsumoto, 1990), although not by others that show no change in position (Shaw & Murray, 1974).

Studies addressing function of the two bands also conflict. Bach and Hull (1998) found no difference in band strain on internal rotation, whereas Lorbach et al. (2010) found that transection of the posterolateral band increased internal rotation on rotational torque at 30° flexion, and was not significantly increased by transecting the anteromedial band.

3.2.4 Combined anterior translation/internal rotation

There is an apparent link between anterior translation and internal rotation of the tibia. Fukubayashi and co-workers (1982) found in a series of cadaver knees that an anterior force of up to 125N applied to the tibia resulted in anterior translation and internal rotation, and that the rotation ceased after the ACL was cut. When the knees were constrained to move only in anterior translation the measured translation was substantially less. In other cadaveric studies, application of a 100N anterior force produced coupled internal rotation (Hollis et al., 1991), and simulated 200N quadriceps contraction caused anterior tibial translation coupled with internal rotation (Li et al., 1999). Internal rotation due to anterior force is not a universal finding, with Lo et al. (2008) showing a 50N anterior force (with a 100N joint compressive force) did not elicit a significant increase in rotation.

Many authors have measured the opposite of this, i.e. anterior translation resulting from applied internal rotation torque; most of these also applied a valgus torque, and they will be reviewed later. Kanamori et al. (2000) measured an anterior translation on internal rotation torque (10N·m) that increased significantly after ACL transection. Two studies investigated tibial translation with internal rotational torque and joint compression force. Lo and colleagues (2008) found no significant increase in anterior translation on a 5N·m rotational torque, although it was at the same level as with a 50N anterior force. Oh et al. (2011) found that anterior translation upon large internal rotational torque (17N·m, with an 800N compressive force) doubled after ACL transection, and concluded that internal rotation torque loads the ACL due to anterior tibial translation.

The issue of coupled anterior translation and internal rotation is clearly the major kinematic issue in ACL reconstruction research, so it is well to discuss this here. Anterior force causes anterior translation that is increased if the tibia is allowed to internally rotate. We propose that pure anterior translation is possible with a low load in the ACL, but with higher load the ACL tethers the medial tibial condyle, and if unconstrained produces internal rotation. (While Nordt et al. (1999) suggested that the increased resistance of medial compared to lateral structures gives rise to internal rotation in this case, and we agree that these structures must allow rotation, Fukubayashi et al. (1982) showed loss of internal rotation when only the ACL was cut.) An imaginary horizontal line across both tibial condyles would then translate anteriorly initially, then with a larger load may appear to translate anteriorly, but would actually diverge laterally. This case is illustrated in Figure 1(a).

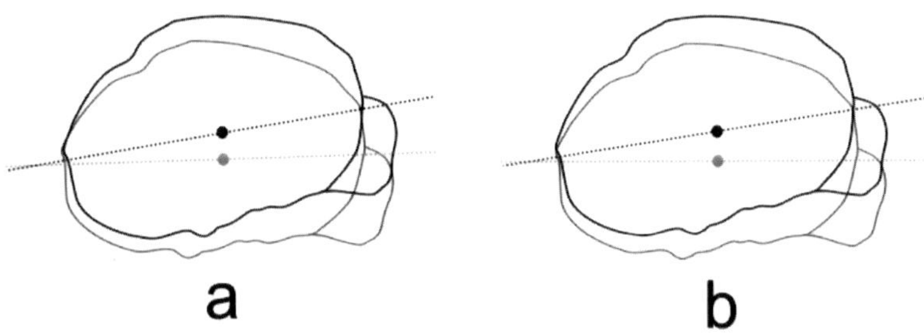

Fig. 1. The articular surface of the proximal tibia, having undergone (a) anterior translation and internal rotation around a central axis, and (b) pure internal rotation around a medially placed axis

Internal rotation torque causes internal rotation, and appears to cause a measurable anterior translation. But neither Kanamori et al. (2000) nor Oh et al. (2011) measured rotation with translation constrained. Fukubayashi et al. (1982) showed that pure anterior translation was restricted compared to anterior translation with unconstrained internal rotation, and it will be seen in 3.2.5 that valgus rotation is greater with internal rotation allowed than constrained. We know of no other studies that have measured rotation this way, so we hesitate to call rotation and translation coupled. Furthermore we know of no explanation of coupled translation that allows us to understand why it occurs. But the effect appears to be greater with ACL deficiency, and as such it is something better to be understood. We think the published data are consistent with a simpler interpretation provided by Lipke et al. (1981), Mannel et al. (2004) and Matsumoto (1990), in that ACL transection causes a medial shift of the rotational axis. Figure 1(a) shows the result of anterior translation and internal rotation about a central axis, but it also looks like the tibia has rotated about an axis just medial to its medial border; Figure 1(b) shows the end result of such a rotation. We ask whether it is possible to detect the difference between these two tibial movements on an actual knee. As the centre of the tibia in Figure 1(b) is travelling along an arc, it should come to rest slightly more medially than in Figure 1(a). Results of studies in vivo (DeFrate et al., 2006) and in vitro (Li et al., 2007; Seon et al., 2010; Van de Velde et al., 2009) show that transection or rupture of the ACL increases medial tibial translation. So the ACL-deficient knee appears to either combine anterior translation, internal rotation and medial translation, or the more parsimonious alternative of internally rotating about a medially shifted axis.

This also concurs with Reuben and colleagues' (1989) conclusion that ACL deficiency causes anterior translation "about a pivot point that is medially based". Translation around a pivot, or axis, is of course rotation.

We suggest that the ACL prevents the *wrong sort* of rotation, that being potentially any rotation about an axis to which the knee is not accustomed. In this case, the ACL appears to prevent anterior translation of the medial tibial condyle, that is rotation about a medial axis.

3.2.5 Valgus rotation

The knee joint is most restricted in motion in the coronal plane, but interesting findings have emerged from studies involving the application of torque in this plane. Inoue and co-workers (1987) subjected a series of canine knees to 0.6N·m valgus-varus torques and measured the resultant rotations with internal-external rotation and anterior-posterior translation first constrained, then unconstrained. Valgus-varus rotation was increased by 220% in the latter case, valgus being coupled with internal rotation and varus with external rotation, and anterior-posterior translation was effectively zero. The effects of ACL transection on these findings were again dependent on constraint: in the constrained state the valgus range increased by 10%, but by 186% when unconstrained, and both valgus and varus were coupled with anterior translation. These results are corroborated by those of Hollis et al. (1991), who found coupled internal and external rotation with applied valgus and varus torques, respectively.

3.2.6 Combined internal rotation/valgus rotation – the 'pivot shift'

Internal rotation and valgus torques are commonly combined in a clinical test for ACL function called the *pivot shift*, which, subject to variations, consists of the application of these torques such that the lateral tibial condyle subluxes anteriorly in extension, and then with flexion the condyle abruptly slides posteriorly at around 30° (Galway & MacIntosh, 1980). Galway and MacIntosh (1980) described the subluxation as involving the whole tibia, but predominantly the lateral condyle was involved.

The usefulness of the clinical pivot shift test as an indicator of ACL deficiency is beyond the scope of this review. It continues to be of biomechanical interest due to an association between a positive test and poorer outcome after ACL reconstruction (Jonsson et al., 2004), although Noyes et al. (1991) found too much operator subjectivity in the movements produced to recommend the manual pivot shift as an objective test.

To better understand the biomechanics of the pivot shift, studies have measured knee kinematics while subjecting cadaveric knees to combined torques to simulate the manoeuvre. Markolf et al. (1995) showed that the combination of internal rotation/valgus torque (10N·m/10N·m) increased ACL force, whereas varus torque with either internal or external rotation did not. Kanamori et al. (2000) showed that anterior translation in the ACL-deficient knee resulting from a 10N·m internal rotation torque increased when that torque was combined with a 10N·m valgus torque; also ACL forces were greater with the combined torque. The most consistent finding in the ACL-deficient knee is an increase in anterior translation, where internal rotation was either not measured (Herbort et al., 2010; Yagi et al., 2002; Zantop et al., 2007), was found to be unchanged (Diermann et al., 2009; Seon et al., 2010) or increased (Kondo et al., 2010; Yamamoto et al., 2004). Studies have also sought to uncover the role of the ACL bands on combined internal rotation/valgus torque. On combined torque (5N·m/10N·m), Gabriel et al. (2004) calculated greater force borne by the anteromedial band than the posterolateral at 15 and 30° flexion, with a greater posterolateral band contribution at 15°, and Wu et al. (2010) found no difference in load borne by either band at 0°, and greater load borne by the anteromedial band at 30°. This is consistent with a picture of lessening posterolateral band contribution to resistance to combined rotation and valgus as flexion increases, and that by 30° the force in the anteromedial band is larger. So it is interesting to note that Zantop and colleagues (2007) found greater anterior translation on combined torque (4N·m/10N·m) when the posterolateral band was cut, compared to the anteromedial band, at 0 and 30° flexion.

The results of kinematic studies suggest that the function of the ACL, even in response to combined torques, is to limit anterior tibial translation. Such findings have led Diermann et al. (2009) to conclude:

To assess the rotational instability of the knee joint during the clinical examination, the observer needs to quantify rather the anterior tibial translation of the tibia than the internal tibial rotation of the tibial head.

So rotational instability is evinced not by rotation but by translation. These results are similar to those seen in 3.2.3. In Lane and co-workers' (1994) cadaveric transection study, which found no increase in internal rotation, the pivot shift test was positive. This was supported by Reuben and colleagues' (1989) findings, with pivot shift-like motion of the knee in the absence of recorded internal rotation change. Lane et al. (1994) concluded that the pivot shift reflected increased anterior translation in the presence of normal rotation.

An alternative explanation is that what is observed in the pivot shift sign is internal rotation about a medially-shifted axis. This was concluded by Matsumoto (1990), who located the rotation axis in cadaveric ACL-deficient knees as lying at the site of the medial collateral ligament, and recalls the findings of Lipke et al. (1981) and Mannel et al. (2004) (3.2.3). Galway and MacIntosh's (1980) description of the phenomenon (above) certainly looks to describe a rotation. Bull et al. (2002) too described a translation and rotation, but both about a medial axis. Noyes et al. (1991) measured the kinematics of an ACL- (and medial collateral ligament-) deficient cadaveric knee subjected to the pivot shift test by 11 orthopaedic surgeons. They recorded concurrent anterior translation and internal rotation, but the amount of movement depended on technique: for example, if initial internal rotation was increased then the medial tibial condyle projected less anteriorly than did the lateral. Musahl et al. (2011) showed that ACL-deficiency (1) increased lateral tibial condyle anterior translation, and (2) changed medial condyle movement from posterior translation to anterior. Why there is a seeming reluctance to describe an instability pattern where the lateral condyle subluxes anteriorly more than the medial as a rotation is unclear. We believe that measuring anterior translation and internal rotation, the latter about a central tibial axis, has led to some researchers as treating these as separate.

3.2.7 In vivo external forces – quadriceps load and body weight

Quadriceps load

Because in extension the quadriceps femoris muscles, acting via the patellar ligament, exert an anterior force on the tibia, contraction of the quadriceps is seen to load the ACL. In higher degrees of flexion the patellar ligament pulls the tibia posteriorly and this effect is lost. Studies using cadaveric knees (Bach & Hull, 1998; DeMorat et al., 2004; Renström et al., 1986) have shown that simulated quadriceps activity significantly increases ACL strain with the knee in up to 60° of flexion, and that ACL force peaks around 30° flexion (Li et al., 1999;

Li et al., 2004). This was corroborated by in vivo studies, showing that actual quadriceps contraction causes ACL strain increases to 30° flexion (Beynnon et al., 1992), and that ACL-deficient knees show increased anterior translation on quadriceps contraction in the same range (Bach & Hull, 1998; Barrance et al., 2006; DeMorat et al., 2004).

Studies examining the behaviour of the two bundles of the ACL on quadriceps contraction have shown equal band strain throughout flexion range (Bach & Hull, 1998; Wu et al., 2010).

Weight-bearing

It is clear that ligament function in the knee is sensitive to weight-bearing status. This has meaning beyond the laboratory: what obtains on the clinician's couch may not obtain on the street. Cadaveric studies have measured anterior translation with the knee unloaded and loaded with a compressive force. Hsieh and Walker (1976) found that a 98N load reduced anteroposterior translation, and Ahmed et al. (1987) showed a decreased range of anterior translation in the presence of a 900N preload, and a decrease in ACL strain with compression. In contrast, Torzilli et al. (1994) found anterior translation of the tibia in response to a joint compressive load (up to 444N), as did Oh et al. (2011), who found translation coupled with internal rotation with a compressive load of 800N. These findings were corroborated in vivo: Beynnon et al. (1997) and Fleming et al. (2001) found an increase in ACL strain with the simple change from non-weight-bearing to weight-bearing. Weight-bearing may increase ACL loading due to the posteroinferior slope of the proximal tibial surface (Hashemi et al., 2008) inducing an anterior shift on tibiofemoral compression (Fleming et al., 2001; Torzilli et al., 1994).

These indings can then help to explain the coupling of internal rotation with other movements. In 3.2.5 the application of valgus-varus torque was seen to induce coupled internal-external rotation (Inoue et al., 1987). The effect of these torques can now be seen in terms of weight-bearing through the lateral and medial condyles, respectively. Valgus torque opposes the lateral femoral and tibial condyles, and due to the slope of the tibial condyle there is relative posterior translation of the femoral condyle i.e. internal tibial rotation. Varus loading would then oppose the medial condyles, causing external tibial rotation. This is supported by Inoue's results following ACL transection: both valgus and varus torques resulted in anterior tibial translation. That the slope is greater on the lateral side (Hashemi et al., 2008) may help to explain the internal rotation found on compressing the knee joint (Meyer & Haut, 2008).

4. Anterior cruciate ligament injury and reconstruction

Loss of function of the ACL leads to kinematic changes that threaten the well-being of the knee and patient, and that may call for surgical reconstruction to combat them. But replacing a native ligament in order to replicate its function, when that function is not completely known, necessitates ongoing evaluation of the kinematics before and after surgery.

4.1 Kinematics of the ACL-deficient knee

In section 3 results of studies were discussed where the kinematics of ACL-deficient knees, both cadaveric and in living patients, were studied where external influences such as simulated weight-bearing and muscle forces were controlled. Studies have also been conducted where those influences were less controlled, in which living patients performed weight-bearing activities closer to normal everyday function, especially gait. These studies are beyond the scope of this review, not due to relevance but complexity: the kinematics of the ACL-deficient knee in walking will be a result of both the deficiency as well as the person's responses to that deficiency.

4.2 Kinematics of the ACL-reconstructed knee

Reconstruction of the ACL typically replaces the ligament with a graft from either a central strip of patellar ligament or one or more hamstring tendons. Studies addressing the kinematics of the ACL-reconstructed knee, comparing reconstructed knees with ACL-intact, and -deficient knees have increased our understanding of the success of attempts to restore knee function after injury. Given the lack of clarity of just what ACL deficiency causes, unsurprisingly these studies have also thrown up questions that remain unanswered.

Given the primacy of the ACL in resisting anterior translation on anterior force, this function has been a focus of ACL reconstruction research. Yoo et al. (2005) investigated the kinematics of reconstructed cadaveric knees under anterior force (130N) and simulated quadriceps load (400N). Anterior translation was restored to intact levels at flexion greater than 30°, but at 30° or less the translation was greater than the intact state.

The effects of reconstruction on knee rotation have of course been another focus. In an in vivo study, Nordt et al. (1999) measured internal and external rotation on rotational torque (5N·m) on ACL-reconstructed knees and compared values with the uninjured side. Internal rotation was decreased and external rotation increased in the reconstructed knees, leading the authors to conclude that internal rotation had been over-constrained. Yoo et al. (2005) did not apply a torsional load but they did measure rotation on anterior force (130N) and quadriceps load (400N). Interestingly internal rotation showed no difference between ACL-intact and -deficient knees, but was decreased in reconstructed compared to intact knees. This again suggested an over-constraint to internal rotation. On a combined internal rotation/valgus torque (10N·m/10N·m) in a cadaveric study, Woo et al. (2002) found that reconstructed knees showed reduced anterior translation compared to the deficient state, but increased compared to the intact state. Woo and coworkers thus suggested that reconstruction was unable to adequately limit rotational laxity, but with these few studies we see evidence of decreased and increased laxity associated with internal rotational torques.

So with problems with rotational laxity, alternative methods have been sought to improve results. One possible problem with the standard ACL reconstruction procedure is that the graft is somewhat vertical, with the femoral end just lateral to the summit of the roof of the intercondylar notch, and obliquity may affect rotational stability (Yamamoto et al., 2004). A potential improvement is a more laterally placed femoral tunnel to increase the obliquity of the graft. (As this reflects the original femoral attachment of the ligament better this has been termed an "anatomic" reconstruction (e.g. Kondo et al., 2011), but as this is also used to describe the effect of a double bundle reconstruction (e.g. Yamamoto et al., 2004) we will use the term *laterally placed*.) The notch with the knee in extension is open posteriorly, so the summit of the roof is anterior. With the knee in the surgical position of flexion, the summit is at the top of view, or at 12 o'clock, and the lateral wall of the notch in the right knee merges with the posterior articular cartilage at 9 o'clock (Seon et al., 2011). So the standard femoral placement is at 11 o'clock (Markolf et al., 2002); from the previous paragraph at least Woo et al. (2002) and Yoo et al. (2005) used the 11 o'clock position. Another effort to mimic the natural anatomy is the double bundle method, where anteromedial and posterolateral bands of the original ligament are replaced separately (Zaricznyj, 1987).

Effect of femoral tunnel site

In a study to compare a laterally placed single bundle reconstruction with the ACL-deficient state, Lie et al. (2007) compared anterior translation and internal rotation in cadaveric knees before and after ACL transection and after reconstruction (in the half-past 10 position). They also varied the graft tension, and examined its effect on kinematics. Anterior translation on anterior force (150N) was reduced from the deficient state up to that of the intact state with increasing graft tension. The pivot shift test was simulated by applying a "specific and unique combination of loads", meaning the results cannot be replicated but the combination of loads was kept constant for each knee. Increasing graft tension again reduced anterior translation, but not internal rotation.

Markolf and colleagues (2002) tested the laxity and ligament graft forces in a series of cadaveric knees with femoral attachment sites at the 10, 11 and 12 o'clock positions. Anterior translation on a 200N anterior force was not affected by tunnel position, and neither was graft force (on 100N anterior force or 5 and 10N·m internal-external rotational and valgus-varus force), between full extension and full flexion.

Seon et al. (2011) compared single bundle in vivo reconstructions with femoral attachments at 11 o'clock ("high") and 10 o'clock ("low"). Both methods reduced anterior translation on 100N anterior force to the same degree, agreeing with Markolf et al. (2002). The main departure from both Markolf et al. (2002) and Lie et al. (2007) was that the low group showed significantly less internal rotation on 10N·m torque than the high group, and without preinjury or contralateral knee range data, the authors declared this result "better".

Single (standard) versus double

Yagi et al. (2002) compared an anatomic double bundle method with a single bundle (11 o'clock) method in a series of cadaveric knees. The double bundle method led to increased anterior translation on a 134N anterior force at 0 and 30° flexion, compared to the intact state, but this translation was significantly less than for the single bundle reconstruction. Ligament force measured was at the intact level for the double bundle method and significantly greater than for the single bundle method up to 60° flexion, and the forces measured in the single bundle were less than in the intact state up to 30°. Single and double bundle reconstructions were both unable to reduce anterior translation on combined internal rotation/valgus torque (5N·m/10N·m), but the double bundle method reduced it more. Kondo et al. (2010) performed a similar study. Both reconstructions showed significant decreases from deficient values in anterior translation on 90N anterior force, with the double bundle method showing significantly less translation, and values were not compared with the intact state. On 5N·m internal rotation torque the double bundle method reduced internal rotation to intact levels, but the single bundle method did not. On combined internal rotation/valgus torque (1N·m/5N·m), both reconstructions lowered anterior translation. Under the combined torque, only the double bundle method reduced internal rotation, but to below intact levels i.e. internal rotation on pivot shift was over-constrained, but not on internal rotation torque.

Single (lateral) versus double

Several studies have attempted to compare the effectiveness of one development over the other i.e. laterally placed single bundle versus double bundle. Yamamoto et al. (2004)

compared a series of cadaveric knees in the ACL-intact, -deficient and –reconstructed (laterally placed [10 o'clock] single bundle and "anatomical" double bundle) states. Anterior translation on 134N anterior force was restored to normal levels in the double bundle method, and was greater than in the intact state in the single bundle method at 60 and 90° flexion. Forces borne by the two ligament grafts reflected these results, those in the single bundle graft being lower than in the intact state at 60 and 90°. Combined internal rotation/valgus torque (5N·m/10N·m) produced anterior translation that was reduced to intact levels by both methods, and graft forces measured were the same with each method. Combined torque produced internal rotation that was restored to intact levels by both methods at 15°, and was greater with both methods at 30°. These results suggest that a single bundle reconstruction may achieve the same rotational stability as a double bundle reconstruction, with a shift in the femoral tunnel location.

Bedi et al. (2010) compared anterior translation of the tibia on anterior force and mechanized pivot shift in cadaveric knees in the ACL-intact, -deficient (including of menisci) and reconstructed states. The reconstruction methods were double bundle and single bundle, the femoral tunnel for the latter being placed in between the tunnel sites for former. They measured movement of the lateral and tibial condyles and a central point independently. Both reconstructions restored translation to the intact level on anterior force (68N). Both reconstructions reduced lateral condyle movement during a "mechanized pivot shift" (torques not given), but the double bundle method reduced it more.

Seon et al. (2010) compared anterior and medial translation and internal rotation ranges in a series of cadaveric knees in the intact, deficient and reconstructed (single [half-past 10] and double bundle) states. They found reconstruction reduced anterior translation on anterior force (134N), simulated quadriceps load (400N) and combined internal rotation/valgus torque (5N·m/10N·m) from the deficient state, but the single bundle method did not reduce translation back to the intact level. Tibial medial translation was increased in the deficient state and was reduced to the intact level by both methods. Internal rotation on quadriceps load was reduced from the intact level by both reconstruction methods, more so with the double bundle, and the double bundle method reduced internal rotation on combined torque compared to the intact state. So although anterior tibial translation was improved with the double bundle method, this method also appears to have over-constrained internal rotation.

In an in vivo patient study comparing laterally placed single bundle and double bundle reconstructions, Aglietti et al. (2010) found an increase in anterior translation on 134N anterior force with the single bundle method, but only at 1- and 2-year follow-up. This reflects the findings of Seon et al. (2010) and Yamamoto et al. (2004), and is a useful reminder that the post-operative phase is only the start of an actual ACL reconstruction.

Hemmerich et al. (2011) compared internal rotation range on internal rotation torque (indexed to body weight) before and after single (10.30) or double bundle in vivo reconstruction. Although internal rotation in the deficient knee was shown to be increased at 0° (and not 30°) flexion, the only significant change in rotation after reconstruction was an over-constraint in the double bundle knees at 30°.

Standard single versus lateral single versus double

Kondo et al. (2011) compared translation and rotation in cadaver knees in the ACL-intact, -deficient, and –reconstructed (single bundle [11 o'clock], laterally-placed single bundle [10.30], and double bundle) states. While all reconstructions restored anterior translation on anterior force (90N) to intact levels, there were differences in rotation. The single bundle (11 o'clock) method was unable to decrease the internal rotation range on internal rotation torque (5N·m) to intact levels, unlike the laterally-placed single bundle and double bundle methods. A mechanized pivot shift test, delivering combined internal rotation/valgus torque (1N·m/5N·m), showed no changes to rotation, even in the deficient state (presumably due to lower rotational torque). Interestingly though, the combined torque caused an anterior translation that was (a) increased in deficient knees, (b) normal in the 11 o'clock single bundle reconstruction, and (c) decreased (i.e. over-constrained) in the laterally-placed single bundle and double bundle reconstructions.

So overall the laterally placed and double bundle methods may improve anterior translation but over-constrain internal rotation, when the specific nature of the rotational function of the ACL is unclear. It is useful at this point to look more closely at some of these data. Kondo et al. (2011) showed that laterally placed single bundle and double bundle reconstructions restored anterior translation on anterior force to normal levels, but over-constrained anterior translation on simulated pivot shift. There was no general over-constraint on rotation, as internal rotation range on rotational torque was normal. If pivot shift does measure anterior translation due to internal rotation, it would appear that the ACL has a greater role in restraining this anterior translation, as there was no over-constraint in translation on anterior force. Anterior translation should therefore be greater on pivot shift after transection than *an equivalent* anterior force, but we know of no models that allow calculation of an anterior force resulting from an internal rotation torque in the knee.

Bedi et al. (2010) showed mean measurements of movement of different parts of the tibia, and while many of these means were not statistically significantly different, they did derive from only five knees, and the pattern of differences provides us with a possible alternative explanation to Kondo and others' (2011) results. In the ACL-intact state, Bedi et al. (2010) showed that the pivot shift test elicited a zero mean anterior-posterior shift for the central point, with a posterior shift of the medial condyle and an anterior shift of the lateral condyle. In terminology appropriate to a situation where the degree of movement is dependent on position, the tibia rotated around a roughly central axis (Fig. 2(a)). The deficient state (again, the menisci were excised) showed anterior shift of the three measured points, lateral > central > medial, i.e. the tibia rotated around a medially placed axis (Fig. 2(b)). The change from posterior to anterior movement of the medial condyle on pivot shift was also shown in Musahl and coworkers (2011) results (3.2.6). The single bundle reconstruction showed movement of roughly equal magnitude of medial and lateral condyles, posteriorly and anteriorly respectively, but greater than in the intact state. That is, the tibia rotated about a central axis but with greater range than the intact state (Fig. 2(c)). Finally, the double bundle reconstruction led to posterior movement of the medial condyle and the central point (medial > central) and the lateral condyle moved anteriorly, i.e. rotated around a laterally placed axis (Fig. 2(d)). In this way Kondo and colleagues' (2011) posterior translation may have been less an over-constraint than a response to a shifted axis.

5. Future research

Over the last 30 or more years there has been much written about the ACL and its function and treatment, and although results of treatment are overall very good, it is surprising that there is still so much confusion regarding the role of the ligament, and there is no meaningful consensus statement about what precisely surgery should be trying to mimic.

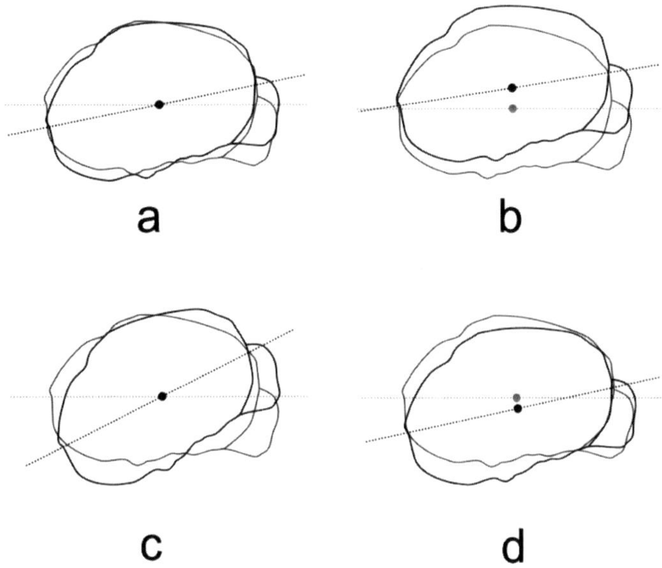

Fig. 2. The articular surface of the proximal tibia, having undergone internal rotation around an axis positioned (a) centrally, (b) medially, (c) centrally, but with greater range than (a), and (d) laterally.

One issue that we believe stands in the way of such consensus is a black and white atmosphere of false dichotomies encouraged by the *statistically significant/non-significant* divide, almost as if, for example, any increase in rotational laxity after ACL injury is the same as any other. What is required is a series of larger high-powered studies where meaningful estimates of laxities can be made. It is quite conceivable that reconstruction can never be perfect, but that a residual laxity is tolerable following reconstruction. But a statistical test with sufficient power to show a statistically significant, yet minor, difference results in a conclusion of abnormality; one where *n* is low enough and/or variance is high enough to mask a larger difference indicates that the situation is normal. We believe that a goal of reconstruction research should be, after stoically accepting that there will be an intact-reconstructed difference, to estimate that difference with confidence intervals and then to determine its clinical significance. Otherwise too much influence is placed in statistical inferences, with not enough in biological ones.

The data in the literature are consistent with a change to knee joint kinematics resulting from a change in position of the axis of knee joint rotation following ACL injury, and possibly also reconstruction. Just as an increase or decrease in rotational range may oppose articular regions not accustomed to opposing each other, and thereby initiate degenerative changes, so too may a change in position of the axis of rotation. We are embarking on research to investigate the range of offset-axis rotation, and the effect on that range of ACL transection. We believe this research will extend current knowledge and thinking that is focussed on central axis rotation, and possibly registers change in axis as increase in translation.

6. Conclusion

The ACL is considered a bipartite ligament, consisting of anteromedial and posterolateral bands, a description that contradicts some sound anatomical research and will live on undaunted. But the ligament is large and complex and there are sound functional reasons for overlooking such quibbles.

A much more significant issue is the function of the ACL. There is no clear understanding of the function of the ACL beyond a role in restricting anterior motion of the tibia, and any brief statement of function either does not aspire to great accuracy or claims unwarranted certainty. Without doubt the ligament opposes anterior translation in response to an anterior force, but any effect on internal tibial rotation, especially about a centrally-placed axis, appears small and variable. Perhaps if injury to the ACL were not quite so frequent and/or disabling the discussion might end there. But less than ideal outcomes from reconstructive surgery, and an association of poor outcomes and a positive pivot shift test, indicate an issue with rotational stability.

But the nature of that instability is poorly characterized. In 1981 it was reasonably argued that ACL deficiency causes a shift in axis of internal rotation, and results since support this, yet 30 years later there is still a tacit rejection of this notion and a continued presumption that rotation always occurs around an axis passing centrally through the tibia.

Given that the ACL does restrict anterior translation and may or may not restrict internal rotation, it is interesting that post-reconstruction kinematics show increased laxity on translation and not enough on rotation. Restoration of function and avoidance of joint degeneration are important enough goals to require that our descriptions of function are as accurate as possible. But despite evidence that reconstruction may over-constrain internal rotation, the principle of *less is good so even less is better* is sometimes invoked in the goal to simply reduce internal rotation range.

We suggest that, just as ACL deficiency may alter the position of the axis of internal-external rotation, reconstruction may have effects on rotational axis location that we do not understand, and we provide a possible explanation for some of the kinematic changes seen after reconstructive surgery. This speculative explanation has too few data to give this confident support, but we believe that axis position on injury and reconstruction deserve more scientific investigation.

7. Acknowledgement

We wish to thank Mr Tavik Morgenstern, School of Medical Sciences, for his assistance with the figures.

8. References

Abbott, L. C., Saunders, J. B. D. M., Bost, F. C. & Anderson, C. E. (1944). Injuries to the ligaments of the knee joint. *Journal of Bone and Joint Surgery*, Vol. 26, No. 3, (July 1944), pp 503-521, ISSN 1535-1386

Aglietti, P., Giron, F., Losco, M., Cuomo, P., Ciardullo, A. & Mondanelli, N. (2010). Comparison between single- and double-bundle anterior cruciate ligament reconstruction. A propspective, randomized, single-blinded clinical trial. *American Journal of Sports Medicine*, Vol. 38, No. 1, (January 2010), pp 25-34, ISSN 0363-5465

Ahmed, A. M., Hyder, A., Burke, D. L. & Chan, K. H. (1987). In-vitro ligament tension pattern in the flexed knee in passive loading. *Journal of Orthopaedic Research*, Vol. 5, No. 2, pp 217-230, ISSN 1554-527X

Amis, A. A. & Dawkins, G. P. C. (1991). Functional anatomy of the anterior cruciate ligament. Fibre bundle actions related to ligament replacements and injuries. *Journal of Bone and Joint Surgery*, Vol. 73B, No. 2, (March 1991), pp 260-267, ISSN 0301-620X

Andriacchi, T. P., Briant, P. L., Bevill, S. L. & Koo, S. (2006). Rotational changes at the knee after ACL injury cause cartilage thinning. *Clinical Orthopaedics and Related Research*, Vol. 442, (January 2006), pp 39-44, ISSN 0009-921X

Andriacchi, T. P., Mündermann, A., Smith, R. L., Alexander, E. J., Dyrby, C. O. & Koo, S. (2004). A framework for the *in vivo* pathomechanics of osteoarthritis at the knee. *Annals of Biomedical Engineering*, Vol. 32, No. 3, (March 2004), pp 447-457, ISSN 0090-6964

Bach, J. M. & Hull, M. L. (1998). Strain inhomogeneity in the anterior cruciate ligament under application of external and muscular loads. *Journal of Biomechanical Engineering*, Vol. 120, No. 4, (August 1998), pp 497-503, ISSN 0148-0731

Bach, J. M., Hull, M. L. & Patterson, H. A. (1997). Direct measurement of strain in the posterolateral bundle of the anterior cruciate ligament. *Journal of Biomechanics*, Vol. 30, No. 3, (March 1997), pp 281-283, ISSN 0021-9290

Barrance, P. J., Williams, G. N., Snyder-Mackler, L. & Buchanan, T. S. (2006). Altered knee kinematics in ACL-deficient non-copers: a comparison using dynamic MRI. *Journal of Orthopaedic Research*, Vol. 24, (February 2006), pp 132-140, ISSN 1554-527X

Bedi, A., Musahl, V., O'Loughlin, P., Maak, T., Citak, M., Dixon, P. & Pearle, A. D. (2010). A comparison of the effect of central anatomical single-bundle anterior cruciate ligament reconstruction and double-bundle anterior cruciate ligament reconstruction on pivot-shift kinematics. *American Journal of Sports Medicine*, Vol. 38, No. 9, (September 2010), pp 1788-1794, ISSN 0363-5465

Berns, G. S., Hull, M. L. & Patterson, H. A. (1992). Strain in the anteromedial bundle of the anterior cruciate ligament under combination loading. *Journal of Orthopaedic Research*, Vol. 10, No. 2, (March 1992), pp 167-176, ISSN 1554-527X

Beynnon, B., Howe, J. G., Pope, M. H., Johnson, R. J. & Fleming, B. C. (1992). The measurement of anterior cruciate ligament strain *in vivo*. *International Orthopaedics*, Vol. 16, No. 1, (March 1992), pp 1-12, ISSN 0341-2695

Beynnon, B. D., Johnson, R. J., Fleming, B. C., Peura, G. D., Renstrom, P. A., Nichols, C. E. & Pope, M. H. (1997). The effect of functional knee bracing on the anterior cruciate ligament in the weightbearing and nonweightbearing knee. *American Journal of Sports Medicine*, Vol. 25, No. 3, (June 1997), pp 353-359, ISSN 0363-5465

Blankevoort, L., Huiskes, R. & de Lange, A. (1988). The envelope of passive knee joint motion. *Journal of Biomechanics*, Vol. 21, No. 9, pp 705-720, ISSN 0021-9290

Brantigan, O. C. & Voshell, A. F. (1941). The mechanics of the ligaments and menisci of the knee joint. *Journal of Bone and Joint Surgery*, Vol. 23, No. 1, (January 1941), pp 44-66, ISSN 1535-1386

Bull, A. M. J. & Amis, A. A. (1998). Knee joint motion: description and measurement. *Journal of Engineering in Medicine*, Vol. 212, No. 5, pp 357-372, ISSN 0954-4119

Bull, A. M. J., Earnshaw, P. H., Smith, A., Katchburian, M. V., Hassan, A. N. A. & Amis, A. A. (2002). Intraoperative measurement of knee kinematics in reconstruction of the anterior cruciate ligament. *Journal of Bone and Joint Surgery*, Vol. 84B, No. 7, (September 2002), pp 1075-1081, ISSN 0301-620X

Butler, D., Noyes, F. & Grood, E. (1980). Ligamentous restraints to anterior-posterior drawer in the human knee. A biomechanical study. *Journal of Bone and Joint Surgery*, Vol. 62A, No. 2, (March 1980), pp 259-270, ISSN 1535-1386

Chaudhari, A. M., Briant, P. L., Bevill, S. L., Koo, S. & Andriacchi, T. P. (2008). Knee kinematics, cartilage morphology, and osteoarthritis after ACL injury. *Medicine and Science in Sports and Exercise*, Vol. 40, No. 2, (February 2008), pp 215-222, ISSN 0195-9131

Clark, J. M. & Sidles, J. A. (1990). The interrelation of fiber bundles in the anterior cruciate ligament. *Journal of Orthopaedic Research*, Vol. 8, No. 2, (March 1990), pp 180-188, ISSN 1554-527X

DeFrate, L. E., Papannagari, R., Gill, T. J., Moses, J. M., Pathare, N. P. & Li, G. (2006). The 6 degrees of freedom kinematics of the knee after anterior cruciate ligament deficiency: an in vivo imaging analysis. *American Journal of Sports Medicine*, Vol. 34, No. 8, (August 2006), pp 1240-1246, ISSN

DeMorat, G., Weinhold, P., Blackburn, T., Chudik, S. & Garrett, W. (2004). Aggressive quadriceps loading can induce noncontact anterior cruciate ligament injury. *American Journal of Sports Medicine*, Vol. 32, No. 2, (March 2004), pp 477-483, ISSN 0363-5465

Desrochers, J., Amrein, M. A. & Matyas, J. R. (2010). Structural and functional changes of the articular surface in a post-traumatic model of early osteoarthritis measured by atomic force microscopy. *Journal of Biomechanics*, Vol. 43, No. 16, (December 2010), pp 3091-3098, ISSN 0021-9290

Diermann, N., Schumacher, T., Schanz, S., Raschke, M. J., Petersen, W. & Zantop, T. (2009). Rotational instability of the knee: internal tibial rotation under a simulated pivot shift test. *Archives of Orthopaedic and Trauma Surgery*, Vol. 129, No. 3, (March 2009), pp 353-358, ISSN 0936-8051

Elias, S. G., Freeman, M. A. R. & Gokcay, I. (1990). A correlative study of the geometry and anatomy of the distal femur. *Clinical Orthopaedics and Related Research*, Vol. 260, (November 1990), pp 98-103, ISSN 0009-921X

Fleming, B. C., Renstrom, P. A., Beynnon, B. D., Engstrom, B., Peura, G. D., Badger, G. J. & Johnson, R. J. (2001). The effect of weightbearing and external loading on anterior cruciate ligament strain. *Journal of Biomechanics*, Vol. 34, No. 2, (February 2001), pp 163-170, ISSN 0021-9290

Fukubayashi, T., Torzilli, P. A., Sherman, M. F. & Warren, R. F. (1982). An *in vitro* biomechanical evaluation of anterior-posterior motion of the knee. Tibial displacement, rotation, and torque. *Journal of Bone and Joint Surgery*, Vol. 64A, No. 2, (February 1982), pp 258-264, ISSN 1535-1386

Furman, W., Marshall, J. L. & Girgis, F. G. (1976). The anterior cruciate ligament. A functional analysis based on postmortem studies. *Journal of Bone and Joint Surgery*, Vol. 58A, No. 2, (March 1976), pp 179-185, ISSN 1535-1386

Fuss, F. K. (1989). Anatomy of the cruciate ligaments and their function in extension and flexion of the human knee joint. *American Journal of Anatomy*, Vol. 184, No. 2, (February 1989), pp 165-176, ISSN 1553-0795

Gabriel, M. T., Wong, E. K., Woo, S. L. Y., Yagi, M. & Debski, R. E. (2004). Distribution of in situ forces in the anterior cruciate ligament in response to rotatory loads. *Journal of Orthopaedic Research*, Vol. 22, No. 1, (January 2004), pp 85-89, ISSN 1554-527X

Galway, H. R. & MacIntosh, D. L. (1980). The lateral pivot shift: a symptom and sign of anterior cruciate ligament insufficiency. *Clinical Orthopaedics and Related Research*, Vol. 147, (March-April 1980), pp 45-50, ISSN 0009-921X

Girgis, F. G., Marshall, J. L. & Al Monajem, A. R. S. (1975). The cruciate ligaments of the knee joint. Anatomical, functional and experimental analysis. *Clinical Orthopaedics and Related Research*, Vol. 106, (January-February 1975), pp 216-231, ISSN 0009-921X

Harner, C. D., Baek, G. H., Vogrin, T. M., Carlin, G. J., Kashiwaguchi, S. & Woo, S. L. Y. (1999). Quantitative analysis of human cruciate ligament insertions. *Arthroscopy*, Vol. 15, No. 7, (October 1999), pp 741-749, ISSN 0749-8063

Harner, C. D., Livesay, G. A., Kashiwaguchi, S., Fujie, H., Choi, N. Y. & Woo, S. L. Y. (1995). Comparative study of the size and shape of human anterior and posterior cruciate ligaments. *Journal of Orthopaedic Research*, Vol. 13, No. 3, (May 1995), pp 429-434, ISSN 1554-527X

Hashemi, J., Chandrashekar, N., Gill, B., Beynnon, B. D., Slauterbeck, J. R., Schutt, R. C., Mansouri, H. & Dabezies, E. (2008). The geometry of the tibial plateau and its influence on the biomechanics of the tibiofemoral joint. *Journal of Bone and Joint Surgery*, Vol. 90A, No. 12, (December 2008), pp 2724-2734, ISSN 1535-1386

Hemmerich, A., van der Merwe, W., Batterham, M. & Vaughn, C. L. (2011). Knee rotational laxity in a randomized comparison of single- versus double-bundle anterior cruciate ligament reconstruction. *American Journal of Sports Medicine*, Vol. 39, No. 1, (January 2011), pp 48-56, ISSN 0363-5465

Herbort, M., Lenschow, S., Fu, F. H., Petersen, W. & Zantop, T. (2010). ACL mismatch reconstructions: influence of different tunnel placement strategies in single-bundle ACL reconstructions on the knee kinematics. *Knee Surgery, Sports Traumatology, Arthroscopy*, Vol. 18, No. 11, (November 2010), pp 1551-1558, ISSN 0942-2056

Hollis, J. M., Takai, S., Adams, D. J., Horibe, S. & Woo, S. L. Y. (1991). The effects of knee motion and external loading on the length of the anterior cruciate ligament (ACL): a kinematic study. *Journal of Biomechanical Engineering*, Vol. 113, No. 2, (May 1991), pp 208-214, ISSN 0148-0731

Hollister, A. M., Jatana, S., Singh, A. K., Sullivan, W. W. & Lupichuk, A. G. (1993). The axes of rotation of the knee. *Clinical Orthopaedics and Related Research*, Vol. No. 290, (May 1993), pp 259-268, ISSN 0009-921X

Hsieh, H. & Walker, P. (1976). Stabilizing mechanisms of the loaded and unloaded knee joint. *Journal of Bone and Joint Surgery*, Vol. 58A, No. 1, (January 1976), pp 87-93, ISSN 1535-1386

Inderster, A., Benedetto, K. P., Künzel, K. H., Gaber, O. & Balyk, R. (1993). Fiber orientation of anterior cruciate ligament: an experimental morphological and functional study, part I. *Clinical Anatomy*, Vol. 6, No. 1, pp 26-32, ISSN 0897-3806

Inoue, M., McGurk-Burleson, E., Hollis, J. M. & Woo, S. L. Y. (1987). Treatment of the medial collateral ligament injury. I: The importance of anterior cruciate ligament on the varus-valgus knee laxity. *American Journal of Sports Medicine*, Vol. 15, No. 1, (January 1987), pp 15-21, ISSN 0363-5465

Jonsson, H., Riklund-Åhlström, K. & Lind, J. (2004). Positive pivot shift after ACL reconstruction predicts later osteoarthrosis. 63 patients followed 5-9 years after surgery. *Acta Orthopaedica Scandinavica*, Vol. 75, No. 5, (October 2004), pp 594-599, ISSN 0001-6470

Kanamori, A., Woo, S. L. Y., Ma, C. B., Zeminski, J., Rudy, T. W., Li, G. & Livesay, G. A. (2000). The forces in the anterior cruciate ligament and knee kinematics during a simulated pivot shift test: a human cadaveric study using robotic technology. *Arthroscopy*, Vol. 16, No. 6, (September 2000), pp 633-639, ISSN 0749-8063

Katouda, M., Soejima, T., Kanazawa, T., Tabuchi, K., Yamaki, K. & Nagata, K. (2011). Relationship between thickness of the anteromedial bundle and thickness of the posterolateral bundle in the normal ACL. *Knee Surgery, Sports Traumatology, Arthroscopy*, DOI: 10.1007/s00167-011-1417-0, ISSN 1433-7347, Retrieved from <http://www.springerlink.com/content/891717442h52384g/>

Kondo, E., Merican, A. M., Yasuda, K. & Amis, A. A. (2010). Biomechanical comparisons of knee stability after anterior cruciate ligament reconstruction between 2 clinically available transtibial procedures. Anatomic double bundle versus single bundle. *American Journal of Sports Medicine*, Vol. 38, No. 7, (July 2010), pp 1349-1358, ISSN 0363-5465

Kondo, E., Merican, A. M., Yasuda, K. & Amis, A. A. (2011). Biomechanical comparison of anatomic double-bundle, anatomic single-bundle, and nonanatomic single-bundle anterior cruciate ligament reconstructions. *American Journal of Sports Medicine*, Vol. 39, No. 2, (February 2011), pp 279-288, ISSN 0363-5465

Kurosawa, H., Walker, P. S., Abe, S., Garg, A. & Hunter, T. (1985). Geometry and motion of the knee for implant and orthotic design. *Journal of Biomechanics*, Vol. 18, No. 7, pp 487-499, ISSN 0021-9290

La Fortune, M., Cavanagh, P., Sommer, H. & Kalenak, A. (1992). Three-dimensional kinematics of the human knee during walking. *Journal of Biomechanics*, Vol. 25, No. 4, (April 1992), pp 347-357, ISSN 0021-9290

Lane, J. G., Irby, S. E., Kaufman, K., Rangger, C. & Daniel, D. M. (1994). The anterior cruciate ligament in controlling axial rotation. An evaluation of its effect. *American Journal of Sports Medicine*, Vol. 22, No. 2, (March 1994), pp 289-293, ISSN 0363-5465

Lehmkuhl, L. & Smith, L. (1983). *Brunnstrom's Clinical Kinesiology*, (4th edition), FA Davis, ISBN 0803655290, Philadelphia

Levangie, P. & Norkin, C. (2001). *Joint Structure and Function: a Comprehensive Analysis*, (3rd edition), MacLennan & Petty, ISBN 0864331657, Eastgardens

Li, G., Papannagari, R., DeFrate, L. E., Yoo, J. D., Park, S. E. & Gill, T. J. (2007). The effects of ACL deficiency on mediolateral translation and varus-valgus rotation. *Acta Orthopaedica*, Vol. 78, No. 3, pp 355-360, ISSN 1745-3674

Li, G., Rudy, T. W., Sakane, M., Kanamori, A., Ma, C. B. & Woo, S. L. Y. (1999). The importance of quadriceps and hamstring muscle loading on knee kinematics and in-situ forces in the ACL. *Journal of Biomechanics*, Vol. 32, No. 4, (April 1999), pp 395-4000, ISSN 0021-9290

Li, G., Zayontz, S., Most, E., DeFrate, L. E., Suggs, J. F. & Rubash, H. E. (2004). In situ forces of the anterior and posterior cruciate ligaments in high knee flexion: an in vitro investigation. *Journal of Orthopaedic Research*, Vol. 22, No. 2, (March 2004), pp 293-297, ISSN 1554-527X

Lie, D. T. T., Bull, A. M. J. & Amis, A. A. (2007). Persistence of the mini pivot shift after anatomically placed anterior cruciate ligament reconstruction. *Clinical Orthopaedics and Related Research*, Vol. 457, (April 2007), pp 203-209, ISSN 0009-921X

Lipke, J. M., Janecki, C. J., Nelson, C. L., McLeod, P., Thompson, C., Thompson, J. & Haynes, D. W. (1981). The role of incompetence of the anterior cruciate and lateral ligaments in anterolateral and anteromedial instability. *Journal of Bone and Joint Surgery*, Vol. 63A, No. 6, (July 1981), pp 954-960, ISSN 1535-1386

Livesay, G. A., Fujie, H., Kashiwaguchi, S., Morrow, D. A., Fu, F. H. & Woo, S. L. Y. (1995). Determination of the *in situ* forces and force distribution within the human anterior cruciate ligament. *Annals of Biomedical Engineering*, Vol. 23, No. 4, (July 1995), pp 467-474, ISSN 0090-6964

Lo, J. H., Müller, O., Wünschel, M., Bauer, S. & Wülker, N. (2008). Forces in anterior cruciate ligament during simulated weight-bearing flexion with anterior and internal rotational tibial load. *Journal of Biomechanics*, Vol. 41, No. 9, pp 1855-1861, ISSN 0021-9290

Lorbach, O., Pape, D., Maas, S., Zerbe, T., Busch, L., Kohn, D. & Seil, R. (2010). Influence of the anteromedial and posterolateral bundles of the anterior cruciate ligament on external and internal tibiofemoral rotation. *American Journal of Sports Medicine*, Vol. 38, No. 4, (April 2010), pp 721-727, ISSN 0363-5465

Mannel, H., Marin, F., Claes, L. & Dürselen, L. (2004). Anterior cruciate ligament rupture translates the axes of motion within the knee. *Clinical Biomechanics*, Vol. 19, No. 2, (February 2004), pp 130-135, ISSN 0268-0033

Markolf, K. L., Burchfield, D. M., Shapiro, M. S., Shepard, M. F., Finerman, G. A. M. & Slauterbeck, J. L. (1995). Combined knee loading states that generate high anterior cruciate ligament forces. *Journal of Orthopaedic Research*, Vol. 13, No. 6, (November 1995), pp 930-935, ISSN 1554-527X

Markolf, K. L., Gorek, J. F., Kabo, J. M. & Shapiro, M. S. (1990). Direct measurement of resultant forces in the anterior cruciate ligament. An *in vitro* study performed with a new experimental technique. *Journal of Bone and Joint Surgery*, Vol. 72A, No. 4, (April 1990), pp 557-567, ISSN 1535-1386

Markolf, K. L., Hame, S., Hunter, D. M., Oakes, D. A., Zoric, B., Gause, P. & Finerman, G. A. M. (2002). Effects of femoral tunnel placement on knee laxity and forces in an anterior cruciate ligament graft. *Journal of Orthopaedic Research*, Vol. 20, No. 5, (September 2002), pp 1016-1024, ISSN 1554-527X

Markolf, K. L., Mensch, J. S. & Amstutz, H. C. (1976). Stiffness and laxity of the knee - the contributions of the supporting structures. A quantitative *in vitro* study. *Journal of Bone and Joint Surgery*, Vol. 58A, No. 5, (July 1976), pp 583-594, ISSN 1535-1386

Markolf, K. L., Park, S., Jackson, S. R. & McAllister, D. R. (2009). Anterior-posterior and rotatory stability of single and double-bundle anterior cruciate ligament reconstructions. *Journal of Bone and Joint Surgery*, Vol. 91A, No. 1, (January 2009), pp 107-118, ISSN 1535-1386

Martelli, S. & Pinskerova, V. (2002). The shapes of the tibial and femoral articular surfaces in relation to tibiofemoral movement. *Journal of Bone and Joint Surgery*, Vol. 84B, No. 4, (May 2002), pp 607-613, ISSN 0301-620X

Matsumoto, H. (1990). Mechanism of the pivot shift. *Journal of Bone and Joint Surgery*, Vol. 72B, No. 5, (September 1990), pp 816-821, ISSN 0301-620X

Matsumoto, H., Seedhom, B. B., Suda, Y., Otani, T. & Fujikawa, K. (2001). Axis location of tibial rotation and its change with flexion angle. *Clinical Orthopaedics and Related Research*, Vol. 371, (February 2001), pp 178-182, ISSN 0009-921X

Meyer, E. G. & Haut, R. C. (2008). Anterior cruciate ligament injury induced by internal tibial torsion or tibiofemoral compression. *Journal of Biomechanics*, Vol. 41, No. 16, (December 2008), pp 3377-3383, ISSN 0021-9290

Murray, M. M. (2009). Current status and potential of primary ACL repair. *Clinics in Sports Medicine*, Vol. 28, No. 1, (January 2009), pp 51-61, ISSN 0278-5919

Musahl, V., Bedi, A., Citak, M., O'Loughlin, P., Choi, D. & Pearle, A. D. (2011). Effect of single-bundle and double-bundle anterior cruciate ligament reconstructions on pivot-shift kinematics in anterior cruciate ligament- and meniscus-deficient knees. *American Journal of Sports Medicine*, Vol. 39, No. 2, (February 2011), pp 289-295, ISSN 0363-5465

Nordin, M. & Frankel, V. H. (1989). Biomechanics of the knee, In: *Basic Biomechanics of the Musculoskeletal system*, Nordin, M. and Frankel, V. H., pp. 115-134, Lea & Febiger, ISBN 0-8121-1227-X, Philadelphia.

Nordt, W. E., Lotfi, P., Plotkin, E. & Williamson, B. (1999). The in vivo assessment of tibial motion in the transverse plane in anterior cruciate ligament-reconstructed knees. *American Journal of Sports Medicine*, Vol. 27, No. 5, (September 1999), pp 611-616, ISSN 0363-5465

Norwood, L. A. & Cross, M. J. (1979). Anterior cruciate ligament: functional anatomy of its bundles in rotatory instabilities. *American Journal of Sports Medicine*, Vol. 7, No. 1, (January 1979), pp 23-26, ISSN 0363-5465

Noyes, F. R., Grood, E. S., Cummings, J. F. & Wroble, R. R. (1991). An analysis of the pivot shift phenomenon. The knee motions and subluxations induced by different examiners. *American Journal of Sports Medicine*, Vol. 19, No. 2, (March 1991), pp 148-155, ISSN 0363-5465

Noyes, F. R., Mooar, P. A., Matthews, D. S. & Butler, D. L. (1983). The symptomatic anterior cruciate-deficient knee. Part I: the long-term functional disability in athletically active individuals. *Journal of Bone and Joint Surgery*, Vol. 65A, No. 2, (February 1983), pp 154-162, ISSN 1535-1386

Odensten, M. & Gillquist, J. (1985). Functional anatomy of the anterior cruciate ligament and a rationale for reconstruction. *Journal of Bone and Joint Surgery*, Vol. 67A, No. 2, (February 1985), pp 257-262, ISSN 1535-1386

Oh, Y. K., Kreinbrink, J. L., Ashton-Miller, J. A. & Wojtys, E. M. (2011). Effect of ACL transection on internal tibial rotation in an in vitro simulated pivot landing. *Journal of Bone and Joint Surgery*, Vol. 93A, No. 4, (February 2011), pp 372-380, ISSN 1535-1386

Øiestad, B. E., Holm, I., Aune, A. K., Gunderson, R., Myklebust, G., Engebretsen, L., Fosdahl, M. A. & Risberg, M. A. (2010). Knee function and prevalence of knee osteoarthritis after anterior cruciate ligament reconstruction. A prospective study with 10 to 15 years of follow-up. *American Journal of Sports Medicine*, Vol. 38, No. 11, (November 2010), pp 2201-2210, ISSN 0363-5465

Renström, P. A., Arms, S. W., Stanwyck, T. S., Johnson, R. J. & Pope, M. H. (1986). Strain within the anterior cruciate ligament during hamstring and quadriceps activity. *American Journal of Sports Medicine*, Vol. 14, No. 1, (January 1986), pp 83-87, ISSN 0363-5465

Reuben, J. D., Rovick, J. S., Schrager, R. J., Walker, P. S. & Boland, A. L. (1989). Three-dimensional dynamic motion analysis of the anterior cruciate ligament deficient knee joint. *American Journal of Sports Medicine*, Vol. 17, No. 4, (July 1989), pp 463-471, ISSN 0363-5465

Sakane, M., Fox, R. J., Woo, S. L. Y., Livesay, G. A., Li, G. & Fu, F. H. (1997). *In situ* forces in the anterior cruciate ligament and its bundles in response to anterior tibial loads. *Journal of Orthopaedic Research*, Vol. 15, No. 2, (March 1997), pp 285-293, ISSN 1554-527X

Sanfridsson, J., Ryd, L., Svahn, G., Fridén, T. & Jonsson, K. (2001). Radiographic measurement of femoral rotation in weight-bearing: the influence of flexion and extension in the knee on the extensor mechanism and angles of the lower extremity in a healthy population. *Acta Radiologica*, Vol. 42, No. 2, pp 201-217, ISSN 0284-1851

Scanlan, S. F., Chaudhari, A. M. W., Dyrby, C. O. & Andriacchi, T. P. (2010). Differences in tibial rotation during walking in ACL reconstructed and healthy contralateral knees. *Journal of Biomechanics*, Vol. 43, No. 9, (June 2010), pp 1817-1822, ISSN 0021-9290

Segawa, H., Omori, G. & Koga, Y. (2001). Long-term results of non-operative treatment of anterior cruciate ligament injury. *Knee*, Vol. 8, No. 1, (March 2001), pp 5-11, ISSN 0968-0160

Seon, J. K., Gadikota, H. R., Wu, J. L., Sutton, K., Gill, T. J. & Li, G. (2010). Comparison of single- and double-bundle anterior cruciate ligament reconstructions in restoration of knee kinematics and anterior cruciate ligament forces. *American Journal of Sports Medicine*, Vol. 38, No. 7, (July 2010), pp 1359-1367, ISSN 0363-5465

Seon, J. K., Park, S., Lee, K. B., Seo, H. Y., Kim, M. S. & Song, E. K. (2011). In vivo stability and clinical comparison of anterior cruciate ligament reconstruction using low or high femoral tunnel positions. *American Journal of Sports Medicine*, Vol. 39, No. 1, (January 2011), pp 127-133, ISSN 0363-5465

Shaw, J. A. & Murray, D. G. (1974). The longitudinal axis of the knee and the role of the cruciate ligaments in controlling transverse rotation. *Journal of Bone and Joint Surgery*, Vol. 56A, No. 8, (December 1974), pp 1603-1609, ISSN 1535-1386

Siu, D., Rudan, J., Wevers, H. & Griffiths, P. (1996). Femoral articular shape and geometry: A three-dimensional computerised analysis of the knee. *Arthroplasty*, Vol. 11, No. 2, (February 1996), pp 166-173, ISSN 1532-8406

Smith, P., Refshauge, K. M. & Scarvell, J. (2003). Development of the concepts of knee kinematics. *Archives of Physical Medicine and Rehabilitation*, Vol. 84, No. 12, (December 2003), pp 1895-1902, ISSN 0003-9993

Soudan, K., Auderkercke, R. & Martens, M. (1979). Methods, difficulties and inaccuracies in the study of human joint mechanics and pathomechanics by the instant axis concept. Example: The knee joint. *Journal of Biomechanics*, Vol. 12, No. 1, pp 27-33, ISSN 0021-9290

Steckel, H., Starman, J. S., Baums, M. H., Klinger, H., Schultz, W. & Fu, F. H. (2007). Anatomy of the anterior cruciate ligament double bundle structure: a macroscopic evaluation. *Scandinavian Journal of Medicine & Science in Sports*, Vol. 17, No. 4, (August 2007), pp 387-392, ISSN 0905-7188

Takai, S., Woo, S. L. Y., Livesay, G. A., Adams, D. J. & Fu, F. H. (1993). Determination of the in situ loads on the human anterior cruciate ligament. *Journal of Orthopaedic Research*, Vol. 11, No. 5, (September 1993), pp 686-695, ISSN 1554-527X

Torzilli, P. A., Deng, X. & Warren, R. F. (1994). The effect of joint-compressive load and quadriceps muscle force on knee motion in the intact and anterior cruciate ligament-sectioned knee. *American Journal of Sports Medicine*, Vol. 22, No. 1, (January 1994), pp 105-112, ISSN 0363-5465

Van de Velde, S. K., Gill, T. J. & Li, G. (2009). Evaluation of kinematics of anterior cruciate ligament-deficient knees with use of advanced imaging techniques, three-dimensional modeling techniques, and robotics. *Journal of Bone and Joint Surgery*, Vol. 91A, Supplement 1, pp 108-114, ISSN 1535-1386

Wang, C. J., Walker, P. S. & Wolf, B. (1973). The effects of flexion and rotation on the length patterns of the ligaments of the knee. *Journal of Biomechanics*, Vol. 6, No. 6, (November 1973), pp 587-596, ISSN 0021-9290

Woo, S. L. Y., Kanamori, A., Zeminski, J., Yagi, M., Papageorgiou, C. & Fu, F. H. (2002). The effectiveness of reconstruction of the anterior cruciate ligament with hamstrings and patellar tendon. A cadaveric study comparing anterior tibial and rotational loads. *Journal of Bone and Joint Surgery*, Vol. 84A, No. 6, (June 2002), pp 907-914, ISSN 1535-1386

Wroble, R. R., Grood, E. S., Cummings, J. F., Henderson, J. M. & Noyes, F. R. (1993). The role of the lateral extraarticular restraints in the anterior cruciate ligament-deficient knee. *American Journal of Sports Medicine*, Vol. 21, No. 2, (March 1993), pp 257-263, ISSN 0363-5465

Wu, J. L., Seon, J. K., Gadikota, H. R., Hosseini, A., Sutton, K. M., Gill, T. J. & Li, G. (2010). In situ forces in the anteromedial and posterolateral bundles of the anterior cruciate ligament under simulated functional loading conditions. *American Journal of Sports Medicine*, Vol. 38, No. 3, (March 2010), pp 558-563, ISSN 0363-5465

Wünschel, M., Müller, O., Lo, J. H., Obloh, C. & Wülker, N. (2010). The anterior cruciate ligament provides resistance to externally applied anterior tibial force but not to internal rotational torque during simulated weight-bearing flexion. *Arthroscopy*, Vol. 26, No. 11, (November 2010), pp 1520-1527, ISSN 0749-8063

Yagi, M., Wong, E. K., Kanamori, A., Debski, R. E., Fu, F. H. & Woo, S. L. Y. (2002). Biomechanical analysis of an anatomic anterior cruciate ligament reconstruction. *American Journal of Sports Medicine*, Vol. 30, No. 5, (September 2002), pp 660-666, ISSN 0363-5465

Yamamoto, Y., Hsu, W. H., Woo, S. L. Y., Van Scyoc, A. H., Takakura, Y. & Debski, R. E. (2004). Knee stability and graft function after anterior cruciate ligament reconstruction. A comparison of a lateral and an anatomical femoral tunnel placement. *American Journal of Sports Medicine*, Vol. 32, No. 8, (December 2004), pp 1825-1832, ISSN 0363-5465

Yoo, J. D., Papannagari, R., Park, S. E., DeFrate, L. E., Gill, T. J. & Li, G. (2005). The effect of anterior cruciate ligament reconstruction on knee joint kinematics under simulated muscle loads. *American Journal of Sports Medicine*, Vol. 33, No. 2, (February 2005), pp 240-246, ISSN 0363-5465

Zantop, T., Herbort, M., Raschke, M. J., Fu, F. H. & Petersen, W. (2007). The role of the anteromedial and posterolateral bundles of the anterior cruciate ligament in anterior tibial translation and internal rotation. *American Journal of Sports Medicine*, Vol. 35, No. 2, (February 2007), pp 223-227, ISSN 0363-5465

Zaricznyj, B. (1987). Reconstruction of the anterior cruciate ligament of the knee using a doubled tendon graft. *Clinical Orthopaedics and Related Research*, Vol. 220, (July 1987), pp 162-175, ISSN 0009-921X

Zatsiorski, V. M. (2002). *Kinetics of Human Motion*, Human Kinetics, ISBN 0880116765, Champaign

17

Biomechanical Assessments in Sports and Ergonomics

Pascal Madeleine, Afshin Samani, Mark de Zee and Uwe Kersting
Physical Activity and Human Performance, Center for Sensory-Motor Interaction (SMI)
Dept. of Health Science and Technology, Aalborg University
Denmark

1. Introduction

Sportsmen as well as workers are subject to contract musculoskeletal injuries. For instance, shoulder injuries are frequent in relation to physical activity in sports and at work with overhead or repetitive arm movements (Hume et al, 2006). Common injuries for the shoulders are for instance rotator cuff injury and impingement syndrome. Rotator cuff injury/impingement syndrome may occur after unaccustomed high intensity repetitive movements (e.g., swimming) or low load repetitive work (e.g., deboning work). The risk of musculoskeletal damage is correlated to the physical and psychological attributes of the performed movement. The known physical external risks include a fixed erected posture, repetitive arm movement, heavy load, insufficient rest, temperature and static posture (Madeleine, 2010). Moreover, internal individual risk factors such as anthropometry (age, height and body mass for instance), gender, physical capacities (muscle force, endurance and fitness for instance) and personality also play a role in these injuries. Psychological risk factors including e.g., stress and pain behaviour are also recognised as important in relation to physical activity. Some sports-related overload injuries are relatively easy to diagnose while an important part of work-related musculoskeletal disorders (MSD) often remains undiagnosed. Thus, despite important scientific efforts the pathophysiology behind most MSD is still unknown. MSD are often accompanied by sensory manifestations such as muscle fatigue and pain located in muscles, tendons, cartilage and ligaments (Madeleine, 2010).

Biomechanical analyses have to date contributed to enhance our knowledge of the underlying causes of movement (McGinnis, 2005). This is supported by the fact that the sole use of observation methods correlate weakly with quantitative biomechanical measures. Biomechanics has indeed enabled a precise quantification of motor strategies in order to optimize, maintain or develop high level human performances while preventing MSD in sports and ergonomics (McGinnis, 2005). This is exemplified by the general agreement concerning the important role of the muscles of the shoulder girdle in the development of rotator cuff injury/impingement syndrome (Escamilla et al, 2009). Thus, biomechanical assessments of human performance contribute to delineate damageable load patterns to the musculoskeletal system in relation to physical activity (Madeleine, 2010). The development of sensor and recording technology has also contributed to the democratisation of biomechanical assessments to a larger part of the population. This is demonstrated by the expansion of objective performance assessment in leisure sports, e.g., running shoes mounted with accelerometer and GPS for the detection of the running distance, speed and running path. This evolution is also remarkable in ergonomics with a number of newly developed devices enabling long lasting physical recording.

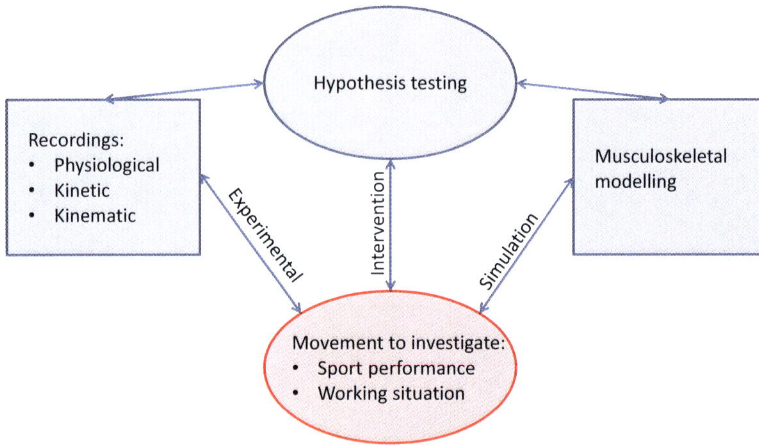

Fig. 1. Scientific approaches to test a hypothesis in experimental, intervention and simulation setup in sports and ergonomics

Usually the extracted variables during a biomechanical analysis will both provide temporal, load and position information. These variables can then be examined in relation to muscle fatigue development as it is suggested to be a precursor of injuries (Madeleine, 2010). This chapter will focus on single bipolar and multi-channels surface electromyography (EMG) or mechanomyography (MMG). The muscle activation pattern provides key information about the onset and the level of muscle activation (muscular load) as well as insight into muscle coordination. Kinetic recordings are primordial for the quantitative assessment of reaction forces and/or pressure distribution profile. Kinematics recordings are performed by means of accelerometer/gyroscope, angular sensor and optical imaging systems and provide information of the movement pattern. The kinetic and kinematics recordings are often combined to estimate joint load (energy, work and power) using an inverse dynamics approach. Further, new trends in biomechanical data analysis like e.g., non-linear dynamics are becoming more common (Madeleine & Madsen, 2009; Rathleff et al, 2010). Finally, biomechanical modelling for the estimation of the musculoskeletal load is becoming more popular in known motor tasks (Erdemir et al, 2007) as modelling approaches enable the assessment of e.g., rescaling of ergonomics or sports equipment. EMG, kinetic and kinematics recordings are used as input or as a validation tool to the applied models investigating human movement (Fig. 1).

Biomechanical measurements can be made in laboratory or field settings (McGinnis, 2005). Advanced measurements including 3D kinematics are easier to perform in a laboratory. The core of the body literature within biomechanics consists of data recorded in laboratories. This has undeniable advantages as the experimenter can use the battery of available methods to assess human movement in what may be considered as an ideal recording environment. Electrical noise affecting EMG recording, location of force platform and cameras for kinetic and kinematics recordings, lights resulting in ghost markers and temperature can be controlled in laboratories. Therefore, laboratory studies usually provide data of high reliability and validity. A number of factors related to the physical environment like the type of movement and some psychosocial factors such as perceived time pressure can indeed be controlled in a laboratory setting (Madeleine et al, 2008a). However, laboratory recording also have limitations as the recording environment is changed; the athlete or worker is not performing in his or her real environment (a pitch for a football game or a slaughterhouse for a butcher). The investigated motor task under laboratory conditions usually simulates some attributes of the motor task of interest. The attached equipment consisting of for instance EMG electrodes, accelerometers, reflective markers as well as the presence of cameras and experimenters can modify the movement measured. In order to circumvent this, the subjects are usually asked to perform a number of trials prior to the recording sessions to get familiarised with the mounted equipment and the laboratory setting.

Field or in-situ measurements enable the biomechanical assessment of the real task. However, researchers might not have the possibility of using advanced equipment for biomechanical assessment due to limited portability and fragility of these devices. Moreover, the quality of the recordings may be altered by many noise sources (electrical, light and temperature) and by the presence of other competitors/workers, coaches or audience. The planning of such recordings should therefore be made very cautiously. In ergonomics, kinematics recordings from video recordings and inclinometers are made in real working conditions (Hansson et al, 2006; Madeleine & Madsen, 2009). In sports, timing devices and 2D video recordings are often collected in relation to physical activity (McGinnis, 2005). Such assessments do most likely not interfere with the performance of the worker or athlete. Here too, the current new technological era combining wireless EMG systems and inertial & magnetic measurement systems is an interesting alternative in ambulatory field settings. It may therefore be expected that advanced biomechanical measurements will be performed more and more in field settings as the athlete or worker is placed in the real environment.

The aim of this chapter is to report the existing biomechanical recordings and non-invasive analysis methods of human movement. The focus is directed towards physiological, kinetic and kinematics recordings during muscular fatigue development and in presence of injuries. Further, the existing technology and analysing methods are discussed in relation to examples in sports and ergonomics used to delineate basic aspects of human movement. Computer simulation and modelling approaches based on inverse dynamics will also be presented.

2. Physiological recordings

Physiological assessments are often used to assess the physical and muscular load during physical activity using heart rate, EMG and MMG recordings. EMG and MMG recordings are more relevant in relation to biomechanics as these signals reflect the muscle force produced during movement. The electrical and mechanical activity of a contraction muscle can thus be investigated in sports and ergonomics. The recordings and analysis of EMG and MMG data in fresh, fatigued and injured conditions provide important insight into adaption mechanisms. Such an understanding is required for the interpretation of the changes in the motor control and the validation of computer simulation and modelling.

2.1 Surface electromyography

The application of EMG has become a standard method in biomechanics since J.V. Basmajian published his book "Muscles alive - their functions revealed by electromyography". The EMG signal represents the electrical activity of the sum of active motor units and reflects indirectly the produced muscle (DeLuca, 1997; McGinnis, 2005; Winter, 1990). Given the properties of EMG, it is now considered as an integral part of biomechanical assessments in relation to physical activity. EMG recordings are employed to delineate changes in muscle activation during force exertion, muscle fatigue or musculoskeletal injuries.

2.1.1 Origin and detection of the surface electromyography signal

A motor unit is comprised of a motor neuron, the axon of the motor neuron and all the muscle fibres innervated by the neuron. The train of the motor unit action potentials (MUAPs) travels through the muscle, fat and skin tissues before being recorded as EMG by a pair of bipolar electrodes on the surface of the skin. The tissues act as a low-pass filter on the electrical potentials; therefore, EMG is comprised of the summed effect of several MUAPs which have been low-pass filtrated. There is an approximately linear relationship between isometric muscular force and so-called integrated EMG (explained later in this section). Moreover, EMG is well-suited for studying the muscle activation profile and global muscle properties such as the amplitude of a contraction. Thus, EMG assessments are valuable as they can reveal muscle fatigue development as well as altered activation profile within a muscle or among muscles in relation to muscle injuries.

It should be noted that a number of factors may alter the quality of the EMG recordings including electrical noise (50/60 Hz from electrical lines), cross-talk from adjacent muscles, anatomical properties of the muscle, electrode locations, muscle length changes as well as type of contraction (isometric or anisometric). EMG is usually recorded using classic bipolar surface electrodes. The electrodes are aligned (inter-electrode distance 2 cm) on abraded ethanol-cleaned skin along the direction of the muscle fibres. The electrodes are placed with respect to anatomical landmarks (Hansson et al, 1992; Hermens et al, 2000). A reference electrode is usually placed over a non-electrically active location. Prior to digitisation the EMG signals are usually pre-amplified/amplified (close to the recording site), band-pass filtered (e.g., 5-500 Hz) and sampled at a frequency higher than 1 kHz. A/D conversion is performed with a 12/16 bit acquisition board. For further details see Standards for Reporting EMG Data in the Journal of Electromyography and Kinesiology.

2.1.2 Processing and interpretation of the electromyogram signal

In sports and ergonomics the EMG processing starts with the extraction of relevant features from the raw EMG signal and continues with data reduction by fitting the outcome to a statistical model. There are a number of methods to process EMG in this respect, and all of them reflect all or some of the main characteristics of the exposure: onset, duration, level and repetitiveness. The applied methodologies of the EMG processing can be categorised into linear and nonlinear approaches. The linear approaches simply assume that EMG is the output of a linear system which has been stimulated with a random process whereas the nonlinear approaches do not rely on this assumption. The advantage of linear approaches is that the processing methods are very well-established and understood whereas the nonlinear approaches face some technical difficulties such as a need for long time-series, the spurious effect of the noise and the curse of dimensionality.

The relevant linear features can be extracted by amplitude and frequency-oriented methods. The amplitude features are extracted from rectified EMG. Rectified data undergo a moving or weighted averaging over a suitable time window.
The choice of the duration of the time window is a compromise between demands on consistency and bandwidth of the signal. The most commonly adopted duration is 100 ms but it is usual to take shorter or considerably longer windows if the contraction is performed more rapidly or slowly (up to 1-2 s.). This is strongly dependent on the degree of the stationarity of the signal. Typical amplitude features are the average rectified value (ARV, mean of rectified values), the integrated EMG (IEMG, the linear envelopment of the EMG signal) and the root mean square (RMS, mean of squared signal). In the frequency domain the features are derived from the frequency spectrum of the EMG signal (DeLuca, 1997). Typical examples of these features are the mean power frequency (MNF or MPF) and median power frequency (MDF). The number of zero crossings of the raw EMG per time unit has also been shown to be associated with the MNF and MDF (Hägg, 1991).
The absolute EMG amplitude depends on a large number of individual factors acting as confounding variables which may invalidate any inter-subject comparison. The normalisation of the EMG signal has been suggested to minimize the effect and inter-subject variability (Mathiassen et al, 1995). The normalisation of the EMG relates all measurements to the electrical activity of the muscles involved in a particular condition. The task is very often a maximum voluntary contraction (MVC). However, there are situations where a reliable and safe MVC is difficult to obtain, for example when the MVC is obtained from upper trapezius or in injured subjects. In such cases the normalisation can be performed using a standardised reference contraction. In the MVC case the EMG amplitude is reported in percentage of maximal voluntary electrical activation (% MVE). Alternatively, if the normalisation is performed with respect to a reference contraction, the EMG amplitude is reported in percentage of the reference voluntary electrical activation (% RVE). The normalisation procedure also induces variance and mask potential differences (Jackson et al, 2009). This point becomes more significant if the healthy subjects are compared with the patient group. (van Dieën et al, 2003).
The amplitude normalisation of the EMG amplitude should not be mixed with normalisation in time performed to investigate cyclic tasks such as the gait cycle. Cyclic tasks consist of a particular temporal pattern repeated over time. However, the repetitions are not exactly identical in length. To achieve a consistent time profile for the cycles, its time profile is slightly expanded or squeezed using an interpolation algorithm. After equalizing the cycle duration to 100% of the stride for gait, the time can be reported as a percentage of the cycle duration. This procedure is defined as the normalisation in time.
During a fatiguing contraction the amplitude of EMG gradually increases while the EMG spectrum is compressed towards lower frequencies. Temporal and spectral changes in the EMG signal are attributed to variations in muscular and neural mechanisms (Madeleine & Farina, 2008). Muscular mechanisms consist of a decrease in muscle fibre conduction velocity, an increase in duration and a decrease in amplitude of the intracellular action potential while neural mechanisms include additional motor unit recruitment, changed motor unit discharge rates (DeLuca, 1997), probably due to reflex inhibition from small diameter muscle afferents (Gandevia, 2001), and motor unit substitution (Westgaard & De Luca, 2001). For example, it has been shown that the endurance time can be fairly predicted by the slope of the MNF or MDF initial drop. However, one of the drawbacks is that the decreasing slope tends to be inconsistent at load levels below approximately 20% MVE (Hansson et al, 1992).

The idea of applying nonlinear time-series processing grew in different fields (Chen, 1988; Roerdink et al, 2006) as discerning deterministic chaos and noise became important. The analysis of deterministic chaos provides information on the system complexity and can explain a complex behaviour using a low-dimensional model (Fraser, 1989). The algorithm for nonlinear processing was developed in the seventies and eighties and has received noticeable attention in biomedical signal processing a decade later. However, in ergonomics and sport only a few studies have utilised the methods despite a promising potential (Granata & Gottipati, 2008; Madeleine & Madsen, 2009; Søndergaard et al, 2010).

Nonlinear methods can potentially be used to investigate the variability of the exposure. The linear methods do not reveal proper information about the true structure of variability (Buzzi et al, 2003; Slifkin & Newell, 1999). Alternatively, nonlinear methods provide some information on the occurrence of recurrent patterns throughout the same time-series (Webber Jr & Zbilut, 2005) and attain further insight into the structural variability of the exposure. The approximate and the sample entropy are probably the most common indices of complexity (or irregularity) applied to process the EMG. It is worth noting that a change in the complexity may or may not be associated with a change in amplitude; thus, in theory the complexity may independently change from the amplitude.

A number of studies reported a loss of complexity in physiological data among patients or elderly people (Lipsitz, 2006; Madeleine et al, 2011; Sung et al, 2005). Therefore, it could be expected that an intact and healthy system would be characterised by a higher complexity compared with patients and elderly people. Although there has been some criticism on this general statement (Slifkin & Newell, 1999), the higher complexity of the EMG may be inferred as a diversity in the paradigm of the motor unit activation. The diversity may delineate a beneficial phenomenon because continuous activity of the same motor units may damage them (Hägg & Åström, 1997). As an alternative some studies argue for a "complexity trade-off" meaning that the loss of the complexity in one part of the system will be compensated by gaining the complexity in some other parts. This has been reported in some experimental studies as well (Rathleff et al, 2010).

As a subcategory of the nonlinear approaches the recurrence quantification analysis (RQA) has been used to detect changes in EMG due to fatigue. The method even over-performed the conventional spectral and amplitude analysis (Felici et al, 2001). Some modelling studies have verified that the RQA can provide some information on the conduction velocity and the degree of synchronization of the motor units (Farina et al, 2002).

2.1.3 High density surface EMG

As mentioned earlier, the bipolar EMG is recorded over one spot on the muscle. This gives a poor representation of the whole muscle activity. Additionally, the bipolar EMG has a very poor spatial selectivity which hinders the decomposition of the EMG into MUAPs.

Due to new advancement in technology it is now possible to record the EMG over a large part of the muscle from several channels simultaneously. Figure 2 shows an example of high-density EMG recorded over the upper trapezius during bilateral shoulder abduction. This gives a more comprehensive representation compared to the bipolar EMG, and the decomposing of the EMG signal seems feasible by utilizing advanced processing techniques. The EMG is recorded from several channels which compose a grid of electrodes over the surface of the muscle.

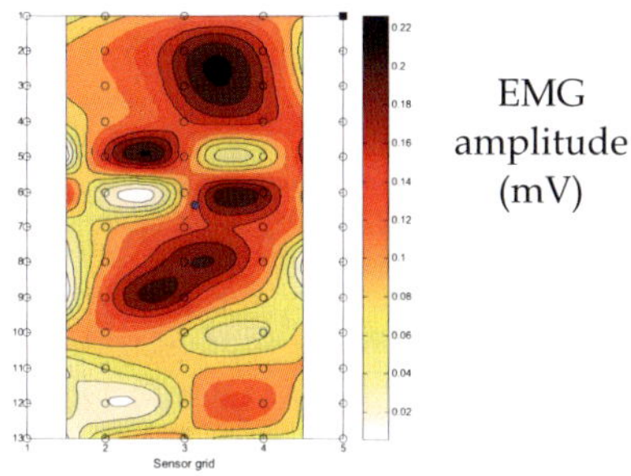

Fig. 2. Example of a high density surface electromyography amplitude map (root mean square values) recorded over upper trapezius

A more detailed spatial selectivity may not be urgently needed in ergonomics and sport, but an improved representation may give some valuable global information to quantify the exposure (Samani et al, 2010). For example, estimating the amplitude indices gives a two-dimensional image of the activity of a muscle. The topological properties of the image may indicate changes in exposure. The centre of the gravity and the modified entropy have been shown to be affected by fatigue and pain development (Farina et al, 2008; Madeleine et al, 2006).

2.1.4 Muscular synergy

The notion of a synergy implies teamwork among the elements of a system; for example, the muscles work together to perform a physical task. This requires the muscles to be coupled as the agonist and antagonist. The quantification of the degree of the coupling between the involved muscles may provide for prognoses of an unhealthy activation pattern (Escamilla et al, 2009). The information theory provides some processing tools which can quantify the coupling and common information between the EMG signals recorded from the involved muscles in a task. This has been done rarely in this kind of context (Madeleine et al, 2011); for example, the mutual information detects both linear and nonlinear dependencies so it can reveal the functional connectivity between the influential elements.

Some studies have described a complex task only by using a few components which are called muscle synergy. These studies utilize different methods of data reduction such as the PCA, non-negative matrix factorization and independent component analysis to find out the minimum number of components which describe the whole task in an optimal way. Using this approach they try to find out how the central nervous system chooses a particular strategy to perform a motor task (Tresch, 2006).

However, some other studies define the synergy in a more elaborate framework. According to them not all co-varying elements work in a synergy, but the co-variation should i) contribute to the same task (sharing) ii) compensate for the error interactively (flexibility) and iii) be task dependent. If co-varying elements meet all these requirements, they are working in a synergy (Latash, 2008). To translate this understanding of synergy into practice the framework of uncontrolled manifold (UCM) has been introduced (Scholz & Schöner, 1999). The UCM assumes that the central nervous system selects a subspace (a manifold) in the space of the controlling elements in which the performance is optimum. Then it arranges co-variations among the elements in such a way that their variation has relatively little effect on the performance. This means that the variation is mostly confined to the UCM. This approach has been applied to functional tasks; however, the method has never been applied to ergonomics and sport applications.

2.2 Mechanomyography

MMG recordings can be regarded as an alternative non-invasive method to EMG enabling the study of muscle excitation-contraction coupling in vivo. MMG most likely reflects the intrinsic mechanical activity of muscle contraction (Orizio, 1993). MMG has been widely used to assess e.g.,, signal-force relationship, muscle fatigue, post exercise muscle soreness, muscle pain as well as neuromuscular diseases.

2.2.1 Origin and detection of the mechanomyogram signal

Despite the fact that the MMG signal has been known for more than two centuries (Wollaston, 1810), the mechanisms of its generation are still not fully understood. Slow bulk movement of the muscle, excitation into ringing of the muscle at its own resonance frequency, and pressure waves due to dimensional changes of the active muscle fibres generate oscillations recorded as the MMG signal (Orizio, 1993). Recent studies have confirmed that MMG mainly originates from muscle fibre displacement underlining a bending mode due to contraction (Cescon et al, 2008; Farina et al, 2008). The MMG may reflect motor unit recruitment, discharge rate, synchronisation and, to some extent, factors which affect the physical muscle milieu, such as intra-muscular pressure, stiffness, and osmotic pressure (Orizio, 1993). The exact contribution of changes in the physical muscle milieu to the MMG signal is not known but it seems less important compared with neural and muscular factors.

Similar to EMG, MMG is usually analysed as an interference signal during voluntary contraction. Its characteristics are determined by all active muscle fibres as linear or non-linear (Orizio et al, 1996) summation of the individual contributions.

Over the last decades different types of transducers have been applied to detect MMG signals, including piezoelectric contact sensor, microphones, accelerometers, and laser distance sensors. The different transduction modes inherent to these sensors result in MMG signals having different temporal and frequency characteristics (Orizio, 1993). Piezoelectric contact sensors are mostly obsolete due their weight, and the applied pressure to obtain a mechanical coupling dampens the recorded MMG signal. Condenser microphones acting as a displacement meter are still used from time to time but they also require a coupling, e.g., air or gel between the muscle and the microphone (Watakabe et al, 2001). Further, the volume of the air-chamber influences the amplitude and the frequency content of the recorded MMG signal. Accelerometers reflecting the acceleration of body surface vibration are currently the most applied sensors for MMG recording due to their small weight and size, easy attachment, and high reliability (Watakabe et al, 2003). Microphones are considered more reliable than accelerometers for the assessment of the MMG signal during dynamic contractions even though accelerometers can be used during dynamic muscle action (Kawczynski et al, 2007). More recently laser displacement sensors have also been used to study muscle dimensional changes without additional inertial load. However, light accelerometers (< 5 g) do not interfere with muscle surface dynamics and provide accurate MMG recordings (Watakabe et al, 2003). Accelerometers are still considered as the golden standard for MMG recordings as the outcome signal is measured in physical units (ms^{-2}) enabling comparison between different studies.

MMG assessment has followed EMG development, i.e. from single channel and multi-channel MMG recordings (Cescon et al, 2004; Madeleine et al, 2007) enabling to report the topography of the activation profile. Sensors are placed over the bulk of the muscles of interest and are attached to the skin using double adhesive tape. The placement of the sensors is preferably defined in relation to anatomical landmarks. Orizio (1993) recommends sensors with a linear transmission within a [1- 800 Hz] frequency range. The sampling frequency is in general set to 1 or 2 kHz as it enables comparison with EMG recordings. A/D conversion is performed with a 12/16 bit acquisition board. Multi-channel recordings have mainly been performed using a light micro-machined accelerometer size (typically with the following specifications: weight < 5 g and linear transmission [DC-100 Hz]). The accelerometers are arranged in a complete or incomplete grid to cover the muscle of interest. The inter-accelerometer distance is defined in relation to anatomical landmarks.

2.2.2 Processing and interpretation of the mechanomyogram signal

The analysis of the MMG signals mostly consists of the extraction of linear features. The linear features (see section 2.1.2) are related to the computation of amplitude and frequency estimators. RMS/ARV and MNF/MDF values are computed over a 0.5-1 s epoch without overlapping. Absolute amplitude and frequency estimators are normalised with respect to the values obtained at 100% MVC (short duration contractions) or during a reference contraction. Amplitude normalisation is also common as it may reduce inter-subject variability of the estimators due to e.g., skin fold thickness or muscle size. However, the normalisation procedure can also mask the variability between groups and changes during sustained contraction (Madeleine et al, 2002; van Dieën et al, 1993). The normalisation of temporal and frequency MMG estimators can result in a lack of changes over time and spatial dependency (Madeleine & Farina, 2008).

Moreover, it should be noted that the spectral contents of the MMG signal also undergo changes during sustained contraction in the power spectral variance (2nd order moment) and skewness (3rd order moment) indicating a complex modification of the shape of the power spectrum (Madeleine et al, 2007). These changes are most likely due to the additional motor unit recruitment of motor units during fatigue development and to the non-linear summation of motor unit contributions to the MMG signal (Orizio et al, 1996). Amplitude and frequency estimator values are averaged to decrease the amount of data and to obtain values corresponding to, e.g.,, 0-100% of the time to task failure or endurance time.

Muscle fatigue development is usually characterised by a shift of the MMG spectrum towards lower frequencies and an increase of the MMG amplitude (Orizio, 1993; Orizio et al, 2003). However, the relationship between temporal and spectral MMG changes and the underlying physiological phenomenon related to fatigue is still not fully understood. A number of factors including the type, intensity and duration of exercise as well as fibre type composition, recruitment pattern, level of training and environmental conditions such as temperature influence the MMG signals (Orizio, 1993). Temporal and spectral changes in the MMG signal follow the changes observed in the EMG signal attributed to variations in muscular and neural mechanisms (Madeleine & Farina, 2008). In presence of delayed onset muscle soreness and acute muscle pain, the amplitude of the MMG is reported to increase (Kawczynski et al, 2007; Madeleine & Arendt-Nielsen, 2005). This increase can be explained by a larger twitch force needed to maintain a constant force output and/or a change in muscle stiffness due to repetitive eccentric exercise.

Most of the studies assessing muscle fatigue development have used a single sensor for MMG recordings (Orizio et al, 2003). This can lead to erroneous interpretation of MMG changes in the time and frequency domain (Cescon et al, 2004). For instance, during sustained contraction the reported changes in EMG amplitude topographical maps are associated to the dependence of fibre membrane properties on fibre location into the muscle, inhomogeneous motor unit recruitment and substitution (Farina et al, 2008). This redistribution is also found in the MMG RMS and MNF maps during sustained contraction in the upper trapezius muscle (Madeleine & Farina, 2008). This emphasises the potential of two-dimensional multi-channel MMG recordings to delineate heterogeneities in muscle activation during both short and sustained contractions (Cescon et al, 2008; Farina et al, 2008; Madeleine et al, 2007). Similar to EMG, a non-linear approach has been used to characterize the distribution of the activation profile. For that purpose, modified entropy has been computed from multi-channel MMG recordings (Madeleine et al, 2007). Heterogeneities reported in the upper trapezius MMG activation maps depict different degrees of activation of muscle regions as well as changes in contractile properties, muscle architecture and irregular effect of dampening including cross-talk from adjacent muscles (Orizio et al, 2003). The various extents of spatial MMG changes among subjects may explain the controversial results already reported during static contractions (Madeleine et al, 2002; Mathiassen et al, 1995). Interestingly, a heterogeneous MMG activation pattern is positively correlated with time to task failure underling functional relevance in the upper trapezius (Madeleine & Farina, 2008). A variable activation pattern could also contribute to avoiding the development of MSD as a higher variability in motor strategies is reported in healthy subjects compared with patients with chronic neck-shoulder pain (Madeleine et al, 2008b).

3. Kinetic recordings

Kinetics is the term given to forces generating movement. Internal forces are generated by e.g., muscle activation, ligaments and joints while external forces are issued from the ground or external loads. The internal forces are in most cases extremely difficult or even impossible to measure and are normally estimated by using computer model (see part 5). The external forces, on the other hand, can be recorded by various types of sensors and analysed in many ways. The recordings and analysis of kinetic data are of great importance as it enables a sound interpretation of the mechanisms involved in movement strategies (McGinnis, 2005; Nigg & Herzog, 2007).

3.1 Force sensor types

In biomechanical applications, forces are mainly quantified using strain gauge, piezoelectric or capacitive transducers. Strain gauge is the most common type of force transducers. Strain gauge measurement relies on the fact that structures subjected to external forces deform (see Part 3.2). Such deformation results in a change in length called strain. The change leads to changes in electricial properties of the material that can be measured. Resistive and piezoresistive transduction modes are by far the most common when using electrical type strain gauges. Resistive strain gauges usually consist of a wire or a foil bonded to an insulated substrate. The strain causes a change in resistance connected to a bridge circuit ideally consisting of four resistors (active and dummy/Poisson strain gauge) enabling temperature compensation, cross-talk diminution and increased sensitivity. Strain gauges are often used in sports and ergonomics applications (Komi, 1990; Madeleine et al, 1999; McGorry et al, 2003) as they enable reaction force measurement during movement (knife, pedals) and in vivo stress and strain measurements (bone or tendon). The advantages of resistive strain gauges are numerous including high accuracy, high sensitivity, low cost, portability, eases of use as well as the possibility to record static and dynamic loads. However, they also have drawbacks including the need for calibration, a limited range of measure, a risk of damage (e.g., by chock), the cross-talk as well as temperature and pressure sensitivity. Piezoelectric sensors require deformations of the atomic structure within a block of special crystalline material (e.g., quartz). The deformation of the quartz crystalline structure changes the electrical characteristics altering the electric charge. Such a change is then translated via a charge amplifier into a signal proportional to the applied force. Piezoelectric sensors are especially sensitive and reliable for dynamic force recordings over a wide range of measure. Drift changes preventing static recordings and costs are the main drawbacks of piezoelectric sensors. Capacitive transducers consist of two electrically conducting plates parallel to each other. These two plates are separated by a space filled dielectric material (non-conductive elastic material). The application of a force will produce a change in the thickness of the dielectric inversely proportional to the measured current. Capacitors are often used for the assessment of the pressure distribution or of the force between two surfaces (see part 3.3). After amplification, forces and moments are sampled at frequencies (≥ 100 Hz) corresponding to a multiple of the sampling frequency used for EMG. Force recordings are often made to, e.g.,, determine task failure in relation to physical activity, set a level of contraction in relation to MVC and to assess force steadiness or size of variability (Kawczynski et al, 2007; Madeleine et al, 2002; Svendsen & Madeleine, 2010).

3.2 Force platforms

Force platforms are probably the most important devices for assessment of performance in a biomechanics laboratory. Force platforms are integrated in walkways and/or handles. Force platforms can be used based on piezoelectric, Hall effect and strain gauge sensing technology. Force platforms are rectangular with force transducers (resistive or piezoresistive strain gauges) mounted in each corner resulting in four coordinate systems. Force platforms using strain gauges are the most suitable for balance or postural studies, are cheaper and can be custom-built. Force platforms are generally mounted on a flat and rigid support to obtain suitable forces during human movement. For postural studies, this is less critical since shear forces have low magnitude. The construction of force platform with force transducers enables the determination of the resulting forces in two horizontal and one vertical component. In accordance with the International Society of Biomechanics (ISB), F_x is the friction force in the direction of movement (anterior-posterior for gait), F_y is the normal contact force in the vertical direction and Fz is the friction force in the direction perpendicular to movement (medio-lateral for gait). The devices are providing resultant forces. The vertical component describes the change in momentum of the centre of mass of the subject in the vertical direction. The anterior-posterior and medial-lateral components correspond to the two other horizontal directions (anterior-posterior and medial-lateral). The reaction forces are expressed in absolute values and/or with respect to the subject's body weight during e.g., jump or pole-vault.

Furthermore, force measurements in the four corners of a force platform can be used to determine the moments M_x, M_y and M_z produced by F_x, F_y and Fz at the origin of the force platform coordinate system (centre of the force platform). The use of Newton's laws of motion enables the computation of the displacement of the centre of pressure. The displacement of the centre of pressure in the anterior-posterior direction (CoP_x) can be roughly estimated by dividing the moment of rotation in the medio-lateral direction by the force in the vertical direction (Winter, 1990). It is important to note that the computation of the CoP is only accurate as long as the exerted vertical force is higher than 0 N (typically 25 N). The digitisation process after amplification enables off-line analysis of impact and active forces from the ground reaction forces measured during locomotion (walking or running) over a number of trials in relation to, e.g.,, footwear (Kersting et al, 2005). The rate of force development is also often computed in relation to explosive force exertion. The displacement of the CoP is often also quantified by computing for instance the sway amplitude, sway path, size of variability and power spectral density function in normal or altered sensory conditions (Baratto et al, 2002; Madeleine et al, 2004; Madeleine et al, 2011). Recently, the combination of linear and non-linear analyses (approximate and/or sample entropy) has gained some attention. The methods depict subtle changes in the dynamics of biomechanical time series. Non-linear analysis provides new insight into the dynamics of force control by underlining important changes in sitting postural control (Søndergaard et al, 2010), patients (Roerdink et al, 2006) and gender effects (Svendsen & Madeleine, 2010).

3.3 Pressure sensors

Expressing the ratio between an exerted force over a known area, pressure measurement is providing key information for the assessment of pressure distribution between two surfaces like for instance foot and shoe. The type of sensors used for measuring the pressure distribution is similar to the ones for sensing force (see part 3.1). The sensor types used most often are capacitor, conductor and pressure sheet (Nigg & Herzog, 2007). Capacitor elements are integrated in pressure distribution mats or insoles consisting of a matrix of m × n stripes of conducting material. Multiplexing techniques are usually applied to assess the force acting on each element. The construction of the conductor sensors is similar to capacitor one (three layers are used), the applied force or pressure is determined as a change in the resistance due to the deformation of the conductive elastomers using Ohm's law. The pressure sheet or foil (fuji foil) is made of two sheets separated by a layer containing microcapsules with a colouring agent. The obtained colour intensity can then be analysed (optical density) in relation to, e.g.,, endurance sports after total knee replacement (Kuster et al, 2000). However, the latter solution does not enable reliable dynamic measurements.

Pressure distribution measurements are often made in sports (saddle, shoe insole, ski-boot shaft) and ergonomics (handgrip, seat comfort). Some recent examples encompass the assessments of plantar pressure distribution measurements during normal gait, among elite rugby league athletes and tennis players during the first serve on various surfaces (Girard et al, 2010; Gurney et al, 2008; Gurney et al, 2009). It is worth noting that these devices are in general rather costly, not very flexible and only measure normal forces. Most commercial pressure mapping systems are now versatile and can be used in a wide number of applications in sports and ergonomics such as handgrip, foot-ware and sitting. These devices can provide real-time information recorded in 3D during both static and dynamic movement. Pressure, force and area profile can be analysed by obtaining e.g., isobar distribution and path of the centre of force enabling a 3D quantification of loading pattern during human movement.

4. Kinematics recordings

The image series presented by Muybridge (e.g. Muybridge, 1984) are, likely, the most cited reference dealing with assessments of segmental motion in human or animal movement. One possible reason for this may be that we still use photogrammetric techniques to a large extent. This becomes particularly obvious when looking across all continents where most biomechanics research facilities consider a, typically 3D, camera system as part of their standard measurement equipment. While Muybridge never provided quantitative analyses on segmental movement derived from his image series, the approach in itself is regarded highly relevant as minimum constraints are put on the subjects.

4.1 Accelerometers and gyroscopes

Accelerometers have been used widely in various areas of biomechanics (see also part 2.2). They are typically small, light and can be mounted to equipment or the human body itself. When mounted to equipment such as rackets or bats they can be used to describe the movement of the tool itself, identify phases within a certain technique as well as characterize vibrations elicited by, e.g.,, impacting an object (Andrew et al, 2003). They have also been used to characterize shock transmission to and within the human body in order to characterize internal loads. In most applications they were attached to the skin and held in place by tape and/or elastic straps (Shung et al, 2009). Data from skin-mounted accelerometers are, despite their inherent precision, sometimes difficult to interpret as their fixation is critical due to the fact that soft tissue movement does not generally follow that of the underlying skeleton. This may not be a problem if the soft tissue vibrations in itself are the object of the measurement (Boyer & Nigg, 2006) but make data interpretation difficult if accelerometry is used to infer on skeletal movement or loading.

Some research groups have mounted accelerometers directly to the bone to overcome these restrictions (Lafortune et al, 1995a). However, such solutions are not generally applicable due to ethical reasons. Most importantly, they may serve to validate other approaches of measurement. One example is a study where bone-mounted accelerometer signals were compared to skin-mounted devices to assess tibial shock during running. Of the five subjects used in this study some showed good agreement between signals recorded by both methods while others displayed non-coherent results. This indicates the non-systematic effects introduced by soft tissue movement and sensor attachment which underlines the necessity to be cautious with interpretations and generalisations. However, the authors found that after applying a frequency correction method the skin-mounted accelerometers can be used to estimate shock transmitted to the tibia (Lafortune et al, 1995b). Additional work from the same group (Lafortune & Hennig, 1991) clearly demonstrated the effect of rotational movement and gravity on measured accelerations, further complicating interpretation. However, with regard to the context used as an example here, it was repeatedly shown that accelerometers attached to the tibia of a runner give reasonable estimates of the impact peak of the ground reaction force and therefore an easily applicable method to evaluate the effects of footwear or running style. Parameters typically extracted are maximum amplitude, acceleration rate, the timing of these values with respect to, e.g.,, initial contact of the object of interest, the frequency of elicited vibrations or other measures derived from the frequency spectrum of the signal.

An area where accelerometers can be used very well is as a trigger signal in high velocity movements (Andrew et al, 2003) where the amplitude is of minor importance (Kersting et al,

2005). They also find numerous applications in the field of activity monitoring as accelerometer signals can be utilised to infer of body position in static or slow movements as well as identify counts and rates of repetitive movements, i.e., estimate the number of loading cycles. Such data sets can be recorded over long time periods and algorithms have been presented to extract activity profiles for various groups of subjects or workers over long time intervals (Hansson et al, 2006; Rosenbaum et al, 2008).
Gyroscopes are sensors which measure angular velocity. They exist in one-dimensional as well as multidirectional configurations and are similarly easy to apply as accelerometers. They are often used in combination with accelerometers, magnetic or other sensors and provide estimates for movement of segments in a kinematic chain (Brodie et al, 2008; Greene et al, 2010) using e.g., Kalman filter technique (Luinge & Veltink, 2005). A considerable advantage of this approach is that one can measure full body kinematics in virtually any environment (Cloete & Scheffer, 2010). Despite very promising developments in this area there are still limitations to the precision of such devices such that laboratory measurements are still considered superior (Roetenberg et al, 2007).

4.2 Angular sensors

Angular movement sensors are, in many cases, implemented as uniaxial goniometers which allow for a direct measure of a joint's excursion. Limitations are that joint excursion can only be assessed in a single plane with such devices. Another requirement for precise measurements is that there should not be any parallax which gives an inherent problem when assessing joints with shifting axes as it is known, e.g.,, for the knee joint. There are various suggested mechanical solutions to compensate for parallax or tissue deformations in specifically constructed goniometers, i.e., for a specific joint (Hennig et al, 1998). To overcome this limitation, flexible two-dimensional angular sensors have been introduced which connect to fixation blocks by a flexible wire. If a joint allows for movement about two degrees-of-freedom its excursions can be fully covered. The flexible connection of the two mounting blocks is independent of translational movement such that variability in mounting the device or any parallax with regard to the joint axis would not affect angular measures. However, any information about translational movement will be lost. Most protocols where goniometers are employed require a reference measurement in an anatomically defined position to account for variations in mounting. After subtracting this offset, parameters such as the extremes of joint excursions can be derived. Joint angle can be expressed in relation to key events characterizing the motion and the range of movement or rate of movement can be extracted.
To the authors' perception, goniometers are easy to use and allow for immediate feedback if required. Their limitations should be kept in mind when designing a study using such devices. One example from research on running mechanics comparing two goniometer approaches is given by Hennig et al. (Hennig et al, 1998). It was shown that an in-shoe goniometer gave smaller amplitudes and angular velocities of movement about the subtalar joint axis while providing less variability from step to step. This study underlines the importance of using the best suitable device when investigating kinematic descriptors of motion. Another example is given by one of the authors (Kersting, 2011) where goniometer and accelerometer measurements where used in combination.
Inclinometers measure the angle against the gravity field by containing a mechanism similar to our vestibular system. They are highly precise and can be used to monitor posture and relatively slow movements as they are limited with regard the frequency of the motion

under consideration. In contrast to goniometers, which typically measure the relative angle of two adhering segments inclinometers determine the absolute segment orientation in space. By combining an inclinometer and goniometer it becomes easy to imagine a setup where, e.g.,, pelvis inclination and hip and knee flexion-extension can be used to monitor indicators for e.g., lower back loading in lifting tasks (Morlock, 2000). In ergonomics, statistical descriptors such as 10th, 50th and 90th percentile are computed to express the properties of the exposure (Hansson et al, 2006).

4.3 Optical imaging systems

Optical systems are the most commonly used devices in laboratory-based movement analysis. In its simplest form, a one-camera system can be used to analyse the movements which are mainly executed in one plane, i.e., which are 2D. The camera could be any digital video camera with sufficient resolution in time and space, depending on the movement under consideration. Its imaging plane should be parallel to the main plane of the movement under investigation. Typically, a recording of a known distance aligned within this plane is sufficient for generating a calibration (Madeleine & Madsen, 2009; Nolan & Lees, 2007). The ratio of pixels on the digital image to the reference distance is then used to calculate a scaling factor. Depending on the quality of the lens and the required precision, lens correction files may be used to compensate for lens errors. Some software packages allow for using point grids during calibration which also allow for a lens correction. In certain cases a four point calibration grid can be used if, e.g.,, the camera cannot be set up in a parallel plane. Up to a certain angular deviation, the distortion can be compensated when assessing e.g., jump performances at international competitions with cameras set up on the stands of a stadium.

Walking and running are the classical examples of two-dimensional movement analysis (van Woensel, 2011). Further applications from sports science are athletic jumps where 2D video analyses have been used. From these recordings joint angles and angular velocities can be derived. Another easily accessible parameter is the location and velocity of the body's centre of mass, which can be used for estimates of energetic changes in certain phases of carrying out a sports technique. The analysis of athletic jumps or gymnastics movements may be used as examples for applying this technique (Arampatzis & Bruggemann, 1999).

The extension of this approach is a multi-camera setup which allows to record objects from several perspectives. By reference to a calibration recording the method of direct linear transformation can be applied to reconstruct the position of a point in space from a minimum of two camera perspectives (Abdel-Aziz & Karara, 1971). Such setups are nowadays realised using several synchronised video cameras which can be sampled by up to 10 000 Hz at spatial resolutions of up to 4 Megapixels. Each camera is typically equipped with its own light source and an optic filter to suppress reflections from items other than a number of retro-reflective markers which are fixed to anatomically defined locations on a person's or animal's body. Marker occlusion can make the analysis of segmental movement difficult. The above mentioned advances in camera technology allow for residuals of less than 0.5 mm in a typical gait laboratory setting.

The analysis of human gait may be considered as one of the most common applications of laboratory based video systems with simultaneous measurement of ground reaction force as described above. Several studies have established their repeatability and reliability with addressing issues such as marker placement and data processing (Laroche et al, 2011). Numerous examples can be found where these methods build a major contribution in clinical decision making or allow for the assessment of operation techniques or other interventions (Beaulieu et al, 2010). Within ergonomics research field, the motion capture system is commonly used to analyse the exposure variation and motor variability. Particularly, the size of cycle-to-cycle variability is of relevance in relation to injuries (Madeleine et al, 2008a).

A continued problem in this area are the errors introduced by mainly skin movement artefacts, especially when it comes to inverse dynamics analyses where deformations and noise may produce substantial deviations of marker motion from the movement of the underlying skeleton. Various approaches have been suggested to apply optimisation procedures to account for the named error source (Andersen et al, 2009; Charlton et al, 2004). The results from these studies are promising and will, presumably, soon become standard in most camera-based methods for motion measurement.

When using video systems outdoors the use of reflective markers is often not possible such that manual digitization becomes necessary. Recently, new active filtering methods have been implemented and become commercially available now, which seem to allow for the use of retro-reflective markers outdoors in full sunlight.

Other approaches are active marker systems where each marker is a made up out of a small light source, typically a light-emitting diode. The effects of muscle fatigue development and MSD injury have been assessed during repetitive hammering tasks using such system (Cote et al, 2005). In some cases, the higher demand in applying the markers due to cable connections may be overcome by a reduced requirement for manual editing work during the tracking process. It may depend on the specific research question and environment to decide which system is most suitable for a planned experiment.

Finally, from the area of computer graphics more and more marker-less tracking systems have sprung off (Corazza et al, 2006) which have partly been validated with respect to high-resolution laboratory based systems (Rosenhahn et al, 2006). Results are very promising, while there is still a gap in resolution between marker-less and marker based systems.

Parameters derived from 3D motion capture are, obviously, rotational and translational measures about all six kinematic degrees of freedom. Mathematically, there are various approaches of describing 3D rotations (Woltring, 1994). While it is, theoretically, equivalent to use attitudes, Euler angles or helical axes it was suggested to relate to anatomical terminology when joint motion in humans is concerned (Madeleine et al, 1999). To unify the systems used for kinematic (and kinetic) data reporting, similarly making parameters comparable across studies, standards were proposed supported by the ISB (Wu et al, 2002; Wu et al, 2005). Similar to kinetic analysis, non-linear approaches have been employed to reveal e.g., complexity and dimensionality changes in relation to human movement (Buzzi et al, 2003; Madeleine & Madsen, 2009; Rathleff et al, 2010; Søndergaard et al, 2010). Kinematic data together with external reaction forces are typically used as input to biomechanical modelling approaches as they are described in the following section.

5. Modelling musculoskeletal load

As already mentioned the quantification of the mechanical loads on the human body in e.g., working situations and sports situations is of interest. However, in experimental sessions it is normally only possible to assess external loads on the body while the internal loads on muscles and joint remain unknown. Joint moments are regularly calculated via an inverse dynamics approach using motion capture and measured external forces. This will not give information on individual muscle forces and joint reaction forces. The only feasible way to obtain these parameters is to make use of advanced musculoskeletal models based on the laws of physics. Traditionally the methods behind musculoskeletal modelling fall into two categories, inverse dynamics and forward dynamics, which are opposite approaches. For a complete overview of the different modelling methods see the review by Erdemir et al. (Erdemir et al, 2007). In this paragraph the focus will be on musculoskeletal modelling based on inverse dynamics.

In inverse dynamics solutions the movement and external forces are input into the musculoskeletal model. Normally, the system has many more muscles than strictly necessary to balance the joint degrees of freedom. The solution of the muscle recruitment problem is therefore subject to the so-called redundancy problem. One of the common ways is that the muscles in the model are recruited by an optimality criterion minimizing fatigue. Mathematically the optimization problem can be stated as follows:

Minimize **f**

$$G(\mathbf{f}^{(M)}) \tag{1}$$

Subject to

$$\mathbf{Cf} = \mathbf{d} \tag{2}$$

$$f_i^{(M)} \geq 0, \qquad i \in \left\{1,\ldots,n^{(M)}\right\} \tag{3}$$

where G is the objective function of the recruitment strategy stated in terms of the muscle forces, $\mathbf{f}^{(M)}$. Subsequently G will be minimised with respect to all unknown forces in the problem, $\mathbf{f}=[\mathbf{f}^{(M)\,T}\ \mathbf{f}^{(R)\,T}]^T$, which are divided into muscle forces, $\mathbf{f}^{(M)}$, and joint reactions, $\mathbf{f}^{(R)}$. Equation (2) is the dynamic equilibrium equation, which enter into the optimization problem as constraints. **C** is the coefficient-matrix for the unknown forces, and the right-hand side, **d**, contains all known applied loads and inertia forces. The last constraint (3) indicates that muscles can only pull, and not push.

The choice of the objective function has always been debated in the literature. Basically the objective function has to reflect the strategy our central nervous system would choose for recruiting our muscles for a given task. Many of the objective functions have been reviewed by Tsirakos et al. (Tsirakos et al, 1997). The most successful criteria so far are the functions of the normalised muscle forces, $f_i^{(m)}/N_i$, where N_i is some measure of the muscle strength, which can be made dependent on the working conditions of the muscle (i.e. force-length relationship and force-velocity relationship). It has been shown that a criterion of minimization of muscle effort gives good results for a set of skilled movements like cycling and gait (Prilutsky and Zatsiorsky, 2002), but it also implies that that these kind of models are limited to the so-called skilled movements. In sports and in working situations there are though many of those skilled movements available to analyse.

Rasmussen et al. (2001) showed that many of the criteria are asymptotically equivalent to a minimum fatigue criterion, the so-called min/max criterion, where there is a maximum cooperation between the muscles, which can be written as follows:

Minimize

$$\max_i\left(\frac{f_i^{(M)}}{N_i}\right) \tag{4}$$

Subject to

$$\mathbf{Cf} = \mathbf{d} \tag{5}$$

$$f_i^{(M)} \geq 0, \qquad i \in \left\{1,\ldots,n^{(M)}\right\} \tag{6}$$

This min/max criterion, which is effectively a minimum fatigue criterion, is a useful criterion for sport performance and ergonomic design optimization. It will enable us to compare the minimal muscle effort necessary in many situations, which would otherwise require enormous experimental resources.

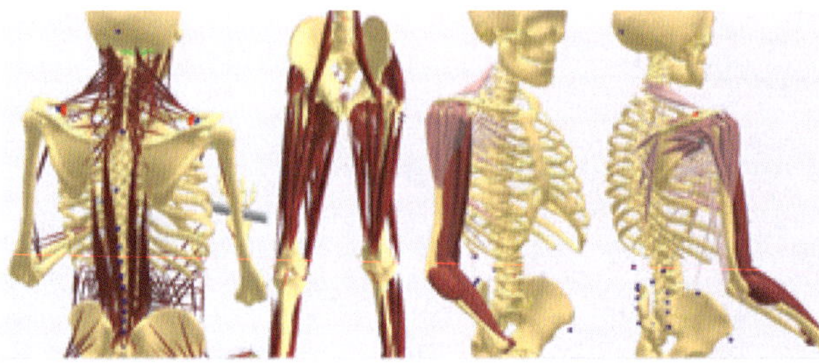

Fig. 3. Example of musculoskeletal models built in the AnyBody Modeling System.

The min/max criterion has been implemented in the AnyBody Modeling System (Damsgaard et al, 2006), which was originally developed at Aalborg University. Several musculoskeletal models (Fig. 3.) are available in the public domain AnyScript Model Repository (www.anyscript.org). An application within ergonomics investigated the influence of seat pan inclination and friction on muscle activity and spinal joint forces using a full-body model of the musculoskeletal system (Rasmussen et al, 2009). By a systematic change of the inclination and friction in the model one gets an impression of the complex relationship between changing these variables and the muscle activity and spinal joint forces. One of the main findings was that the combination of high friction and a backwards inclining seat pan will maximize the spinal forces while minimizing the muscle activity. This means that the seated posture that minimizes the fatigue and hence may be experienced as more comfortable also maximizes the spinal load.

Simulations give the possibility of changing the parameters in a systematic way while monitoring an output measure as a function of those parameters. An example could be to find the optimum position of the saddle for a cyclist while minimizing the muscle activity for a given power output. However, this would require a person-specific model of the athlete if this would be used in elite sports. But with the enormous development going on in the imaging field it is anticipated that person-specific modelling will be feasible in the near future which would make it very attractive for optimizing performance for an individual athlete.

6. Conclusion

The present chapter presents in a concise manner the existing and novel approaches for biomechanical assessments of human movement. Only the combination of physiological, kinetic and kinematic recordings provide a full picture of the musculoskeletal loads in relation to physical activity. Experimental and computational approaches are thus extremely valuable to assess and improve human performances without increasing the risk of injury.

7. Acknowledgment

The authors are grateful to Danish Agency for Science, Technology and Innovation, Det Obelske Familiefond and Gigtforeningen for partly supporting the present work.

8. References

Abdel-Aziz, Y.I., Karara, H.M. (1971). Direct Linear Transformation from Comparator Coordinates into Object Space Coordinates in Close-Range Photogrammetry. *Symposium on Close-Range Photogrammetry*, pp. 1-18.

Andersen, M.S., Damsgaard, M., Rasmussen, J. (2009). Kinematic Analysis of Over-Determinate Biomechanical Systems. *Computer Methods in Biomechanics and Biomedical Engineering*, Vol. 12, No. 4, pp. 371-384.

Andrew, D.P., Chow, J.W., Knudson, D.V., Tillman, M.D. (2003). Effect of Ball Size on Player Reaction and Racket Acceleration during the Tennis Volley. *Journal of Science Medicine and Sports*, Vol. 6, No. 1, pp. 102-112.

Arampatzis, A., Bruggemann, G.P. (1999). Mechanical Energetic Processes during the Giant Sswing Exercise before Dismounts and Flight Elements on the High Bar and the Uneven Parallel Bars. *Journal of Biomechanics*, Vol. 32, No. 8, pp. 811-820.

Baratto, L., Morasso, P.G., Re, C., Spada, G. (2002). A New Look at Posturographic Analysis in the Clinical Context: Sway-Density versus Other Parameterization Techniques. *Motor Control*, Vol. 6, No. 3, pp 246-270.

Beaulieu, M.L., Lamontagne, M., Beaule, P.E. (2010). Lower Limb Biomechanics during Gait do not Return to Normal Following Total Hip Arthroplasty. *Gait & Posture*, Vol. 32, No. 2, pp. 269-273.

Boyer, K.A., Nigg, B.M. (2006). Muscle Tuning during Running: Implications of an Un-Tuned Landing. *Journal of Biomechanical Engineering* , Vol. 128, No. 6, pp. 815-822.

Brodie, M.A., Walmsley, A., Page, W. (2008). Dynamic Accuracy of Inertial Measurement Units during Simple Pendulum Motion. *Computer Methods in Biomechanics and Biomedical Engineering*, Vol. 11, No. 3, pp. 235-242.

Buzzi, U.H., Stergiou, N., Kurz, M.J., Hageman, P.A., Heidel, J. (2003). Nonlinear Dynamics Indicates Aging Affects Variability during Gait. *Clinical Biomechanics*, Vol. 18, No. 5, pp. 435-443.

Cescon, C., Madeleine, P., Farina, D. (2008). Longitudinal and Transverse Propagation of Surface Mechanomyographic Waves Generated by Single Motor Unit Activity. *Medical & Biological Engineering & Computing*, Vol. 46, No. 9, pp. 871-877.

Cescon, C., Farina, D., Gobbo, M., Merletti, R., Orizio, C. (2004). Effect of Accelerometer Location on Mechanomyogram Variables during Voluntary, Constant-Force Contractions in Three Human Muscles. *Medical & Biological Engineering & Computing*, Vol. 42, No. 1, pp. 121-127.

Charlton, I.W., Tate, P., Smyth, P., Roren, L. (2004). Repeatability of an Optimised Lower Body Model. *Gait & Posture*, Vol. 20, No. 2, pp. 213-221.

Chen, P. (1988). Empirical and Theoretical Evidence of Economic Chaos. *System Dynamics Review*, Vol. 4, No. 1, , pp. 81-108.

Cloete, T., Scheffer, C. (2010). Repeatability of an Off-The-Shelf, Full Body Inertial Motion Capture System during Clinical Gait Analysis. *Conference Proceedings IEEE Engineering in Medicine and Biology Society*, Vol. 1557, No. 170, pp. 5125-5128.

Corazza, S., Mundermann, L., Chaudhari, A.M., Demattio, T., Cobelli, C., Andriacchi, T.P. (2006). A Markerless Motion Capture System to Study Musculoskeletal Biomechanics: Visual Hull and Simulated Annealing Approach. *Annals of Biomedical Engineering*, Vol. 34, No. 6, pp. 1019-1029.

Côté, J.N., Raymond, D., Mathieu, P.A., Feldman, A.G., Levin, M.F. (2005). Differences in Multi-Joint Kinematic Patterns of Repetitive Hammering in Healthy, Fatigued and Shoulder-Injured Individuals. *Clinical Biomechanics*, Vol. 20, No. 6, pp. 581-590.

Damsgaard, M., Rasmussen, J., Christensen, S.T., Surma, E., de Zee, M. (2006). Analysis of Musculoskeletal Systems in the AnyBody Modeling System. *Simulation Modelling Practice and Theory*, Vol. 14, No. 8, , pp. 1059-1070.

DeLuca, C.J. (1997). The Use of Surface Electromyography in Biomechanics. *Journal of Applied Biomechanics*, Vol. 13, No. 2, pp. 135-163.

Erdemir, A., McLean, S., Herzog, W., van den Bogert, A.J. (2007). Model-Based Estimation of Muscle Forces Exerted During Movements. *Clinical Biomechanics*, Vol. 22, No. 2, pp. 131-154.

Escamilla, R.F., Yamashiro, K., Paulos, L., Andrews, JR. (2009). Shoulder Muscle Activity and Function in Common Shoulder Rehabilitation Exercises. *Sports Medicine*, Vol. 39, No. 8, pp. 663-685.

Farina, D., Li, X., Madeleine, P. (2008). Motor Unit Acceleration Maps and Interference Mechanomyographic Distribution. *Journal of Biomechanics*, Vol. 41, No. 13, pp. 2843-2849.

Farina, D., Fattorini, L., Felici, F., Filligoi, G. (2002). Nonlinear Surface EMG Analysis to Detect Changes of Motor Unit Conduction Velocity and Synchronization. *Journal of Applied Physiology*, Vol. 93, No. 5, pp. 1753-1763.

Farina, D., Leclerc, F., Arendt-Nielsen, L., Buttelli, O., Madeleine, P. (2008). The Change in Spatial Distribution of Upper Trapezius Muscle Activity is Correlated to Contraction Duration. *Journal of Electromyography and Kinesiology*, Vol. 18, No. 1, pp. 16-25.

Felici, F., Rosponi, A., Sbriccoli, P., Filligoi, G., Fattorini, L., Marchetti, M. (2001). Linear and Non-Linear Analysis of Surface Electromyograms in Weightlifters. *European Journal of Applied Physiology*, Vol. 84, No. 4, pp. 337-342.

Fraser, A.M. (1989). Information and Entropy in Strange Attractors. *IEEE Transactions on Information Theory*, Vol. 35, No. 2, pp. 245-262.

Gandevia, S.C. (2001). Spinal and Supraspinal Factors in Human Muscle Fatigue. *Physiological Reviews*, Vol. 81, No. 4, pp. 1725-1789.

Girard, O., Micallef, J.P., Millet, G.P. (2010). Effects of the Playing Surface on Plantar Pressures During the First Serve in Tennis. *International Journal of Sports Physiology and Performance*, Vol. 5, No. 3, pp. 384-393.

Granata, K.P., Gottipati, P. (2008). Fatigue Influences the Dynamic Stability of the Torso. *Ergonomics*, Vol. 51, No. 8, pp. 1258-1271.

Greene, B.R., McGrath, D., O'Neill, R., O'Donovan, K.J., Burns, A., Caulfield, B. (2010). An Adaptive Gyroscope-Based Algorithm for Temporal Gait Analysis. *Medical & Biological Engineering & Computing*, Vol. 48, No. 12, pp. 1251-1260.

Gurney, J.K., Kersting, U.G., Rosenbaum, D. (2009). Dynamic Foot Function and Morphology in Elite Rugby League Athletes of Different Ethnicity. *Applied Ergonomics*, Vol. 40, No. 3, pp. 554-559.

Gurney, J.K., Kersting, U.G., Rosenbaum, D. (2008). Between-Day Reliability of Repeated Plantar Pressure Distribution Measurements in a Normal Population. *Gait & posture*, Vol. 27, No. 4, pp. 706-709.

Hägg, G.M., Åström, A. (1997). Load Pattern and Pressure Pain Threshold in the Upper Trapezius Muscle and Psychosocial Factors in Medical Secretaries with and without Shoulder/Neck Disorders. *International Archives of Occupational and Environmental Health*, Vol. 69, No. 6, pp. 423-432.

Hägg, G. (1991). Comparison of Different Estimators of Electromyographic Spectral Shifts during Work when Applied on Short Test Contractions. *Medical and Biological Engineering and Computing*, Vol. 29, No. 5, , pp. 511-516.

Hansson, G.A., Stromberg, U., Larsson, B., Ohlsson, K., Balogh, I., Moritz, U. (1992). Electromyographic Fatigue in Neck/Shoulder Muscles and Endurance in Women with Repetitive Work. *Ergonomics*, Vol. 35, No. 11, pp. 1341-1352.

Hansson, G.A., Arvidsson ,I., Ohlsson, K., Nordander, C., Mathiassen, S.E., Skerfving, S., Balogh, I. (2006). Precision of Measurements of Physical Workload during Standardised Manual Handling. Part II: Inclinometry of Head, Upper Back, Neck and Upper Arms. *Journal of Electromyography and Kinesiology*, Vol. 16, No. 2, pp. 125-136.

Hennig, E.M., Moering, H., Milani, T. (1998). Measurement of Rearfoot Motion during Running with an In-Shoe Goniometer Device. *Proceeding of the Third North American Congress on Biomechanics*. No. 1, pp. 323-324.

Hermens, H.J., Freriks, B., Disselhorst-Klug, C., Rau, G. (2000). Development of Recommendations for SEMG Sensors and Sensor Placement Procedures. *Journal of Electromyography and Kinesiology*, Vol. 10, No. 5, pp. 361-374.

Hume, P.A., Reid, D., Edwards, T. (2006). Epicondylar Injury in Sport - Epidemiology, Type, Mechanisms, Assessment, Management and Prevention. *Sports Medicine* , Vol. 36, No. 2, pp. 151-170.

Jackson, J.A., Mathiassen, S.E., Dempsey, P.G. (2009). Methodological Variance Associated with Normalization of Occupational Upper Trapezius EMG using Submaximal Reference Contractions. *Journal of electromyography and kinesiology*, Vol. 19, pp. 416-427.

Kawczynski, A., Nie, H., Jaskolska, A., Jaskolski, A., Arendt-Nielsen, L., Madeleine, P. (2007). Mechanomyography and Electromyography during and after Fatiguing Shoulder Eccentric Contractions in Males and Females. *Scandinavian Journal of Medicine & Science in Sports* , Vol. 17, pp. 172-179.

Kersting, U.G. (2011). Regulation of Impact Forces during Treadmill Running. *Footwear Science*, Vol. 3, No. 1, pp. 59-68.

Kersting, U.G., Janshen, L., Bohm, H., Morey-Klapsing, G.M., Bruggemann, G.P. (2005). Modulation of Mechanical and Muscular Load by Footwear during Catering. *Ergonomics*, Vol. 48, No. 4, pp. 380-398.

Komi, P.V. (1990). Relevance of In Vivo Force Measurements to Human Biomechanics. *Journal of Biomechanics* , Vol. 23, pp. 23-34.

Kuster, M.S., Spalinger, E., Blanksby, B.A., Gachter, A. (2000). Endurance Sports after Total Knee Replacement: A Biomechanical Investigation. *Medicine and Science in Sports and Exercise*, Vol. 32, No. 4, pp. 721-724.

Lafortune MA, Hennig EM. (1991). Contribution of angular motion and gravity to tibial acceleration. *Medicine and Science in Sports and Exercise*, Vol. 23, No. 3, pp. 360-363.

Lafortune, M.A., Lake, M.J., Hennig, E. (1995a). Transfer Function between Tibial Acceleration and Ground Reaction Force. *Journal of Biomechanics*, Vol. 28, No. 1, , pp. 113-117.

Lafortune, M.A., Henning, E., Valiant, G.A. (1995b). Tibial Shock Measured with Bone and Skin Mounted Transducers. *Journal of Biomechanics,* Vol. 28, No. 8, pp. 989-993.

Laroche, D., Duval, A., Morisset, C., Beis, J.N., d'Athis, P., Maillefert, J.F., Ornetti, P. (2011). Test-Retest Reliability of 3D Kinematic Gait Variables in Hip Osteoarthritis Patients. *Osteoarthritis and Cartilage,* Vol. 19, No. 2, pp. 194-199.

Latash, M.L. (2008). *Synergy.* ,Oxford University Press, ISBN 0195333160, NYC, NY, USA.

Lipsitz, L.A. (2006). Aging as a Process of Complexity Loss. In: *Complex Systems Science in Biomedicine.J.Y.* Kresh, (Ed.), pp. 641-654: Springer.

Luinge, H.J., Veltink, P.H. (2005). Measuring Orientation of Human Body Segments Using Miniature Gyroscopes and Accelerometers. *Medical and Biological Engineering and Computing*, Vol. 43, No. 2, pp. 273-282.

Madeleine, P. (2010). On Functional Motor Adaptations: From the Quantification of Motor Strategies to the Prevention of Musculoskeletal Disorders in the Neck-Shoulder Region. *Acta Physiologica*, Vol. 199, pp. 1-46.

Madeleine, P., Madsen, T.M.T. (2009). Changes in the Amount and Structure of Motor Variability during a Deboning Process Are Associated with Work Experience and Neck–Shoulder Discomfort. *Applied Ergonomics*, Vol. 40, No. 5, , pp. 887-894.

Madeleine, P., Farina, D. (2008). Time to Task Failure in Shoulder Elevation Is Associated to Increase in Amplitude and to Spatial Heterogeneity of Upper Trapezius Mechanomyographic Signals. *European Journal of Applied Physiology*, Vol. 102, No. 3, pp. 325-333.

Madeleine, P., Arendt-Nielsen, L. (2005). Experimental Muscle Pain Increases Mechanomyographic Signal Activity during Sub-Maximal Isometric Contractions. *Journal of Electromyography and Kinesiology*, Vol. 15, No. 1, pp. 27-36.

Madeleine, P., Nielsen, M., Arendt-Nielsen, L. (2011). Characterization of Postural Control Deficit in Whiplash Patients by Means of Linear and Nonlinear Analyses–A Pilot Study. *Journal of Electromyography and Kinesiology* , Vol. 21, No. 2, pp. 291-297.

Madeleine, P., Voigt, M., Mathiassen, S.E. (2008a). The Size of Cycle-to-Cycle Variability in Biomechanical Exposure among Butchers Performing a Standardised Cutting Task. *Ergonomics*, Vol. 51, No. 7, pp. 1078-1095.

Madeleine, P., Mathiassen, S.E., Arendt-Nielsen, L. (2008b). Changes in the Amount of Motor Variability Associated with Experimental and Chronic Neck-Shoulder Pain during a Standardised Repetitive Arm Movement. *Experimental Brain Research*, Vol. 185, pp. 689-698.

Madeleine, P., Samani, A., Binderup, A., Stensdotter, A.K. (2011). Changes in the Spatio-Temporal Organization of the Trapezius Muscle Activity in Response to Eccentric Contractions. *Scandinavian Journal of Medicine & Science in Sports*, Vol. 21, pp. 277-286.

Madeleine, P., Tuker, K., Arendt-Nielsen, L., Farina, D. (2007). Heterogeneous Mechanomyographic Absolute Activation of Paraspinal Muscles Assessed by a Two-Dimensional Array during Short and Sustained Contractions. *Journal of Biomechanics*, Vol. 40, pp. 2663-2671.

Madeleine, P., Prietzel, H., Svarrer, H., Arendt-Nielsen, L. (2004). Quantitative Posturography in Altered Sensory Conditions: A Way to Assess Balance Instability in Patients with Chronic Whiplash Injury. *Archives of Physical Medicine and Rehabilitation.* , Vol. 85, No. 3, pp. 432-438.

Madeleine, P., Farina, D., Merletti, R., Arendt-Nielsen, L. (2002). Upper Trapezius Muscle Mechanomyographic and Electromyographic Activity in Humans during Low Force Fatiguing and Non-Fatiguing Contractions. *European Journal of Applied Physiology.* , Vol. 87, No. 4-5, pp. 327-336.

Madeleine, P., Lundager, B., Voigt, M., Arendt-Nielsen, L. (1999). Shoulder Muscle Co-Ordination during Chronic and Acute Experimental Neck-Shoulder Pain. An Occupational Pain Study. *European Journal of Applied Physiology.* , Vol. 79, pp. 127-140.

Madeleine, P., Leclerc, F., Arendt-Nielsen, L., Ravier, P., Farina, D. (2006). Experimental Muscle Pain Changes the Spatial Distribution of Upper Trapezius Muscle Activity during Sustained Contraction. *Clinical Neurophysiology*, Vol. 117, pp. 2436-2445.

Madeleine, P., Jorgensen, L.V., Søgaard, K., Arendt-Nielsen, L., Sjøgaard, G. (2002). Development of Muscle Fatigue as Assessed by Electromyography and Mechanomyography during Continuous and Intermittent Low-Force Contractions: Effects of the Feedback Mode. *European Journal of Applied Physiology*, Vol. 87, No. 1, pp. 28-37.

Mathiassen, S.E., Winkel, J., Hägg, G.M. (1995). Normalisation of Surface EMG Ampltude from the Upper Trapezius Muscle in Ergonomic Studies - A Review. *Journal of Electromyography and Kinesiology*, Vol. 5, No. 4, pp. 197-226.

McGinnis, P.M. (2005). *Biomechanics of Sport and Exercise*, Human Kinetics, ISBN 9780736051019, Champaign, IL, USA.

McGorry, R.W., Dowd, P.C., Dempsey, P.G. (2003). Cutting Moments and Grip Forces in Meat Cutting Operations and the Effect of Knife Sharpness. *Applied Ergonomics*, Vol. 34, No. 4, pp. 375-382.

Morlock, M.M. (2000). Determination of the in Vivo Loading of the Lumbar Spine with a new Approach Directly at the Workplace- First Results for Nurses. *Clinical Biomechanics*, Vol. 15, pp. 549-558.

Muybridge, E. (1984). *The Male and Female Figure in Motion.* Dover Publication Inc., ISBN 0486247457, Toronto, Canada.

Nigg, B.M., Herzog, W. (2007). *Biomechanics of the Musculo-Skeletal System*, John Wiley & Sons, ISBN 9780470017678, NYC, NY, USA.

Nolan, L., Lees, A. (2007). The Influence of Lower Limb Amputation Level on the Approach in the Amputee Long Jump. *Journal of Sports Science*, Vol. 25, No. 4, pp. 393-401.

Orizio, C. (1993). Muscle Sound: Bases for the Introduction of a Mechanomyographic Signal in Muscle Studies. *Critical Review in Biomedical Engineering*, Vol. 21, No. 3, , pp. 201-243.

Orizio, C., Gobbo, M., Diemont, B., Esposito, F., Veicsteinas, A. (2003). The Surface Mechanomyogram as a Tool to Describe the Influence of Fatigue on Biceps Brachii

Motor Unit Activation Strategy. Historical Basis and Novel Evidence. *European Journal of Applied Physiology*, Vol. 90, No. 3-4, , pp. 326-336.

Orizio, C., Liberati, D., Locatelli, C., De Grandis, D., Veicsteinas, A. (1996). Surface Mechanomyogram Reflects Muscle Fibres Twitches Summation. *Journal of Biomechanics*, Vol. 29, No. 4, pp. 475-481.

Prilutsky, B.I., Zatsiorsky, V.M. (2002). Optimization-based models of muscle coordination. *Exercise and Sport Sciences Reviews*, Vol 30, No 1, pp. 32–38.

Rasmussen, J., Tørholm, S., de Zee, M. (2009). Computational Analysis of the Influence of Seat Pan Inclination and Friction on Muscle Activity and Spinal Joint Forces. *International Journal of Industrial Ergonomics*, Vol. 39, No. 1, pp. 52-57.

Rasmussen, J., Damsgaard, M., Voigt, M. (2001). Muscle Recruitment by the Min/Max Criterion - A Comparative Numerical Study. *Journal of Biomechanics*, Vol. 34, No. 3, pp. 409-415.

Rathleff, M.S., Olesen, C.G., Moelgaard, C.M., Jensen, K., Madeleine, P., Olesen, J.L. (2010). Non-Linear Analysis of the Structure of Variability in Midfoot Kinematics. *Gait & Posture*, Vol. 31, No. 3, pp. 385-390.

Roerdink, M., De Haart, M., Daffertshofer, A., Donker, S.F., Geurts, A.C.H., Beek, P.J. (2006). Dynamical Structure of Center-of-Pressure Trajectories in Patients Recovering from Stroke. *Experimental Brain Research*, Vol. 174, No. 2, pp 256-269.

Roetenberg, D., Slycke, P.J., Veltink, P.H. (2007). Ambulatory Position and Orientation Tracking Fusing Magnetic and Inertial Sensing. *IEEE Transactions on Biomedical Engineering*, Vol. 54, No. 5, pp. 883-890.

Rosenbaum, D., Brandes, M., Hardes, J., Gosheger, G., Rodl, R. (2008). Physical Activity Levels after Limb Salvage Surgery are not Related to Clinical Scores-Objective Activity Assessment in 22 Patients after Malignant Bone Tumor Treatment with Modular Prostheses. *Journal of Surgical Oncology*, Vol. 98, No. 2, pp. 97-100.

Rosenhahn, B., Brox, T., Kersting, U.G., Smith, A.W., Gurney, J.K., Klette, R. (2006). A System for Marker-Less Motion Capture. *Kuenstliche Intelligenz*, Vol. 20, No. 1, , pp. 46-52.

Samani, A., Holtermann, A., Søgaard, K., Madeleine, P. (2010). Active Biofeedback Changes the Spatial Distribution of Upper Trapezius Muscle Activity during Computer Work. *European Journal of Applied Physiology. Vol. 110, No. 2, pp. 415-423.*

Scholz, J.P., Schöner, G. (1999). The Uncontrolled Manifold Concept: Identifying Control Variables for a Functional Task. *Experimental Brain Research*, Vol. 126, No. 3, pp. 289-306.

Shung, K., de Oliveira, C.G., Nadal, J. (2009). Influence of Shock Waves and Muscle Activity at Initial Contact on Walk-Run Transition Evaluated by Two Models. *Journal of Applied Biomechanics*, Vol. 25, No. 2, pp. 175-183.

Slifkin, A.B., Newell, K.M. (1999). Noise, Information Transmission, and Force Variability. *Journal of Experimental Psychology: Human Perception and Performance*, Vol. 25, No. 3, pp. 837-851.

Søndergaard, K.H.E., Olesen, C.G., Søndergaard, E.K., de Zee, M., Madeleine, P. (2010). The Variability and Complexity of Sitting Postural Control are Associated with Discomfort. *Journal of Biomechanics*, Vol. 43, No. 10, pp. 1997-2001.

Sung, P.S., Zurcher, U., Kaufman, M. (2005). Nonlinear Analysis of Electromyography Time Series as a Diagnostic Tool for Low Back Pain. *Medical Science Monitor : International Medical Journal of Experimental and Clinical Research*, Vol. 11, No. 1, pp. 1-5.

Svendsen, J.H., Madeleine, P. (2010). Amount and Structure of Force Variability during Short, Ramp and Sustained Contractions in Males and Females. *Human Movement Science*, Vol. 29, pp. 35-47.

Tresch, M. (2006). Matrix Factorization Algorithms for the Identification of Muscle Synergies: Evaluation on Simulated and Experimental Data Sets.

Tsirakos, D., Baltzopoulos, V., Bartlett, R. (1997). Inverse Optimization: Functional and Physiological Considerations Related to the Force-Sharing Problem. *Critical Reviews in Biomedical EngineerinG*, Vol. 25, No. 4, pp. 371-407.

van Dieën, J.H., Cholewicki, J., Radebold, A. (2003). Trunk Muscle Recruitment Patterns in Patients with Low Back Pain Enhance the Stability of the Lumbar Spine. *Spine*, Vol. 28, No. 8, pp. 834-841.

van Dieën, J.H., Vrielink, H.H.E.O., Housheer, A.F., Lotters, F.B.J., Toussaint, H.M. (1993). Trunk Extensor Endurance and its Relationship to Electromyogram Parameters. *European Journal of Applied Physiology*, Vol. 66, No. 5, pp. 388-396.

van Woensel, W.C. (2011). A Perturbation Study of Lower Extremity Motion During Running. *Journal of Applied Biomechanics*, Vol. 8, No. 1, pp. 30-47.

Watakabe, M., Mita, K., Akataki, K., Ito, K. (2003). Reliability of the Mechanomyogram Detected with an Accelerometer during Voluntary Contractions. *Medical & Biological Engineering & Computing*, Vol. 41, No. 2, pp. 198-202.

Watakabe, M., Mita, K., Akataki, K., Itoh, Y. (2001). Mechanical Behaviour of Condenser Microphone in Mechanomyography. *Medical & Biological Engineering & Computing*, Vol. 39, No. 2, pp. 195-201.

Webber Jr, C.L., Zbilut, J.P. (2005). *Recurrence Quantification Analysis of Nonlinear Dynamical Systems*. In M. A. Riley & G. C. Van Orden (Eds.), Tutorials Incontemporary Nonlinear Methods for the Behavioral Sciences (pp. 26-94). Retrieved March 1, 2005, from http://www.nsf.gov/sbe/bcs/pac/nmbs/nmbs.jsp

Westgaard, R.H., De Luca, C.J. (2001). Motor Control of Low-Threshold Motor Units in the Human Trapezius Muscle. *Journal of Neurophysiology*, Vol. 85, No. 4, pp. 1777-1781.

Winter, D.A. (1990). *Biomechanics and Motor Control of Human Movement*. New York,Wiley Interscience Publication.

Wollaston, W.H. (1810). On the Duration of the Muscle Action. *Philosophical Transactions of the Royal Society B*, Vol. 1.

Woltring, H.J. (1994). 3-D Attitude Representation of Human Joints: A Standardization Proposal. *Journal of Biomechanics*, Vol. 27, No. 12, pp. 1399-1414.

Wu, G., van d, H., Veeger, H.E., Makhsous, M., Van, R.P., Anglin, C., Nagels, J., Karduna, A.R., McQuade, K., Wang, X., Werner, F.W., Buchholz, B. (2005) ISB Recommendation on Definitions of Joint Coordinate Systems of Various Joints for the Reporting of Human Joint Motion-Part II: Shoulder, Elbow, Wrist and Hand. *Journal of Biomechanics*, Vol. 38, No. 5, pp. 981-992.

Wu, G., Siegler, S., Allard, P., Kirtley, C., Leardini, A., Rosenbaum, D., Whittle, M., D'Lima, D.D., Cristofolini, L., Witte, H., Schmid, O., Stokes, I. (2002). ISB Recommendation on Definitions of Joint Coordinate Systems of Various Joints for the Reporting of Human Joint Motion-Part I: Ankle, Hip, and Spine. *Journal of Biomechanics*, Vol. 35, No. 4, pp. 543-548.

18

Biomechanics of the Neck

Haibin Chen[1], Liying Zhang[1,2], Zhengguo Wang[1],
King H. Yang[2] and Albert I. King[2]
[1]*State Key Laboratory of Trauma, Burns, and Combined Injury*
Institute of Surgery Research & Daping Hospital
Third Military Medical University
[2]*Bioengineering Center*
Wayne State University
[1]*PR China*
[2]*USA*

1. Introduction

From a mechanical and structural point of view, the human neck is a very complex mechanism, containing vital neurologic, vascular, and respiratory structures as well as the cervical vertebrae and spinal cord. The incidence of neck injuries in traffic accidents appears to be relatively low compared to for instance head injuries, except for specific accident configurations like a rear end collision where more than 50% of the injuries appear to be in the neck area. However, the vehicle injury priority rating data indicated that neck injuries became the fifth most important injury category (after head, face, chest and abdomen). Knowledge on the mechanism causing neck injuries is still rather limited. Therefore, various biomechanical models (i.e. animal/human models and numerical models), injury mechanisms and injury tolerance of the neck will be presented in this chapter.

2. Neck biomechanics models

2.1 Animal models

2.1.1 Goat in vivo model

An in vivo goat model (Cavanaugh et al., 2006; Chen et al., 2005; Lu et al., 2005a, 2005b) was developed to investigate the injury threshold of cervical facet joint capsules (FJC) in vivo. The method incorporated a custom-fabricated testing frame for facet joint loading, a stereoimaging system, and a template-matching technique to obtain single afferent response. The C5 articular process was then pulled via a computer-controlled actuator at a rate of 0.5 mm/sec to simultaneously stretch the C5-6 capsule, record sensory nerve activity due to stretch and record strain by tracking targets on the capsule. In these studies Lu et al (2005b) demonstrated a quantitative relationship between capsule sensory discharges and applied capsule stretch from cervical facet joints. Neural responses of all mechanosensitive units showed statistically significant correlations (all $P<<0.05$) with both capsular load ($r^2 = 0.744 \pm 0.109$) and local strain ($r^2 = 0.868 \pm 0.088$). Most of the capsular neural receptors responded in the physiologic range of capsule stretch and fired at strains of $(10.2 \pm 4.6)\%$

that typically do not signal pain. However, higher capsular strains of (47.2 ± 9.6)% triggered discharges from higher threshold receptors which were most likely from nociceptors. Nociceptors transmit signals to the central nervous system to signal pain. Afterdischarges were reported in these goat studies after capsular strains of (45.0 ± 15.1)% and may be related to tissue injury and release of inflammatory mediators into the surrounding tissue. These changes may lead to central sensitization of pain pathways in the spinal cord which may lead to persistent or chronic whiplash pain.

2.1.2 Rat in vivo model

A rat model was used by Quinn et al (2007) who conducted a study to quantify the structural mechanics of the cervical facet capsule and define the threshold for altered structural responses in this ligament during distraction. Tensile failure tests were performed using isolated C6/C7 rat facet capsular ligaments (n = 8); gross ligament failure, the occurrence of minor ruptures and ligament yield were measured. Gross failure occurred at (2.45 ± 0.60)N and (0.92 ± 0.17)mm. However, the yield point occurred at (1.68 ± 0.56)N and (0.57 ± 0.08)mm, which was significantly less than gross failure ($P < 0.001$ for both measurements). Maximum principal strain in the capsule at yield was (80 ± 24)%. Energy to yield was (14.3 ± 3.4)% of the total energy for a complete tear of the ligament. Ligament yield point occurred at a distraction magnitude in which pain symptoms begin to appear in vivo in the rat.

Findings presented here suggest a relationship between structural damage of the facet capsular ligament and potential mechanisms of pain for subfailure distraction. Quinn et al (2007)'s data show ligament yield at a significantly lower distraction than gross failure. While these subfailure distractions may not produce visible ligament tears, detection of the ligament's altered structural response may provide an indication of an injury sufficient to elicit sustained nociceptor firing, pain symptoms, and persistent activity in the nervous system. Given the evidence that painful joint distractions begin near ligament yield, this study may suggest that the physiologic range of the facet joint is actually limited to prior to yield. This mechanical study provides a framework for future in vivo studies in determining a mechanical threshold for persistent pain, and also provides data for quantitative scaling to other animal models and to the human. These findings provide mechanical definition of altered ligament behavior corresponding with a loading condition known to produce pain, linking mechanical damage and persistent pain for the first time.

2.2 Human models

2.2.1 Human cadaveric models

A bench-top trauma sled was used to apply four intensities of whiplash trauma to human cadaveric cervical spine specimens and to measure resultant intervertebral rotations using high-speed cinematography (Grauer & Panjabi, 1997). Objectives were to determine the cervical spine levels most prone to injury from whiplash trauma and to hypothesize a mechanism for such injury. Six occiput to T1 (or C7) fresh cadaveric human spines were studied. Physiologic flexion and extension motions were recorded with a motion analysis system by loading up to 1.0 N m. Specimens then were secured in a trauma sled, and a surrogate head was attached. Flags were fixed to the head, and individual vertebrae were monitored with high-speed cinematography (500 frames/sec). Data were collected for 12 traumas in four classes defined by the maximum sled acceleration. The trauma classes were 2.5 G, 4.5 G, 6.5 G, and 8.5 G (G: acceleration of gravity). In the whiplash traumas, the peak intervertebral rotations of C6-C7 and C7-T1 significantly exceeded the maximum physiologic extension of all trauma classes studied. The maximum extension of these lower levels occurred significantly before full neck extension. The upper cervical levels were consistently in flexion at the time of maximum lower level extension. It was concluded that in whiplash, the neck forms an S-shaped curvature, with lower level hyperextension and upper level flexion. A subsequent C-shaped curvature with extension of the entire cervical spine produced less lower level extension.

2.2.2 Volunteer models

The volunteers sat on a seat mounted on a sled that simulated actual car impact acceleration (Ono et al., 1997). Impact speeds (4, 6, and 8 km/h), seat stiffness, neck muscle tension, and alignment of the cervical spine were selected for a parametric study of the head-neck-torso kinematics and cervical spine responses. The effects of these parameters were studied without the headrest. Muscle activity was measured with surface electromyography. The cervical vertebrae motions were recorded by cineradiography (90 frames/sec radiograph) and analyzed to quantify the rotations and translations of cervical vertebrae during impact. Furthermore, the motion patterns of cervical vertebrae during impact were compared with the normal motions. A subject's muscles in the relaxed state did not affect the head-neck-torso kinematics on rear-end impact. The ramping-up motion of the subject's torso was observed, caused by the inclination of the seat back. An axial compression force occurred. The lower cervical vertebral segments extended and rotated before the motions of the upper segments. These motions were beyond the normal physiologic cervical motions, which could trigger the facet joint injury mechanism. In addition, the more rigid the seat cushion, the greater the axial compression force. In contrast, the torso rebounding caused by the softer seat cushion tended to intensify the shearing force applied to the upper vertebrae. It was also deduced that the initial posture of the cervical spine affected the impact responses of head and neck markedly. Based on the differences in the alignment of the cervical spine between male and female occupants, it was deduced that the female neck injury incidence may be higher than that of the male, because the female cervical spine takes the kyphosis position more often than does the male cervical spine.

2.3 Numerical models

2.3.1 Two-joint neck models

Two-joint neck models were proposed in the 1970's and 1980's (Bowman & Robbins, 1972; Seemann et al., 1984; Bosio and Bowman, 1986; Wismans et al., 1987). These are relatively simple models in which the head, neck and torso were linked by two pivots or ball-socket joints, depending on whether the model was 2-D or 3-D. The upper joint was normally located near the occipital condyles, and the lower joint was usually situated near the first thoracic (T1) vertebra. Although fairly simple, these models contributed greatly to the analysis of the global kinematics of the head-neck complex during frontal, lateral and oblique impacts, over the past 30 years. For example, Wismans et al. (1987) used this type of model to simulate the head-neck motion. In these studies, the neck was modeled as a rigid body, and the geometrical and mechanical properties of the joints were determined based on those test data. Performance requirements for future dummy neck designs were also defined by means of this model. Similar models have been proposed as well by Bosio & Bowman (1986), except an extensible neck was used instead of a rigid one. In these two studies, model validations were performed in the -Gx and +Gy directions. A nonlinear joint stiffness and a neck elongation stiffness were found to be necessary to obtain satisfactory simulation results. Very similar models were also used to perform a parametric study by Bowman & Robbins (1972) to investigate the injury mechanism of the human neck in frontal impact, as well as to test another theory by Seemann et al. (1984), who proposed that some volunteers "locked" their neck joints in anticipation of sled firing. Because two-joint models were originally developed for describing the global motion of the head and neck relative to the torso, they were not adequate to describe vertebral kinematics and cervical soft tissue deformation. It is apparent that more detailed models would be needed.

2.3.2 Multi-body (MB) neck models

MB neck models were the second category of numerical models of the human cervical spine. In these models, the head and vertebrae were modeled as rigid bodies, while the soft tissues were modeled as either nonlinear viscoelastic intervertebral joints or by a detailed arrangement of spring-damper elements to represent the intervertebral discs, ligaments, facet joints, and muscles. For instance, De Jager et al. (1994) developed a MADYMO-based 3-D MB model of the head-neck based on the model of Deng & Goldsmith (1987). In this model, the rigid head and vertebrae were connected by linear viscoelastic intervertebral joints and nonlinear elastic muscle elements. A sensitivity analysis was also performed in this study, and it was found that head mass, joint stiffness and damping coefficients for rotational deformations had a major influence on model response. Subsequently, De Jager et al. (1996) developed a more detailed version of this model, in which linear viscoelastic discs, nonlinear viscoelastic ligaments, frictionless facet joints and contractile muscles were simulated. Model responses to 15-G frontal and 7-G lateral impacts were validated against volunteer data. This model was then modified by Van der Horst et al. (1997) who included more muscles, and divided the muscles into segments to simulate muscle curvature. Volunteer frontal impact data at reduced G-levels were used for model validation.

2.3.3 FE neck models

In the past 20 years, several FE models of the human cervical spine were developed by Camacho et al (Kleinberger, 1993; Dauvilliers et al., 1994; Camacho et al., 1997; Kumaresan et al., 1997; Yang et al., 1998; Halldin et al., 2000; Chancey et al., 2003; Meyer et al., 2004). Because FE models allowed for a more detailed and realistic representation of the neck geometry and its material behavior, more detailed neck injury mechanisms could be studied using this kind of model.

The first FE neck model presented at The STAPP Car Crash Conference was made by Kleinberger (1993). In this model, the geometries of the vertebrae and the skull were highly simplified, and the atlanto-occipital articulation was represented by a pin joint. Only the model responses to axial stiffness and neck versus head angle curve during an 8-G frontal sled test were compared with experimental data. No detailed validations were conducted at that time.

Dauvilliers et al. (1994) proposed another FE neck model, which was also fairly simple by current standards. In this model, each vertebra consisted of only 12 solid elements, and spring-damper elements were used to simulate the major ligaments. The model responses were compared to volunteer kinematics during frontal and lateral impacts. Head accelerations responses of the model matched the experimental data fairly well; However, the head displacement and angle data were not close to the reference data. One limitation of this model was that muscles which could have a significant influence on model response during frontal and lateral impacts were not simulated.

Kumaresan et al. (1997) presented a set of detailed FE models of a one-year old, three-year old, and six year old pediatric human cervical spine from C4 to C6 vertebrae. Although their study only focused on the pediatric neck, the development and validation of the adult FE model were also provided. Compared to other neck models, this model had complicated geometries and consisted of several very detailed anatomical structures, such as the endplate, uncovertebral joint and synovial fluid. The adult model flexibilities under quasi-static loading conditions were validated against experimental data. However, this model only simulated 3 vertebrae; and thus head-neck response during impact could not be simulated. For modeling the pediatric neck, it has been found that the inclusion of the local geometry and material property changes produced higher changes in the flexibilities than pure structural scaling. This finding emphasized the need to consider the local geometry and material property changes to better predict the biomechanical responses of the pediatric human cervical spine.

Camacho et al. (1997) proposed an FE head-neck model to investigate the dynamic responses of the head and neck to near-vertex head impact. In this model, highly simplified rigid vertebrae were connected by nonlinear spring elements, the stiffness of which was measured from quasi-static flexion-extension tests. To simulate head impact, a deformable head was defined and linked to the C1 vertebra. Strictly speaking, their model should be classified as a MB neck model coupled with an FE head model. The results showed that this model could accurately predict resultant neck forces, resultant head forces and accelerations measured in cadaveric near-vertex head impact tests with impact surfaces at -15 deg, 0 deg and +15 deg with respect to the horizontal. Although the model produced higher neck forces than the validation corridors during the latter portions of the simulations, the authors explained that this was because at that time some of the cadaveric specimens had suffered cervical spine injuries, and thus possessed decreased load carrying capacity. This model was also used to estimate human neck tensile tolerance (Chancey et al., 2003), but no further validations were conducted.

Yang et al. (1998) developed a detailed FE neck model the geometry of which was taken from an MRI. It incorporated a previously developed head and brain model, so that head-neck response could be simulated during impact. All the bony structures, articular surfaces, relevant ligaments and intervertebral discs were described. It should be noted that it was the first model that included the ligaments in the upper vertebrae (Occiput-C2). Near-vertex head impact test data with impact surface at 0° deg to the horizontal and cadaveric rear impact sled test data were used to validate the model. Model responses matched the experimental data fairly well. However, for the rear impact, only head kinematics from the model and test were compared. Although model results of facet capsule stretch percentage were presented, such results have not been validated as yet due to the limited experimental data available. The validated model has also been integrated into a skeleton torso model to study the neck response during head-torso-airbag interaction.

Another FE head-neck complex model was developed by Halldin et al. (2000), who attempted to use the model to evaluate a new car roof design concept. This was also a fairly detailed model, slightly smaller in size than the model developed by Yang et al. (1998). Component compression tests and near-vertex head impact tests with impact surface at

-15 deg, 0 deg, and +15 deg to the horizontal were used to validate the model. Most of the model responses matched the experimental data fairly well.

Meyer et al. (2004) presented another detailed FE head-neck complex model. Because the aim of their study was not to reproduce bony fracture, but to simulate more moderate lesions, the vertebrae were modeled by rigid shell elements. The major contribution of this model was the model validation procedure. The model responses were validated against volunteer and/or cadaveric impacts in frontal, lateral, oblique, and rear directions. Moreover, frequency domain information was also taken into account to improve model responses. To the best of our knowledge, this was the first time researchers validated the FE neck model in both the time and frequency domains.

3. Neck injury mechanisms

Because the neck is a slender column that can be subjected to a variety of bending loads in association with an axial load, the injury modes can be classified as compression, tension-extension, tension-flexion, compression-extension, compression-flexion, and lateral bending.

3.1 Compression injuries

These injuries result from crown impacts to the head which produce a high compressive load on the neck accompanied by bending loads that can depend on the initial orientation of the head, initial configuration of the neck, and surface friction. They are not common automotive injuries but can occur in ejections and rollovers. The compression comes from the mass of the body following the head, which is stopped by a resisting surface.

In order to understand the injury mechanisms of this kind compression loading, this chapter summarizes a numerical investigation of factors affecting cervical spine injuries during rollover crashes by Hu et al (2008). In fact, rollover crashes are the most hazardous vehicular crashes to the human cervical spine. The incidence rate of AIS 3+ (AIS: Abbreviated Injury Scale) cervical spine injuries in rollovers was nearly 4 times that occurring in frontal and side crashes (Yoganandan et al., 1989). The cervical spine was also the third most commonly injured body region during rollovers after the head and thorax (Hu et al, 2005), and injuries to the cervical spine may often lead to permanent disabilities.

Previous experimental (Bahling et al., 1990) and numerical (Hu, 2007) studies have shown that cervical spine injuries in rollovers were mainly caused by the inertia of the occupant's torso compressing the head into the roof/ground, which is often referred to as "the diving mechanism." In the past 3 decades, several cadaveric experiments were conducted to investigate cervical spine injuries under diving type of impacts. The injury mechanism under sagittal plane loading (combined compression and flexion/extension) is reasonably well understood, and many important and widely acknowledged conclusions have been drawn, including: (1) neck injury mechanisms are dependent on the neck orientation and impact direction, (2) padding will add constraints to the head which, in turn, will increase the risk of neck injury, and (3) if the neck can escape from the direction of impact momentum, the risk of neck injury will be greatly reduced.

However, during rollovers, the centrifugal force tends to maintain a belted occupant erect with his/her head upward and outboard (Bahling et al., 1990), thus it is common that an impact to the occupant's head would come from the upper and lateral sides of the vehicle. Therefore, a combined lateral bending, compression, and flexion/extension could be a very common neck loading mode during rollovers. Because of the complex nature of rollover crashes, there is no typical rollover scenario that can be specified easily (Hu et al, 2007). To investigate the neck injury mechanism under this complex combined loading condition, multiple experiments under different loading directions have to be conducted to mimic different rollover scenarios. Because of the difficulty in securing test samples and the high cost associated with performing cadaveric experiments, this research strategy needs to be modified. With recent advancement in computing technology and software, numerical modeling could provide a cost-effective way to perform this type of research. Recently, several published finite element (FE) human head-neck models (Camacho et al., 1997; Halldin et al., 2000; Zhang et al., 2005) have been validated under diving type of impact conditions, but until now none has simulated the combined lateral bending and loading in the sagittal plane–a loading condition similar to real rollover scenarios. Furthermore, although many risk factors have been identified in previous studies to be associated with cervical spine injuries, no study has systematically analyzed those factors. Therefore, Hu et al. (Hu et al., 2008) carried out a study to investigate neck responses under various complex loading conditions similar to real-world rollover scenarios using a detailed FE head-neck model. The effects of changing the coefficient of friction (COF), impact velocity, padding material thickness and stiffness, and muscle force on the risk of neck injuries were analyzed in 16 different impact orientations based on a Taguchi array of design of experiments.

In summary, the following primary simulation results were found: (1) Impact velocity is the most important factor in determining the risk of cervical spine fracture ($P = 0.000$). (2) Decreases in the COF between the head and impact surface can effectively reduce the risk of cervical spine fracture ($P = 0.038$). (3) If the COF is not 0, an impact with lateral force component could sometimes increase the risk of cervical spine fracture; and the larger the angle of the impact surface, the more important it becomes to reduce the COF to protect the neck. (4) Soft ($P = 0.033$) and thick ($P = 0.137$) padding can actually decrease the neck fracture risk, which is in contrast to previous experimental data. Furthermore, Hu et al. (2008) concluded that a careful selection of proper padding stiffness and thickness, along with a minimized COF between the head and impact surface or between the padding and its supporting structure, may simultaneously decrease the risk of head and neck injuries during rollover crashes.

3.2 Tension-extension injuries

Tension-extension loading is common and is responsible for a group of injuries including whiplash, hangman's fractures, and structural injury to the anterior column of the spine. Tension-extension loading can occur in three primary ways:

- Fixation of the head with continued forward displacement of the body. This occurs commonly in unbelted occupants hitting the windshield and as a result of falls and dives.
- Inertial loading of the neck following an abrupt forward acceleration of the torso, as would occur in a rear-end collision (whiplash mechanism (Chen et al., 2009)).
- Forceful loading below the chin directed postersuperiorly (as in a judicial hanging).

Herein, this chapter summarizes research aimed at providing some kinematics responses and injury mechanisms of the neck in the rear-end collision.

3.2.1 Neck kinematics responses in the rear-end collision

Yang and King (2003) carried out a study to document the kinematics of the neck during low-speed rear-end impacts. In a series of experiments reported by Deng et al. (2000), a pneumatically driven mini-sled was used to study cervical spine motion using six cadavers instrumented with metallic markers at each cervical level, a 9-accelerometer mount on the head, and a tri-axial accelerometers on the thorax. A 250-Hz x-ray system was used to record marker motion while acceleration data were digitized at 10,000 Hz. Results show that, in the global coordinate system, the head and all cervical vertebrae were primarily in extension during the entire period of x-ray data collection. In local coordinate systems, upper cervical segments were initially in relative flexion while lower segments were in extension. Facet joint capsular stretch ranged from 17% to 97%. In the vertical direction, the head and T1 accelerated upward almost instantaneously after impact initiation while there was delay for the head in the horizontal direction. This combination was the result of a force vector which was pointed in the forward and upward direction to generate an extension moment. Upward ramping of the torso was larger in tests with a 20-deg seatback angle. The study concluded that the kinematics of the neck is rather complicated and greatly influenced by the large rotations of the thoracic spine. Significant posterior shear deformation was found, as evidenced by the large facet capsular stretch. Although the neck forms a "mild" S-shaped curve during whiplash, using its shape as an injury mechanism can be misleading because the source of pain is likely to be located in the facet capsules.

3.2.2 Axial compression hypothesis

In volunteer tests, McConnell et al (1993) found that a vertical acceleration can be measured during a low speed rear-end impact. This ramping up phenomenon was due to the straightening of the spine or the mechanical interaction between the seatback and the torso. This same phenomenon was also reported in a high-speed X-rays study of the neck for volunteers subjected to rear impact forces (Matsushita et al, 1994) and in Hybrid II dummy tests by Viano (1992). However, the measured vertical acceleration and movement were rather small and McConnell et al later reported it to be insignificant compared to that measured horizontally (McConnell et al, 1995).

Although the vertical acceleration may seem small, it plays a significant role in the cervical spine biomechanics. The head generally possesses about 4.5 kg of inertial mass. Even a small acceleration could generate a significant compressive force at the neck. In a rear-end impact, the car seat pushes (shears) the torso forward while the neck is subjected to this axial compression. Based on this observation, Yang and Begeman (1996) proposed a new hypothesis to explain the rear-end neck injury mechanism stating that axial compression can cause loosening of ligaments and make it easier for the cervical facet joint capsule and other tissues to be injured. Because these injuries occur in soft tissues, this new theory explains why there is generally no objective evidence.

The facet joint geometry of the cervical spine also plays an important role. In frontal impacts, the upper vertebra will shear anteriorly, relative to the lower vertebra. By observing the anatomy of the facet joints, it is evident that contact of the facet joints can protect against excessive frontal shear. However, in a rear-end impact, the lower vertebra shears anteriorly, the facet joint offers no protection to such a motion. This can be the reason that the rate of neck injury is much lower in frontal impacts of the same or even higher severity.

To test this hypothesis, an in vitro experiment was designed to investigate the theory that axial compression reduces the shear stiffness when the cervical spine is moved due to a rear-end impact (Yang et al., 1997).

Cervical spine specimens from C1-T1 were dissected from the entire spine. The C1 vertebra was fixed to an aluminum plate with screws. The other end (T1) was potted in epoxy and attached to a six-axis load cell. Two LED markers were attached to each vertebral body from C2-C7. One additional LED maker was attached to the frame of the Instron as reference. During the test, the actuator moves upward to simulate the seat back pushing from behind.
Five tests were done for each specimen. In the first test, the T1 was moved anteriorly to stimulate a rear-end impact for 20 mm displacement at a quasi-static speed of 0.04 mm/s. In the next four tests, an axial compression of 44.5 N, 89.0 N, 133.5 N and 178 N of dead weight were applied through a cable-pulley system. The same procedure as in the first test was then reported. Shear stiffness values were calculated from the load cell and motion data.
Result showed that shear stiffness values were reduced significantly with increased axial compression. Based on the total shear force vs the shear deflection data for a typical C5-C6 motion segment, it can be clearly seen that the shear stiffness decreased as the applied axial compression increased. The shear force vs deflection curves were nonlinear due to coupling rotations of vertebrae. The shear stiffness, defined as the final linear portion of the force-deflection curve, was reduced significantly with increased axial compression. For example, for the C2-C3 portion of the specimen No. 715, shear stiffness was only 50% of that without axial preload (Table 1).

	Stiffness (N/mm)			
	C2-C3	C3-C4	C4-C5	C5-C6
No preload	14.9	9.0	10.9	18.6
178 N preload	7.5	4.5	6.3	5.0

Table 1. Shear stiffness values calculated at each vertebra level (Specimen No. 715)

It should be noted that in previous typical static tests, the shear stiffness is expected to increase as the axial compression increase. Yang (1997)'s experimental data show the opposite trend. This explain why the neck injury rate is higher in a rear-end impact than that of a frontal impact. The axial compression presented in rear-end impact reduce the shear stiffness of the cervical spine and make it easier to be injured. Dynamic tests can give researchers more insight into the neck injury mechanism. Those data can be useful in the design of new equipment such as head restraints to protect the neck from rear-end impact injury.

3.2.3 Axial pretorque hypothesis

Whiplash victims who had their head turned at impact have more severe and persistent symptoms than patients who were facing forward (Sturzenegger et al., 1994; Sturzenegger et al., 1995). These findings have prompted biomechanical studies using human cadaveric necks to investigate why a head-turned posture increases injury potential. Dynamic rear-impact tests of prerotated ligamentous spines (occiput-T1) produce increased neck flexibility (interpreted as injury) in extension, lateral bending and axial rotation (Panjabi et al., 2006). Though concentrated in the lower cervical spine, these "injuries" were not isolated to particular spinal ligaments. Detailed measurements of the strain field in the facet capsule have also shown that a head-turned posture generates higher capsular strains than a neutral head posture, but the quasi-static loads applied during those tests were limited to pure flexion/extension moments and did not include the axial compression or posterior shear present during whiplash loading (Winkelstein et al, 2000). Thus the question of how a head-turned posture combined with multiaxial whiplash loads affects facet capsular ligament strain has yet to be answered.

For this reason, Siegmund et al. (2008) used human cadaveric motion segments to: (1) quantify the intervertebral kinematics and facet capsule strains under whiplash-like loads in the presence of an initial axial rotation, and (2) compare the capsule strains generated by these combined loads to the previously-published strains needed to injure these ligaments in isolated shear failure (Siegmund et al, 2001). Their overall hypothesis was that capsular strains during this simulated whiplash exposure are similar to those needed to injure the capsular ligament (Siegmund et al, 2008).

According to Siegmund et al. (2008), thirteen motion segments were used from 7 women donors (50 ± 10 years). Axial pretorques (±1.5 N m), axial compressive preloads (45, 197, and 325 N), and quasi-static shear loads (posteriorly-directed horizontal forces from 0 to 135 N) were applied to the superior vertebral body to simulate whiplash kinematics with the head turned. Three-dimensional displacements of markers placed on the right facet capsular ligament were used to estimate the strain field in the ligament during loading. The effects of pretorque direction, compression, and posterior shear on motion segment motion and maximum principal strain in the capsule were examined using repeated-measures analyses of variance.

Results showed that axial pretorque affected peak capsule strains more than axial compression or posterior shear. Peak strains reached 34%±18% and were higher for pretorques toward rather than away from the facet capsule (i.e., head rotation to the right caused higher strain in the right facet capsule).

Similarly, based on a validated intact head to first thoracic vertebra (T1) computational model, parametric analysis was used to assess effects of increasing axial head rotation between 0° and 60° and increasing impact severity between 8 and 24 km/h on facet joint capsule strains (Storvik et al., 2011). Rear impacts were simulated by horizontally accelerating the T1 vertebra. Characteristics of the acceleration pulse were based on the horizontal T1 acceleration pulse from a series of simulated rear impact experiments using full-body post mortem human subjects. Joint capsule strain magnitudes were greatest in ipsilateral facet joints for all simulations incorporating axial head rotation (i.e., head rotation to the left caused higher ligament strain at the left facet joint capsule). Strain magnitudes increased by 47%–196% in simulations with 60° head rotation compared to forward facing simulations. These findings indicate that axial head rotation prior to rear impact increases the risk of facet joint injury.

3.2.4 Facet joint impingement hypothesis

Ono et al. (1997) and Yoganandan et al. (1998) both proposed a facet joint impingement hypothesis. Specifically, Ono et al (1997) theorized that the facet synovium or a portion of the facet capsule could be trapped between the facet joint surfaces and pinched, causing pain. However, there is no biomechanical evidence that the capsule is loose enough to be trapped between the facet joint and even if it was trapped, evidence is lacking to show that nociceptors are present in the synovium or the trapped portion of the capsule that is indeed set off by the pressure. Kaneoka et al (1999) hypothesized that the center of rotation moved superiorly during a whiplash and caused the tip of the inferior facet (of the upper vertebra) to impact the superior facet surface (of the lower vertebra). This proposition that compression of the facet surfaces can produce pain is probably untenable since cartilage is devoid of nociceptors and there is no neurophysiological evidence that the nociceptors in the subchondral bone can be made to fire by this presumed compression.

3.2.5 Transient pressure gradient hypothesis

Aldman (1986) proposed a neck injury hypothesis for rear impact which states that injuries to the nerve root region in the cervical spine are a result of transient pressure gradients in the spinal canal during rapid neck extension (Svensson et al., 2000). In experimental neck trauma research on animals, pressure gradients were observed and indications of nerve cell membrane dysfunction were found in the dorsal root ganglia (DRG) of the cervical spine ganglia. The experiments covered neck extension, flexion and lateral bending. A theoretical model in which fluid flow was predicted to cause the transient pressure gradients was developed and a neck injury criterion based on Navier-Stokes Equations was applied on the flow model. The theory behind the Neck Injury Criterion indicates that the neck injury occurs early on in the rearward motion of the head relative to the torso in a rear-end collision. Thus the relative horizontal acceleration and velocity between the head and the torso should be restricted during the early head-neck motion to avoid neck injury. The flaw in this theory is that the observed transient pressure should affect all DRG's in the neck but whiplash pain is generally limited to the lower cervical spine. Furthermore, injury to nerve roots leads to radiculopathy (pain in the extremities) and not pain in the neck.

3.3 Tension-flexion injuries

These are relatively uncommon because complaints of chronic or persistent neck pain by belted occupants involved in frontal crashes are rare. In very severe frontal crashes, atlanto-occipital and C2/C3 separation can occur. Thomas & Jessop (1983) produced these injuries in subhuman primates that were fully restrained and were subjected to a frontal deceleration of 120 G.

3.4 Compression-extension injuries

These injuries can occur to unrestrained front seat occupants involved in a frontal crash. When the head impacts the windshield, the neck is placed into extension and compression simultaneously. Such occupants are likely to sustain fracture of one or more spinous processes as well as symmetrical lesions of the pedicles, facets, and laminae. If there is a fracture-dislocation, the inferior facet is displaced posteriorly and upward and appears to be more horizontal than normal on X-ray (Viano & King, 1997).

3.5 Compression-flexion injuries

Wedge compression fractures of the vertebral bodies are the results of a combination of a flexion bending moment and compressive loading of the vertebral motion segment resulting in greater compressive stresses and failures in the anterior of the vertebral body. This type of injury is classified as compression-flexion and may be produced by compressive loading of the head, with or without actual head rotation.

3.6 Lateral bending injuries

Lateral bending occurs when there is a side or oblique impact. This is usually accompanied by shear and axial loading. Injuries characteristic of this type of loading are lateral wedge fractures of the vertebral body and fractures to the posterior elements on one side of the vertebral column. Avulsion of the brachial plexus can also occur. When the neck is subjected to twisting, unilateral facet dislocations or unilateral locked facets are seen (Moffat et al.,

1978). However, pure torsional loads on the neck are rarely encountered in automotive crashes.

4. Neck injury tolerance

There is no widely accepted tolerance for the various loading modes on the neck. The reasons for this inability to set tolerance levels are many. The spine is a multisegmented column with nonlinear structural properties. Its geometry is complex, it produces large strains at physiologic loading, and its constituent elements have nonlinear material properties. Cervical injury mechanisms have been shown to be sensitive to the initial position of the neck, the direction of loading, the degree of constraint imposed by the contact surface, and possibly the rate of loading. These factors are in addition to the normal biological variation in the strength of human tissue and the level of injury we are willing to tolerate. For example, serious neck problems are not encountered in frontal crashes unless the G-level of impact is very high. However, in rear-end collisions, long-term neck pain can result, even though the impact is of low level.

4.1 Tolerance of the neck in flexion-extension

There is ample evidence that the neck can take a fairly high frontal deceleration without injury. Ryan (Ryan, 1962), using himself as a test subject, withstood a 23-G impact without injury. He was wearing a single belt with tighteners. Ewing et al. (1969) conducted volunteer tests at 10 G and reported only belt contusions from the military harness used. Head accelerations at the mouth mount reached (38:6 ± 6:8) G. Similar tests with male volunteers performed by Cheng et al. (1979) reached a maximum sled deceleration of 10 G with no reported injuries. However, in the same series, only one of three female volunteers was willing to reach the 10-G level. The main reason given for discontinuing the tests was the intolerable whipping of the head due to weakness in the neck. Volunteer test results reported by Mertz & Patrick (1967, 1971) are the most frequently cited and widely used. The only volunteer was Prof. Patrick himself. He withstood a flexion moment of 59.4 N m (Newton-meters) with neck pain. This was defined as the pain threshold. At 87.8 N m, he had an immediate onset of pain and prolonged soreness. This was defined as a flexion injury threshold.

Many cadaveric studies on neck flexion have been reported. Lange (1971) produced a variety of neck injuries at high levels of sled deceleration in both frontal and rear-end impacts. The injuries were above human tolerance, and the only reason for citing this paper is to emphasize the fact that the observed "disc ruptures" were, in fact, disc separations from the endplates or transvers cleavage through the centre of the disc, accompanied by rupture of the longitudinal ligaments.

4.2 Tolerance of the neck in extension

A large number of studies has been conducted to study the problem of whiplash-associated disorders (WAD). These were mostly at low impact levels aimed at understanding the causes of neck pain resulting from minor rear-end crashes. On the other hand, there were the studies by Clemens & Burow (1972), who created disc injuries that were frequently associated with anterior longitudinal ligamentous rupture. There were also some joint capsular tears and bony fractures. Because of the overly severe input used (approximate sled acceleration of 25 G), it was not possible to establish a threshold for any of the injuries that were documented. Returning to the work of Mertz & Patrick (1967, 1971), we find that the static limit for Prof. Patrick was 23.7 N m and the average static limit from 10 volunteers was 21.2 N m. Their dynamic results show that the moment tolerated at the base of the skull was 16.7 N m for Prof. Patrick. The proposed noninjurious limit is 47.4 N m or twice the static limit of Prof. Patrick, and the proposed ligamentous injury limit is 57 N m. This limit is based on ligamentous damage to a small cadaver at 33.4 N m, which when scaled to the size of Prof. Patrick was 57 N m. The scaling method used was proposed by Mertz & Patrick (1967). These limits may be too high for neck pain associated with whiplash. Pain can occur without any visible damage to the soft tissue. Microscopic examination of the tissue may be necessary to establish a basis for whiplash-induced pain.

4.3 Tolerance of the neck in lateral bending

There do not appear to be much tolerance data of the neck in lateral bending. Analysis of volunteer data obtained by Ewing et al. (1977) by Wismans & Spenny (1983) show that there were no obvious injuries from runs made at 5 to 10 G. These tests resulted in a lateral bending moment of 20 to 60 N m and lateral rotations of 52 deg. Cadaveric studies have been conducted by Kallieris et al. (1987) simulating three-point belted near-side occupants. The 58 cadavers tested ranged in age from 19 to 65 years and the impact speeds were between 40 and 60 km/h. A variety of injuries, ranging from AIS 1 soft tissue damage to AIS 3 or higher bony fractures were found, frequently at the C6 level. The maximum head resultant acceleration for these tests was 163 G. Far-side lateral impacts were studied by Horsch et al. (1979) and by Kallieris & Schmidt (1990). When an in-board shoulder beltwas used, some AIS 1 cervical injuries were found in both studies. However, in the older cadavers used by Horsch et al. (1979), they found transverse clefts of cervical discs as described above. It is not clear whether the tolerance values from this study are valid or not. The delta V for the Horsch experiments was between 33 and 37 km/h. In the second study by Kallieris & Schmidt (1990), the cadavers used were younger and only AIS 1 injuries were found for a delta V of 50 km/h.

5. Conclusions

Neck injuries can range from mild to catastrophic. Generally, the injuries involving the spinal cord at the higher cervical levels are life threatening whereas those at the lower levels can result in paralysis. To injure the cord, it is necessary to disrupt the alignment or integrity of the cervical column. Burst fractures of cervical vertebral bodies can propel fragments into the cord and cause permanent cord damage. Subluxation of one vertebra over another decreases the size of the spinal canal, again causing cord damage. It is not necessary to sever the cord to produce quadriplegia. If the cord is impacted or crushed temporarily, sufficient damage can be done to paralyze the extremities. In the upper cervical area, separation of the atlas from the occiput is generally a fatal injury. Other life-threatening injuries to the upper column are multiple fractures of the arches of C1 and fractures through the pars interarticularis of C2 (hangman's fracture). Milder forms of cervical injury include the so-called whiplash syndrome caused by a rear-end collision. Although clinical literature frequently describes it as a real injury, the picture is confused by a multitude of claims of an injury for which the etiology is unknown.

This chapter summarized research aimed at providing some biomechanical characteristics of the neck in a form that will be useful in the design of protective systems and in the development of societal strategies to reduce the number of cervical spine injuries. To this end, various biomechanical models (i.e. animal/human models and numerical models), injury mechanisms and injury tolerance of the neck were presented.

Much work remains to be done. Improvements in numerical models of neck dynamics has been dramatic and remains promising. Future research to develop injury prevention strategies that capitalize on these results will be required. Understanding the effects of the spinal musculature, tensile neck injuries, and the unique features of the pediatric spine also remain as goals for the next decade.

6. Acknowledgements

This work was supported by grants from the National Natural Science Foundation of China (No. 30928005), the Chongqing Natural Science Foundation of China (No. CSTC2009BB5013), and the Third Military Medical University Research Foundation of China (No. 2009XHG16).

7. References

Aldman, B (1986). An Analytical approach to the impact biomechanics of head and neck. Proc.30th AAAM Conf., pp. 439-454.

Bahling, GS.; Bundorf, RT. & Kaspzyk, GS. (1990). Rollover and drop tests – The influence of roof strength on injury mechanics using belted dummies, *Proc. 34th Stapp Car Crash Conference*, Vol. 34, (October 1990), pp. 101-112, ISSN 0148-7191.

Bosio, AC. & Bowman, BM. (1986). Simulation of head-neck dynamic response in -Gx and +Gy. *Proc. 30th Stapp Car Crash Conference*, Vol. 30, (October 1986), pp. 345-378, ISSN 0148-7191.

Bowman, BM. & Robbins, DH. (1972). Parameter study of biomechanical quantities in analytical neck models. *Proc. 16th Stapp Car Crash Conference*, Vol. 16, (November 1972), pp. 14-44, ISSN 0585-086X.

Camacho, DL.; Nightingale, RW.; Robinette, JJ.; Vanguri, SK.; Coates, DJ. & Myers, BS. (1997). Experimental flexibility measurements for the development of a computational head-neck model validated for near-vertex head impact. *Proc. 41 Stapp Car Crash Conference*, Vol. 41, (November 1997), pp. 473-486, ISSN 0148-7191.

Cavanaugh, JM.; Lu, Y.; Chen, C. & Kallakuri, S. (2006). Pain generation in lumbar and cervical facet joints. *J Bone Joint Surg Am*, Vol. 88 Suppl 2, (April 2006), pp. 63-67, ISSN 0021-9355.

Chancey, VC.; Nightingale, RW.; Ee, CA.; Knaub, KE. & Myers, BS. (2003). Improved estimation of human neck tensile tolerance: Reducing the range of reported tolerance using anthropometrically correct muscles and optimized physiologic initial conditions. *Proc. 47th Stapp Car Crash Conference*, Vol. 47, (October 2003), pp. 135-153, ISSN 1532-8546.

Chen, C.; Lu, Y.; Cavanaugh, JM.; Kallakuri, S. & Patwardhan, A. (2005). Recording of neural activity from goat cervical facet joint capsule using custom-designed miniature electrodes. *Spine*, Vol. 30, (June 2005), pp. 1367-1372, ISSN 1528-1159.

Chen, HB.; Yang, KH. & Wang, ZG. (2009). Biomechanics of whiplash injury. *Chin J Traumatol*, Vol. 12, No. 5, (October 2009), pp. 305-314, ISSN 1008-1275.

Cheng, R.; Mital, NK.; Levine, RS. & King, AI. (1979). Biodynamics of the living human spine during−Gx impact acceleration. *Proc. 23rd Stapp Car Crash Conference*, Vol. 23, (February 1979), pp. 723-764, ISSN 0585-086X.

Clemens, HJ. & Burow, K. (1972). Experimental investigations on injury mechanisms of cervical spine at frontal and rear-front vehicle impacts. *Proc. 16th Stapp Car Crash Conference*, Vol. 16, (November 1972), pp. 76-104, ISSN 0585-086X.

Dauvilliers, F., Bendjellal, F., Weiss, M., Lavaste, F. & Tarriere, C. (1994). Development of a finite element model of the neck. *Proc. 38th Stapp Car Crash Conference*, Vol. 38, (November 1994), pp. 77-91, ISSN 0148-7191.

Deng, YC. & Goldsmith, W. (1987). Response of a Human Head/Neck/Upper-Torso Replica to Dynamic Loading-II Analytical/Numerical Model. *Journal of Biomechanics*, Vol. 20, No. 5, (February 1987), pp. 487-497, ISSN 0021-9290.

Deng, B.; Begeman, PC.; Yang, KH., Tashman, S. & King, AI. (2000). Kinematics of human cadaver cervical spine during low speed rear-end impacts. *Proc. 44th Stapp Car Crash Conference*, Vol. 44, (November 2000), pp.171-188, ISSN 1532-8546.

Ewing, CL.; Thomas, DJ.; Patrick, LM.; Beeler, GW. & Smith, MJ. (1969). Living human dynamic response to−Gx impact acceleration II, accelerations measured on the head and neck. *Proc. 13th Stapp Car Crash Conference*, Vol. 13, (December 1969), pp. 400–415, ISSN 0585-086X.

Ewing, CL.; Thomas, DJ.; Lustik, L.; Muzzy, WH.; Willems, GC. & Majewski, P. (1977). Dynamic response of the human head and neck to CGy impact acceleration. *Proc. 21st Stapp Car Crash Conference*, Vol. 21, (October 1977), pp. 547–586, ISSN 0585-086X.

Grauer, JN. & Panjabi, MM. (1997). Whiplash produces an S-shaped curvature of the neck with hyperextension at lower levels. *Spine*, Vol. 22, (November 1997), pp. 2489-2494, ISSN 0362-2436.

Halldin, PH.; Brolin, K.; Kleiven, S.; Holst, HV.; Jakobsson, L. & Palmertz, C. (2000). Investigation of conditions that affect neck compression-flexion injuries using numerical techniques. *Proc. 44th Stapp Car Crash Conference*, Vol. 44, (November 2000), pp. 127-138, ISSN 1532-8546.

Horsch, JD.; Schneider, DC.; Kroell, CK. & Raasch, FD. (1979). Response of belt restrained subjects in simulated lateral impact. *Proc. 23rd Stapp Car Crash Conference*, Vol. 23, (February 1979), pp. 69–104, ISSN 0585-086X.

Horst, MJ.; Thunnissen, JG.; Happee, R.; Haaster, RM. & Wismans, JS. (1997). The influence of muscle activity on head-neck response during impact. Proc. 41st Stapp Car Crash Conference, Vol. 41, (November 1997), pp. 487–508, ISSN 0148-7191.

Hu, JW.; Lee, JB. & Yang, KH. (2005). Injury patterns and sources of non-ejected occupants in trip-over crashes: a survey of NASS-CDS database from 1997 to 2002. *In: 49th Association for the Advancement of Automotive Medicine Annual Conference*, Vol. 49, (September 2005), pp. 119–132, ISSN 1540-0360.

Hu, JW.; Chou, CC. & Yang, KH. (2007). A weighted logistic regression analysis for predicting the odds of head/face and neck injuries during rollover crashes. *In: 51st Association for the Advancement of Automotive Medicine Annual Conference*, Vol. 51, (November 2007), pp. 363–379, ISSN 1540-360.

Hu, JW.; Yang, KH.; Chou, CC. & King, AI. (2008). A numerical investigation of factors affecting cervical spine injuries during rollover crashes. *Spine*, Vol. 33, No. 23, (November 2008); pp. 2529-2535, ISSN 1528-1159.

Jager, MD.; Sauren, A.; Thunnissen, J. & Wismans, J. (1994). A three-dimensional head-neck model: Validation for frontal and lateral impacts. *Proc. 38th Stapp Car Crash Conference*, Vol. 38, (November 1994), pp. 93-109, ISSN 0148-7191.

Jager, MD.; Sauren, A.; Thunnissen, J. & Wismans, J. (1996). A Global and a Detailed Mathematical Model for Head-Neck Dynamics. *Proc. 40th Stapp Car Crash Conference*, Vol. 40, (November 1996), pp. 269–281, ISSN 0148-7191.

Kallieris, D. & Schmidt, G. (1990). Neck response and injury assessment using cadavers and the US-SID for far-side lateral impact of rear seat occupants with inboardanchored shoulder belts. *Proc. 34th Stapp Car Crash Conference*, Vol. 34, (October 1990), pp. 93–100, ISSN 0148-7191.

Kaneoka, K.; Ono, K.; Inami, S. & Hayashi, K. (1999). Motion analysis of cervical vertebrae during whiplash loading. *Spine*, Vol. 24, No. 8, (April 1999), pp. 763-769, ISSN 0362-2436.

Kleinberger, M. (1993). Application of Finite Element Techniques to the Study of Cervical Spine Mechanics. *Proc. 37th Stapp Car Crash Conference*, Vol. 37, (November 1993), pp. 261-272, ISSN 0148-7191.

Kumaresan, S.; Yoganandan, N. & Pintar, FA. (1990). Finite element analysis of the cervical spine: a material property sensitivity study. *Clin Biomech*, Vol. 14, No. 1, (January 1999), pp. 41-53, ISSN. 0268-0033

Lu, Y.; Chen, C.; Kallakuri, S.; Patwardhan, A. & Cavanaugh, JM. (2005a). Development of an in vivo method to investigate biomechanical and neurophysiological properties of spine facet joint capsules. *Eur Spine J*, Vol. 14, No. 16, (August 2005a), pp.565-572, ISSN 0940-6719.

Lu, Y.; Chen, C.; Kallakuri, S.; Patwardhan, A. & Cavanaugh, JM. (2005b). Neurophysiological and biomechanical characterization of goat cervical facet joint capsules. *J Orthop Res*, Vol. 23, No. 4, (July 2005b), pp. 779-787, ISSN 0736-0266.

Matsushita T.; Sato TB.; Hirabayashi K. & Fujimura S. (1994). X-ray study of the human neck motion due to head inertial loading. *Proc. 39th Stapp Car Crash Conf*, Vol. 39, (November 1994), pp.55-64, ISSN 0148-7191.

Svensson, MY.; Ola, B.; Johan, D.; Hans, AH.; Yngve, H.; Per, L.; Anders, S. & Anette, S. (2000). Neck injuries in car collisions- a review covering a possible injury mechanism and the development of a new rear-impact dummy. *Accident Analysis and Prevention*, Vol. 32, No. 2, (March 2000), pp.167-175, ISSN 0001-4575.

McConnell, WE.; Howard, RP.; Guzman, HM.; Bomar, JB.; Raddin, JH.; Benedict, JV. & Smith, HL. (1993). Analysis of human test subject kinematic responses to low velocity rear end impacts. *Society for Automobile Engineers*, (March 1993), pp.21–30, ISSN 0418-7191.

McConnell, WE.; Howard, RP.; Van, PJ.; Krause, R.; Guzman, HM.; Bomar, JB.; Raddin, JH.; Benedict, JV. & Hatsell, CP. (1995). Human head and neck kinematics after low velocity rear-end impacts-understanding 'whiplash'. *Proc. 39th Stapp Car Crash Conf*, Vol. 39, (November 1995), pp. 215-238, ISSN 0148-7191.

Mertz, HJ. & Patrick, LM. (1967). Investigation of the kinematics and kinetics of whiplash. *Proc. 11th Stapp Car Crash Conference*, Vol. 11, (November 1967), pp.267–317, ISSN 0585-086X.

Mertz, HJ. & Patrick, LM. (1971). Strength and response of the human neck. *Proc. 15th Stapp Car Crash Conference*, (February 1971), pp. 207–255, ISSN 0585-086X.

Meyer, F.; Bourdent, N.; Deck, C.; Willinger, R. & Raul, JS. (2004). Human Neck Finite Element Model Development and Validation against Original Experimental Data. *Proc. 48th Stapp Car Conference*, Vol. 48, (November 2004), pp. 177-206, ISSN 1523-8546.

Moffat, EA.; Siegel, AW. & Huelke, DF. (1978). The biomechanics of automotive cervical fractures. *Proc. Conf. AAAM, 22nd*, Vol. 22, pp. 151–168.

Myers, BS. & Winkelstein, BA. (1995). Epidemiology, classification, mechanisms, and tolerance of human cervical spine injuries. *In: Critical Reviews in Bioengineering*, Vol. 23, (March 1995), pp. 307–410, ISSN 0278-940X.

Ono, K.; Kaneoka, K.; Wittek, A. & Kajzer, J. (1997). Cervical injury mechanism based on the analysis of human cervical vertebral motion and head-neck-torso kinematics during low speed rear impacts. *Proc. 41st Stapp Car Crash Conference*, Vol. 41, (November 1997), pp. 339-356, ISSN 0148-7191.

Panjabi, MM.; Ivancic, PC. & Maak, TG. (2006). Multiplanar cervical spine injury due to head-turned rear impact. Spine, Vol. 31, No. 4, (February 2006), pp. 420–429, ISSN 1528-1159.

Quinn, KP. & Winkelstein, BA. (2007). Cervical facet capsular ligament yield defines the threshold for injury and persistent joint-mediated neck pain. *J Biomech*, Vol. 40, No. 10, (October 2007), pp. 2299-2306, ISSN 0021-9290.

Ryan, JJ. (1962). Human crash deceleration tests on seat-belts. *Aerosp. Med*, Vol. 3, (February 1962) pp. 167–174, ISSN 0001-9402.

Seemann, MR.; Lustick, LS. & Frisch, GD. (1984). Mechanism for control of head and neck dynamic response. *Proc. 28th Stapp Car Crash Conference*, Vol. 28, (October 1984), pp. 207-222, ISSN 0148-7191.

Siegmund, GP.; Davis, MB.; Quinn, KP.; Hines, E.; Myers, BS.; Ejima, S.; Ono, K.; Kamiji, K.; Yasuki, T. & Winkelstein, BA. (2008). Head-turned postures increase the risk of cervical facet capsule injury during whiplash. *Spine*, Vol. 33, No. 15, (July 2008), pp. 1643-1649, ISSN 1528-1159.

Siegmund GP.; Myers BS. & Davis MB. (2001). Mechanical evidence of cervical facet capsule injury during whiplash: a cadaveric study using combined shear, compression, and extension loading. *Spine*, Vol. 26, No. 19, (October 2001), pp. 2095–2101, ISSN 0362-2346.

Storvik, SG. & Stemper, BD. (2011). Axial head rotation increases facet joint capsular ligament strains in automotive rear impact. *Med Biol Eng Comput*, Vol. 49, No. 2, (February 2011), pp. 153-161, ISSN 1741-0444.

Sturzenegger, M.; DiStefano, G. & Radanov, BP. (1994). Presenting symptoms and signs after whiplash injury: the influence of accident mechanisms. *Neurology*, Vol. 44, No. 4, (April 1994), pp. 688–693, ISSN 0028-3878.

Sturzenegger, M.; Radanov, BP. & Di Stefano, G. (1995).The effect of accident mechanisms and initial findings on the long-term course of whiplash injury. *J Neurol*, Vol. 242, No. 7, (July 1995), pp. 443–449, ISSN 0340-5354.

Viano, DC. (1992). Influence of seatback angle on occupant dynamics in stimulated rear-end impacts. *SAE* , Vol. 242, (September 1992), pp. 177–217, ISSN 0148-7191.

Winkelstein, BA.; Nightingale, RW. & Richardson, WJ. (2000). The cervical facet capsule and its role in whiplash injury: a biomechanical investigation. *Spine,* Vol. 25, No. 10, (May 2000), pp. 1238–1246, ISSN 0362-2346

Wismans, J. & Spenny, DH. (1983). Performance requirements for mechanical necks in lateral flexion. *Proc. 27th Stapp Car Crash Conference,* Vol. 27, (October 1983), pp.137–148, ISSN 0148-7191.

Wismans, J.; Philippens, M.; Oorschot, Ev.; Kallieris, D. & Mattern, R. (1987). Comparison of human volunteer and cadaver head-neck response in frontal flexion. *Proc. 31st Stapp Car Crash Conference,* Vol. 31, (November 1987), pp.1-13, ISSN 0148-7191.

Yang, KH.; Zhu, F.; Luan, F.; Zhao, L. & Begeman, PC. (1998). Development of a finite element model of the human neck. *Proc. 42nd Stapp Car Crash Conference,* Vol. 42, (November 1998), pp. 1-11, ISSN 0148-7191.

Yang, KH. & Begman, PC. (1996). A proposed role for facet joints in neck pain in low to moderate speed rear end impacts. Part I: Biomechanics. *In: 6th Injury Prevention Through Biomechanics Symposium, WSU,* Vol. 6, (May 1996), pp. 59-63, ISSN 1028-6586.

Yang, KH.; Begeman, PC.; Muuser, M.; Niederer P. & Walz, F. (1997). On the Role of Cervical Facet Joints in Rear End Impact Neck Injury Mechanisms. *SAE,* Vol. 6, (February 1997), pp. 59-63, ISSN 0148-7191.

Yang KH. & King AI. (2003). Neck kinematics in rear-end impacts. *Pain Res Manage,* Vol. 8, No. 2, (Summer 2003), pp. 79-85, ISSN 1203-6765.

Yoganandan, N.; Haffner, M. & Maiman, DJ. (1989). Epidemiology and injury biomechanics of motor vehicle related trauma to the human spine. *Proc. 33rd Stapp Car Crash Conference,* Vol. 33, (October 1989), pp. 79-85, ISSN 0148-7191.

Yoganandan, N.; Pintar, FA. & Klienberger M. (1998). Cervical spine vertebral and facet joint kinematics under whiplash. *J Biomech Eng,* Vol. 120, No. 2, (April 1998), pp. 305-307, ISSN 0148-0731.

Zhang, QH.; Teo, EC. & Ng, HW. (2005). Development and validation of a CO-C7 FE complex for biomechanical study. *J Biomech Eng,* Vol. 127, No. 5, (October 2005), pp. 729–735, ISSN 0148-0731.

Permissions

The contributors of this book come from diverse backgrounds, making this book a truly international effort. This book will bring forth new frontiers with its revolutionizing research information and detailed analysis of the nascent developments around the world.

We would like to thank Asst. Prof. Dr. Vaclav Klika, for lending his expertise to make the book truly unique. He has played a crucial role in the development of this book. Without his invaluable contribution this book wouldn't have been possible. He has made vital efforts to compile up to date information on the varied aspects of this subject to make this book a valuable addition to the collection of many professionals and students.

This book was conceptualized with the vision of imparting up-to-date information and advanced data in this field. To ensure the same, a matchless editorial board was set up. Every individual on the board went through rigorous rounds of assessment to prove their worth. After which they invested a large part of their time researching and compiling the most relevant data for our readers. Conferences and sessions were held from time to time between the editorial board and the contributing authors to present the data in the most comprehensible form. The editorial team has worked tirelessly to provide valuable and valid information to help people across the globe.

Every chapter published in this book has been scrutinized by our experts. Their significance has been extensively debated. The topics covered herein carry significant findings which will fuel the growth of the discipline. They may even be implemented as practical applications or may be referred to as a beginning point for another development. Chapters in this book were first published by InTech; hereby published with permission under the Creative Commons Attribution License or equivalent.

The editorial board has been involved in producing this book since its inception. They have spent rigorous hours researching and exploring the diverse topics which have resulted in the successful publishing of this book. They have passed on their knowledge of decades through this book. To expedite this challenging task, the publisher supported the team at every step. A small team of assistant editors was also appointed to further simplify the editing procedure and attain best results for the readers.

Our editorial team has been hand-picked from every corner of the world. Their multi-ethnicity adds dynamic inputs to the discussions which result in innovative outcomes. These outcomes are then further discussed with the researchers and contributors who give their valuable feedback and opinion regarding the same. The feedback is then collaborated with the researches and they are edited in a comprehensive manner to aid the understanding of the subject.

Apart from the editorial board, the designing team has also invested a significant amount of their time in understanding the subject and creating the most relevant covers. They scrutinized every image to scout for the most suitable representation of the subject and create an appropriate cover for the book.

The publishing team has been involved in this book since its early stages. They were actively engaged in every process, be it collecting the data, connecting with the contributors or procuring relevant information. The team has been an ardent support to the editorial, designing and production team. Their endless efforts to recruit the best for this project, has resulted in the accomplishment of this book. They are a veteran in the field of academics and their pool of knowledge is as vast as their experience in printing. Their expertise and guidance has proved useful at every step. Their uncompromising quality standards have made this book an exceptional effort. Their encouragement from time to time has been an inspiration for everyone.

The publisher and the editorial board hope that this book will prove to be a valuable piece of knowledge for researchers, students, practitioners and scholars across the globe.

List of Contributors

Antonio Boccaccio and Carmine Pappalettere
Dipartimento di Ingegneria Meccanica e Gestionale, Politecnico di Bari, Italy

Valery B. Kokshenev
Departamento de Física, Universidade Federal de Minas Gerais, Belo Horizonte, Brazil

Per Christiansen
University of Aalborg, Department of Biotechnology, Chemistry, and Environmental Engineering, Sohngaardsholmsvej 57, DK-9000 Aalborg, Denmark

Miroslav Holeček, Petra Kochová and Zbyněk Tonar
Department of Mechanics, Faculty of Applied Sciences University of West Bohemia, Pilsen, Department of Histology and Embryology, Faculty of Medicine in Pilsen, Charles University in Prague, Pilsen, Czech Republic

K. Engel
German Sport University Cologne, Germany

R. Herpers
Bonn-Rhine-Sieg University of Applied Sciences, Germany

U. Hartmann
University of Applied Sciences Koblenz, Germany

Rami K. Korhonen
Department of Applied Physics, University of Eastern Finland, Kuopio, Finland

Simo Saarakkala
Department of Medical Technology, University of Oulu, Oulu, Finland
Department of Diagnostic Radiology, University of Oulu and Oulu University Hospital, Oulu, Finland

Elizabeth Crane, David Childers, Geoffrey Gerstner and Edward Rothman
University of Michigan, U.S.A

Antonio Pérez-González, Carmen González-Lluch, Joaquín L. Sancho-Bru, Pablo J. Rodríguez-Cervantes and José L. Iserte-Vilar
Universitat Jaume I, Spain

Shihab Asfour and Moataz Eltoukhy
Department of Industrial Engineering, University of Miami, USA

Antonio Pérez-González, Marta C. Mora, Beatriz E. León, Margarita Vergara, José L. Iserte, Pablo J.
Rodríguez-Cervante, Antonio Morales and Joaquín L. Sancho-Bru
Universitat Jaume I, Spain

Václav Klika and František Maršík
Institute of Thermomechanics, v.v.i., Academy of Sciences of Czech Republic, Czech Republic

Václav Klika
Dept. of Mathematics, FNSPE, Czech Technical Univerzity in Prague, Czech Republic

Valery B. Kokshenev
Departamento de Física, Universidade Federal de Minas Gerais, Belo Horizonte, Brazil

Timo Rantalainen and Adam Klodowski
Department of Mechanical Engineering, Lappeenranta University of Technology, Department of Health Sciences, University of Jyväskylä, Finland

Masaya Hirashima
Graduate School of Education, The University of Tokyo, Japan

Andrew R. Lammers and Ulrich Zurcher
Cleveland State University, USA

Christopher D. S. Jones
School of Medical Sciences, Australia

Paul N. Grimshaw
School of Mechanical Engineering, University of Adelaide, Adelaide, Australia

Pascal Madeleine, Afshin Samani, Mark de Zee and Uwe Kersting
Physical Activity and Human Performance, Center for Sensory-Motor Interaction (SMI), Dept. of Health Science and Technology, Aalborg University, Denmark

Haibin Chen, Liying Zhang and Zhengguo Wang
State Key Laboratory of Trauma, Burns, and Combined Injury, Institute of Surgery Research & Daping Hospital, Third Military Medical University, PR China

Liying Zhang, King H. Yang and Albert I. King
Bioengineering Center, Wayne State University, USA